THE COMPLETE GUIDE TO WOMEN'S HEALTH

BRUCE D. SHEPHARD, M.D., F.A.C.O.G., graduated Phi Beta Kappa from the University of California, Berkeley, in 1966. He earned his M.D. degree from the University of California School of Medicine in San Francisco in 1970. Since 1976 he has maintained a private practice in Tampa, Florida, where he also serves on the clinical faculty of the University of South Florida College of Medicine. Dr. Shephard is a Fellow of the American College of Obstetricians and Gynecologists, a Diplomate of the American Board of Obstetrics and Gynecology, and a member of the American Medical Writers Association.

CARROLL A. SHEPHARD, R.N., PH.D., is currently a psychologist in private practice in Tampa. She has been involved in health education for women and children and has taught childbirth preparation, parenting classes, and maternal and child nursing. Other areas of interest include health psychology and marriage and family counseling. Dr. Shephard received her B.S. in nursing from the University of Florida and her Ph.D. from the University of Miami in Florida.

Bruce and Carroll are the proud parents of three children: Chris, age twenty; Carl, age seventeen; and Lizzy, age twelve.

THE COMPLETE GUIDE TO WOMEN'S HEALTH

THIRD REVISED EDITION

Bruce D. Shephard, M.D., F.A.C.O.G.
and
Carroll A. Shephard, R.N., Ph.D.

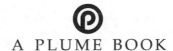

A PLUME BOOK

Note to the Reader

The ideas, procedures, and suggestions contained in this book are not intended as a substitute for consulting with your physician. All matters regarding your health require medical supervision.

PLUME
Published by the Penguin Group
Penguin Books USA Inc., 375 Hudson Street, New York, New York 10014, U.S.A.
Penguin Books Ltd, 27 Wrights Lane, London W8 5TZ, England
Penguin Books Australia Ltd, Ringwood, Victoria, Australia
Penguin Books Canada Ltd, 10 Alcorn Avenue, Toronto, Ontario, Canada M4V 3B2
Penguin Books (N.Z.) Ltd, 182–190 Wairau Road, Auckland 10, New Zealand

Penguin Books Ltd, Registered Offices: Harmondsworth, Middlesex, England

Published by Plume, an imprint of Dutton Signet, a division of Penguin Books USA Inc.
First Plume Printing (Revised Edition), June, 1985
First Plume Printing (Second Revised Edition), December, 1990
First Plume Printing (Third Revised Edition), February, 1997

10 9 8 7 6 5 4 3 2 1

PHOTO & ILLUSTRATION CREDITS

Photo on page 344 and illustrations in Chapter 16, Pregnancy, reprinted with the permission of Wyeth-Ayerst Laboratories.

Illustrations on page 42 and photo on page 43 reprinted with the permission of Wisconsin Pharmacal Company.

Illustration on page 297 reprinted with the permission of Richard Wolf Medical Instruments Corporation.

Lori Hoffman was the photographer for the following pages:
1, 18, 75, 123, 133 (top), 136, 146, 147, 150, 153, 175, 179, 191, 196, 218, 222, 231, 245, 253, 254, 260, 323, 333, 335, 337, 358, 362, 363 (bottom), 364, 369, 392, 407, 443, 482.

Joe Traina was the photographer for the following pages:
38, 65, 93, 94, 95, 98, 99, 102, 105, 106, 114, 117, 128, 129, 130, 133 (bottom), 134, 145, 149, 162, 167, 172, 177, 185, 186, 217, 219, 235, 289, 318, 341, 359, 404, 428, 526, 527.

Manuel M. Chavez was the photographer for the following pages:
2, 7, 21, 31, 63, 110, 113, 119, 120, 126, 127, 131, 132, 135, 143, 151, 152, 171, 183, 233, 291, 295, 302, 354, 355, 360, 361, 363 (top), 367, 378, 422.

REGISTERED TRADEMARK—MARCA REGISTRADA

LIBRARY OF CONGRESS CATALOGING-IN-PUBLICATION DATA

Shephard, Bruce D.
  The complete guide to women's health / Bruce D. Shephard
and Carroll A. Shephard. — 3rd rev. ed.
    p. cm.
  Includes bibliographical references and index.
  ISBN 0-452-27792-2
  1. Gynecology—Popular works. 2. Obstetrics—Popular works.
3. Women—Health and hygiene. I. Shephard, Carroll A.
II. Title.
RG121.S533 1997
618—dc20

96-26960
CIP

Printed in the United States of America
Set in Palatino
Designed by Julian Hamer

Dedicated to our parents

Madelyn R. Shephard, 1914–1979

Richard G. Shephard

Georgianna C. Swanson

Eldon C. Swanson, M.D., 1908–1989

and to our great kids, Chris, Carl, Lizzy, and little Dianna

Contents

Tables

Preface

This book was written for you and for all women who wish to participate more actively and more knowledgeably in their own health care.

Until fairly recently, health care meant, for most women, a visit to the doctor when there was a medical problem. Health care meant finding a "good" doctor who would make the right medical decisions for his or her patient. Today this concept is being challenged as more and more women are discovering that, even without a medical background, they can learn to use a vast amount of information about their own health care. The intention is not to replace medical care but to shift some emphasis for maintaining good health from the medical professional to the individual.

The emergence of "women's health" in the 1990s has made health information ever more accessible. But a second megatrend—the rise of "managed health care"—has made it even more critical for women to be able to use that information wisely. Put simply, "managed care" means medicine now is run strictly as a business. The payers—employers and insurance companies—facing rising health costs have reorganized the health care system through the formation of health maintenance organizations (HMOs) and preferred provider organizations (PPOs). Today, 100 million Americans are enrolled in these organizations, which seek to reduce the most costly aspects of health care, like hospitalization and surgery, while emphasizing wellness strategies and patient education. Under managed care, a woman can expect to have less access to her own physician and may be required to go through the primary-care physician in order to see specialists like OB/GYNs. In this new marketplace, it's all the more important for women to be informed consumers, to make health care decisions wisely, and to use self care appropriately.

Readers of this book will be interested to know that self care has always been a major aspect of our guide, which uses symptom-diagnosing flow charts for dozens of common ailments. Our intent is to go beyond clarifying the medical facts. We also hope to help you decide when to avoid certain services, such as tests, medicines, and surgery. But when you do need these services, we'll try to explain how to use them wisely to keep you well now and in the future.

Bruce D. Shephard, M.D., F.A.C.O.G.
Carroll A. Shephard, R.N., Ph.D.

August 1996

Doctors Bruce and Carroll Shephard can be reached by writing to 4302 North Habana Avenue, Suite 300, Tampa, Florida 33607. We welcome your comments and suggestions for future editions of this book.

Acknowledgments

The mammoth task of rewriting this book could not have been done without the able assistance of our editors at Plume, Alexia Dorszynski and Deb Brody. We very much appreciate their insightful comments, patient editing, and, above all, their concern for the many issues affecting the health care of women.

Our first writing of this book would not have been possible without the cooperation and support of many other people. Shirley M. Miller, our initial editor, gave us constructive guidance throughout the formulation of our first edition. Charles Mendez and the Mariner Publishing Company provided the support essential to the initial publication of this book. Terry Peterson and Joseph Traina helped in the preparation of the initial drawings and photographs for the book. Warren Chandler, our medical illustrator, contributed some excellent drawings on cosmetic surgery. Carole Cheeley, R.N., provided creative suggestions for the manuscript's preliminary draft. We also want to acknowledge the help of G. D. Searle and Co., Wyeth-Ayerst Laboratories, and Parke-Davis, a division of Warner-Lambert Company, for permission to reproduce several illustrations appearing in the book.

It isn't easy to keep abreast of all the current changes in medicine. We wish to thank Pamela Van Hine and her staff at the Resource Center of the American College of Obstetricians and Gynecologists for their help. Celio Guerriere, M.D., and John Favata, M.D., also provided valuable new information in their areas of expertise, cosmetic surgery and emergency medicine.

Typing and compiling a manuscript of this length and detail is trying at best. We want to thank Linda Pollack, Priscilla Adkins, Lauren Hodgson, Rebecca Hancock, and Suzanne Chipollini for their detailed and helpful assistance. We also want to thank the operating room, newborn nursery, labor and delivery, and postpartum staffs at St. Joseph's Women's Hospital. Special thanks go to our staff, especially Janet Valenti and Allison Waddington, for their support during the work on this revised third edition.

Many friends made this update possible through their cooperation and unique help. The support and friendship of Richard and Bonnie Hoffman is much appreciated. Lori Hoffman, Carrie Jones, Tammy Gonzalez, Karen Taylor, Christine Perkins, Doritha Poole, and Minnie Dennard also deserve a special thanks. Diane Ballota, Linda Gentry, Susan Ellet, Vicki Geiss, Linda Hughes, Diane Fultz, Carol Lieber, Joanne Edwards, Judy, Tracy, and Kim Hankerson, Nancy and Holly Barber, Karen Myers, Pam Corbett, and Margo Connelly all contributed toward making this revision possible. Richard and Joanne Swanson helped in providing information in their areas of interest. Steven Lieber, D.M.D., Susan Fallieras, Malinda Gray, Marion Reid, Jane Owry, Etta Breit, and Carole Guerriere all helped with initial manuscript preparation. We also appreciate the patience and understanding of our children while we were endlessly "working on the book."

Finally, and most important, we want to thank our patients, who gave us the inspiration to write in the first place and kept us motivated to pursue this project to the end.

Bruce D. Shephard, M.D., F.A.C.O.G.
Carroll A. Shephard, R.N., Ph.D.

August 1996

Consultants

We very much appreciate the kindness of our various colleagues (listed alphabetically below) who reviewed select portions of the manuscript dealing with their particular areas of expertise. Their comments and suggestions were an invaluable contribution toward making the book accurate, complete, and up-to-date.

John S. Breen, M.D.
  Private Practice in Infectious Diseases
  Diplomate, American Board of Internal
    Medicine
  Tampa, Florida

Sexually transmitted
  diseases

Denis Cavanaugh, M.D., F.A.C.O.G.
  Professor of Obstetrics and Gynecology
  Director of Gynecologic Oncology
  H. Lee Moffitt Cancer Center and
    Research Institute
  Tampa, Florida

Cancer of the female
  reproductive system

Carole Cornell, R.N., B.S.
  Assistant Director of Surgical Services
  Tampa General Hospital
  Tampa, Florida

Hospital care before
  and after surgery

Kathleen J. Dolan, R.N., M.S.
  Chairperson
  Parent-Child Nursing
  Samuel Meritt–St. Mary's College
    Intercollegiate Nursing Program
  Oakland, California

Pregnancy and
  childbirth

Charles R. Engle, R.Ph.
  Eckerd Drugs
  Tampa, Florida

Drugs

Nicholas G. Fallieras, M.D.
  Fellow, American College of Obstetricians
    and Gynecologists
  Tampa, Florida

Pregnancy and
  childbirth

Dianne Swanson Gaines, M.S., P.T.
  Registered Physical Therapist
  College of Health Professions
  University of Florida
  Gainesville, Florida

Joint and back
  problems and
  physical fitness

Grace Lau, R.D., L.D., C.D.E.
  Registered Dietician
  Diabetes Management Program
  St. Joseph's Hospital
  Tampa, Florida
	Nutrition

Lorraine Kushner, M.A., L.M.H.C.
  Fellow, American College of Childbirth
    Educators
  ASPO/Lamaze
  Tampa, Florida
	Pregnancy and
	  childbirth

Norman R. Miller, Ph.D.
  Psychologist in private practice
  Tampa, Florida
	Depression, nervousness,
	  and anxiety

Marilyn Myerson, Ph.D.
  Assistant Professor, Women's Studies
    Program
  Director, Division of Interdisciplinary
    Social Studies
  University of South Florida
  Tampa, Florida
	Female sexuality

Frank C. Riggall, M.D., F.A.C.O.G.
  Medical Director
  Medical Center of Advanced
    Reproductive Technology
  Sandlake Hospital
  Orlando, Florida
	Pregnancy, childbirth,
	  and infertility

William N. Spellacy, M.D., F.A.C.O.G.
  Professor and Chairman
  Department of Obstetrics and Gynecology
  University of South Florida
    College of Medicine
  Tampa, Florida
	High-risk pregnancy

John R. Tagler, R.Ph.
  MEDCO
  Tampa, Florida
	Drugs

Susan H. Tagler, R.Ph.
  MEDCO
  Tampa, Florida
	Drugs

Kathleen E. Toomy, M.D.
  Assistant Professor of Pediatrics
  Division of Genetics
  Children's Hospital
  National Medical Center
  Washington, D.C.
	Genetics

Barry S. Verkauf, M.D., F.A.C.O.G.
  Associate Professor of Obstetrics and
    Gynecology
  University of South Florida
    College of Medicine
  Tampa, Florida
	Infertility, hormone
	  problems

Foreword

The 1990s could be characterized as a time of massive availability of and desire for information. We read about medical breakthroughs in magazines and newspapers as well as hear about them on the radio and on television. Even our computers now provide us with a plethora of data and opinions. The problem is not how to obtain the information, but rather how to interpret it and what to do about issues of concern.

Like the previous editions, the third edition of *The Complete Guide to Women's Health* is a very comprehensive, readable, and reliable reference for those who have questions regarding women's health and for those who may be confused by information from other sources. It deals with controversial and emotion-laden topics from a very objective as well as supportive perspective. The tables are concise, the format is easy to read, and the chapters are well organized. Of special note is the section "What Your Symptoms Mean," which provides a concise description and evaluation of and recommendation for many specific health concerns.

The updates for the new edition are especially beneficial. In the six years since the second edition, new forms of contraception have become available to women in America. These as well as the traditional methods are well described in terms of their use, risks, and effectiveness. Some changes have been made in the practice of obstetrics both in and out of the hospital. These issues are important updates for those who have questions regarding the current management of pregnancy, labor, and delivery. During this decade the use of the laparoscope has been expanded in gynecology. The new techniques and procedures that can be performed, sometimes on an outpatient basis, are addressed.

This third edition of *The Complete Guide to Women's Health* is one that is beneficial to both the medical and the lay communities. For the former, it provides for educated patients who can understand the causes or treatments available for a specific problem as well as how to preserve good health. And for the lay reader, it is an excellent guide for determining if a problem is serious enough to merit medical or surgical intervention. It is a superb information source for health issues of concern to women and those who care about them throughout their lives.

Constance J. Bohon, M.D.
President, The Jacobs Institute of Women's Health

THE COMPLETE
GUIDE TO
WOMEN'S HEALTH

HEALTH STRATEGIES FOR WOMEN

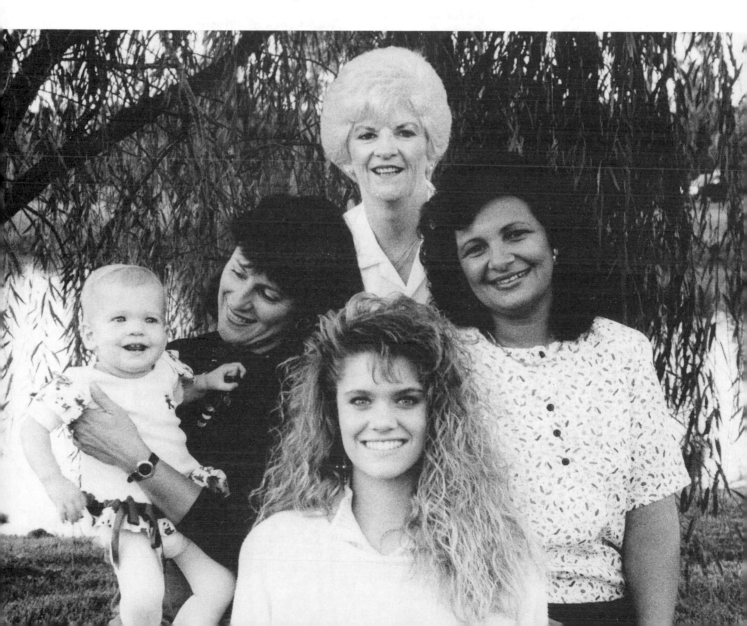

CHAPTER 1

Choosing the Right Doctor or Other Health Professional

How Do I Choose the Right Doctor?

This may be the wrong question to ask. Do you still *have* a choice? That is the real question in the 1990s. Common sense tells us that good medical care depends upon a trusting patient-

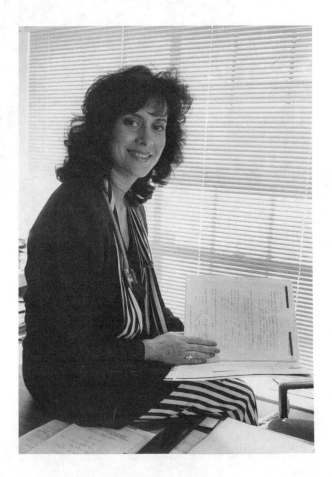

doctor relationship. But economic sense now drives the cost-ridden health care system. The principal payers in this system, employers and insurance companies, now have more to say about access to doctors—including YOUR doctor—than ever before. Often this means you must choose an M.D. from an approved list or pay more to see your own physician if his or her name is not on the list. This chapter is designed to help you make such decisions—now, before an emergency arises and you have to accept whatever care, good or bad, that is available. Although in many parts of the country there are reliable cost-saving alternatives to the doctor—nurse midwives and nurse practitioners, about whom we will talk before this chapter ends—we will concentrate first on demystifying the M.D.

Four Types of Physician

Most women who want a doctor as their primary health care provider choose from four types of physician: the general practitioner (often called a G.P.), the family practitioner, the internist, or the obstetrician-gynecologist (referred to by some people as an OB-GYN, pronouncing each letter separately). Each of these doctors attended medical school for four years and each must pass an exam in order to be licensed to practice in his or her state. The educational differences among these doctors lie in their postgraduate training.

A *general practitioner* (the G.P.) is either an M.D. (Doctor of Medicine) or a D.O. (Doctor of Osteopathy) whose knowledge of obstetrics (which deals with women during pregnancy and childbirth) and gynecology (the study of the functions and diseases of the female organs) may be limited, because these areas of study are now electives in most medical schools. The first postgraduate year, formerly called "internship," may or may not include a period of study in obstetrics and gynecology. In fact, in some states, this postgraduate training has been abolished as a requirement for state licensure.

The *family practitioner* is a new form of specialist who is replacing the G.P. in many parts of the country. The three years of training following medical school includes a minimum of three months of obstetrics and gynecology. Both the G.P. and the family practitioner are oriented as primary care physicians to treat the entire family. They generally do not perform surgery but will refer patients to surgeons or other specialists if special problems arise. These generalists may also make referrals for obstetrical and gynecological care.

The *internist*, a specialist in internal medicine, has three or more years in postgraduate training with possibly three months in obstetrics and gynecology. In addition, the internist may have a subspecialty in one of many areas of study: the heart (cardiology), the joints (rheumatology), the digestive system (gastroenterology), and so on. Again, if a medical condition outside the expertise of the internist occurs, he or she will refer patients to a qualified specialist. The internist may or may not perform routine gynecology checkups; that's something you'll need to ask.

The *obstetrician-gynecologist* takes three to four years of specialty training after medical school, including roughly eighteen months of obstetrics and eighteen months of gynecology. Similar to the internist, the OB-GYN may take subspecialty training in areas such as high-risk pregnancy or gynecological cancer. Obstetrician-gynecologists, who often provide primary care for women because of the declining numbers of general practitioners, also guide patients to the right health professional when serious medical problems occur.

Alternative Health Professionals

As health care costs continue to rise in the 1990s, *physician extenders*—especially nurse-midwives and nurse practitioners—will become more visible providers of women's health care because they can save you money without your having to sacrifice quality of care. These alternative health care providers, who usually work under the supervision of a physician, may be the right choice for the woman who is in general good health. Both perform routine breast and pelvic exams and provide excellent contraceptive counseling. And both are usually trained to send you to the appropriate physician if unusual medical problems develop. Be aware, however, that their educational backgrounds vary.

A certified nurse-midwife (CNM) is a registered nurse who has taken at least one year of additional specialized training in a program approved by the American College of Nurse-Midwives. The CNM usually works closely with

an obstetrician and is trained to provide complete obstetrical care including delivery in uncomplicated pregnancies. Currently over 4,000 certified nurse-midwives are practicing in all fifty states. These professionals typically work in hospitals, birth centers, health maintenance organizations, and private practices.

Registered nurses in many states can train to become family or gynecology nurse practitioners through specialized training programs ranging from a few months up to nearly two years. The programs consist of a formal curriculum leading to either a certificate or Master's degree in nursing. Nurse practitioners can order diagnostic procedures under the supervision of a physician. There is also emphasis on social, psychological, and preventive health in their training.

Another type of health provider, the lay midwife, is sometimes confused with the certified nurse-midwife. Lay midwives include at least two groups—"granny midwives" who traditionally have assisted at childbirth in areas where medical care has been unavailable and a younger, more radical group who have been staunch proponents of home birth. Historically the lay midwife has depended upon hand-to-hand passage of information and experience to get her training and has tended to have little formal education. However, some states now license lay midwives and have established training programs.

Questions to Consider When Selecting a Health Professional

In addition to educational differences, health professionals vary in personality, ability, and style as much as professionals do in every field. In the beginning stages of choosing among them, you should consider these basic questions:

1. Does your health plan limit your choice of doctors to a "list" or panel? If it does, and you choose an M.D. not on the panel, what will it cost? (Some insurance plans cover up to 80% for certain services by nonpanel physicians.)
2. Would you feel more comfortable with a male or female health professional? Some women believe that only another woman will fully grasp their problems. As of 1994, 75% of gynecologists are males, but the

availability of female doctors is increasing. In 1994, 57% of OB-GYNs in training were females.

3. Is age an important factor to you? Some young women prefer a younger physican since he or she is more likely to share their views, particularly of contemporary lifestyles. Older women may prefer more mature physicians for the same reason.

4. Do you have a diagnosed medical problem (say, heart disease)? If so, then the applicable specialist (in this case, a cardiologist) may be the wisest choice as your health professional.

5. Are you planning to become pregnant in the future? You might want to choose the obstetrician-gynecologist who can ultimately provide maternity services as well as fill your current gynecological needs.

6. Does your physician have staff privileges at the hospital of your choice? This is something to keep in mind, for example, if you are planning to have a baby and have a preference as to where you will deliver.

7. Do you prefer to see primarily one physician or would you rather have the services of several who are part of a group? Solo practice, a rapidly declining option, represents perhaps the last vestige of traditional American medicine. Group practices, meanwhile, have increased in (economic) popularity and range in size from two- to three-person groups to large practices of ten, twenty, or more physicians.

Group Practice vs. Solo Practice

The solo practitioner, who may be a G.P. or specialist, has no partners or organizational affiliation. He or she may be your sole source of medical help if you live in a rural area. Some women prefer the solo physician because they feel strongly about seeing the same physician with each office visit and establishing an intimate doctor/patient relationship. In most cases, even if you choose a group practice, you can usually elect to schedule your planned office visits with one specific member of the group. In emergencies, however, whether you are seen by the group or the solo practitioner, you may be

seen by a doctor who is a stranger to you if your own physician is sick or on vacation or otherwise not available.

There are two types of group practice. One is simply a group of the same kind of specialist—an OB-GYN group, for example. The other is a group composed of several major specialties, perhaps including one or more obstetrician-gynecologists. In group practices, physicians share coverage for weekends and nights with their colleagues, thus enabling individual physicians to have more time off. Insurance companies—the "managed care" people—(see Chapter 2) like group practices because they allow them to pool office expenses and administrative costs. The multispecialty group offers the additional advantage of more comprehensive care because the several specialists can offer various perspectives on medical problems. If you do select a group practice, remember that the larger the group, the less likely your own doctor in the group will be on call on any given night or weekend when you might need him or her.

. . . If You Have a Choice

There are three basic criteria from which to view a health care provider: availability, amiability, ability. The "three As," as we call them, apply to physicians as well as other health professionals.

Availability

Access to a doctor depends partly on the size, organization, and type of practice the doctor has. Be sure you understand the scope of a doctor's practice in terms of your own needs or possible future needs. Some doctors, for example, limit their practices to gynecology and infertility; it would be stressful, for example, to develop a sound relationship with such a physician only to have to change doctors when you become pregnant. Sometimes, however, such a change is happily necessary when your earlier visits were made for infertility problems that have been solved.

If you are considering a group practice, you'll need to ask how the "on call" schedule operates, as it varies widely. Obviously, a doctor in a solo or small group practice will be more readily available to you than one in a large group practice.

Access to specialist physicians has changed recently and in a very basic way under "managed care." As we'll discuss in the next chapter, many insurance plans as well as a growing number of plans that operate under Medicare and Medicaid use "gatekeepers." These health professionals, who are typically primary-care physicians (PCPs), work for or with the particular insurance company in question. The gatekeeper's function is to decide, based on certain medical criteria established within the insurance company, whether your medical problem requires referral to a specialist or can be handled by the PCP. Your insurance plan determines whether you must see a gatekeeper before having access to specialists for a variety of medical problems from migraines to vaginal infections.

Amiability

Amiability means an attitude that leads to a comfortable doctor/patient relationship. Your psychological and emotional needs determine what you seek in a doctor/patient relationship. If you have strong beliefs about certain issues, such as contraception, abortion, rooming-in, or breast-feeding, it is essential to find a physician who shares at least some of these beliefs. You should be completely comfortable in being yourself with your physician without worrying that his or her personal value judgments will influence how he or she provides for your care. Amiability is a factor that is difficult to evaluate prior to meeting the physician and one you may have little control over if your insurance plan has a highly restricted physician panel.

Ability

The most difficult quality to judge—ability—is also the most important. As in any profession, there is a spectrum of skill and judgment. Most doctors specialize—that is, they limit their practice to one area of medicine. However, specialization does not automatically mean the doctor has had additional supervised training in that area unless he is board-certified. This additional attainment, board-certification, based on written and oral exams, is one measure that a doctor is qualified to practice his or her specialty. You can determine if a physician is board-certified by looking at his or her wall diplomas or stationery, by calling your local county medical society, or by looking in the *Directory of Medical Specialists* available at your public library. Occasionally board-certified specialists will take further training in the form of a fellowship: the internist in cardiology or gastroenterology, the obstetrician in high-risk pregnancy (perinatology) or gynecological cancer, to name a few. Certificates indicating fellowships of one or two years in one of these subspecialties do indicate a significantly greater level of skill and knowledge in that area.

Some consumers feel safe in judging a doctor's ability according to the hospitals in which he or she has staff privileges. The presence of staff privileges means more now than it did just a few years ago. To maintain their accreditation, hospitals now must scrutinize physician performance through "peer review" committees that look at everything from complication rates to cesarean-section rates. The total absence of staff privileges is not a good sign, especially if a large hospital is close to the doctor's office. Most doctors limit their practice to one or two hospitals for convenience. Some hospitals will go out of their way to help you find a doctor—usually one on their staff—through referral services that provide names of qualified physicians. These information bureaus, which are listed in the yellow pages of telephone directories under "physicians," have become a standard marketing technique for many hospitals.

Many people choose a doctor who is recommended by their friends. Be cautious; while it may be possible to assess amiability and attentiveness on the basis of another's experience, assessing medical ability is another matter. A fine cosmetic scar, for instance, says nothing about the judgment required in determining the need for surgery. The advice of a labor-and-delivery or operating room nurse would be a more reliable referral source for an obstetrician or surgeon. Your pediatrician is also a good referral source, but your particular health plan may limit your choice to a physician on the plan's "approved" list. If you go "out of network" to a physician not on that list you may have to pay added out-of-pocket costs that may be considerable if hospitalization or surgery is involved.

Shopping for the right health professional for

your needs is not easy. The highest quality in this marketplace is found only if you take the time and energy to seek it out. Your body and peace of mind deserve your best efforts.

Changing Doctors

What about changing doctors? This is always an option, but it need not be the first step if you are dissatisfied with some aspect of your medical care. Before switching physicians try to bring the problem to your doctor's attention. Most doctors want their patients to be well treated and satisfied with their care. If it is something the doctor can change, like a rude receptionist or long waits in an examining room, let him or her know about it. But if the problem persists or you are just not comfortable with the relationship, it is perfectly okay to seek care elsewhere. Once you decide to make the switch, you don't have to let your physician know or explain why, although you may do so if you feel it will be helpful. You do have the right to a copy of your records. One way to handle this is to sign a release for medical records when you visit your new physician; he or she can use this release to request the records by mail.

CHAPTER 2

Using the Health Care System

You cannot use our health care system wisely or economically if you are unaware of alternative health care services available to you. The last chapter described your choices in health care professionals and explained that their availability to you might be limited by your insurance plan. This chapter will point out your options in health care facilities. Again, your choice of hospitals may be limited by the type of plan you have. These limits on providers and facilities are part of what is called "managed" care: services provided by doctors and/or hospitals in which costs are kept as low as possible through various financial incentives and contractual arrangements. The two best examples of managed care are *HMO*s and *PPO*s. It is important that you understand something about these health care concepts before we go on to discuss the health care facilities themselves.

Health Maintenance Organizations (HMOs)

An HMO is an organization, for profit or non-profit, that provides comprehensive health care for a prepaid fixed fee. The consumer or his or her family joins the HMO by making regular monthly payments. Freedom to select your health care provider may be limited as may your choice of hospitals, depending on the institutions participating in the HMO. However, to increase their consumer popularity, most HMOs now offer a "point-of-service" plan in which out-of-network physicians may be used at an additional cost in the form of deductibles and coinsurance. In 1995, HMOs served 20% of the U.S. population, a remarkable jump from just 4% in 1980. (See Table 1 to find out how to obtain more information on possible HMOs in your area.)

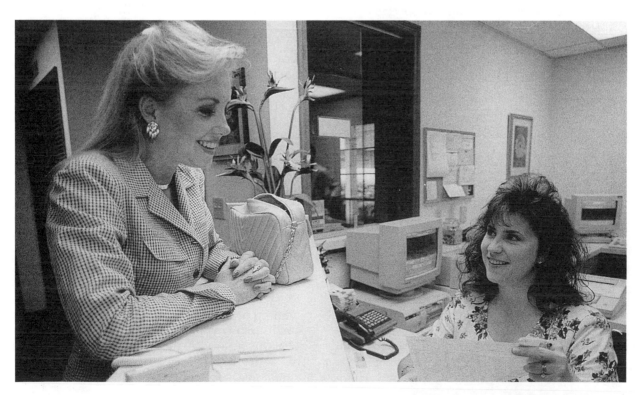

Preferred Provider
Organizations (PPOs)

A PPO is a group of health care providers (doctors and/or hospitals) that contract with employers or insurance companies (so-called third-party payers) to deliver medical care at a discount. The consumer pays on a fee-for-service basis, but a ceiling or maximum charge is established by the employer or insurance company. Employees are given financial incentives in the form of lower copayment or deductibles to use the doctors and hospitals participating in the PPO. PPO enrollees usually do not have to receive care from approved physicians or hospitals (who participate in the PPO by contract), but their out-of-pocket expenses are increased if they don't. The PPO concept is popular with some doctors and hospitals, especially where increased competition is forcing them to make tradeoffs to keep their patients and their markets. Overall, PPOs, which now provide health care for about 20% of Americans, usually limit the choices of doctors somewhat less than HMOs. Like some HMOs (known as *independent practice associations*), physician members of a PPO practice in their individual offices. Both HMOs and PPOs use "gatekeepers"—primary-care physicians who control utilization of health care services such as referrals to specialists or admission to the hospital.

The Hospital

Hospitalization is the costliest part of medical care in terms of your wallet and probably your psyche as well, so you should avoid it when possible. If you can have minor surgery or a series of tests on an outpatient basis, then make every effort to do so.

Of course, there are times when admission to a hospital cannot be avoided. If you are pregnant or you need surgery and you do not have health insurance or a prepaid health plan, consider using a county or university hospital where a sliding-scale fee may be used rather than a flat fee-for-service. When a medical school is affiliated with a hospital, the technical side of care—the lab tests and procedures—is likely to be superior, though the human warmth element may suffer at times. More tests than you actually need may be ordered by a zealous doctor in training. However, you will have close supervision by resident physicians trained with the latest available knowledge. The level of obstetrical care afforded by supervised OB-GYN residents at hospitals affiliated with medical schools is generally very good.

If you must be hospitalized for, say, an elective operation, ask your doctor if you need to be hospitalized the night before surgery; if not, arrange for an "A.M. admission" to save a day's cost. Check on the possibility of an early discharge, too—within twenty-four hours of a normal birth or as early as the third or fourth day following major surgery or a cesarean birth. Sometimes an early discharge can be facilitated by arranging for home care by various home health agencies. While in the hospital, ask about taking your own medications instead of having them supplied by the more costly hospital pharmacy. And question any test or procedure you think is unnecessary, especially if the same test was done recently by another doctor or at another hospital.

The Emergency Room (ER)

Be familiar with the emergency room at your local hospital. The physicians there are often board-certified members of the American College of Emergency Room Physicians. Physicians in other specialties may also elect to work in the ER because it offers shorter hours and fewer business pressures. There has been a recent national trend in ERs to establish "express care," usually available from 10 A.M. to 10 P.M., to treat minor emergencies quickly, with financial rates competitive with those of walk-in clinics. Such centers can also provide immediate referral to a specialist should your problem require it. If you are being treated for a problem by your physician and are not getting better, call him or her prior to going to the ER. He or she may be able to save you both time and money. It isn't economical or medically preferable to use the ER for small problems that can be treated by your regular physician. Whenever possible, ERs should be reserved for serious trauma or emergency situations.

Walk-in Clinics

These "doc-in-the-box" clinics have sprung up to provide medical care at a rate lower than that provided by emergency rooms and with less waiting. These clinics operate on a cash or credit basis and may have to refer you to the emergency room for treatment by a specialist should your problem be serious enough. No physician qualifications except state licensure exist for most such clinics, and they are often staffed by doctors looking for extra income or those just starting out. Unless you are familiar with them and know the staff, walk-in clinics should be the last place to shop for health care. You may end up needing a referral and paying twice for the same problem.

Free Clinics

The Public Health Department's Free Clinics provide general primary care as well as contraceptive counseling and prenatal care. Financial eligibility may be required and a small fee asked for the service. Pregnancy screening and VD (venereal disease) detection and treatment are usually free of charge. Staffing may be by a physician or nurse practitioner. Continuity of care varies, depending on the physician/nurse turnover and continued state and local funding. Referral for specific health problems is provided.

Planned Parenthood

Excellent contraceptive counseling, especially for women with an uncomplicated health history, can be obtained at a reasonable fee at Planned Parenthood centers. This organization also offers pregnancy counseling, abortion and sterilization services, or referral for such services on an outpatient basis. Some branches of Planned Parenthood give special educational programs for marriage, sex education, prenatal care, and a variety of health-related topics. Staffing is variable, consisting of nurse practitioners, physicians, and lay persons.

Women's Clinics for Pregnancy Termination

Pregnancy termination is simply another way of saying abortion. These clinics, which offer free pelvic exams and pregnancy tests as an introductory feature, usually present a single-fee package that includes first-trimester abortion (up to 12 weeks) with pre- and post-abortion counseling, pertinent laboratory tests, and contraceptive counseling. Special problems, such as RH sensitization due to pregnancy, can be treated at the clinic for an extra fee. Local anesthesia as opposed to general anesthesia is usually given, and the procedure is done on an outpatient, short-stay basis usually requiring less than three hours. Some clinics will perform second-trimester abortions (between 12 and 24 weeks) usually in a nearby hospital. Staffing is typically provided by board-certified OB-GYNs, nurse practitioners, and trained counselors. If you are researching this service, inquire not only as to costs but also as to what follow-up care exists. Many physicians are now doing pregnancy terminations in their own offices at fees competitive with these clinics and sometimes with better follow-up care.

Women's Crisis Centers

These centers provide immediate counseling to women in crisis situations, such as rape, divorce, and physical abuse. Frequently free of charge, they depend largely on volunteer services, and as such the quality and experience of counselors varies greatly. Referral services for health problems are usually available.

It bears repeating that the time to look into and even visit the health care facilities in your locale is before you desperately need them. Table 1 lists various resources to help you in your search.

The High Cost of Health Care

During the 1980s, health care settings were increasingly affected by competitive pressures arising from the continued high cost of health care. In the 1990s, the federal government, insurance companies, and businesses will remain the big spenders in the health care arena. All three will attempt to control costs by arrangements with HMOs and PPOs. To date, neither competitive pressures nor government programs have been able to keep the cost of health care from consistently rising faster than the consumer price index. During a time of such medical miracles as in vitro fertilization and laser surgery, the cost of health insurance has climbed out of reach of millions of American women. About 15 million women of reproductive age in the United States have no access to health insurance or public assistance. Among the 3.7 million women who give birth each year, one out of twelve had no maternity coverage, either public or private, in 1991. This was an improvement from 1985, however, when—prior to the expansion of Medicaid coverage—twice as many women were uninsured for their pregnancies. As of 1994, a majority of women of childbearing age have some form of private insurance and nearly all such plans, whether traditional or HMO, offer some maternity coverage. A significant number of U.S. pregnancies are covered under Medicaid, which funded 1.24 million deliveries in 1994, 32% of all births of that year.

Table 1   RESOURCES FOR FINDING HEALTH CARE ALTERNATIVES

1. Local branch of American Nurses Association

2. Local women's organizations, e.g., National Organization for Women

3. Local university, department of women's studies or college of nursing

4. Local medical school, department of internal medicine, family practice, or obstetrics and gynecology

5. Local hospital, department of nursing service or in-service education

6. Local county medical association

7. Local public library

8. Classified section of newspaper or phone book

9. Local branch, Planned Parenthood Association

10. Local Public Health Department

11. Group Health Association of America, Inc.
    Communication and Information Department
    1129 20th Street, N.W., Suite 600
    Washington, D.C. 20036
        (This organization will provide information about HMOs in your area.)

12. American College of Nurse-Midwives
    818 Connecticut Avenue, N.W., Suite 900
    Washington, D.C. 20006

13. Association of Women's Health Obstetric
        and Neonatal Nurses
    700 14th Street, N.W., Suite 600
    Washington, D.C. 20005

CHAPTER 3

Understanding Female Anatomy and Its Functioning

Figure 1
External female anatomy.

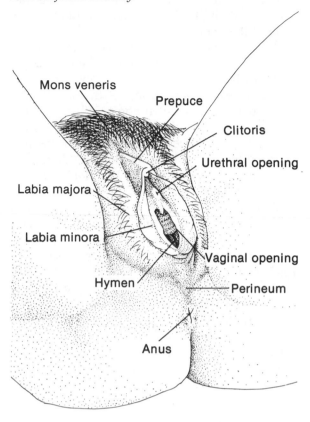

The women's movement has encouraged greater individual responsibility for health and body awareness. In the past (and still in the present for some) the natural urge for self-exploration in childhood was inhibited, and women often learned to ignore their sexual organs. Not so much anymore. Many women openly discuss, among friends or in women's groups, their concerns about their body functioning. They can choose from among a great many books that explain female anatomy and sexuality. Self-examination, too, is a way many women are learning. We hope this chapter will increase your knowledge of basic female anatomy and physiology and will make you more comfortable with the terms used by your clinician.

The easiest way to examine yourself is with a mirror, which should be at least four or five inches wide. Plan for a few private moments to look at yourself and identify your external genitalia, or sexual organs. You can squat, or lie on your back with your head and knees elevated, or sit on the edge of a chair. If you have a full-length mirror, you might be able to position yourself in front of it. In any case, find a position that is comfortable and relaxing to you.

The External Female Anatomy

This is the area you can see in your mirror (see Figure 1). As you read about each organ, remember that individual differences in size, shape, and coloration are normal and may be due to racial factors, childbirth, or genetic factors. If you have any doubts or questions, consult your clinician.

The *mons veneris* is the triangular area of fatty tissue that covers the pubic bone. Pubic hair, usually coarse and curly, covers the mons and may continue up to your naval. The thickness and amount of hair varies greatly. Pubic hair makes its appearance during adolescence as the result of an increased output of sex hormones.

The *vulva* is the name of the entire outer area of a woman's genital-urethral organs. The vulva includes the labia majora (large lips), labia minora (small lips), the clitoris, the urethral opening, and the vaginal opening.

The *labia majora* are two soft folds of outer skin that cushion and protect the vaginal opening. Like skin elsewhere in the body, they are covered with hair and sebaceous (oil) glands. As a woman becomes older, these lips become more flaccid, or looser; after childbirth they may no longer completely cover the labia minora.

The *labia minora* are small, sensitive lips just

inside the labia majora. They play an important role in sexual activity, becoming engorged during excitation, thus providing a tighter grip around the penis.

As you separate the labia majora, you will see the *clitoris* at the top of the folds where the larger and smaller lips come together. The *prepuce*, or clitoral foreskin, sits on top of the smaller lips and looks like a small triangle. When you feel the small rounded clitoris with your finger, you will find it to be very sensitive. With manipulation, it becomes stiff and enlarged, filling with blood during sexual activity, similar to the engorgement of the male penis.

Directly below the clitoris is a small dark "dimple" called the *urethral opening*, which is the opening through which you urinate. The *urethra* is the canal through which urine is passed from the bladder.

Below the urethral opening is the *hymen* or its remnants. The hymen is the thin fibrous tissue that partially covers the vagina, leaving a small opening for vaginal or menstrual discharge. This opening can be stretched or torn through such athletic activities as horseback riding or bicycle riding or through initial intercourse. The tearing of the hymen may cause bleeding, which will stop by itself, and possibly some discomfort. Since the hymen is highly elastic, the use of a lubricant (K-Y Jelly) during initial sexual activity almost always allows an intact hymen to stretch gradually without much physical trauma. After the hymen is stretched or torn, small folds of tissue, called *hymenal tags*, may remain. Rarely, the hymen may cover the entire vaginal opening (called an *imperforate hymen*), blocking normal intercourse as well as trapping menstrual blood within the vagina. This condition requires correction about the time of the onset of puberty; the procedure is a simple surgical one easily done on an outpatient basis.

The *perineum* is the area below the vagina and above the anus. If you have given birth, you may observe small thin scars here from a procedure called an *episiotomy*. This procedure involves making a small cut (and then repairing it with stitches) in the perineum during delivery to prevent tearing of the vaginal muscles into the anus. The *anus* is the opening into the rectum. After childbirth, small skin tags may be present around the anus, the result of stretching and pressure during pregnancy and the delivery process. These skin tags are remnants of previous hemorrhoids and are quite common.

The Internal Female Anatomy

The internal female organs are normally "felt" by the clinician during the pelvic examination, which will be discussed in Chapter 4. Figure 2 shows you the location of each of these organs, which include the vagina, cervix, uterus, Fallopian tubes, and ovaries.

The *vagina*, an elastic organ similar to a tiny tunnel, connects the cervix (opening of the uterus) to the outside of your body. The vagina varies in length from three to five inches. Sometimes called the *birth canal*, the vagina can expand during childbirth to five inches in width. The length of the vagina does not affect the ease of delivery or sexual enjoyment. Unless the hymen is intact, inserting one or two fingers into the vagina will not cause discomfort. The vagina should feel soft, moist, and pliable. The vagina lies between the bladder (above) and the rectum (below) (see Figure 7). Using a flashlight and a plastic speculum, available from your gynecologist or local women's self-help group, you may better visualize the vagina in your mirror. As you insert your fingers into the vagina, you may touch something hard and dimpled which feels similar to the tip of your nose. This is the *cervix*, or mouth of the uterus. If you have an intrauterine device (IUD), the string may be felt in the vagina, but the IUD itself should be located above the cervix. The cervical opening is very small; thus tampons are prevented from being pushed up into the uterus. Two glands, called *Bartholin's glands*, open into the vagina, one gland on either side, near the hymen and produce a thin mucus that helps to lubricate the vagina. These glands are not visible on the outside unless blockage of the gland opening occurs, producing a cyst or infection.

The *uterus*, a shiny, pink, pear-shaped, muscular organ, is designed to nourish and support the developing fetus. It is normally about the size of a fist. An amazingly versatile organ, the uterus stretches to many times its size during pregnancy and contracts its powerful muscles to begin the birth process. The inner lining of the uterus, called the *endometrium*, is composed of

Figure 2 *Internal female anatomy.*

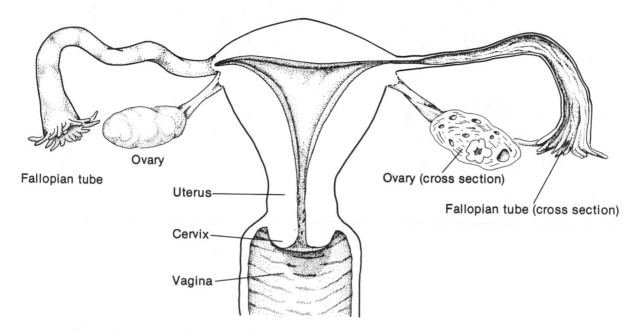

Fallopian tube

Ovary

Uterus

Cervix

Vagina

Ovary (cross section)

Fallopian tube (cross section)

soft, blood-enriched tissue that sloughs (drops off or sheds) each month during your menstrual period. The uterus has three openings: two upper openings into the Fallopian tubes and one lower opening (cervix) into the vagina. The top portion of the uterus, called the *fundus*, is what nurses and doctors are feeling when they push on your stomach following childbirth. The only time you can normally feel your uterus is at this time, too. For the first few days after delivery you can push on your abdomen with your hand and feel a hard, round ball about the size of a grapefruit.

Women often think of the *Fallopian tubes* as the pathway of the egg into the uterus. It is sometimes forgotten that it is here, in one of the two Fallopian tubes, where embryonic life begins. The sperm, after successfully negotiating its trip up the vagina, cervix, and uterus, meets the egg (called an *ovum*) in the upper portion of one Fallopian tube, and fertilization takes place. During the six-day journey it takes for the fertilized egg to migrate down the tube, specialized cells along the passageway maintain and protect the egg, as they wave it on its way to the uterus.

The two *ovaries*, one located on either side of the uterus adjacent to the opening of each Fallopian tube, produce the sex hormones estrogen and progesterone. These are the major female hormones that stimulate the development of fe-

male characteristics during puberty and make reproduction possible. The eggs (ova) are also housed here and number about 400,000 at the time of puberty, although only one out of every thousand ova will be used in a woman's lifetime. The process of *ovulation*, the release of a matured egg from the ovary, will be discussed later in this chapter.

The Breasts

Probably no other part of a woman's anatomy is as obvious as the breasts, yet many women know very little about them. The breasts function both as milk producers following childbirth and as organs of sexual stimulation. Breast tissue contains essentially fat cells and a network of milk-producing glands (see Figure 3). The fat cells, unlike the general fat elsewhere in the body, are a specific type which grow in response to the increase in sex hormones during adolescence. Breast development starts in a girl anywhere from one to two years before she begins to menstruate. The size of one's breasts is determined largely by genetic factors and depends on the amount of fatty tissue present. Breasts respond to normal cyclic hormonal changes and may swell or feel tender just before a menstrual

Figure 3
Normal breast anatomy.

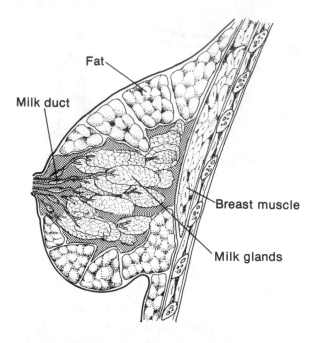

Fat

Milk duct

Breast muscle

Milk glands

period. A slight difference in the size of the two breasts is also normal.

The pinkish-red or brownish portion around the nipple of each breast is called the *areola*. The color of the areola is usually darker in pregnant women and in women who have had children. The nipple may protrude from the areola or lie flat. Cold temperature, sexual stimulation, or breast-feeding may cause the nipples to become temporarily more erect. You may see small bumps surrounding the areola; these are sebaceous (oil) glands that lubricate the nipple during nursing. Small hairs sometimes arise from the follicles in the areola, a perfectly normal situation.

Self-examination of the breasts

It is essential that you examine your breasts each month to detect possible breast cancer in its early stages. Breast cancer is the leading cause of death due to cancer among women and is also the most common cause of death in American women between the ages of forty and forty-five. With rare exception, these tumors are painless; and without a routine self-examination, their presence may go undetected. (See Appendix E.)

The best time to examine your breasts is right after your period. Sometimes just before or during your period, your breasts may feel more tender or thickened. For this reason, breast examination, either by you or your clinician, is most reliable when performed just after a period rather than the week before. If you are past menopause, pick a particular day of the month, say the first, mark it on your calendar, and make your breast examination each month on this day.

First, look at your breasts in a mirror. Any retraction, discharge, scaling, or other skin changes around the nipple may be an early sign of breast cancer. Any breast bulging, dimpling, or redness should be noted and reported to your clinician. Do your breasts seem symmetrical, with both nipples at the same level? Do both nipples look the same? Raise your hands above your head and repeat the same observation. This helps to expose the lower surface of the breasts and makes it easier to see any changes in shape or contour.

The next step is to palpate your breasts, that is, to examine them by feeling them in a certain way. Here is how to do it. Because you can more easily detect irregularities of the breast tissue by letting the breast tissue flatten against the chest wall, simply lie down on the floor, on a bed or sofa, or perhaps in the bathtub. As you examine, for example, your left breast, raise your left arm above your head, resting your left hand behind your head. Placing a small pillow or towel under your shoulders may help you in this examination of the breast tissue. Gently feel your left breast with the fingers of your right hand, beginning around the nipple, pressing lightly with your fingers. Move your fingers in widening circles or slightly back and forth so that you systematically cover the entire breast. What you are feeling for is a lump or thickness. Repeat this examination with your left arm lying down by your side. Pay special attention to the area between the nipple and the armpit as this is one of the most common locations of tumors. To examine your right breast, simply reverse the procedure, with your right hand behind your head, and so on. Check each nipple for possible discharge by gently squeezing it between your thumb and forefinger. Ask your clinician or the nurse to demonstrate this technique to you. They may have special teaching materials, such as videotapes or pamphlets, for your use.

Regular self-examinations help you to know

what your breasts feel like normally. With practice you will be able to detect any lump, thickness, or irregularity that may appear.

Hormonal Changes During a Woman's Life Cycle

The word *menses*, which means the same as menstrual period, comes from the Latin word *mensis*, meaning "month." The menstrual cycle averages 28 days in length, with normal variation ranging from 21 to 35 days. Menstrual bleeding is traditionally considered the beginning of the menstrual cycle. Times of emotional and physical stress can delay or speed up the start of the menstrual cycle. Breast-feeding may delay the resumption of menstruation, perhaps for several months after delivery, even after you have stopped breast-feeding.

What causes menstruation?

Menstruation is a complicated hormonal process initiated by the brain hormones LH (luteinizing hormone) and FSH (follicle-stimulating hormone), both of which come from the pituitary gland, at the base of the brain. LH and FSH start the process by stimulating the ovaries to produce their own hormones, estrogen and progesterone. The hypothalamus, also located in the brain, regulates the release of FSH and LH from the pituitary gland. This helps explain the effect of psychological stress on the menstrual cycle since the hypothalamus is considered a principal emotional center in the brain. If you are overly upset, the message gets to the hypothalamus; the hypothalamus contacts the pituitary gland, and your menstrual cycle may arrive early or be delayed.

The first half of the menstrual cycle is dominated by the production of FSH by the pituitary. This hormone is responsible for the maturation of the egg in one of the ovaries prior to ovulation. The maturing egg is located in a special part of the ovary called the follicle; this follicle secretes estrogen. Each month estrogen stimulates the growth of a whole new uterine lining (endometrium) in which a fertilized egg can implant itself. Approximately halfway through the menstrual cycle, LH causes the release of the egg

from its follicle. This release is called *ovulation* and it may be accompanied by a brief, sharp pain on one side of the abdomen. An increase in vaginal mucus discharge or slight spotting may also occur near the time of ovulation.

The second, or postovulatory, half of the menstrual cycle is characterized by increasing levels of both estrogen and progesterone, which some authorities believe are responsible for many of the symptoms of premenstrual tension. After releasing its egg, the ovarian follicle is called the *corpus luteum*, which continues to secrete hormones. The released egg enters one of the Fallopian tubes, usually on the same side that ovulation occurred, and begins its six-day journey to the uterus. Fertilization must take place during this time period. Rarely, a fertilized egg may implant in the tube, causing a *tubal*, or *ectopic*, *pregnancy*. If the egg isn't fertilized, it disintegrates and is released in the menstrual blood.

The corpus luteum stops producing estrogen and progesterone at the end of the cycle if conception has not occurred. As the hormone levels drop, the blood supply ceases to nourish the uterine lining and menstrual bleeding begins. The low production of estrogen eventually acts as a stimulus for pituitary production of FSH to begin the next menstrual cycle. In the absence of fertilization, the corpus luteum normally recedes, leaving only a small scar on the surface of the ovary. Occasionally it may persist as a small cyst for several weeks or months, accounting for one of the most common causes of mild pelvic pain in women.

How does fertilization occur?

Fertilization, or conception, occurs with the union of one egg and one sperm in the Fallopian tube. The male testes continuously produce sperm, and millions of sperm leave the penis upon ejaculation during intercourse. The sperm quickly "swim" up through the cervix and the uterus to the tiny entrance into the tubes. Pregnancy begins when the sperm and the egg unite (see Figure 4).

What happens if fertilization occurs?

When conception takes place, the hormone production of the last half of the menstrual cycle is

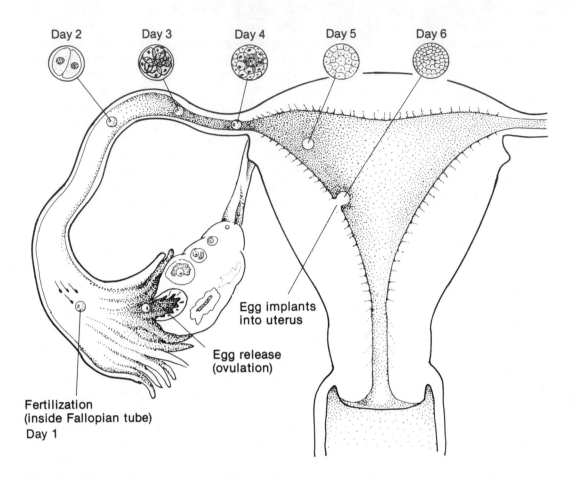

Day 2   Day 3   Day 4   Day 5   Day 6

Egg implants
into uterus

Egg release
(ovulation)

Fertilization
(inside Fallopian tube)
Day 1

Figure 4   *The first six days of life. Fertilization results when a sperm from the male unites with an egg from the female. If fertilization occurs, division of the egg begins. It then takes about six days for the fertilized ovum to travel through the tube and reach the uterus where the mass of cells implants into the uterine lining. Modified with permission of Parke-Davis, division of Warner-Lambert Company* (Female Reproductive Organs—in Health and Illness, *1978).*

changed. With implantation of the fertilized egg about one week after ovulation, the *placenta*, which is the organ for receiving oxygen and nutrients and discharging waste products, begins to develop. The developing placenta soon produces HCG (human chorionic gonadotropin), sometimes known as the pregnancy hormone, which prevents the cyclic hormonal changes of menstruation from taking place. It acts as a stimulus to the corpus luteum to continue its production of estrogen and progesterone for the first three months of pregnancy, after which production is taken over by the placenta. HCG is the hormone measured in all pregnancy tests.

During this time twinning may occur in one of two ways. Fraternal twins will result if the woman produces two eggs within the same month and they are fertilized by two different sperm. Identical twins result from the splitting of a single fertilized egg in the first few weeks of development. The chance of having twins is about one in ninety. Fraternal twins are more common than identical twins by a ratio of about two to one. It is not clear which factors make a woman susceptible to having identical twins; however, a slight increase in the frequency of fraternal twins has been linked with increasing maternal age, large family size, and a family history of twins, especially involving the maternal side of the family.

The ovaries rest during pregnancy, with no stimulation of follicles or ovulation taking place. Menstruation resumes within the first three months following delivery in about 85% of women. The remaining 15% usually begin menstruating again in the next four to six months.

At what age does menstruation begin?

A girl experiences her first period, called the *menarche*, usually at about the age that her mother did. The average age of menarche today is about twelve years, although it is common to find menarche beginning anywhere between the ages of ten to fourteen. If a woman has not started to menstruate by the age of sixteen, she should consult a physician for evaluation.

The menstrual cycle is usually irregular for the first two years or so. Many initial periods may be *anovulatory* (no ovulation) while the adolescent body matures and hormone production becomes more regular. The anovulatory cycles prevent pregnancy from occurring in a young girl until her body and bone structure are sufficiently mature. If she is engaging in sexual activity, however, and if pregnancy is not desired, a method of birth control should be considered because there is no certainty that each successive period will be anovulatory.

How do you know when you are ovulating?

The basal body temperature (BBT) chart is a way commonly used to determine the time of ovulation. The basal body temperature refers to the temperature of your body at rest. To determine your BBT, take your temperature *immediately* upon awakening every day. This means *before* you get out of bed. Record your temperature from a special thermometer used for this purpose on a chart supplied by your physician or pharmacist. (This procedure is discussed in more detail in Chapter 6.) There is a slight but definite elevation of your BBT at the time of ovulation. The rise is caused by the production of progesterone at ovulation and usually measures no more than 0.4 to 1.0 degree Fahrenheit. This rise in temperature persists until the progesterone production stops prior to menstruation. If you become pregnant, your temperature will stay at the higher level. Infertility caused by failure to ovulate can be determined by use of the BBT. Figure 9 shows examples of different temperature chart patterns. Cervical mucus charting, as discussed in Chapter 6, is another method used for determining ovulation.

Some women experience "middle pain" (*mittel-schmerz*) each month around the time of ovulation. This brief, sharp pain felt on one side (or the other) of the lower abdomen occurs just as the egg is released from the surface of the ovary (ovulation).

How does menopause occur?

Anovulatory cycles, similar to those in adolescents, usually start around forty-five years of age and are due to declining production of hormones by the ovaries. The premenopausal years, called the *climacteric*, usually span a four- to six-year period; it takes this long for the ovaries to stop producing hormones. The age a woman experiences menopause, while bearing no relationship to the woman's age of menarche, is closely correlated with the age that her mother stopped having periods.

The first indication that the ovaries are slowing down is menstrual irregularity. Periods usually become lighter and less frequent with some variation from month to month. A woman is considered to have reached menopause when she has not had a period for twelve consecutive months.

As the ovaries gradually stop production of estrogen, the pituitary produces increasing amounts of FSH and LH in a futile attempt to stimulate estrogen production by the ovary. Some authorities believe these high levels of FSH and LH account for certain menopausal symptoms, such as hot flashes and night sweats. For many years following menopause, the ovaries continue to produce small amounts of estrogen as well as minute amounts of male sex hormones (androgens), accounting for the slight hair growth noticed by some women at this time.

When Should You Talk to Your Child About Sexuality?

The earlier an honest, open line of communication is established, the easier it is. Through the mass media—television, music, movies, tapes, magazines, and books—children inevitably see and hear a great deal about sex early in life. Sex is used to sell entertainment and products, makes headlines in the news, and is the explicit subject of many popular songs. Much of a child's

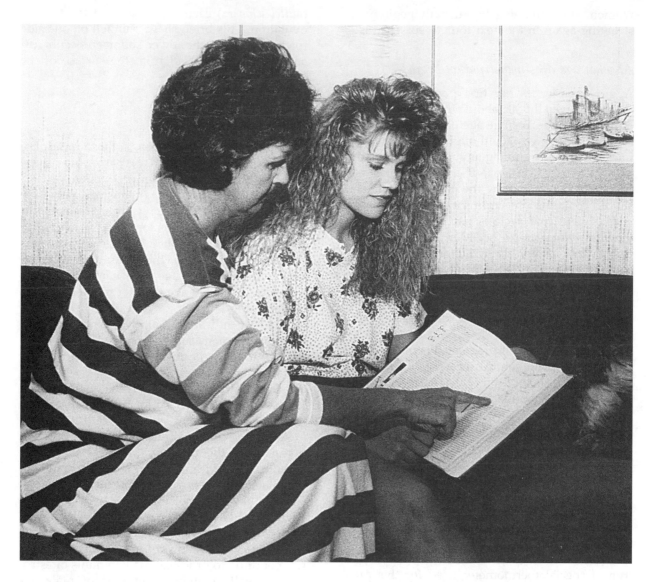

learning about sexuality takes place gradually and informally.

Children are curious about different aspects of sexuality at different ages. Preschoolers ask questions about gender differences and the names and functions of parts of the body. They become curious about childbirth, asking such questions as "How does the baby get out?" (That question is asked much earlier than "How does the baby get in?") It is important to answer these questions when they are asked. A number of studies have shown that adolescent girls who have been given an honest and accurate education in human sexuality become unintentionally pregnant much less often than girls who have not. They are also more likely to postpone sexual relations longer than their uninformed sisters.

Discussion of sexuality also helps to safeguard your child from child molestation, providing knowledge about appropriate boundaries for allowable "touching." Teenagers usually have questions about values, impulses, and pressures surrounding sex that they feel are too personal to ask a school nurse or sex-education teacher. Ideally, these questions should be dealt with at home; in an era of rampantly growing rates of sexually transmitted diseases and teenage pregnancy, it is important for young people to have their facts straight.

It is a good idea to prepare your son or daughter for puberty so they will not be surprised when menstruation or "wet dreams" suddenly occur. Both of these events signify fertility, and children need to be aware of their sexual responsibilities. Planning a mother-daughter or father-son talk between the ages of nine and eleven is recommended. It may be helpful to have both parents participate; this provides an excellent opportunity to teach family religious values. Breast self-examination should also be discussed with young girls so they can be exposed to the idea, even though routine breast exams are not recommended until age twenty. Hygiene can also be discussed. Good communication started at this age will leave your son or daughter comfortable enough to return to you for further questions or resolution of suspected fears during their teenage years.

Education departments at local hospitals often offer group "girl talks," which use videotapes that present helpful information covering topics from sexually transmitted diseases to contraception. Be certain to familiarize yourself with the content of your child's school health education so you know what he or she has been taught. After puberty, it is wise to offer your son or daughter a chance for a question-and-answer session. Let them know you are always available to answer questions or make clarifications as they encounter new information from their peer group. An excellent resource that discusses the social and psychological challenges facing young girls today can be found in *Reviving Ophelia: Saving the Selves of Adolescent Girls* by Mary Pipher (Ballantine Books, 1995).

CHAPTER 4

Getting the Most Out of Your Office Visit

Most women feel reluctant and a little fearful about their initial visit to a gynecologist or other health professional. The pelvic examination is often an unnerving intrusion of privacy even in longstanding doctor/patient relationships. This emotional and physical discomfort can be diminished if you know what to expect. This chapter provides a step-by-step guide to the exam and offers specific suggestions to help you get the most out of your office visit.

Making Your Appointment

Evaluate your needs before making an appointment. If your problem is not urgent, schedule your appointment between menstrual periods. If you unexpectedly start your period prior to a scheduled exam, check with your doctor to see if you need to reschedule. Otherwise you may spend your time and money on two visits, one for a checkup and the other for a Pap smear. Do not douche or use a vaginal cream for at least twenty-four hours before your appointment; you may be washing away important clues to diagnosing some vaginal conditions. Having intercourse prior to your visit does not in any way affect the doctor's exam. If your reason to see the doctor will not require an exam, try to handle the problem with a phone call.

Medical Records

You have a legal right to see your medical records at any time. Hospital records are usually more detailed than office records and are thus more useful to a physician unfamiliar with your health history. Three aspects of hospital charts are usually well documented. These are the nurses' progress notes, the operative note (what was found and what was done), and the pathology report, which reflects the findings at surgery. For obstetrical patients, the labor-and-delivery record contains the essential information about previous childbirths. In requesting your records from other doctors' offices, it is particularly important to obtain these portions of the hospital record.

Patients often assume that medical records are detailed and complete. Unfortunately this is not so. You can keep a record of any symptoms or findings you have with much more accuracy than is usually documented in the records. Your keeping your own record is a good idea especially if pelvic abnormalities are found. From the examination, your doctor should be able to provide you with information about abnormal cysts, swellings, or tumors to the centimeter. Because written information about your medical history may be sketchy, it is important to verbally recount your history to your doctor in addition to requesting that records be sent to your doctor.

The Pre-Exam Interview

Physicians and other health care providers are taught to take a medical history according to a prescribed format. In practice this format is considerably shortened depending on the time allotted and the severity of the problem. Physician assistants may take a more thorough history than do physicians. More often than not, a diagnosis is made from a careful history rather than from the physical exam. In preparing for an initial office visit, it is helpful if you have a written record of your health history. At the back of this book a Health History Profile checklist is provided (see Appendix A). The checklist emphasizes women's health problems and is designed to cover most of the questions you are likely to be asked. Table 2 shows what general areas of information the Health History Profile covers.

You can either make photocopies of the blank Health History Profile checklist directly from the one at the back of this book; or you can tear it out of the book and perhaps make some blank

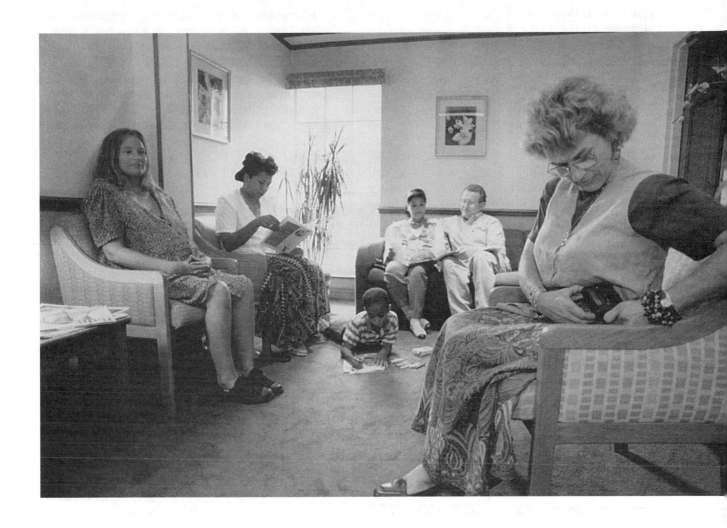

Table 2 AREAS OF INFORMATION COVERED BY THE HEALTH HISTORY PROFILE*

Area of Information	Comment
1. Current problems	1. Are there specific concerns or problems that you want to discuss with your clinician?
2. Menstrual history	2. Are your periods regular? Any unusual bleeding or pain?
3. Contraceptive history	3 What birth control method(s) have you used? Any problems or side effects?
4. Pregnancy history	4. Be sure to mention any complications of pregnancy or childbirth you have experienced.
5. Previous conditions	5. Include any past illnesses requiring medical treatment.
6. Previous hospitalizations	6. Include any previous surgery.
7. Family history	7. It is especially important to include any family history of breast cancer, high blood pressure, or diabetes.
8. Medication history	8. Include your drug allergies and side effects you have experienced.

* The complete Health History Profile checklist appears in the back of this book (Appendix A).

copies of it, to use one for each different doctor you visit who asks for this information. You can thus take more time before your appointment to prepare this information carefully for your doctor, and you will also be able to check out things that may not come to mind immediately in the doctor's office, like family history. The more accurate the information is that you give your doctor, the better able he or she is to evaluate your health problem. After you have completed the Health History Profile, you may want to make a copy of the completed form and keep it for your own records to use in the future. You can bring the completed form with you at the time of your office visit.

Before, rather than after, your pelvic exam, make clear your reason for coming so that your doctor will be alert for your specific concern. If your problem has been a chronic one, be certain to explain why it concerned you enough to make the appointment at this particular time. If the reason for your visit is a second opinion about a problem, you may wish to keep this to yourself until after the examination to see if your second doctor's diagnosis confirms the first doctor's opinion. Your doctor should know that you are selective about your care. If the problem is something you feel is not directly related to the gynecological area, mention it. Gynecologists are the principal physicians for many women and can readily treat simple nongynecological problems. For more serious or chronic ailments, inquire about a referral to a specialist.

The Gynecological Exam

Most gynecologists do a modified form of the complete physical examination. This includes determination of weight and blood pressure, a urinalysis, and a blood count as well as examination of the skin, throat, neck, chest, heart, breasts, abdomen, and pelvis. There is some controversy about the benefits of the complete physical exam, especially in individuals under forty. The American Cancer Society now recommends that women without any symptoms should have breast and pelvic exams every three years between age twenty and forty and annually after age forty (see Table 3). Pap smear recommendations are very general. Many physicians believe annual Pap smears are very important, as

the number of precancerous conditions and early cancers of the cervix remains high. In addition to annual Pap smears, most gynecologists recommend continuing the yearly checkup regardless of age to examine for other medical conditions, especially if the gynecologist is the woman's primary physician. Table 3 also suggests a time schedule for other recommended medical procedures, based on your age and medical history. Discuss with your doctor those areas mentioned in Table 3 that apply to you.

The breast exam

More than 90% of palpable breast cancers are detected through self examination. In Chapter 3 we described how you can do this simple, quick exam yourself. You should learn how to do this procedure and perform it on a regular basis. When the clinician examines your breasts, point out any areas that concern you. You may want to ask for a demonstration of the breast self-exam at this time also. (See Appendix E.) Fortunately, the vast majority of breast masses detected are benign.

The pelvic exam

The self-pelvic and self-Pap exams are not as convenient or as easy to do compared to the breast self-exam. For this reason, it can be done more reliably by a doctor or nurse who has the experience to differentiate normal from abnormal. Because of normal changes throughout the menstrual cycle, changes brought about by childbirth, and individual variation, there is a wide spectrum of what is considered normal pelvic findings. The nurse or family practitioner will often refer a questionable normal finding to an OB-GYN specialist for clarification. A nurse or female assistant is almost always present to assist during the pelvic exam for medical-legal reasons and to provide you with empathetic support.

It is important to urinate just prior to the pelvic exam, both for your own comfort and so that your doctor won't misdiagnose a full bladder as a cyst. (You may have just given a urine specimen to the nurse or a lab assistant, but after a long waiting-room wait you may have the urge to urinate again. Don't hesitate to do so.) Before the exam, you are usually given a drape sheet or examining gown. The purpose of the drape

Table 3   AMERICAN CANCER SOCIETY GUIDELINES FOR CANCER-RELATED CHECKUPS*

Exam and/or Procedure	Age 20 to 40	Age 40 and Over	Exceptions (Higher-Risk Women Who May Need More Frequent Testing)
General checkup including breast and pelvic exam as well as exam of skin, mouth, thyroid, and lymph nodes	Every 3 years	Every year	See exceptions below; women at risk for uterine (endometrial) cancer (see Table 69) should have an endometrial tissue sample (biopsy) at menopause
Breast self-exam	Every month	Every month	
Pap test	All women who are, or who have been, sexually active, or have reached age 18, should have an annual Pap test and pelvic examination. After a woman has had three or more consecutive satisfactory normal annual examinations, the Pap test may be performed less frequently at the discretion of her physician.		Higher risk for cervical cancer (see Table 66)
Breast X-ray (mammogram)	Not applicable	Every 1 to 2 years starting age 40; every year after age 50	Higher risk for breast cancer (see Table 60)
Guaiac slide test (to check for blood in stool)	Not applicable	Every year after age 50	Higher risk for colon or rectal cancer (personal or family history of polyps in the rectum or colon or of cancer in the rectum or colon; personal history of ulcerative colitis)
Sigmoidoscopy (procto exam—see glossary)	Not applicable	Every 3 to 5 years after age 50	Higher risk for colon or rectal cancer (personal or family history of polyps in the rectum or colon or of cancer in the rectum or colon; personal history of ulcerative colitis)
Endometrial tissue sample	Not applicable	At menopause if high-risk**	

* Guidelines set forth by the American Cancer Society for women without symptoms as revised, 1987. The A.C.S. recommends that you talk with your doctor to see how these guidelines relate to you.
** History of infertility, obesity, failure to ovulate, abnormal uterine bleeding, or estrogen therapy.

sheet is to cover your lower abdomen and thighs to help preserve your remaining modesty—not to cover up what the physician is doing. If you prefer, the drape can be arranged to permit eye contact with the doctor. However, if the gown is objectionable to you and you are wearing a slip, ask if you can wear your own slip instead of the gown.

Pelvic examining tables have metal stirrups (sometimes plastic covered) for resting your heels while you slide your hips down to the edge of the table. Let your knees spread apart comfortably and relax as much as possible. The more relaxed your abdominal and vaginal muscles, the more comfortable and thorough will be the exam. To facilitate relaxation, ask your doctor to let you know what he or she is doing during each step of the exam.

The pelvic exam consists of four steps, which should take no more than a few minutes to complete. In the first step, the external genitalia, or vulva, is inspected, including the labia majora, labia minora, clitoris, urethral opening, and outer vagina. You may want to request that your examiner clarify any questions you have concerning your anatomy by use of a mirror. Point

Figure 5
View of cervix and vagina during the pelvic examination.

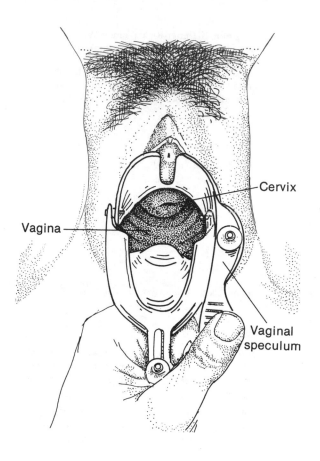

Cervix

Vagina

Vaginal speculum

Figure 6
Obtaining a Pap smear.

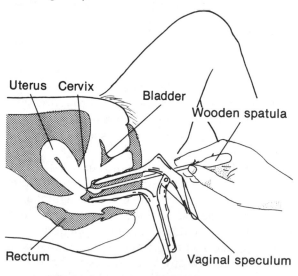

Uterus Cervix

Bladder

Wooden spatula

Rectum

Vaginal speculum

out areas of irritation or lesions you have noticed. Because of the rich suppy of nerve endings of the vulva, a very small area may be the source of a lot of discomfort to you but may go unnoticed by the physician. The pelvic support provided by your vaginal muscles is tested next; childbirth may have caused some normal stretching and loss of support, especially in women who have had large babies or more than three children. The clinician inserts one or two fingers into the vagina and presses down while you are asked to strain or cough to bring out any bulge or muscle weakness in the upper or lower vagina (*cystocele* or *rectocele*). Be sure to mention if you have noticed any vaginal protrusion, loosening of the vaginal muscles during sex, or some loss of bladder control.

The second step in the exam involves insertion of a plastic or metal speculum and is called the *speculum exam*. If a metal speculum is used, don't hesitate to request that it first be warmed. This insertion is done by slowly introducing the closed speculum into the vagina. After insertion, the speculum is opened just wide enough to permit the doctor to see the cervix and upper vagina (see Figure 5). Aside from pressure or mild discomfort, any pain or pinching you may experience indicates either inflammation or an impatient examiner. Let your doctor know if his or her technique is not a gentle one.

The primary purpose of the speculum part of the exam is to do the Pap test (see Figure 6). This painless test, named for its inventor, Dr. George Papanicolaou, involves gently scraping the cervix with a small wooden or plastic spatula to collect cells, which are smeared on a glass slide and then sprayed with a fixative. The slide is then sent to a cytology laboratory for microscopic examination of the cell characteristics. A few days later, the doctor receives a report indicating whether the cells are normal, atypical, or malignant (see Chapter 37 for a fuller explanation of Pap test results). Fortunately, abnormalities detected by this test are usually due to inflammation (vaginitis) and not to cancer. Usually, precancerous changes in the cells show up several years before actual invasive cancer develops in the tissues. Regular checkups, therefore, practically insure against development of a life-threatening cervical cancer. Most authorities recommend that an initial exam, including a Pap smear, be done on a woman by the age of eighteen or at the beginning of sexual activity, whichever is earlier.

Another purpose of the speculum exam is to diagnose various vaginal and cervical inflammatory conditions, some of which are infectious and most of which produce more discharge than usual. If your problem concerns a vaginal infection, a *wet prep* may be done. This is a slide preparation obtained from secretions of the vagina for microscopic examination. If you are concerned about the possibility of a venereal infection, a *transgrow* culture, a standard test for gonorrhea, may be done. You have to ask for this test specifically in most doctors' offices. The test is accomplished by swabbing a sample of cervical secretions with a cotton-tipped applicator onto a culture plate, which is then sent to a bacteriology lab. It takes up to seventy-two hours for the results of the test because it takes that long for the bacteria to grow on the culture medium. In general, other types of vaginal cultures for monilia (yeast) or nonspecific bacteria have little practical value in the diagnosis and treatment of most vaginal infections.

The speculum exam provides other information, too. The diagnosis of miscarriage is made exclusively from the speculum exam. If miscarriage has occurred, the cervical opening will be dilated and there will be evidence that tissue has been passed. Also, if ovulation has occurred within the last day or two, it is theoretically possible to detect this occurrence from the speculum exam. At ovulation there will be clear, copious mucus present and the mouth of the cervix will be widened. Previous pregnancy affects the appearance of the cervix; the cervical opening will be widened and the amount of glands on the surface will be increased. This normal increase in glands accounts for the slightly greater amount of vaginal secretions in women who have been pregnant. The pill may produce this effect as well. IUD placement, if an IUD is present, is also checked at the time of the speculum exam.

The third step of the woman's pelvic exam involves evaluation of the uterus, tubes, and ovaries and is called the *bimanual exam*. The physician removes the speculum and inserts two fingers into the vagina alongside the cervix while the other hand presses the lower abdomen and directs the pelvic organs toward the examining fingers (see Figure 7). Using this method, the

Figure 7
Side view of the pelvic examination.

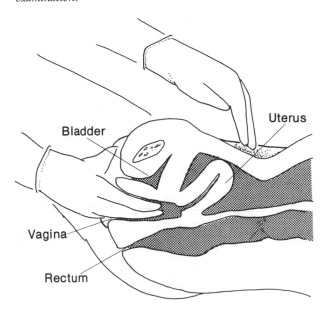

examiner first attempts to outline the uterus to determine its size, contour, position, and consistency. The interior of the uterus, that is, the uterine cavity, cannot be evaluated by this exam. Uterine size varies with age and childbirth. Adolescents and women beyond the menopause will normally have a smaller uterus than women in the childbearing years. With succeeding pregnancies the uterus enlarges. Physicians sometimes refer to the size of a uterus by using the equivalent size during pregnancy as a reference point. For example, a "six-weeks size uterus" would be about two cubic inches in size. After several pregnancies, the uterus may become as large as six-weeks size as a result of the hypertrophy, or stretching process, after childbirth. A uterus larger than six-weeks size would be considered enlarged. Even if no periods have been missed, pregnancy is considered a possibility since the apparent last menstrual period may actually have been due to bleeding resulting from the implantation of the fertilized egg.

If your doctor feels that you have a significantly enlarged uterus, you may be able to feel it with your hand by the following procedure. While the doctor is examining you through the vagina, have him or her elevate the uterus with the examining fingers and ask him or her to place your hand over the lower abdomen where he or she is feeling the uterus. If you can easily

Figure 8
Side view showing the pelvic examination with a retroverted uterus. A rectal examination will allow a more complete evaluation of the uterus.

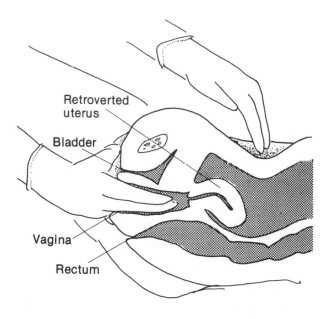

Retroverted uterus

Bladder

Vagina

Rectum

feel the uterus in this manner, this usually confirms that the uterus is indeed enlarged. This procedure may be difficult in some individuals because of pain, immobility of the uterus, or "backward tilting" of the uterus.

Abnormalities in uterine contour or shape are unusual. They most often represent either a growth, such as a small fibroid, or a variation in the embryonic formation of the uterus. These variations are completely harmless except that they may occasionally give rise to problems in pregnancy and childbirth.

Because the uterus is mobile, its position can change according to your activity. In the past, it was mistakenly thought that a tilted, or retroverted, uterus (see Figure 8) could cause a miscarriage or infertility; however, this position is now known to be a normal variation. The uterus has various muscular and fibrous supports. During childbirth these supports may be weakened or stretched so that the uterus sits just slightly lower in the vaginal canal. This change, called *descensus* or *prolapse*, is usually minimal and requires no treatment.

After the uterus is felt by the examiner, the ovaries and tubes are examined, first on one

side and then on the other. The same bimanual technique described above is used. This is the most difficult part of the pelvic exam for the doctor and patient alike, and it will be helpful if you relax your abdominal muscles as much as possible. It may help to take deep breaths in and out through your mouth to help you relax. In many individuals it is not really possible for the examiner to distinctly palpate (feel) the Fallopian tubes and ovaries as separate structures, especially after the menopause, because then these structures become smaller. The examiner is mainly concerned with any abnormal enlargement of the ovary-tube complex, which is normally felt on exam as a single structure measuring up to approximately one cubic inch. The Fallopian tubes are rarely involved in cancer and more commonly are associated with infectious diseases. Like the uterus, the ovaries and tubes do not normally swell during a normal menstrual cycle.

If you feel any tenderness during the bimanual exam, tell the examiner. It will help your doctor to know if you have more discomfort than is usual for you. Compared to the uterus, the ovaries are normally more sensitive to pressure produced by the exam.

The final step in the pelvic exam is known as the *rectovaginal exam*. Most women, during this step of the exam, experience some discomfort; you can decrease this discomfort by bearing down or straining. This part of the exam involves a variation of the bimanual techniques described above. The examiner places one finger in the rectum and leaves the other in the vagina. The purpose is to examine the rectum and the area between the rectum and vagina called the *cul-de-sac*. The rectal exam may detect hemorrhoids, polyps, or colon cancer (a rare occurrence). A rectal exam is sufficent in examining adolescents or others where only a small hymenal opening is present. Because the doctor can reach higher than through the vaginal route alone, greater palpation of the ovaries is possible. If you have hemorrhoids, ask your doctor to omit the rectovaginal exam.

You may wonder about what your doctor can actually determine about you from the pelvic exam and what conditions cannot be determined from the exam. Table 4 outlines and answers some of the questions you may be thinking about in this respect.

Table 4   WHAT CAN MY DOCTOR TELL FROM A PELVIC EXAM?

Question	Yes	No	Comment
If I am pregnant?	X		Not always reliable until after six weeks from last menstrual period; cysts are occasionally confused with pregnancy; pregnancy test is needed for confirmation.
If I have an intact hymen?	X		
If I am a virgin?		X	Unless hymen is intact.
If my external anatomy is normal?	X		
If I have a vaginal odor?		X	Rarely apparent in most situations.
If I have had a baby?	X		Cervix (mouth of uterus) is enlarged; usually episiotomy scar or scars are seen.
If I have had a miscarriage or abortion?		X	Occasionally the cervix is slightly enlarged, indicating previous pregnancy.
If I masturbate?		X	
If I have gonorrhea?		X	A laboratory test (culture) is the only way to confirm the diagnosis.
If I have a vaginal infection?	X		
If I have venereal warts?	X		
If I have had sex recently?	X		If a slide test of vaginal secretions is done, sperm are often seen.
If I can have an orgasm?		X	
If I can get pregnant?		X	The majority of causes of infertility cannot be detected by exam alone; several tests are usually required.
If I can deliver a baby normally?		X	Most women have normal vaginal deliveries. Little can be accurately predicted about whether you will need a cesarean section.
If I get pregnant, am I likely to have premature labor, a miscarriage, or a breech birth?		X	This cannot be predicted by examination alone except in rare instances.
If my uterus, or womb, is enlarged?	X		
If my cervix is inflamed?	X		
If my vaginal muscles are loose?	X		
If my bladder is "dropped"?	X		
If there is weakness or decreased support of vaginal muscles?	X		
If my uterus is "dropped," or prolapsed?	X		
If I need hormones?	X		This is recognized when the vagina is very dry and the vaginal wall tissues appear extremely thin.
If I have a pregnancy in my tube?		X	This requires surgery to confirm.
If my tubes are blocked or scarred?		X	This diagnosis is presumptive; only by certain tests or surgery can this condition be confirmed.
If I have a spastic colon?		X	Diagnosis is made by X-ray and history.
If I have endometriosis?		X	Confirmation by surgery is required.
If I have cancer?		X	Diagnosis can be suspected but biopsy is required to prove.
If my periods are heavy?		X	
If I have fibroids?		X	This common diagnosis is always a presumptive one.

The Post-Exam Interview

If no abnormalities are found, you may be told "everything is fine." However, if you came to the office with specific symptoms unexplained by the exam, you should not leave without a clear understanding of your condition and plans for follow-up care. It is not always possible for doctors to be completely sure that the exam is normal. Unless a definite problem can be determined, the doctor may recommend a follow-up exam rather than starting treatment without a definite diagnosis. For example, stool may be confused with a pelvic tumor; in this case, your doctor may suggest an enema before your next visit. If some doubts exist in your mind about your exam, questions you may want to ask are:

1. Is my uterus enlarged?
2. Is there a question of pregnancy?
3. Is an ovary enlarged?
4. Is there any inflammation of the cervix?
5. Is anything abnormal?

You should know before leaving the office:

1. Are any tests to be scheduled and, if so, what are they for?
2. Could follow-up be handled without an office visit?

If any treatment is planned, ask these questions:

1. Is any printed literature available? If not, ask your physician to make a simple drawing to facilitate your understanding of the problem. Some physicians have audiovisual cassettes for their patients on various subjects such as surgical procedures.
2. If medication is prescribed: What are the actions and side effects? How will the prescribed medication react with any other medication I may be taking? When should I or should I not take the medication, for example, on an empty stomach, with food, or not with certain foods? Is free sample medication available? All physicians are visited regularly by pharmaceutical representatives who leave samples of all the commonly used drugs, including birth control pills.
3. Specifically what is the program of treatment? Are alternative treatments possible? If necessary, get a second opinion, especially if surgery is proposed following an initial visit.

The post-exam interview offers an additional opportunity to evaluate your physician's approach to the doctor/patient relationship and to influence to some extent the course it will take in subsequent visits. Classically doctors have been taught they should have much more authority than is actually necessary. This approach encourages women to become very dependent upon their physicians. Many health professionals now follow more of a patient-participation type model, in which patients actively share in the process of determining their own health needs and alternatives. You are probably best off with a doctor whose approach allows you to participate in decisions involving your health care.

At the close of a patient's visit, doctors often expect pressing, last-minute questions. Even if you don't have such a question, ask one just so you can determine your doctor's willingness to give you the explanations and answers you need.

Leaving the Office

Sometimes you may feel depressed or frustrated when leaving the office. If you do, try to figure out why. Did you ask all the questions you wanted to? Sometimes a patient is too tense to ask all her questions or to understand what the physician has said. Only when the patient is home rethinking the interview or is trying to explain to someone else what the doctor has said does she realize that she is confused. If this happens to you, don't hesitate to call the physician to clarify your information, especially if something new or unexpected is discovered. Sometimes the nurse can simply help you over the phone by looking over your record. Don't be afraid to inquire, repeatedly if necessary, about anything pertaining to your office visit—it is your right and your responsibility to be well-informed.

References for Section One

American College of Obstetricians and Gynecologists, Committee on gynecologic practice, *Committee Opinion* 128. Routine cancer screening, Oct 1993.

Churgay, C. Colorectal cancer screening in women for the primary care practitioner. *The Female Patient* 19:21–36, May 1994.

Legato, M. Health care in the United States: the new focus on women. *The Female Patient* (supplement): 33–39, Feb 1995.

Horton, J., ed. *The Women's Health Data Book—A Profile of Women's Health in the United States.* Washington, D.C.: Jacobs Institute of Women's Health, 1995.

Stotland, N. Pelvic examinations: the patient's perspective. *The Female Patient* 12:63–68, Dec 1987.

Mayer, T. Occasional notes—HMO's: origins and development. *New England Journal of Medicine* 312(9): 590–594, Feb 28, 1985.

What to know before you go HMO. *Changing Times: The Kiplinger Magazine*, Nov 1984.

Lissovoy, G. Preferred provider organizations: today's models and tomorrow's prospects. *Inquiry* 23:7–15, Spring 1986.

American College of Obstetricians and Gynecologists. *Standards for Obstetric-Gynecologic Services*, 7th ed. A.C.O.G., Washington, D.C., 1989.

1987 Summary: national hospital discharge survey. National Center for Health Statistics. *Advance Data,* Sep 28, 1988.

Spitzer, N. Pap screening for teenagers: a life-saving precaution. *Contemporary OB/GYN* 31(1):33–42, Jan 1988.

Freeman, R. Obstetric care in the 1990's: dream or nightmare? *Contemporary OB/GYN* 31(1):106–107, Jan 1988.

Gold, R. Paying for maternity care in the United States. *Family Planning Perspectives* 19(5):109–206, 1987.

American College of Obstetricians and Gynecologists. *Strategies and Options for Improving Access to Maternity Healthcare: The Obstetrician-Gynecologist as Advocate.* Washington, D.C., 1988.

Alan Guttmacher Institute: *Blessed Events and the Bottom Line: Financing Maternity Care in the United States.* New York: A.G.I., 1987.

A WOMAN'S GUIDE TO BIRTH CONTROL

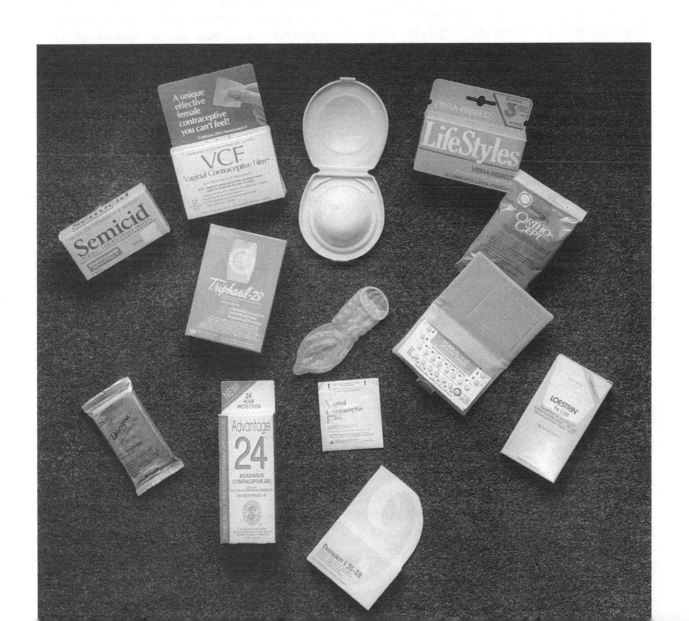

CHAPTER 5

An Overall Look at Birth Control

Contraception is a continuing concern for many women. Despite recent medical advances, a completely safe, effective, and reversible method of birth control has yet to be developed. While no major contraceptive breakthroughs occurred in the 1990s the decade's important developments included the introduction within the United States of two new hormonal contraceptives—Norplant and Depo-Provera—and a new barrier method—the female condom. In addition, the Today vaginal sponge was withdrawn from the market due to the cost of complying with strict government regulations concerning the manufacturing process.

While the focus in the 1970s and early 1980s was on the health risks of the various birth control methods, in the 1990s the health risks of sexual activity itself are at issue. The risk of AIDS has resulted in widespread use of barrier methods, like the latex condom, which probably provides the best protection against this disease of any single contraceptive method. For many couples, contraceptive choice has meant using a combination of methods that maximize effectiveness and protection from sexually transmittable diseases—for instance, use of the pill plus a latex condom or diaphragm.

Four major types of birth control methods are in use today:

1. Natural family planning methods.
2. Barrier methods (condom, diaphragm, etc.)
3. Intrauterine devices (IUDs).
4. Hormonal contraception (pills, Depo-Provera, and Norplant).

In the next four chapters of this section we will discuss each of these major types in some depth; in the last chapter, we will give you information designed to help you select the contraceptive method that is best for you. Regardless of the method or methods you choose, remember that a barrier method (preferably, the condom) is strongly recommended for every couple unless each partner has tested negative for AIDS and the couple has been mutually monogamous for a period of at least six months prior to the testing.

Of the four methods, birth control pills have been the most popular and are used by 30% of married couples in the United States using contraception. Barrier methods, such as the condom, diaphragm, cervical cap, and various spermicides, may soon rival the pill as the most widely used method of birth control. Aside from providing protection from STDs, barrier methods are well suited for couples who plan to have a child within a year or who cannot use hormonal contraception or an IUD for medical reasons. The IUD, although used by only a small percentage of women, continues to be an appropriate choice of birth control for some couples who have completed childbearing. The rhythm method, now expanded and known as natural family planning, has historically been the least frequently used birth control method. These four methods add up to much less than 100% since nearly 50% of married couples now choose a permanent method of birth control (voluntary sterilization). Coitus interruptus, or "withdrawal," in which the man withdraws his penis just prior to ejaculation was used as a contraceptive method much more in past times. Today, coitus interruptus cannot be considered an effective birth control method for a woman who chooses not to conceive.

With the number of new and sometimes conflicting reports in the media about health risks, decreased fertility, or cancer-causing effects of various contraceptive methods, it is often hard for a woman to decide which method is best for her. To help you make this decision, we have divided the process of contraceptive selection into three simple steps, outlined in Table 18 at the end of this section. This chart, along with the information presented throughout this section, will guide you in your choice of the most appropriate method of birth control for your personal needs.

CHAPTER 6

Natural Family Planning

The natural methods of birth control, known collectively as *natural family planning* (NFP), *periodic abstinence*, or the *fertililty awareness* method, owe much of their popularity to women's concerns about the medical hazards of birth control pills and the IUD as well as the high cost of medical care. In fact, natural family planning has now become the third most popular overall method of birth control, after the pill and the various barrier methods. NFP is used by approximately 5% of women using contraception.

All methods of natural family planning depend upon abstaining from intercourse (or using other forms of contraception) during the fertile days of the menstrual cycle. This fertile period includes the days just prior to and after ovulation, which occurs approximately midway between menstrual periods. Ovulation can be determined by the *temperature method*, the *calendar method*, or the *cervical mucus method*, each of which is considered a separate method of NFP.

Keep in mind that any penile-vaginal contact without protection at any time during your fertile days, even though you don't actually have intercourse, allows the possibility, however small, of your becoming pregnant.

The Temperature Method

The temperature method is based on the fact that a woman's basal (resting) temperature (known as basal body temperature (BBT)) drops briefly and then rises half a degree following ovulation. The temperature remains elevated until just before menses begins. Normal resting temperature usually ranges from 96 to 98 degrees and 97 to 98 degrees after ovulation. A rise in temperature that persists for at least three days indicates that ovulation has occurred. Safe days are from the fourth day of sustained temperature rise through the last day of your next period. You should avoid intercourse between the last day of your next period until the temperature again rises for three days in the next cycle (see Figure 9).

Your temperature should be taken and recorded daily, preferably on a special chart, immediately upon your awakening, before you get out of bed. You can purchase a basal body thermometer and temperature charts at a drugstore, to make this method more convenient.

The Calendar Method

Of the three natural family planning methods, the calendar method (sometimes referred to as the "rhythm method") is the most cumbersome and least used, largely because it depends on a woman having regular, predictable cycles from one month to the next.

Before you can actually use the calendar method as your sole method of birth control, you will need to keep a written record of when each menstrual period begins. You will need to keep a record of the *length* of each cycle, that is, how many days from the start of one period to the start of the next period, for about eight months before beginning to use this method, unless your cycles are perfectly regular. This requirement may be an initial disadvantage because another form of contraception, but not the pill, should also be used during these first eight months. The pill cannot be used because the pill influences your normal pattern of ovulation. Each month, update your record so you are always using your most recent eight months in the calculations you will be using for the calendar method.

The calculations are based on the fact that the interval from ovulation until the beginning of your next period is always 14 days, regardless of cycle lengths. In other words, if you have a short cycle for one month, say 21 days, ovulation should occur on or about day 7 (21 minus 14 days). Day number 1 is always the first day of your period. In a longer cycle, for example 34 days, ovulation occurs on day 20 (34 minus 14 days). Since it is the time before ovulation that can vary in length—postovulation time (that is, from the day of ovulation to the first day of your next period) is always 14 days—you cannot pre-

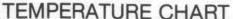

TEMPERATURE CHART

Day of Cycle	1	2	3	4	5	6	7	8	9	10	11	12	13	14	15	16	17	18	19	20	21	22	23	24	25	26	27	28	1	2	3	4	5	6
Day of Month	8/5	8/6	8/7	8/8	8/9	8/10	8/11	8/12	8/13	8/14	8/15	8/16	8/17	8/18	8/19	8/20	8/21	8/22	8/23	8/24	8/25	8/26	8/27	8/28	8/29	8/30	8/31	9/1	9/2	9/3	9/4	9/5	9/6	9/7
Intercourse					X		X			X			X			X			X			X												

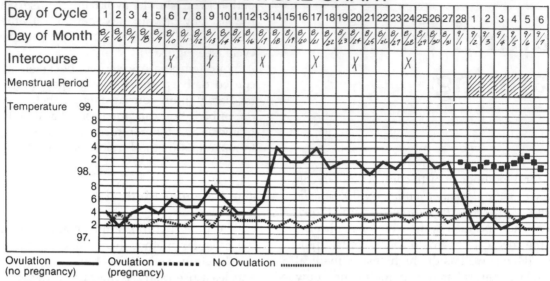

Ovulation ———— (no pregnancy)   Ovulation ●●●●●●●● (pregnancy)   No Ovulation ⋯⋯⋯⋯

Figure 9 *The solid line represents a typical temperature chart pattern for ovulation. The temperature rises after ovulation and remains elevated if pregnancy occurs (thick broken line). The thin broken line represents the pattern you would see if no ovulation occurred. The temperature chart can be used for birth control as a part of "natural family planning" or as a guide to help time intercourse in couples who wish to conceive.*

dict ovulation without a knowledge of previous cycle lengths. Less variation in cycle length means you have a smaller range of possible fertile days and, therefore, fewer days of abstinence. In other words, the more regular your cycle, the better this method will work. If your cycles vary by a week or more in length, this method of birth control may be too risky for you.

Here's how to calculate the fertile days, remembering that day number 1 is always the first day of your period:

1. To determine your *first fertile day*: select the shortest cycle from the previous eight months and subtract 18. The number 18 is derived by using the 14-day interval to pinpoint ovulation and then adding four days to cover sperm survival. For example, if your shortest cycle was 27 days, your first fertile day is number 9 (27 minus 18). This means the first day you should abstain from intercourse during this month is the 9th day of your cycle.
2. To determine your *last fertile day*: select the longest cycle from the previous eight months and subtract 11. The number 11 is

derived by using the 14-day interval to pinpoint ovulation and then subtracting three days to allow for egg survival. For example, if your longest cycle was 32 days, your last fertile day is day number 21 (32 minus 11). This means that the last day you should abstain from intercourse during this month is the 21st day of your cycle. In this example, fertile days would be from the 9th to the 21st day, a total of 13 days.

If you have an unusually long cycle during the preceding eight months, the number of calculated fertile days would increase accordingly. But if your cycles are always about the same length, the number of abstaining days are less and decrease to an absolute minimum of eight days a month for a woman whose cycles are always exactly the same length.

The Cervical Mucus Method (Billings Method)

The cervical mucus method is the latest, least studied, and most controversial method of natural family planning. It depends on a thorough

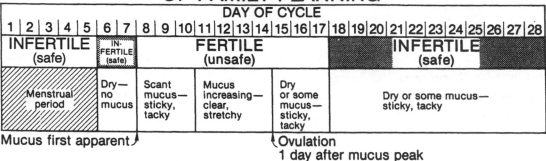

CERVICAL MUCUS METHOD
OF FAMILY PLANNING

DAY OF CYCLE																											
1	2	3	4	5	6	7	8	9	10	11	12	13	14	15	16	17	18	19	20	21	22	23	24	25	26	27	28
INFERTILE (safe)					IN-FERTILE (safe)		FERTILE (unsafe)										INFERTILE (safe)										
Menstrual period					Dry— no mucus		Scant mucus— sticky, tacky			Mucus increasing— clear, stretchy				Dry or some mucus— sticky, tacky			Dry or some mucus— sticky, tacky										

Mucus first apparent ↲   ↳Ovulation
                                1 day after mucus peak

Figure 10 *Intercourse is "safe" during infertile days. During "unsafe," or fertile, days another method of birth control must be used if you have intercourse.*

understanding of your anatomy and menstrual cycle because you predict ovulation by observing and recording daily changes in the amount, consistency, and color of the cervical mucus. To obtain the mucus sample, you can touch the cervix directly, reach inside the vagina, or simply wipe the vulva.

Figure 10 summarizes the cervical mucus changes in a typical cycle. Usually no mucus is present for a few days after your period ends. During these "early dry days," intercourse is safe although there is a small chance of pregnancy due to sperm survival into the first "wet" (fertile) day which follows. A mucous discharge is present within the vaginal opening about six days before ovulation. This is the start of the "wet" days. As ovulation approaches, the mucus changes from cloudy and thick to clear and thin (like raw egg white) and suddenly increases in amount for one or two days. Intercourse should be avoided from the start of your "wet" days until at least three days after the amount of mucus "peaks." Ovulation occurs about twenty-four hours after this mucus peak. After ovulation the mucus decreases in quantity, becomes cloudy and thick again, and may be absent altogether for a few "late dry days" before your next period starts. Strict proponents of the mucus method also recommend abstinence during the menstrual period since mucus cannot be evaluated at this time.

The mucus method is not appropriate or feasible for everyone. Women using foam or other vaginal contraceptives may find it difficult to "read" their cervical mucus. Mucus evaluation is also less reliable in the presence of a vaginal infection, following childbirth, and in women approaching menopause when glandular secretions are less likely to occur according to a cycle.

Combining Natural Methods

Various combinations of natural methods are possible to increase effectiveness or decrease abstinence days, or both. For example, your first fertile day may be determined by the calendar method (subtract 18 from your shortest cycle) and your last fertile day by the temperature or cervical mucus method. This combination decreases the number of days requiring abstinence but may be slightly less effective than the temperature method alone, which permits intercourse only after ovulation. When combining methods, rely on the calendar prediction for your last fertile day whenever you have doubts about interpreting your temperature or mucus pattern, or if you have a cold or vaginal infection which could alter these signs. If you don't use the calendar method, the safest approach when in doubt is to abstain or to use other birth control until you have a clear indication that ovulation has occurred.

Another approach is to combine all three methods (see Figure 11). High rates of effectiveness approaching 91% have been reported in recent studies of this combination, known as the *sympto-thermal method*. Many couples combine barrier contraception with natural family planning on the fertile days of the cycle to allow greater sexual freedom and spontaneity. Al-

Table 5 COMPARISON OF THE THREE NATURAL METHODS OF BIRTH CONTROL

	Temperature	Calendar	Cervical Mucus
Effectiveness*	over 90%	70–85%	over 90%
Number of fertile days (28-day cycle)	12	8	10
Affected by vaginal infection	no	no	yes
Requires regular cycles	no	yes	no
Requires daily record keeping	yes	no**	yes

* Based on a limited number of studies, these rates assume abstinence or use of a barrier method during fertile days.

** Only first day of each cycle.

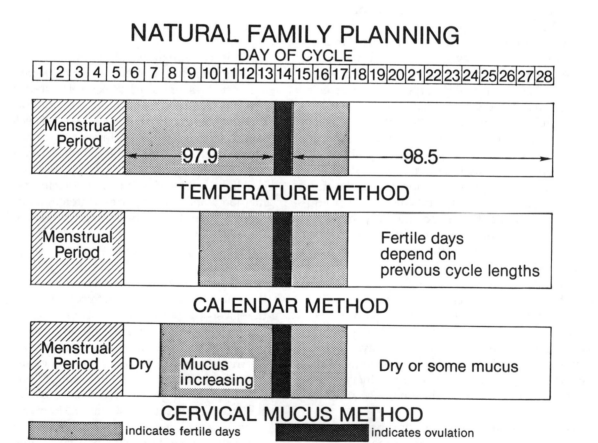

NATURAL FAMILY PLANNING
DAY OF CYCLE

| 1 | 2 | 3 | 4 | 5 | 6 | 7 | 8 | 9 | 10 | 11 | 12 | 13 | 14 | 15 | 16 | 17 | 18 | 19 | 20 | 21 | 22 | 23 | 24 | 25 | 26 | 27 | 28 |

Menstrual Period ←— 97.9 —→ ←— 98.5 —————→

TEMPERATURE METHOD

Menstrual Period — Fertile days depend on previous cycle lengths

CALENDAR METHOD

Menstrual Period — Dry — Mucus increasing — Dry or some mucus

CERVICAL MUCUS METHOD

indicates fertile days   indicates ovulation

Figure 11 *This illustration indicates fertile days in a typical month for each method of natural family planning. By combining the temperature method with either the calendar or cervical mucus method you can reduce the number of abstinence days.*

though medical checkups are not required for this method of contraception, some instruction from a professional or a woman familiar with the techniques involved is often helpful, especially in the beginning.

Advantages and Disadvantages

Although the natural methods are economical, free of medical side effects, and successfully practiced by many women, physicians are often reluctant to recommend them, perhaps partly because of the time required to explain their use. Physicians also point to studies which show NFP to be one of the least effective methods of birth control, averaging less than 80% effectiveness. This high failure rate is due in part to the fact that many women who use natural family planning do not have regular menstrual cycles with clear-cut temperature and cervical mucus discharge patterns. Women who do have regular cycles may use this method with a much higher degree of effectiveness.

Another disadvantage to NFP is the need for time-consuming, almost compulsive, record keeping, which demands a high-level commitment to a method that requires abstinence nearly half of the time. There is one unnatural aspect to natural family planning: if pregnancy does occur, there is a greater chance of fertilizing an overmature egg, one that was released from the ovary several days before fertilization. If this occurs, the chance of a fetal abnormality may be slightly increased.

Table 5 shows a comparison, according to certain factors, of the three rhythm methods discussed here. For more information on natural family planning, contact your local Roman Catholic diocese, your local Planned Parenthood clinic, or the local county health department family planning clinic.

CHAPTER 7

The Diaphragm and Other Barrier Methods

The barrier methods of birth control act in one of two ways: the sperm is either immobilized by a chemical (cream, foam, jelly, or suppository) or mechanically blocked from entering the uterus (diaphragm, condom). In actual practice, the effectiveness of barrier methods varies from 64% to 97%, depending on how carefully the method is used. Remember that the barrier method needs to be applied before there is any penile-vaginal contact. Most studies show lower pregnancy rates with the diaphragm and condom methods than with either foam or suppositories. Contraceptive effectiveness increases tremendously if you combine two barrier methods.

The Diaphragm

The diaphragm is the oldest consistently reliable method of contraception; it was used by women for generations before the introduction of the IUD and the pill. The diaphragm is a soft rubber cuplike device (with a flexible, spring rim) that is used with a sperm-killing (spermicidal) cream or jelly and is inserted into the vagina by the woman or her partner so that it covers the cervix, that is, the entrance to the uterus. You need a prescription to obtain a diaphragm since it must be fitted to your exact size. There are about seven sizes ranging from 60 to 90 millimeters in

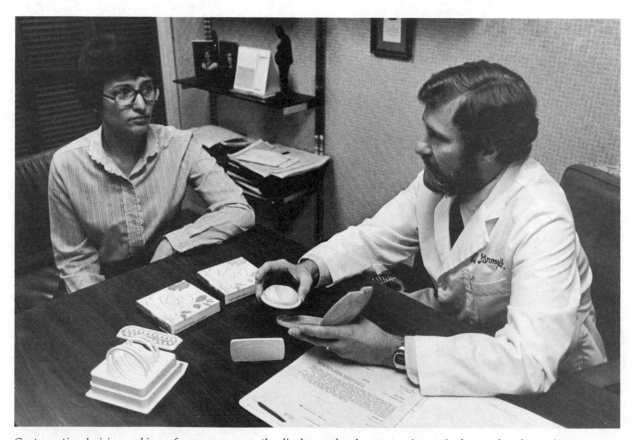

Contraceptive decision making—for some women, the diaphragm has become an increasingly popular alternative.

Figure 12 *Using a diaphragm.*

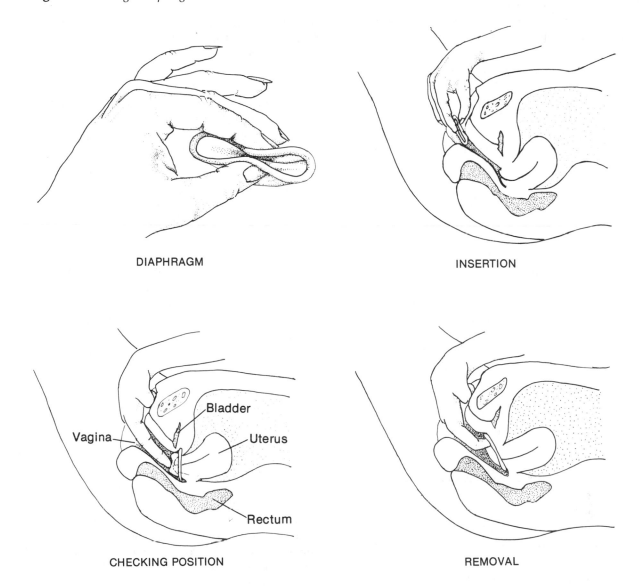

DIAPHRAGM

INSERTION

CHECKING POSITION

REMOVAL

diameter. A snug fit is important: since your vagina will expand slightly during sexual activity, a diaphragm that is too small could become dislodged during intercourse; one that is too large may be uncomfortable. Be sure to have the size of your diaphragm checked every two years and replaced at that time, even if the size has not changed. You are also likely to need a change in size after childbirth, miscarriage, or abortion, or if you have gained or lost over twenty pounds.

Learning the technique of diaphragm insertion takes time and patience (see Figure 12). Try it in the clinician's office and make sure he or she checks your proper placement of the diaphragm when it is initially fitted. You might feel more comfortable having the nurse help insert the diaphragm. During insertion, make sure the diaphragm is directed toward your tailbone, not toward the midback. This prevents positioning the diaphragm in front of (above) your cervix. In most women, the diaphragm slips naturally over the cervix regardless of the direction of insertion. As you finish inserting the diaphragm and you tuck the front of the rim up behind your pelvic bone, proceed to feel the cervix (it feels like the tip of the nose) through the soft, cuplike dome of the diaphragm to confirm that it is positioned correctly.

Instead of using manual insertion (accompanied by pinching the rim of the diaphragm between thumb and forefinger), you may find it helps to use a plastic introducer, which can be included in the prescription for the diaphragm. This method will also make the insertion less messy because the introducer easily guides the diaphragm into the vagina. If any doubt about placement remains (and it often does), come back into the clinician's office with your diaphragm in place to have the position rechecked.

Here are some tips to maximize the effectiveness of diaphragm use:

1. Always use your diaphragm when you have intercourse, even during your period. Be sure to insert the diaphragm before any penile-vaginal contact.
2. You might find it convenient to insert the diaphragm routinely at bedtime. Although the manufacturer's instructions may indicate protection for six hours after the diaphragm, with jelly or cream, is inserted, it is a good idea to use additional cream, jelly, or foam if you have intercourse after an hour or more from the time of insertion.
3. Do not douche or remove the diaphragm for at least six hours after intercourse, or after the last intercourse.
4. Apply additional cream or jelly before each time you have intercourse while the diaphragm is still in place. A plastic applicator for this purpose may be provided along with the diaphragm, if you ask for it, or it may be bought separately at the drugstore.
5. Keep in mind that during intercourse the position most likely to dislodge the diaphragm is that of the woman on top.
6. After use, wash your diaphragm with mild soap and water, rinse and dry it well, and powder it with cornstarch (not talcum powder) to reduce moisture, which may weaken the rubber.
7. Check the diaphragm frequently for tiny, pinpoint holes by holding it up to the light or filling it with water. It is a good idea to have a spare available in case you need it.
8. The diaphragm may be left in place for twenty-four hours. If left for longer periods of time, there is a small chance of developing a vaginal discharge or uterine infection.

The Cervical Cap

Although approved by the FDA in 1988, the Prentif Cavity-Rim, a brand of cervical cap, is still not widely available. The method is used by approximately 200,000 U.S. women. This birth control device is similar to the diaphragm, which blocks the entry of sperm into the uterus. The FDA-approved cap is manufactured in England and has also been available in other countries for many years. Approval followed efforts by women's groups and progress made in U.S. research trials that determined the cap's effectiveness was similar to that of the diaphragm (about 85%).

The small, thimble-shaped rubber cap covers the cervix like a mini-diaphragm and is inserted and removed by the woman. As with the diaphragm, you need a prescription because the cap must be fitted to your size. One advantage of the cervical cap over the diaphragm is that it may be worn for up to forty-eight hours and may be less messy because spermicide, which is used initially, does not have to be reapplied upon repeated intercourse. Other advantages include disassociation of the contraceptive from intercourse (that is, the cervical cap can be inserted at a convenient time, not necessarily just before intercourse), low price, lack of serious side effects, and possible prevention of venereal disease. The main disadvantage appears to be its sometimes difficult insertion and removal, which requires more skill than does insertion of the diaphragm. Also, because of the limited sizes currently available, some women cannot be fitted without a significant risk of dislodgement during intercourse. A possible risk of the cap, still under study, is the development of abnormal Pap smears and associated minor infections in the first few months of use.

To wear the cap, a woman must have normal Pap smears (including a normal smear three months after initial fitting). Contraindications include cancer of the cervix or uterus and infections of the vagina or cervix. The cap must not be used during menses or in the first few weeks following pregnancy or abortion because of a slightly increased risk of toxic shock syndrome during these times.

For more information contact Cervical Cap Ltd., 430 Monterey Avenue, Los Gatos, California 95030; telephone: (408) 395-2100.

The Male Condom

Former Surgeon General C. Everett Koop, M.D., once said the following about AIDS: "The best protection against infection right now, barring abstinence, is the use of a condom." The advice is still true today. The condom's ability to offer some protection against sexually transmitted infections including AIDS accounts for increasing use of this method. The male condom is now the second most popular form of reversible birth control after the pill. According to the Alan Guttmacher Institute, a reproductive-health research organization, the number of unmarried women using condoms doubled between 1982 and 1987 to 2.2 million, or about 16% of the sexually active, fertile female population. Purchases by women now represent 40% of all condoms sold.

The condom, a rubber sheath that fits over a man's erect penis, acts by preventing the sperm from entering the uterus. Of all methods of birth control, the latex condom offers the best protection against venereal disease, including AIDS. Some condoms come lubricated with a spermicide, which provides an additional safeguard against pregnancy and sexually transmitted infections should the semen spill on withdrawal. See Table 6 for help in talking with your partner about the use of a condom. Improper use,

---

Table 6 — HOW TO TALK ABOUT CONDOMS WITH A RESISTANT, DEFENSIVE, OR MANIPULATIVE PARTNER

If the partner says:	You can say:	If the partner says:	You can say:
"You're on the pill. I don't need a condom."	"I'd like to use it anyway. We'll both be protected from infections we may not realize we have."	"What kinds of alternatives?"	"Maybe we'll just pet, or postpone sex for a while."
"I *know* I'm clean (disease-free); I haven't had sex with anyone in X months."	"Thanks for telling me. As far as I know, I'm disease-free, too. But I'd still like to use a condom since either of us could have an infection and not know it."	"This is an insult! Do you think I'm some sort of disease-ridden gigolo?"	"I didn't say or imply that. I care for you, but in my opinion, it's best to use a condom."
"I'm a virgin."	"I'm not. This way we'll both be protected."	"None of my other girlfriends make me use a condom. A *real* woman isn't afraid."	"Please don't compare me to them. A real woman cares about the man she dates, herself, and about their relationship."
"I can't feel a thing when I wear a condom; it's like wearing a raincoat in the shower."	"Even if you lose some sensation, you'll still have plenty left."	"I love you! Would I give you an infection?"	"Not intentionally. But many people don't know they're infected. That's why this is best for both of us right now."
"I'll lose my erection by the time I stop and put it on."	"I'll help you put it on— that'll help you keep it."	"Just this once."	"Once is all it takes."
"By the time you put it on, I'm out of the mood."	"Maybe so, but we feel strongly enough for each other to stay in the mood."	"I don't have a condom with me."	"I do." or "Then let's satisfy each other without intercourse."
"It destroys the romantic atmosphere."	"It doesn't have to be that way."	"You carry a condom around with you? You were planning to seduce me!"	"I always carry one with me because I care about myself. I have one with me tonight because I care about us both."
"Condoms are unnatural, fake, a total turnoff."	"Please let's try to work this out—an infection isn't so great either. So let's give the condom a try. Or maybe we can look for alternatives."	"I won't have sex with you if you want me to use a condom."	"So let's put it off until we can agree." or "OK, then let's try some other things besides intercourse."

Adapted from the article "Cutting the Risks for STDs" by Alan Grieco, Ph.D., which appeared in the March 1987 issue of *Medical Aspects of Human Sexuality*. Reprinted with permission from *Medical Aspects of Human Sexuality*. © Cahners Publishing Company, published July 1989. All rights reserved.

rather than product failure, is the primary reason for the failure of condoms to protect against sexually transmitted disease and pregnancy. Here are some good techniques to follow:

1. Use the condom with each act of intercourse.
2. Use the condom prior to any genital contact.
3. Avoid using oil-based lubricants like petroleum jelly, mineral oil, baby oil, or cold cream, which may weaken latex condoms and make them more likely to break. If additional lubrication is needed, water-soluble lubricants like H-R Lubricating Jelly or K-Y Jelly or Transi-Lube foaming sexual lubricant have been found useful. (None has spermicidal properties, however.)
4. Leave a ½-inch space at the end of the condom to minimize the risk of breakage after ejaculation.
5. After climax, your partner should immediately grasp the condom firmly at the base of the penis to prevent the condom from slipping off, and withdraw promptly, before erection is lost.

The Female Condom

A nonprescription condom for women, marketed under the name Reality, was approved by the FDA in 1993. The Reality condom, the first barrier birth control method for women providing some protection against VD, became generally available in drugstores by late 1994. The device contains two flexible diaphragmlike rings at either end of a soft, loose-fitting polyurethane sheath. It is inserted like a tampon, with the inner ring covering the cervix and the outer ring remaining outside. This disposable condom for women requires no fitting and, like the male condom, is designed to protect against VD as well as prevent pregnancy.

It may take some practice to learn the technique of inserting the Reality condom. Become comfortable with the device and practice inserting the condom before using it with a partner. Here is the technique of insertion:

Figure 13
The female condom. Reprinted with permission of Wisconsin Pharmacal Company.

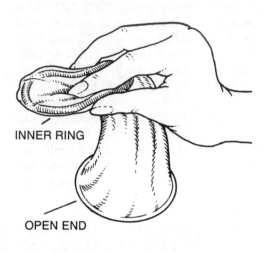

Figure 14
Insertion of the female condom. Reprinted with permission of Wisconsin Pharmacal Company.

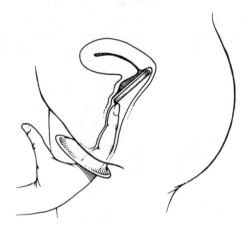

1. Assume a comfortable position; for example, lie down with your legs bent and knees apart or stand with one foot on a chair.
2. Grasp the inner ring of the closed end of the condom (let the open end hang down).
3. With the inner ring squeezed together, insert the ring and vaginal pouch deep into the vagina (the outer ring will hang down slightly outside the vagina).

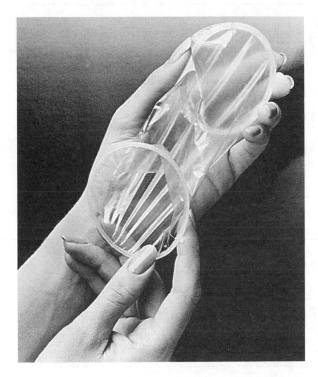

The female condom. Reprinted with permission of Wisconsin Pharmacal Company.

During sex it may be helpful for the woman to guide the penis into the female condom. After intercourse, remove the condom by first squeezing and twisting the outer ring to contain the semen inside the pouch. The condom is not intended for reuse and should be disposed of in the garbage and not flushed down the toilet.

Contraceptive Foam, Cream, Jelly, Suppositories, and Film

These preparations contain spermicides. (Don't confuse them with feminine hygiene products, which are often on the same shelf in your local drugstore.) Cream and jelly products are used with a diaphragm. Foam is often used by itself partly because of its easy application. However, contraceptive effectiveness, as well as protection against VD, is greatly enhanced when the condom is used in addition to these products. Foam is packaged in a pressurized container which comes with either a plastic applicator or a nozzle for direct release of foam into the vagina. If you use an applicator, buy only a refill the next time since the applicator is reusable.

Insert the applicator deep into the vagina to be sure the foam will be ejected close to the cervix. You can do this while you are lying down or squatting or with one leg up on a chair. Foam, unlike vaginal suppositories (Encare, Semicid), which take ten to fifteen minutes to melt or dissolve, is immediately effective. Remember to shake the container before use to enhance foam effectiveness.

A newer product, Vaginal Contraceptive Film, consists of a two-inch square of dissolvable "film," which looks and feels like a thin piece of semitransparent plastic. The film is placed deep in the vagina on the cervix, where it quickly dissolves and releases spermicide. The film must be introduced at least five minutes but not more than an hour and a half prior to intercourse. The Vaginal Contraceptive Film may be somewhat less messy than foam or jelly but has the same disadvantage as contraceptive suppositories: sexual activity must be delayed until the product dissolves. Another new spermicidal product that seeks to avoid this issue is Advantage 24. It can be administered up to twenty-four hours prior to intercourse.

Advantages and Disadvantages

An advantage of the barrier methods is their complete lack of serious side effects. Previously the only adverse reaction was minor irritation or burning from the spermicide or the rubber used in the contraceptive material itself. However, recent studies suggest frequent use of spermicides may damage the vaginal lining, possibly increasing the risk of HIV transmission in some women. No fetal abnormalities or cancer have been associated with any barrier method of contraception. Probably the greatest criticism of barrier contraception is inconvenience—the need to apply the method close to or just before the time of lovemaking.

Table 7 compares the various barrier methods of contraception.

Table 7   COMPARISON OF DIFFERENT
BARRIER METHODS OF BIRTH CONTROL

	Male Condom	Diaphragm	Foam	Suppositories and Tablets	Cervical Cap	Female Condom
Approximate effectiveness in actual use	90%	85%	80%	80%	85%	75%
Effect upon sensation during sex	some de-crease*	little or none**	none**	none**	none**	some decrease
Available over-the-counter	yes	no; cream or jelly is	yes	yes	no; cream or jelly is	yes
Protection against VD	substantial	moderate	minimal-moderate	minimal-moderate	moderate	substantial
Aesthetic considerations	least messy	messy during insertion and removal	tends to be messy	tends to be messy	messy during insertion and removal	minimally messy
Common brand names	many brands	Koromex Ortho	Delfin Emko Koromex	Encare Conceptrol	Prentif Cavity-Rim	Reality

 * Least with animal products (Fourex, Naturalamb).

** Occasional burning or irritation affecting you or your partner may occur from the cream, jelly, foam, or suppository. If the burning or irritation continues, switch to another brand.

CHAPTER 8

Intrauterine Devices

The intrauterine device (IUD) involves the insertion by a clinician of a small object into the uterus (see Figure 15). No one knows exactly how these devices work, but we do know they prevent fertilization. This probably occurs by some type of spermicidal effect or by an action to inhibit sperm transport.

All but one of the IUDs of the early 1980s are unavailable. IUDs like the Lippes Loop, the Saf-T-Coil, and the Copper 7—devices that were popular with millions of women and found safe and effective by the FDA—have been removed from the market by their manufacturers, largely because of the threat of product liability lawsuits. Yet none of these IUDs was associated with the same high rate of serious infection as the Dalkon Shield, the users of which were seven to nine times more likely than nonusers to contract serious infections like pelvic inflammatory disease. However, this is not true of modern IUDs. A 1992 article in the *Lancet*, a highly respected medical journal, reviewed the experience of 22,000 IUD users who are at low risk for sexually transmitted diseases. The researchers concluded these IUD users "do not have excess pelvic inflammatory disease." IUDs will probably make a significant comeback in the late 1990s.

The two IUDs available today are the Progestasert, which releases the hormone progesterone, and the Copper T 380A, an IUD developed by the nonprofit Population Council and first marketed in the United States in 1988 under the name Paragard. The Progestasert must be replaced every year; the Copper T is good for ten years. These devices are best suited for women who are over twenty-five, are in a mutually monogamous stable relationship, have had at least one child, and have no history of pelvic inflammatory disease (see Chapter 24). For such women the risk of IUD-related infection is quite minimal.

The effectiveness of the IUD varies from 98% to 99%. About 20% of women with IUDs will have them removed within one year because of side effects, including painful or heavy periods and uterine or tube infections.

IUD Insertion

Since the placement of an IUD into the uterus of a pregnant woman may cause miscarriage, IUDs are inserted during the last two days of a menstrual period, when pregnancy can be ruled out.

Mild *cramping* is common during and following insertion of the IUD. A transitory fainting reflex occasionally accompanies IUD insertion and may require IUD removal if this symptom is associated with nausea and severe cramping. Such symptoms are more likely to occur in women who have never been pregnant.

Expulsion of the IUD may occur at any time; but if it is going to occur, it usually occurs within

---

Table 8   CONTRAINDICATIONS TO THE IUD

Definite contraindications

1. Suspected or possible pregnancy
2. Suspicious or abnormal Pap smear
3. Past or present history of sexually transmitted infection, including gonorrhea, chlamydia, or syphillis
4. Past or present history of pelvic inflammatory disease (PID)
5. Vaginal bleeding of unknown cause
6. Abnormalities of the cavity of the uterus

Possible contraindications

1. Bleeding between periods
2. Fainting attacks
3. Heart disease involving the heart valves
4. Heavy menstrual flow
5. Diabetes
6. Recent abortion or miscarriage
7. Severe menstrual cramps
8. Multiple sexual partners
9. No previous pregnancy

---

the first month after insertion. During this first month, you might want to use a second method of contraception, such as foam or condoms. Expulsion occurs in 5% to 12% of women using the IUD, most commonly during or after a menstrual period, and occurs more frequently in women who have never been pregnant.

You will be told to check for expulsion by examining your cervix to feel for the IUD string. If you cannot feel it, keep in mind the string often curls up within the uterus, but call your doctor for an appointment just in case. If you can feel the string (but not the IUD itself), the IUD is

Figure 15 *Intrauterine device (IUD). The end of the IUD string extends just past the cervical opening. Modified with permission of G.D. Searle and Co. (The Female Reproductive System. San Juan, Puerto Rico, 1976).*

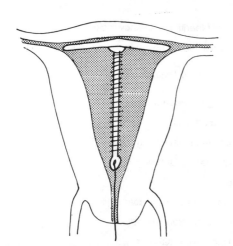

likely to be in place. The most important reason to check yourself periodically is to make sure the IUD itself is not protruding from the cervix since this increases the risk of pregnancy.

Have your doctor or nurse practitioner check the position of the IUD a few weeks after it is fitted and at subsequent checkups. If the string cannot be seen or felt by the examiner, he or she will try to locate the IUD by inserting a small probe within the uterus. An alternate and costlier approach is to obtain an X-ray or sonogram.

Advantages and Disadvantages

The main advantages of IUDs are their high rate of effectiveness and their convenience (no need for abstinence or for diaphragm insertions). The major disadvantages are serious side effects. The overall serious risks associated with the IUD are about the same for women under the age of thirty-five as the risks for the pill. Problems with IUD use are discussed below, and warning signals requiring a call to your clinician are listed in Table 9.

Increased *bleeding* is one of the most common side effects of the IUD. Periods may increase in duration or flow; or, less commonly, bleeding may occur between periods. Excessive bleeding may lead to anemia. These side effects usually subside after the first few months of IUD use.

Increased *menstrual cramping* is a common side effect of IUD use, especially among women who have never been pregnant.[1] Pelvic pain, including painful intercourse, may be a sign of uterine *infection*, particularly when associated with fever, bad-smelling discharge, or spotting between periods. There is a definite increased risk of such infection among IUD users who have multiple sexual relationships or a history of previous tube infections. Treatment of IUD-related infections which most commonly involve the uterus (*endometritis*) consists of antibiotics and usually does not require removal of the device. More severe infections causing low abdominal cramping pain involve the tube or ovary and may require surgery or cause sterility.

Severe, persistent pain immediately after insertion of the IUD, accompanied by the fact that

[1] If menstrual cramping occurs you may want to ask your clinician to prescribe one of the *antiprostaglandin* drugs such as Anaprox, Motrin, or Ponstel (see Chapter 79). These drugs have been approved by the FDA for relief of menstrual cramps. Antiprostaglandin drugs work by blocking the action of prostaglandin, a hormone that plays a major role in causing uterine contractions and cramping and is found in excessive amounts in IUD wearers.

you are unable to feel your IUD string, may indicate perforation of the device through the wall of the uterus. Perforation occurs less than one percent of the time and is usually treated by removal of the IUD by laparoscopy (see glossary).[2]

Pregnancy may occur after an unnoticed expulsion or with the device still in place. In the latter case, miscarriage occurs approximately half of the time if the IUD is not removed and significantly less often when it is removed. Sometimes when the string is not visible and pregnancy is suspected, a sonogram is done to determine if the IUD is within the uterus, outside the uterus (perforated), or not present at all (expelled). Certain complications to both mother and fetus are more frequent if the IUD is retained within the uterus. These complications include delayed miscarriage (up to 20 weeks), premature delivery, stillbirth, and various infections either before or after childbirth. No increase in birth defects is known to occur in women who become pregnant while wearing an IUD. The effects on the fetus of progesterone-medicated IUDs are unknown. Tubal (ectopic) pregnancy has recently been found to be more frequent among IUD users, occurring in one pregnancy out of twenty, as compared to the usual rate of one in eighty.

Table 10 answers some questions you may have about the IUD.

Table 10   QUESTIONS COMMONLY ASKED ABOUT THE IUD

Can I use the IUD if . . .	Yes	No	Comment
I have had a cesarean section?	X		
I have a heart murmur?	X		Use may be contraindicated if murmur is due to rheumatic heart disease or congenital heart disease.
I delivered six weeks ago?	X		Expulsion and perforation rates are slightly higher until at least 8 weeks postpartum.
I had a therapeutic abortion two to three weeks ago?	X		If you were more than 12 weeks pregnant, wait until 6 to 8 weeks after your abortion.
I have an infection of the cervix or an abnormal Pap smear?		X	Wait until after diagnosis and/or treatment is completed for IUD insertion.
I douche or use tampons?	X		

[2] A government-sponsored research project, the Women's Health Study, reported finding an unusual frequency of uterine perforation among IUD users who were breast-feeding. The timing of insertion did not change the perforation risk—those who had IUDs inserted at the time of the six-weeks postpartum checkup were not more likely to experience perforation during lactation than those with later insertions. The increased perforation risk for breast-feeding women may be because the walls of the uterus remain thin during lactation due to lower estrogen levels at this time.

CHAPTER 9

Hormonal Contraception (Birth Control Pills, Depo-Provera, and Norplant)

Birth Control Pills (Oral Contraceptives)

About twelve million American women use oral contraceptives, the most effective and most popular method of birth control presently available. It is estimated that at least 85% of women who wish to avoid pregnancy do not have medical contraindications to the pill and can safely use this form of contraception. Since the mid-1970s, researchers have more precisely identified women at risk to develop serious side effects from the pill. This has led to lower-dose pills and a subsequent wider margin of safety for pill users.

If your doctor recently prescribed birth control pills for you, you may have received a lengthy government pamphlet called a Patient Package Insert (PPI). We will cover the major points covered in the PPI in terms that will help clarify the benefits and risks of these pills.

Considerations Before You Choose the Pill

Most women who take birth control pills are on "combination" pills that contain both estrogen and progesterone. Unless otherwise stated, remarks about the pill in this chapter refer to "combination pills."

Most side effects of the pill are not serious and some are beneficial (see Table 13). Common side effects usually subside after a few menstrual cycles. It usually takes that long for the body to adjust, so it is better not to switch pills during the initial two to three months of use. Adverse reactions to the pill are usually mild, and these, as well as serious effects, are also noted in Table 13.

Cardiovascular complications—i.e., problems involving the heart or blood vessels, such as heart attacks, strokes, and blood clots—are the most serious side effects of the pill and require immediate medical attention. Until recently, most large studies have indicated that users of birth control pills were several times more likely than non-users to develop these complications. Recent research, however, is showing different results. Since about the mid-1980s studies based on the lower-dose birth control pills have shown that health risks in *nonsmoking* pill users are lower than previously believed. Much of the recent data comes from large, long-term projects such as the Royal College of General Practitioners' Oral Contraception Study. The most recent British data indicates no increased mortality among nonsmoking pill users under thirty-five compared to non-users. And from age thirty-five to forty-four, the data indicate that risks for pill users increase only marginally in healthy nonsmoking women. Clearly the vast majority of pill complications in previous studies have been concentrated in one of two groups:

1. Women over thirty-five who smoke and
2. Women over thirty-five with cardiovascular risk factors such as a history of high blood pressure, increased cholesterol, excessive weight gain, or a strong family history of heart disease.

Table 11   ABSOLUTE CONTRAINDICATIONS TO COMBINATION BIRTH CONTROL PILLS

1. Present or previous blood clots including clots in the leg (thrombophlebitis), in the lung (pulmonary embolus), in the brain (stroke or cerebrovascular accident), or in the heart (heart attack or coronary thrombosis). History of angina or chest pain due to heart disease.
2. Present active liver disease such as hepatitis or cirrhosis.
3. Present or previous cancer of the breast, uterus, or liver.
4. Pregnancy—known or suspected.
5. Abnormal or unexplained vaginal bleeding.

Table 12 RELATIVE CONTRAINDICATIONS TO COMBINATION BIRTH CONTROL PILLS

If this risk factor applies to you . . .	You should have . . .	You should probably stop taking the pill if . . .
migraine headaches	checkups* at least every six months; consider neurologist evaluation if headaches persist after stopping pill	headaches increase in frequency or severity
epilepsy	checkups* every six months and periodically by internist	seizures increase in frequency
diabetes (requiring insulin)	checkups* every six months and periodically by internist	insulin control is difficult
high blood pressure	your blood pressure checked within three months initially and then every six months	blood pressure increases
infrequent periods, every three to six months (possible relative infertility)	(see Chapter 78, Menstrual Periods—Infrequent, Short, or Absent)	pregnancy is planned within one to two years
depression	(see Chapter 62, Depression)	severe anxiety or depression develops
vaginitis	a wet smear (office test); glucose tolerance test if repeated yeast infections	yeast infections do not respond to treatment
gallbladder disease	liver function tests annually	tests are abnormal or gallbladder attacks increase in frequency or severity
liver disease	liver function tests annually	tests are abnormal
sickle-cell anemia (see glossary)	a sickle-cell test if unsure whether you have sickle-cell anemia	any worsening of disease, such as bone pain, occurs
family history of heart attacks before age 50	blood cholesterol and triglycerides annually	either of these is abnormally elevated
family history of uterine cancer	a Pap smear semiannually	you have frequent abnormal bleeding on the pill and are over age 35
family history of breast cancer	periodic mammograms (see Chapter 34)	you have an abnormal mammogram, severe cystic breast disease, or a breast biopsy showing atypical cells
jaundice (see glossary) during pregnancy	liver function tests annually	tests are abnormal
diabetes during pregnancy	a glucose tolerance test annually	tests are abnormal
high blood pressure during pregnancy	your blood pressure checked every one to three months initially	blood pressure increases
history of cigarette smoking	or consider having a cardiac treadmill test (stress test) after age 30	you are over age 30 and presently smoke

*by your gynecologist or other primary-care physician.

The increased safety of the current low-dose oral contraceptives was emphasized in a recent committee opinion of the American College of Obstetricians and Gynecologists, which stated that "recent data, when controlled for age, indicate that duration of pill use has no effect on mortality and that age is of less importance than previously thought." Today most nonsmoking women over forty can take the pill safely, provided they are free of cardiovascular risk factors such as diabetes and elevated lipids.

In assessing pill side effects, pill benefits as

well should be kept in mind. Pill users have fewer ovarian cysts, fewer breast cysts, less iron-deficiency anemia, and more regular menstrual cycles. Although the pill is responsible for approximately 10,000 hospitalizations annually in the United States, it *prevents* about 50,000 hospitalizations each year—a net protective effect.

How Birth Control Pills Differ

There are two basic types of pills: the *combination pill* and the *mini-pill*. Ninety-nine percent of the time, doctors prescribe the combination pill. There are presently approximately thirty brands of combination pills on the market, each of which contains estrogen and progesterone. The estrogen component may be ethinyl estradiol or mestranol, while the progesterone component consists of one of several different possible synthetic compounds. It is the specific type and dose of these hormonal components that makes each oral contraceptive pill unique.

The combination pill

The vast majority of combination pills today are "low dose" and contain 20 to 35 micrograms of the hormone estrogen (see Table 14). Most physicians start new patients out on one of these low-dose pills because of their greater safety compared to older pills containing 50 micrograms of estrogen. Overall, low-dose pills are well tolerated by most women, although during the first cycle or so you may experience nuisance side effects, such as nausea or spotting.

All combination oral contraceptives come in packages of 21 or 28 pills. Both packages contain 21 hormone pills. The 28-day pack also contains 7 "blanks," which have no active ingredients. These are reminder pills so that you avoid a break in the pill-taking schedule. You can select whichever type you prefer. Some women find it easier to take 28-day pills because the pills are taken without interruption, presumably with less chance of missing taking a pill on the first day of the next cycle. Some 28-day pills (e.g., Norlestrin Fe 1/50) contain small amounts of iron in the last seven pills. This offers no particular advantage. Women with iron deficiency anemia should be on daily supplemental iron.

The mini-pill

The second type of birth control pill, sometimes called the *mini-pill*, contains only progesterone in each tablet. The advantage of the mini-pill is that it has no estrogen, the hormone believed to be responsible for most serious combination pill side effects. Certain serious side effects, such as blood clots, have not been associated with use of the mini-pill. This pill is sometimes prescribed for women over thirty-five with known risk factors for heart disease, such as smoking or high blood pressure. The three mini-pills currently on the market are Ovrette, Micronor, and Nor-Q-D.

The "morning-after" pill

The "morning-after" pill refers to high-dose estrogen tablets, taken usually in only two doses. This form of contraception is an emergency measure only and must be used within three days of unprotected intercourse. The simplest regimen calls for taking two tablets of the oral contraceptive Ovral and repeating the dose twelve hours later. Another regimen that has been suggested is to use other less-potent birth control pills, such as Lo/Ovral or Nordette, taking four (instead of two) pills each time.

How to Take Birth Control Pills

Complete this checklist before starting to take the combination pill for the first time.

1. You have no *absolute* contraindications to the pill (see Table 11).
2. You have no or only one *relative* contraindication to the pill (see Table 12).
3. You have had a recent breast and pelvic examination as well as a blood pressure check—preferably the exam should take place within a month before starting the pill.

The suggestions below may help you to use the combination pill as effectively as possible.

If you have not had prior intercourse, you can start taking the pill anytime, although starting just after a period is usually most convenient. If you are sexually active, begin your cycle of pills only after a normal period. Take your first pill on the fifth day of your period whether or not

Table 13   POSSIBLE SIDE EFFECTS OF COMBINATION BIRTH CONTROL PILLS

Mild Side Effects

(usually subside in three months):

Nausea (most common)
Weight gain (usually less than five pounds)
Fluid retention
Spotting between periods
Breast tenderness

Moderately Serious Side Effects

(advise physician if any of these symptoms develop; consider switching pills or stopping altogether):

Breast pain, discharge, or engorgement
Rash, itching, or jaundice (see glossary)
Reduced tolerance to contact lenses
Lack of periods
Headaches (may be migraine or related to high blood pressure)
Nervousness
Depression

Serious Side Effects—Danger Signals

(stop pill and contact physician immediately if any of these symptoms occur):

Symptom	Possible Cause
Leg tenderness or swelling	Thrombophlebitis (inflammation of leg vein with possible formation of blood clot)
Sudden chest pain, shortness of breath, coughing up blood	Pulmonary embolus (blood clot in lung sometimes originating in legs) or coronary thrombosis (heart attack—blood clot in heart)
Sudden, partial, or complete loss of vision in an eye	Retinal thrombosis (blood clot in eye)
Sudden weakness, numbness, or inability to move a part of the body; impaired speech, blurred vision, blackouts	Stroke (blood clot in brain)

Possible Beneficial Effects

Decreased menstrual pain, bleeding, and premenstrual tension
Predictable control of menstrual cycle
Fewer breast cysts
Decreased endometriosis
Improved complexion
Decreased rheumatoid arthritis (slight effect)
Less ovarian and uterine cancer
Less pelvic inflammatory disease

the bleeding has stopped. Some pill manufacturers recommend taking the first pill on the Sunday following the onset of your period (however, if your period begins on Sunday, start taking the pills that very same day). In either case, use another birth control method if you have intercourse during the first seven days on the pill—after that, you are protected. Take the

Table 14   COMPARISON OF BIRTH CONTROL PILLS* BY DOSAGE

	Brand Name	Estrogen Dose (Micrograms)	Serious Side Effects	Minor Side Effects	Theoretical Effectiveness
Group I, Medium Dose (50 micrograms of estrogen)	Demulen 1/50	50			
	Nelova 1/50M	50			
	Norethin 1/50M	50			
	Norinyl 1/50	50	Very few	Few	99.7%
	Ortho-Novum 1/50	50			
	Ovcon 50	50			
	Ovral	50			
Group II, Low Dose (Less than 50 micrograms of estrogen)	Brevicon	35			
	Demulen 1/35	35	Similar to	More frequent	99%
	Desogen[2]	30	or possibly	than Group I	
	Jenest 28	35	less fre-		
	Levlen	30	quent than		
	Levora .15/30	30	Group I		
	Loestrin 1/20	20			
	Loestrin 1.5/30	30			
	Lo/Ovral	30			
	Modicon	35			
	Nelova .5/35E	35			
	Nelova 1/35E	35			
	Nelova 10/11	35			
	Nordette	30			
	Norethin 1/35E	35			
	Norinyl 1/35	35			
	Ortho-Cept[2]	30			
	Ortho-Cyclen[2]	35			
	Ortho-Novum 1/35	35			
	Ortho-Novum 10/11	35			
	Ortho-Novum 7/7/7[1]	35			
	Ortho Tri-Cyclen[1,2]	35			
	Ovcon 35	35			
	Tri-Levlen[1]	30/40			
	Tri-Norinyl[1]	35			
	Triphasil[1]	30/40			

* Mini-pill not included.

Recommendations for pill selection: For maximum safety always start with a pill in Group II.

[1] These pills represent a subgroup of low-dose oral contraceptives known as multiphasic or triphasic pills. Rather than containing the same dosage in each pill, multiphasic pills contain three different dosages in each pill pack to simulate the hormonal variation of a normal menstrual cycle. In Ortho-Novum 7/7/7, Ortho Tri-Cyclen, and Tri-Norinyl, the progesterone dosage varies, while the estrogen dosage in each pill is held constant. In Tri-Levien and Triphasil, both the estrogen and progesterone dosages vary.

[2] These pills contain norgestimate or desogestrel, never progestins available since the early 1990s. The possible clinical advantages of these newer products—especially their ability to lower certain lipids in the blood—is under study. As of the mid-1990s, the available research indicates the risks and advantages of each of the Group II pills are about the same. For pill-specific information, discuss current research findings about the pill you are or will be taking with your physician.

pill at the same time each day for a total of 21 days. Then for the next 7 days take no pills (if you have the 21-pill packet) or take pills 22 through 28, which are a different color (if you have the 28-pill packet). During these 7 days a menstrual period usually occurs. After these 7 pill-free days (or days when a different-colored pill is taken in the 28-pill packet), take the first pill of your next packet and begin the sequence again.

If you start the pill following pregnancy, follow these guidelines:

1. *After a normal pregnancy:* It's a good idea to ask your clinician to prescribe the pill for

use two to three weeks after the baby is born; this way you will be protected prior to your six-week checkup in case you have intercourse before this time.

2. *After a miscarriage or therapeutic abortion (up to 12 weeks):* Use of birth control pills should begin immediately since ovulation resumes much more quickly following miscarriage or abortion than after a full-term pregnancy.

3. *After a late therapeutic abortion or late miscarriage (after 12 weeks):* Start one week after the procedure. Ovulation occurs sooner than after a normal pregnancy but not as soon as following early miscarriage or early therapeutic abortion.

If you forget to take a pill, take two pills the next day. The chance of getting pregnant is unlikely. If you lose a pill (for example, if it falls down the sink), you have two alternatives. You could take a pill from another pill package, which you then would not be able to use (except as replacements for future lost pills, until the expiration date for that package); or you could simply take the next pill from your current pack. If you missed two pills in the first two weeks, take two pills on the day you remember and two the next day. If two pills are missed in the third week of the pill pack, start a new package of pills immediately, unless you start your pills on a Sunday. In that case, keep taking a pill every day until Sunday and on Sunday, discard the original pack and start a new package. Whenever you miss two pills, use a backup method of birth control such as condoms for the next seven days.

When to Stop the Pill

If you develop any serious side effects of the pill (see Table 13), you should consult your physician about stopping the pill. If you develop other side effects listed in this table, you may want to switch pills or stay with the same pill for two or three months since many of these symptoms subside on their own. Consult your doctor.

Go off the pills two to three months prior to attempting pregnancy and use another method of birth control such as foam or condoms during this time.

Go off the pills one to two months prior to elective surgery. This will decrease the risk of blood clot complications after surgery as well as blood loss. Use another method of birth control during this time.

Previously, many authorities advised women to go off the pill by age forty. With the wider margin of safety in low-dose birth control pills today, many healthy, nonsmoking women can continue taking the pill into their forties, perhaps even until menopause, if other methods of birth control are unacceptable. For women over thirty-five on the pill, it's especially important to have regular checkups (annual or semiannual) and to have periodic testing of blood sugar and blood cholesterol levels. Women who smoke should start thinking about changing to another method of birth control at age thirty and certainly not take the pill after age thirty-five. Likewise, women who are significantly overweight or who have risk factors for cardiovascular disease should avoid the pill after age thirty-five. Such risk factors include a personal history of high blood pressure, diabetes, or increased cholesterol, as well as a family history of heart disease in a near relative under fifty.

When to Switch Pills—
Common Pill Problems

Fortunately, most pill problems are not serious and subside on their own in two or three months and do not require changing to a different pill. Much has been written about the relationship of the hormonal dosages in the combination pill to specific side effects. However, the particular hormone ratios in each pill have a combined action that is not the same in each woman. Clinicians often use trial and error in switching pills to lessen troublesome side effects. Nevertheless, there are a few useful guidelines to follow when dealing with certain side effects:

Light bleeding or spotting may occur on days when you take the pill, especially during the first three cycles while your body adjusts to the pill. This is known as *breakthrough bleeding*. If the bleeding is heavy, take two pills a day (one in the morning and one before you go to bed) on the pill day when spotting occurs. Take the second pill from a separate packet used for this purpose. If breakthrough bleeding persists after the first few cycles, then try a pill with more estrogen. If you have been using a sub-50 pill, try one with 50 micrograms. With some 50-microgram pills, such as Norlestrin 1/50, it may be possible to control breakthrough bleeding by increasing the amount of progesterone component (switching to Norlestrin 2.5 in this case) while keeping the same dose of estrogen.

An *absent period* is not the same as minimal spotting. Even a single brown spot each month is normal for some women on the pill. Complete absence of a period is more common with the mini-pill and with the sub-50s. This may be corrected by increasing the estrogen dosage in the case of combination pills. Get a pregnancy test if you miss two periods on the pill, even if you have not missed any pills.

Nausea, breast tenderness, or *breast swelling* are characteristic estrogen side effects which may subside or lessen by reducing the amount of estrogen in the pill. These symptoms are a good indication for stepping down to the sub-50s if you currently take a pill with 50 micrograms of estrogen. Premenstrual fluid retention is sometimes reduced by using a pill with less estrogen, but the response to switching pills is less consistent than with the other estrogen-dependent side effects.

The Pill and Pregnancy

Although the risk is very low, several studies have suggested the risk of fetal malformations in women taking hormones, including the pill, *during* the first three months of pregnancy. The risk appears to be somewhat greater for women who took hormones as a diagnostic test for pregnancy, or for treatment of threatened miscarriage, than for those taking birth control pills in early pregnancy. No definite evidence links birth defects or miscarriages to pregnancies conceived immediately *after* going off the pill. A report by the Harvard School of Public Health found no increased risk of fetal malformation in women who became pregnant one month or more after stopping the pill. Some newer evidence indicates a higher frequency of twins when conception occurs within two months of going off the pill.

Previously women were urged to wait six months after going off the pill before attempting pregnancy. This long wait now appears to be unwarranted. A wait of two or three months is sufficient since after that time there appears to be no increased risk of twins or fetal abnormalities. Furthermore, if you become pregnant without menstruating subsequent to your last pill period, it is difficult to determine when you became pregnant because the timing of the first ovulation following your last cycle of pills is often variable. Once your regular menstrual cycle becomes established after you stop the pill, calculation of your due date if pregnancy should occur becomes much more reliable. The due date is especially important for the high-risk mother-to-be.

Does the Pill Cause Infertility?

The overall fertility of pill users and nonusers is identical, regardless of how long a woman is on oral contraceptives. In the first cycle after the pill is stopped, ovulation is sometimes delayed a few weeks, but overall capacity for becoming pregnant is unchanged. In women who have very infrequent periods, the pill may be associated with some difficulty in their becoming pregnant because of their failure to ovulate. It isn't clear whether such delay of ovulation is pill-related or would have occurred anyway. Women who have had infrequent periods prior to pill use are more likely to experience a prolonged delay (six months or more) in the onset of their first period subsequent to stopping the pill. Usually ovulation can be restored, if pregnancy is desired, by taking a so-called fertility drug such as Clomid (see Chapter 13). These ovulation problems affect fewer than 1% of women using the pill.

The Pill and Cancer

There is presently no convincing evidence that oral contraceptives cause any type of cancer in women, although the long-term effects of the pill are not completely known. However, three types of malignancy—breast cancer, uterine cancer, and malignant melanoma (a form of skin cancer)—are associated with increased tumor growth when estrogen is taken. Because the pill contains estrogen, you should not take the pill if you have had any of these types of cancer.

Nearly all clinical studies show no overall increased risk of breast cancer among pill users compared with nonusers. The largest of these re-

Table 15   QUESTIONS COMMONLY ASKED ABOUT BIRTH CONTROL PILLS

Question	Yes	No	Comment
Are all birth control pills equally effective?		X	The mini-pill has a failure rate of about 3% compared to less than 1% for combination pills.
Can the pill stunt growth in a young woman?		X	Not if taken after menstrual periods have begun.
Should I wait two to three months after stopping the pill before planning to get pregnant?	X		The chances of fetal malformations and of twins may be slightly increased if you get pregnant during the first month after stopping the pill.
Can I take the pill if I have varicose veins?	X		Unless they are quite severe, not considered a contraindication.
Should the pill be taken during the months I am breast-feeding?		X	Combination pills may decrease the quantity of breast milk and are usually not prescribed in breast-feeding mothers. The mini-pill, which does not have this effect, may be used instead.
Do I need to take iron while on the pill?		X	Unless you are already anemic.
Are periodic "rest periods" desirable (that is, going off the pill for a length of time)?		X	There are no benefits to "rest periods" and you are exposed to a greater risk of unplanned pregnancy at this time.
Does the pill usually decrease sex drive?		X	There is no clear pattern toward increasing or decreasing sexual feelings or responsiveness.
If my mother took DES during her pregnancy with me, can I take the pill?*	X		While no adverse effects have been reported, routine checkups are advisable approximately every six months.
Is spotting during the first cycle on the pill normal?	X		This light bleeding usually subsides after the first few cycles on pills.
Is facial skin pigmentation which develops while a woman is on the pill improved by switching pills?		X	This pigmentation may occur with different pills regardless of dosage and is made worse by exposure to sunlight.
Should I use a second method of birth control during the first cycle on the pill?	X		Until after the first seven pills are taken; after that you are safe.
Is my fertility increased or decreased after going off the pill?		X	Wait two to three months before attempting pregnancy.

* For more information on DES see Chapter 38.

search projects—a multicenter, ongoing study by the Centers for Disease Control and known as the Cancer and Steroid Hormone Study (CASH)—looked at subgroups of pill users. The CASH study found no increased risk of breast cancer among pill users with long-term use (15 years or more), those with a family history of breast cancer, or those with a history of fibrocystic breast disease, compared with nonusers. Despite these reassuring overall statistics, the matter of whether other subgroups might be at risk remains unclear. For example, when reanalyzing the CASH data by age, women under 35 were found to have a slight increase in developing breast cancer, whereas pill users over 44 had a slight decreased risk. The magnitude of these changes was quite low, and the results have been unconfirmed by other studies (such as a report from New Zealand that found no increased breast cancer risk among young pill users). Certainly more long-term data is needed to fully resolve this issue.

While an association between the pill and breast cancer is presently a hypothetical one, there are now very real data showing that the pill actually protects women from certain other cancers. For example, using the pill cuts the risk of developing uterine cancer by 50% and the risk of cancer of the ovary by 40%. Recognizing these noncontraceptive health benefits, the FDA, as of 1988, has permitted drug manufacturers to include such information in product labeling. Other potential benefits for women using oral contraceptives include less iron-deficiency anemia, less menstrual pain, and more regular periods.

The relationship between long-term pill use and the development of cancer of the cervix is unclear. Most recent studies have failed to confirm an overall increase in the risk of cervical cancer with pill use. However, women who have taken the pill for five years or more have been shown in some studies to have twice the risk of developing cervix cancer or precancerous changes (see Chapter 37). Whether this finding represents cause and effect or merely the association of other cancer risk factors among the population of pill users is not certain.

Depo-Provera (DMPA)

Depo-Provera (depot medroxyprogesterone acetate) is a relatively new and highly effective method of hormonal birth control approved in the United States by the FDA in late 1992. This drug, sometimes abbreviated DMPA, consists of a long-acting form of the hormone progesterone given by injection every three months. DMPA is over 99% effective and has been used by 30 million women worldwide for many years. This "hormone shot" acts primarily by suppressing ovulation and has few side effects, although some women experience headaches, bloating, and mood changes. It has the advantage of not containing the hormone estrogen and, thus, may be the appropriate choice for some women who cannot take the combination pill.

A hallmark side effect of DMPA is that it causes suppression of normal menses. Approximately 50% of women taking DMPA stop having their periods after one year of use and nearly 70% cease to have menses after two years. Such effects are not harmful but may suppress ovulation for up to eighteen months after use. For this reason, DMPA is not recommended for

women who wish to conceive within two years. Irregular spotting or bleeding on and off may occur as well.

DMPA has been well studied and, like the pill, is not associated with an overall increased risk of breast cancer but does protect against endometrial cancer. Long-term DMPA users have been noted to have a slight decrease in bone density, which is reversed upon discontinuation of DMPA. Further study of this concern has been recommended by the FDA.

Although package labeling indicates DMPA is contraindicated in women with a history of blood clots and some forms of vascular disease, many physicians believe DMPA (and other progesterone-only hormonal contraceptives, such as Norplant and the mini-pill) is safe for many such patients. Thus, women over thirty-five who smoke or have high blood pressure or a history of coronary heart disease and cannot take the combination pill may be appropriate candidates for DMPA. Because each woman's medical circumstances are unique, these questions should first be discussed with your physician. The greater prescribing flexibility of DMPA and its high level of convenience make this new hormonal contraceptive an excellent alternative for some women.

Contraceptive Implants (Norplant)

Norplant, a contraceptive implant, was approved by the FDA in 1990. The implant consists of several silastic capsules containing the hormone levonorgestrel, a type of progesterone. The capsules are injected subcutaneously into the skin of the upper arm using local anesthesia in the physician's office. The implants continuously release progesterone, providing highly effective contraception for up to five years. The capsules are then removed in the doctor's office.

Like Depo-Provera, Norplant is a good alternative for patients who cannot take the estrogen-containing combination birth control pill. Norplant may thus be suitable for women with conditions such as high blood pressure or a history of blood clots, but like other hormonal methods is contraindicated in patients with a history of breast cancer, unexplained vaginal bleeding, or possible pregnancy. The implant is also a good choice for patients who are thirty-five and smoke or who have trouble remembering to take the pill reliably. Removal of this implant requires considerable physician experience and skill, and can be tricky, taking up to over an hour in the office. The main side effect of the method, irregular vaginal bleeding, occurs in over 50% of patients during the first year of Norplant use, decreasing to less than a third of patients by the fifth year of use.

CHAPTER 10

Selecting Your Method

We hope you have a good working knowledge about contraception after reading the previous chapters. Now comes the difficult part: selecting the contraceptive method best for you. Your doctor is a good source of specific information. It would be easy to let him or her decide for you, but we think you are the one to make the most appropriate choice. Table 16 summarizes the advantages and disadvantages of the major birth control methods.

Three Steps to Selecting Your Method

There are three essential steps to follow in selecting your birth control method:

1. How *effective* does your chosen method need to be?
2. How *safe* will the method be for you?
3. How *acceptable* is the method for you?

The three-step decision-making process is outlined in Table 18.

Step 1—Effectiveness

Effectiveness here means how well the method keeps you from becoming pregnant. Begin by selecting from Table 17 the method which offers the highest effectiveness required for your needs. Remember that effectiveness is directly related not only to the inherent efficiency of the method (known as *theoretical* effectiveness) but also to how carefully the method is going to be used (known as *use* effectiveness). The theoretical effectiveness and use effectiveness rates are very close for the IUDs and the hormonal method. Note that the widest difference between the theoretical effectiveness rate and the use ef-

fectiveness rate is found with the barrier methods (diaphragm, condom, foam, and cervical cap) and the rhythm methods. To know which end of the effectiveness range for a specific method applies to you, you should add a fudge factor based on your own motivation to consistently use these methods properly. With proper use, the barrier methods or rhythm methods may be nearly as effective as the pill or IUD. The question you need to answer is: How careful and painstaking am I likely to be in using the method I choose? Be honest with yourself. Remember also that effectiveness increases considerably when you use two methods at the same time.

Step 2—Safety

Safety here refers to the health risks involved with the use of each method. There are three separate risks to consider:

1. the risk of side effects and death associated with the method itself (higher for the hormonal methods and the IUD);
2. the risk (medical and death) associated with unexpected pregnancy (or therapeutic abortion) if the method fails (higher for barrier and rhythm methods); and
3. the risk of acquiring sexually transmitted diseases such as AIDS. This risk is lowest when barrier methods are used.

When you add the risk of the method itself and the risk of pregnancy, the combined risk of any one of the four traditional methods (pill, IUD, barrier, and rhythm) in nonsmoking women under age thirty is essentially the same—namely, 1 to 2 deaths per 100,000 women per year. In other words, based on the experience of hundreds of thousands of nonsmoking women, *up to age thirty* your overall risk calculated statistically is similar, regardless of which birth control method you choose. After age thirty, the picture changes in three ways:

1. The risk of death (mortality) in pill users who smoke rises disproportionately with increasing age. This risk is four to seven times the risk compared to that for non-smoking pill users.
2. The mortality risk among pill users who do

Table 16 ADVANTAGES AND DISADVANTAGES OF BIRTH CONTROL METHODS

Method	Advantages	Disadvantages
Pill	almost complete effectiveness; convenient and does not interfere with sexual spontaneity; decreased menstrual blood loss and cramping	not safe for all women; rare serious and numerous minor side effects
IUD	very effective; does not interfere with sexual spontaneity; most convenient method	frequent side effects, especially in women who have not had children; if pregnancy occurs, serious infection or other complications may develop
Barrier (*diaphragm, condom, foam, cervical cap*)	very effective if properly used; no major medical complications; possible prevention against venereal disease	may interfere with sexual spontaneity; may be inconvenient or messy; chance of pregnancy higher than for pill or for IUD
Depo-Provera (DMPA)	highly effective and convenient	menses may stop; requires injection ("shot") every three months
Norplant	highly effective and convenient	irregular bleeding common; may be difficult to remove
Rhythm (*natural family planning*)	no physical side effects; accepted by all religions	high chance of pregnancy; abstinence or back-up method required nearly half of the time; requires diligent record keeping; may be difficult to use if periods are irregular

Table 17 EFFECTIVENESS RATES* FOR VARIOUS BIRTH CONTROL METHODS

Method	Theoretical Effectiveness Rate	Use Effectiveness Rate
Combination pill	99.9%	96% to 99% (97% average)
Cervical cap	94%	83% to 89%
Depo-Provera (DMPA)	99.7%	99.7%
Diaphragm (with spermicide)	97%	80% to 97% (85% average)
Female condom	95%	75%
Foam	97%	71% to 97% (80% average)
IUD	99%	99%
Male condom	97%	64% to 97% (90% average)
Male condom and spermicide	99%	94%
Norplant	99.8%	99.8%
Rhythm (natural family planning)	95% to 99%	53% to 99% (80% average)

* Based on rates reported from various studies.

Table 18   THREE-STEP APPROACH FOR SELECTING YOUR BIRTH CONTROL METHOD

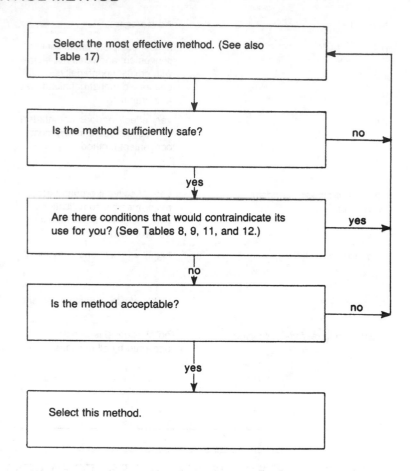

Step 1:   Effectiveness — Select the most effective method. (See also Table 17)

Step 2:   Safety — Is the method sufficiently safe?   no

Are there conditions that would contraindicate its use for you? (See Tables 8, 9, 11, and 12.)   yes

yes

Step 3:   Acceptability — Is the method acceptable?   no

yes

Select this method.

---

* The use of a condom plus spermicide is recommended for all couples unless each partner has tested negative for AIDS and the couple has been mutually monogamous for a period of at least six months prior to the testing.

not smoke increases only slightly between age thirty and age forty. These risks are due largely to risks associated with the method itself.

3. The mortality risk among users of traditional contraception (barrier method and rhythm method) increases somewhat after age thirty to 2 to 4 deaths per 100,000 women per year. These risks are due largely to pregnancy risks from failure of the method.

Step 3—Acceptability

Acceptability is a subjective determination; that is, every person has a different idea of what is acceptable, and this determination is one you must make for yourself. The method selected in the first two steps of this process must now conform to your personal needs for convenience and sexual spontaneity. However, such needs should never, in our opinion, override the higher need for safety in sexual relationships. This means that, except for mutually monogamous relationships in which each member of the couple has previously tested negative for AIDS, a condom plus spermicide should be used universally (even by a woman on the pill) regardless of how "unacceptable" these methods may be to either partner.

Newer Methods of Birth Control

Enormous costs and years of research are involved in the development of new drugs, including contraceptives. Unfortunately the Federal government has not made research into new birth control methods a priority and annually spends about ten cents per capita on contraceptive research. FDA drug testing regulations require extensive animal and human testing, so that most drugs take five to ten years or more before they are approved. Some drugs which are widely used in other countries do not meet the FDA's strict requirements for safety or effectiveness. An example is Depo-Provera, which was not approved in the United States until 1992 despite its worldwide use for birth control for over thirty years in more than 30 million women in ninety different countries. Unfortunately, few other contraceptive innovations can be expected in the next few years. This is largely due to fear of lawsuits, which has discouraged drug companies from introducing newer contraceptive products in the United States.

Resources

For further information on birth control and family planning clinics, contact your local women's center or write to the following:

Planned Parenthood Federation
    of America, Inc.
810 Seventh Avenue
New York, New York 10019

Zero Population Growth, Inc.
1400 Sixteenth Street, N.W., Suite 320
Washington, D.C. 20036

References for Section Two

American College of Obstetricians and Gynecologists *Technical Bulletin* 198. Hormonal contraception, Oct 1994.

American College of Obstetricians and Gynecologists *Technical Bulletin* 164. The intrauterine device, Feb 1992.

American College of Obstetricians and Gynecologists, Committee on adolescent health care, *Committee Opinion* 154. Condom availability for adolescents, Apr 1995.

American College of Obstetricians and Gynecologists, Committee on gynecologic practice, *Committee Opinion* 41. Contraception for women in their later reproductive years, Dec 1985.

Contraception in the later reproductive years: a valid aspect of preventive health care. *Dialogues in Contraception 5* 4(5), Winter 1995.

Connell, E. The female condom—a new contraceptive option. *Contemporary OB/GYN* 20–27, Oct 1994.

Pollack, A. New issues in spermicide use. *Contemporary OB/GYN* 29–39, Technology 1994.

Intrauterine devices and pelvic inflammatory disease: an international perspective. *The Lancet, Clinical Practice* 339:785–788, Mar 28, 1992.

Connell, E. Depot medroxyprogesterone acetate: clinical experience in the United States. *The Female Patient* 19:91–100, Nov 1994.

Connell, E. DMPA: a practical guide. *The Female Patient* 19:75–80, Nov 1994.

Goldzieher, J. Developments in contraception: counseling patients. *The Female Patient* 12:43–51, Dec 1987.

Connell, E. Reevaluating women's contraceptive needs. *Contemporary OB/GYN Special Issue* 32:27–35, Sep 1988.

Schwartz, B. Contraception update. *Williams Obstetrics*, Supplement 11, Mar 1987.

Notelovitz, M. The use of oral contraceptives past the age of 35: bridging the gap. *International Journal of Fertility*, Supplement 33:13–20, 1988.

Carr, B. Starting the new patient on oral contraceptives. *International Journal of Fertility*, Supplement 33: 21–26, 1988.

Speroff, L. Multiphasic and monophasic OCs. *Contemporary OB/GYN Special Issue* 32:124–146, Sep 1988.

Grimes, D. Multiphasic OCs and ovarian cysts. *Contemporary OB/GYN Special Issue* 32:103–114, Sep 1988.

Burnhill, N. *Safety of intrauterine contraceptive devices symposium* 11(3): July–Sep 1989

Soderstrom, R. IUDs require informed consent. *Contemporary OB/GYN Special Issue* 32:115–123, Sep 1988.

Adams, R. How to use a condom. *Medical Aspects of Human Sexuality*: July 1987.

Voeller, B. Mineral-oil lubricants cause rapid deterioration of latex condoms. *Contraception* 39:95–101, 1989.

Zinaman, M. What you should know about natural family planning. *Contemporary OB/GYN Special Issue* 32:69–89, Sep 1988.

Kaufman, D. The effect of different types of intrauterine devices on the risk of pelvic inflammatory disease. *Journal of the American Medical Association* 250:759–762, 1983.

Connell, E. Barrier contraceptives—their time has returned. *The Female Patient* 14(5):66–77, May 1989.

Copper-T 380A IUD marketed in U.S. *FDA Drug Bulletin*, Aug 1988.

Cervical cap approved for contraception. *FDA Drug Bulletin*, Aug 1988.

Medical update—cervical cap returns. *The Female Patient* 13:67, Sep 1988.

Machol, L. A fresh look at barrier contraceptives. *Contemporary OB/GYN* 31(3):132–153, Mar 1988.

Tatum, H. A new IUD offering more copper, better results. *Contemporary OB/GYN Special Issue* 32:36–50, Sep 1988.

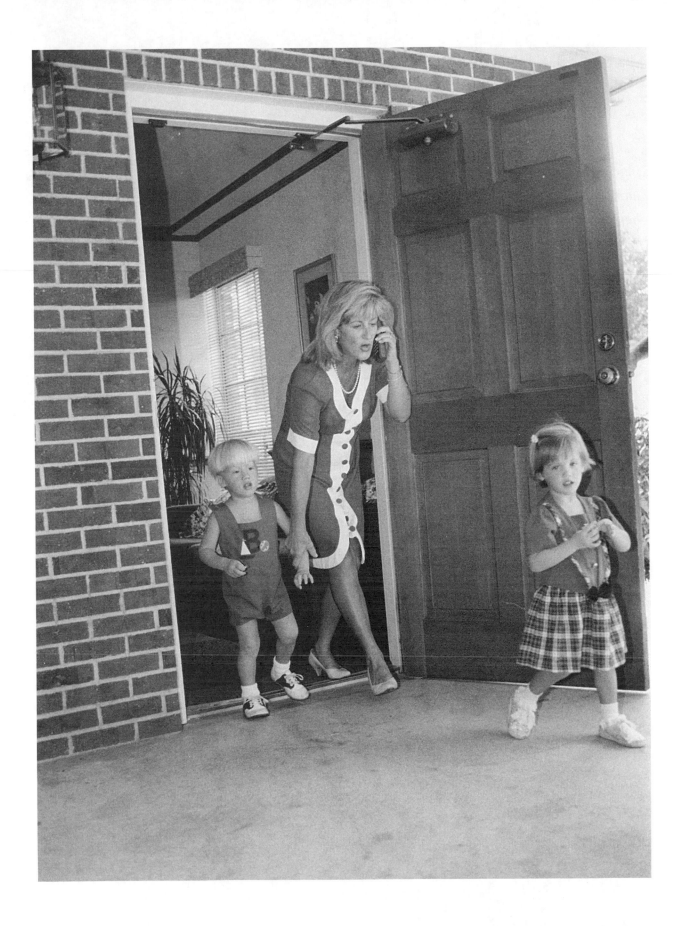

PLANNING
PREGNANCY

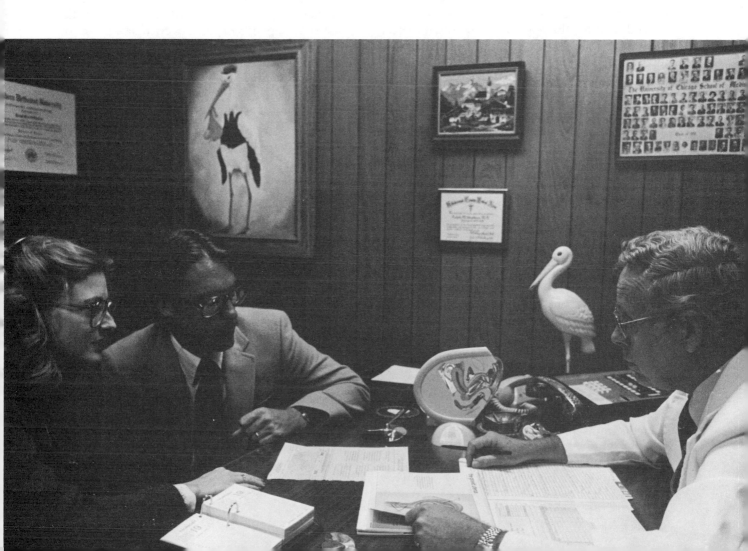

CHAPTER 11

Identifying Birth Defects

Concern with preventing genetic birth defects has grown steadily in the past decade among the general population and health professionals alike. Genetic disease or genetically influenced conditions now account for nearly one-third of infant deaths, and major defects affect about 2.5% of all live-born infants. In all, about 250,000 babies are born with some physical or mental defect every year. Because some diseases, such as cystic fibrosis, Tay-Sachs disease, and sickle-cell anemia (see glossary), may not show up for several months, the real chance of a birth defect is about 5%. Looking at it another way, 95% of infants appear healthy at birth and will not develop major birth defects in later life.

The causes of birth defects range from genetic roots that result in, say, Down syndrome, to underlying environmental influences, like drugs, exposure to radiation, or maternal infection (German measles). Few birth defects have a single, major environmental or genetic cause. Most are believed to result from the interaction of several genes, possibly in combination with subtle environmental influences. As a result, birth defects usually occur irregularly and unpredictably. However, couples with known risk factors, such as a family history of an inherited genetic disease, previous birth of a defective child, or advanced maternal age, often want to know their chance of having a healthy baby. Genetic counseling deals with these and other factors in helping such couples plan their families.

What Is Genetic Counseling?

Genetic counseling is the process of educating couples who want to have children about how some birth defects happen, what the couple's chances are of having a normal baby, and what

alternatives are open to them if they are at risk of having a baby with a birth defect. Genetic counseling uses the science of genetics to help prevent birth defects. If you have a child with a birth defect and/or mental retardation, you would be wise to seek genetic counseling before attempting another pregnancy. Primary-care physicians, such as family practitioners or obstetricians, often provide initial counseling since they are the ones who see the patients first. At times, the medical geneticist and his or her specialized laboratory may be needed as well.

Counseling explains the risks of having a child with a certain disorder and what that disorder means. It also offers the couple alternatives for dealing with the risk. Valuable clues from your medical and family health history can often determine the pattern of inheritance or expected frequency of a certain genetic disorder. After a physical examination and sometimes screening tests that are required to reach a diagnosis, appropriate alternatives can be considered: for example, prenatal testing, adoption, artificial insemination, sterilization. The option selected depends on the severity of a given defect and the risks involved. Fortunately, 95% of the time, couples seeking genetic counseling about a particular disorder can expect reassurance that their baby will not be affected by the disorder in question.

Genes and Chromosomes

You can understand how different disorders may be inherited by looking at the basic body unit—the cell. Every human cell except the sperm cell and egg cell contains 46 chromosomes, each filled with thousands of genes arranged in pairs. Half of each gene pair comes from the egg cell of the mother and half from the sperm cell of the father. Genes contain the material that controls all of our physical features from eye color and ear shape to critical parts of the heart and nervous system. The genetic information carried in genes directs the growth, development, and function of our bodies throughout life. Considering the vast information contained in our genes, it is amazing that mistakes resulting in genetic disorders occur as infrequently as they do. Most people are carriers of a few genes for inherited diseases. However, normal genes most often outweigh the effects of faulty genes. Unless both parents carry the same abnormal genes, the offspring is usually unaffected.

Genetic disorders can be classified into three basic types: chromosomal disorders, single-gene disorders, and multifactorial inheritance.

Chromosomal disorders result from an abnormality in the number or structure of the chromosomes in each cell. These disorders occur during an isolated accident (such as acquiring an extra chromosome) in the development of the fertilized egg. Such chromosomal errors are then transmitted to all other cells from the moment of fertilization. It should be stressed that parents of offspring with a chromosomal defect are almost never the carriers of that defect because chromosomal abnormalities are rarely inherited. The risk of bearing a child with this defect, however, does increase with maternal age.

Most chromosomal errors have serious medical consequences and many result in miscarriage. This is nature's way of handling severely defective embryos. Less often, chromosomal problems result in stillbirth or multiple birth defects. Chromosomal abnormalities of varying severity occur in about one out of two hundred newborns.

In Down syndrome (which used to be called mongolism), the most common chromosomal defect, the affected child has 47 chromosomes in each cell, rather than the normal 46. The disorder causes mental retardation and a typical so-called mongoloid appearance: small head, slanting eyes, and other physical abnormalities. Down syndrome and other chromosomal disorders can be diagnosed prenatally.

Single-gene disorders, hereditary conditions caused by a single defective gene, affect approximately 1% of newborns. According to the laws of genetics, there are three ways in which these defects may be transmitted from generation to generation: dominant inheritance, recessive inheritance, and X-linked inheritance.

With *dominant inheritance* (see Table 19) it takes just one defective gene from either parent to cause a disorder in the offspring. If that faulty gene is passed to the offspring, the faulty gene always dominates the normal counterpart gene from the other parent and causes the child to inherit the defect. Since the child will inherit from the affected parent *either* the normal gene *or* the defective gene, then each child has a 50% chance of inheriting the defect. To understand

Table 19 HOW DOMINANT INHERITANCE WORKS (SINGLE-GENE DISORDERS)

(Only one parent is affected whose single faulty gene (D) dominates its normal counterpart (A).)

Normal Parent   **Affected Parent**

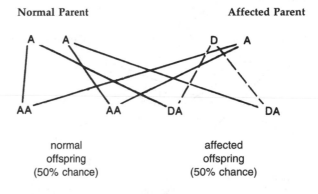

normal offspring (50% chance)   affected offspring (50% chance)

this percentage, you need to picture the genes of each parent in pairs. Let's say one gene of one parent's pair is faulty; the other gene of that same pair is normal. Only one of the gene twosome is passed to the offspring. If the normal gene is passed, the child will be normal. If the faulty (dominant) gene is passed, the child will have a birth defect. This is one of the *laws of inheritance*. Examples of dominantly inherited disorders include hypercholesterolemia (high blood cholesterol), Huntington's disease (progressive nervous system degeneration), and certain forms of dwarfism. At present, very few dominantly inherited disorders can be diagnosed during pregnancy.

Recessive inheritance (see Table 20) requires one defective gene from each of *both* the parents to cause the disorder in the offspring. In the case of *recessive* inheritance, if a person has one normal gene and one defective gene, the normal gene takes precedence over its defective recessive counterpart. This means that this person is not *affected* by the disease but can be a *carrier*, that is, can pass the defect on to offspring. Each child has a 25% chance of inheriting the defect when both parents are carriers. If only one parent is a carrier, the offspring cannot inherit the defect but each child has a 50% chance of being a carrier of the defect. Single-gene defects include many inborn errors of metabolism, so

Table 20   HOW RECESSIVE INHERITANCE WORKS (SINGLE-GENE DISORDERS)

Both parents are usually unaffected and have a normal gene (A), which takes precedence over its faulty recessive counterpart (r).

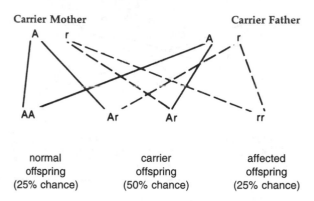

Carrier Mother   Carrier Father

| normal offspring (25% chance) | carrier offspring (50% chance) | affected offspring (25% chance) |

called because they don't allow normal chemical reactions in body cells. Many of these metabolic conditions cause mental retardation or death in early childhood. Examples of recessively inherited disorders include cystic fibrosis (disorder of the mucous and sweat glands), galactosemia (inability to digest milk sugar), phenylketonuria (a biochemical disorder causing mental retardation), sickle-cell disease (severe form of anemia), and Tay-Sachs disease (fatal brain damage). Since this form of inheritance occurs when neither parent seems to be affected (but both are carriers), diagnosis is usually made only after the birth of an affected child. If a child has been diagnosed with one of these disorders, the child's parents may be advised to have an amniocentesis in subsequent pregnancies, because this test can detect about seventy of the four hundred known recessively inherited disorders.

X-linked, or sex-linked, *inheritance* disorders occur when a genetic condition is transmitted through the X chromosome. Normal females have two X chromosomes in each cell. Normal males have one X chromosome and one Y chromosome. In X-linked inheritance, the mother usually carries an abnormal gene on one of the X chromosomes but is usually not affected herself. Each son has a 50% chance of inheriting this

disorder. Each daughter has a 50% chance of being a carrier, like her mother. Examples of X-linked disorders are hemophilia (defect in blood-clotting mechanisms), some forms of muscular dystrophy (progressive muscle wasting), and color blindness. Most X-linked disorders cannot be diagnosed during pregnancy, but amniocentesis does establish the sex of the fetus and consequently whether or not the child could be affected.

Table 21 summarizes the chances of all offspring being a carrier or being affected, according to certain existent conditions, in the three ways that single-gene disorders may be inherited.

Multifactorial inheritance refers to defects resulting from the interaction of faulty genes and possibly a negative environment. The risks for these defects are based on their statistical frequency in the population rather than on laws of inheritance. If you have one affected child, the risk of having another with the same defect is approximately 5%. Certain malformations in this group, including spina bifida (open spine) and anencephaly (failure of brain development), can be diagnosed during pregnancy by amniocentesis. Nearly all other genetic diseases in this category, although they include 90% of all birth defects, cannot be diagnosed by prenatal testing.

Preventing Genetic Disease

Carriers of genetic diseases are not affected themselves but may be at risk for passing a defect to their children. Couples who carry (but are not themselves affected by) harmful traits may thus not be aware of their risk status unless there is an affected relative in the family or they themselves have an affected child. Medical screening tests can presently detect about seventy separate genetic diseases. These tests detect the parents who are the carriers of faulty genes that may lead to a birth defect. Carrier detection has been most widely applied to screening for sickle-cell disease and Tay-Sachs disease because each of these diseases occurs so frequently within a specific population. Ten percent of U.S. blacks are carriers of sickle-cell disease and 3% of Jewish persons of eastern European ancestry are carriers of Tay-Sachs disease. Both of these diseases are transmitted by recessive inheritance and af-

Table 21   CHANCES OF INHERITING SINGLE-GENE DISORDERS

Type of Inheritance	Parent Affected?	Parent Carrier?	Chance of Offspring Being a Carrier	Chance of Offspring Being Affected
Dominant inheritance (1 parent carries faulty gene, 1 parent genetically normal)	yes	no	0%	50%
Recessive inheritance (1 parent carries faulty gene, 1 parent genetically normal)	no	yes	50%	0%
Recessive inheritance (both parents carry same faulty gene)	no (neither)	yes (both)	50%	25%
Sex-linked inheritance (mother carries faulty gene, father genetically normal)	no	yes (mother)	25% (50% of all females, 0% of males)	25% (50% of all males, 0% of females)

fect 25% of the offspring when both parents are carriers.

Another form of genetic screening involves chromosomal analysis called *karyotyping* to search for abnormalities in parental chromosomes. This blood test presently costs about $450 and takes a technician several days to perform, making it impractical for mass screening. As stated previously, most chromosomal defects result from isolated accidents rather than from inheritance. In rare cases, however, parents who are carriers of chromosomal abnormalities may transmit the defect to their offspring. Often the only clue to the person carrying a chromosomal abnormality is a history of reproduction problems. Therefore, couples with a history of any of the following pregnancy-related difficulties should consider chromosomal testing to see if either partner carries abnormal chromosomes:

1. Three or more miscarriages.
2. Two miscarriages plus a child born with a birth defect.
3. Two miscarriages and a stillbirth.
4. Stillbirth where birth defects are present.
5. Infertility if routine tests prove negative.
6. Previous child with a birth defect (some instances).

Some couples who feel they may be at risk undergo these screening tests to detect single-gene or chromosomal defects so they can make informed decisions about pregnancy. If affected, some partners elect to remain childless; others take the risk of having their own child, or they adopt children. Artificial insemination is another option when only the husband is a carrier. The affected couples who do attempt pregnancy often undergo prenatal testing to determine if a given genetic defect is present in the fetus.

Prenatal testing for birth defects

Nearly 90% of birth defects are *not* subject to prenatal diagnosis; that is, it is not possible with 90% of birth defects to determine through a prenatal test whether a birth defect exists. Of the 10% remaining, those most suitable for prenatal diagnosis include:

1. Chromosomal abnormalities (such as Down syndrome).
2. Metabolic disorders (rare).
3. Sex-linked disorders (rare).
4. Specific disorders of the central nervous system (anencephaly, spina bifida).

The four main types of tests that help to diagnose birth defects in pregnancy are sonography, certain blood tests, amniocentesis, and chorionic villus sampling.

Sonography (see Chapter 16), a procedure using sound waves, has in the past ten years become increasingly refined and is capable of diagnosing various abnormalities by sixteen to eighteen weeks of pregnancy and sometimes earlier. It is important to understand that many of these diagnoses cannot be made if the sonogram is performed too early (e.g., six to twelve weeks) in the pregnancy. Also, the type of sonogram used makes a difference. Many fetal abnormalities will not be detected by the basic, *level-one* sonogram that many obstetricians use in their offices to diagnose twins, locate the placenta, or calculate a "due" date. The most complete exam for diagnosing birth defects is known as a *level-two* sonogram. This more detailed and expensive examination of the baby's organs is usually performed around eighteen weeks by a radiologist or perinatologist (see glossary). While it is impractical to perform level-two sonograms on all women, those with a history of certain defects (spina bifida, congenital heart disease, and others) or who have taken drugs in early pregnancy may benefit from having this procedure. The use of routine sonography in pregnancy continues to be debated, but the procedure is considered very safe and useful, and it sometimes detects the unexpected, such as twins.

Blood tests used in diagnosing birth defects include the screening of potential carriers of genetic diseases such as sickle cell disease and Tay-Sachs disease (see above). By far the most widely used blood test for genetic diagnosis is the alpha-fetoprotein (AFP) test, which measures the amount of a fetal protein found both in the mother's blood and in the amniotic fluid. Performed at fifteen to eighteen weeks, this test identifies women at increased risk for having a baby with a neural tube defect (NTD), a group of birth defects that involve the nervous system, including anencephaly (failure of brain formation) and spina bifida (open spine). Such conditions may cause serious neurological impairment, and 95% of the time there is no past family history of these conditions.

The only drawback of the AFP test is that while only 1 to 2 women per 1,000 have a fetus with an NTD, about 50 of these women will have an elevated test value. Although most of these abnormal values are not associated with an abnormal fetus, the only way to find out for sure is to go through further testing. First, the blood test is repeated. If it is abnormal (either high or low), a sonogram is performed to confirm that gestational dates are accurate, since being "off" on dates can result in a falsely high or low AFP value (also, twins give a falsely high value). If dates are confirmed by sonogram and no abnormality is found, an amniocentesis is done to measure AFP levels in the amniotic fluid. A high level of AFP in the amniotic fluid is associated with a 90% chance that the fetus has a neural tube defect. A low level of AFP is also investigated by amniocentesis, and a chromosome evaluation is done since low AFP levels have been associated with a slightly increased risk of Down syndrome and other chromosomal abnormalities. In fact, such blood testing to screen for Down syndrome has become widely used recently, especially when there is a family or personal history of birth defects or when the mother is over thirty-five years of age. While the AFP is the principal blood test involved in this screen, the test's accuracy is improved by measuring (in the same blood sample) two other substances—the hormones human chorionic gonadotropin and estriol. Using the combined results from these three tests—collectively known as Triple Marker Screening or Multiple Marker Screening (MMS)—can improve the overall accuracy of screening for Down syndrome compared to using the AFP blood test alone.

Historically, *amniocentesis*, a procedure to remove a sample of amniotic fluid (the "waters" surrounding the baby), is the best-known prenatal test and can identify more birth defects than any other procedure. Recently, amniocentesis has been performed earlier in pregnancy, at ten to fourteen weeks, without added fetal risks. If subsequent research supports its initial success, "early" amniocentesis may soon replace the later procedure.

Amniocentesis takes about five minutes to perform. Although the risk of fetal injury is practically zero, the chance of spontaneous miscarriage as a direct result of this procedure is approximately 1 out of 300. Other complications, such as infection and bleeding, are rare. Sonography is usually performed prior to amniocentesis to help guide the needle to a "pocket" of fluid away from the placenta. Passing the needle through the placenta is likely to cause leakage of fetal blood cells into the maternal circulation, possibly resulting in complications for Rh negative women. For this reason, even if sonography is used, Rh negative women now receive a small dose of RhoGAM, a drug to prevent complications, after amniocentesis.

Table 22 lists the possible reasons for genetic amniocentesis. A couple should seriously consider having the procedure performed if any of the conditions apply. The most common reason

Table 22 POSSIBLE REASONS FOR AMNIOCENTESIS TO IDENTIFY BIRTH DEFECTS

Possible Reason	Incidence of Birth Defect
Age over 35, especially if over 37	1% to 2%
Three or more miscarriages	less than 1%
Either parent has a known chromosomal abnormality	1% to 100% (average 10%)
The mother has had a chromosomally abnormal child in the past, such as Down syndrome	variable* (average 1% to 2%)
There is a history of Down syndrome (or other chromosomal abnormality) in either parent's family	variable (average less than 1%)
The mother has male relatives with muscular dystrophy, hemophilia, or other sex-linked disorder	25%
Both parents are carriers for or have had a child with a hereditary metabolic disorder (e.g., Tay-Sachs disease)	25%
The mother has had a child with spina bifida (open spine) or anencephaly; or the disorder is present in a close family member (parent or sibling)	3% to 5%

* The recurrence risk in 95% of women who have given birth to a child with Down syndrome is 1% to 2%. In the other 5% of women, either parent may carry an abnormal chromosome which has a recurrence risk of approximately 5% to 10%.

for prenatal amniocentesis is advanced maternal age. As women grow older, they have increased chances for bearing children with chromosomal problems, such as Down syndrome. Advanced paternal age is not nearly as important. The reason for this may be that a man continuously produces sperm throughout his life, whereas a woman is born with the number of eggs she will have throughout life. As the eggs age, chromosomal accidents during ovulation or fertilization may occur with increased frequency. After the age of thirty-five, the risk of Down syndrome and other chromosomal abnormalities increases significantly. There may be some debate as to whether the risk in women between the ages of thirty-five and thirty-nine justifies the procedure; however, taking into account the increased risk of *all* chromosomal abnormalities in this age group—approximately 2%—many authorities believe that amniocentesis is indicated. After age forty, amniocentesis is definitely recommended.

Another common reason for genetic amniocentesis is the previous birth of a child with a chromosomal defect, including Down syndrome. A woman with this history has a 1% to 2% risk for recurrence, regardless of her age. A much higher risk for recurrence—25%—exists for cou-

ples who have children with inherited metabolic disorders where both parents are carriers. Prior to the use of amniocentesis, such carrier parents had two options: to go with the throw of the genetic dice or to remain childless. Now, some of these disorders can be identified by amniocentesis. At this time, practical methods are not available to screen a given individual for all of the known metabolic abnormalities. A person is tested only for the abnormality at risk. In couples who have had children with certain abnormalities of the brain (anencephaly) and spinal column (spina bifida), the woman should undergo amniocentesis, because the recurrence risk for these defects is approximately 5%.[1]

The fourth and newest test for prenatal diagnosis, *chorionic villus sampling* (CVS) or *chorion biopsy*, may rival amniocentesis by the late 1990s as the procedure of choice for diagnosing genetic disorders in early pregnancy. CVS allows doctors to screen for genetic defects as early as the tenth week of pregnancy and gives results within one to two weeks. CVS involves insertion of a small tube through the cervix into the uterus (or this may be accomplished like amniocentesis, by passing a small needle through the abdominal wall into the uterus) to take a sample of the

1 Recently, the number of disorders that can be identified from amniotic fluid studies has been increased using a technique called *DNA analysis*. This new technology now is used to diagnose Duchene's muscular dystrophy, sickle-cell disease, hemophilia, and cystic fibrosis.

chorion, a membrane surrounding the fetus. Cells from the chorion have the same genetic makeup as the fetus. Earlier detection of birth defects by this method is a major advantage over amniocentesis, which is performed near the sixteenth week of pregnancy.

CVS, which is being evaulated by the National Institutes of Child Health and Human Development at seven medical centers, has been performed in over 50,000 pregnancies. The miscarriage rate due to the procedure has been similar to or just slightly higher than that for amniocentesis and has corresponded directly to the experience of the physician with the CVS technique. Long-term effects on growth, development, and intellectual function need to be assessed since CVS has only been used extensively since 1985.

A different approach to prenatal diagnosis involves sampling fetal blood directly from the umbilical cord. This technique, called *umbilical cord sampling* (or *fetal blood sampling*), is always performed by a perinatologist. The procedure tests for a wide range of fetal conditions, and results are rapidly available—in seventy-two to ninety-six hours. Cord sampling is a more invasive technique than amniocentesis and potentially more risky, as it can interfere with blood flowing through the umbilical cord. One indication for using umbilical cord sampling occurs when the decision to have genetic testing is made after the pregnancy has reached close to twenty weeks and rapid results are imperative. Other uses include more accurate diagnosis of certain fetal infections like rubella and toxoplasmosis (see Chapter 20), as well as identification of certain suspected birth defects, such as hemophilia.

Limitations of prenatal tests

The relative rarity of genetic abnormalities even in high-risk populations is a major factor limiting the wider use of amniocentesis for detection of genetic disease. Even if amniocentesis were done on all women over thirty-five, the frequency of Down syndrome, for instance, would be decreased by less than 50% since the *average* maternal age for this condition is less than thirty-four years. For the genetic diseases that can be diagnosed, the options are presently limited by the inability to treat the vast majority of

diseases either in utero (in the uterus) or following childbirth. Consequently, for those few women who have a positive prenatal diagnosis, there are really only two alternatives: abortion or risking the birth of a deformed child. Couples who select abortion often experience depression following termination of the pregnancy. Despite the emotional trauma involved, couples selecting therapeutic abortion may consider this option preferable to the birth of a severely defective child.

Gender preselection

Choice of a girl or a boy may become a parental option by the end of the 1990s. However, techniques enabling sex selection are far from perfect. Scientists have long known that the sex of a child depends on whether a "male" or "female" sperm fertilizes the egg; the sperm carrying the Y chromosome will produce a boy and one bearing the X chromosome is responsible for producing a girl.

Numerous methods of sex determination have been proposed. Popular but unsubstantiated theories in the 1960s emphasized the use of coital timing and baking soda or vinegar douches to enhance the survival of male or female sperm, respectively. The most promising method of sex selection today involves separation of male and female sperm. A technique for sperm separation was originally developed by a reproductive physiologist, Dr. Ronald Ericsson, in 1973. Ericsson's patented method takes advantage of the fact that male and female sperm "swim" at different rates. A sperm race is set up by suspending a drop of semen onto a solution of albumin, a dense fluid found in blood. The technique allows collection of the faster-moving male sperm which swim to the bottom of the albumin-filled glass tube. More recent sperm-separation techniques perfected in Australia and in the United States use a method called flow cytometry in which each sperm is stained and separated according to how much DNA it contains. Slightly more DNA will be present in X sperm. Researchers in sperm separation claim the technique is 75% to 80% successful. While the procedure is currently not widely used except for couples at risk for X-linked inheritance disorders, such as hemophilia, by the twenty-first century sperm sepa-

Table 23   INFORMATION ABOUT COMMON BIRTH DEFECTS

Name	Frequency of Occurrence	Risk of Recurrence	Detectable in Pregnancy	Genetic Classification
Anencephaly (failure of brain development)	1:1000	1:20	yes (amniocentesis; sonography)	multifactorial
Cleft lip and/or palate	1:1000	1:20	no	multifactorial
Clubfoot	1:1000	1:30	no	multifactorial
Congenital heart disease	1:1000	1:50	sometimes (sonography)	multifactorial
Congenital hip dislocation	1:1000	1:25	no	multifactorial
Cystic fibrosis	1:2500	1:4	yes (amniocentesis)	single gene
Down syndrome	1:650 (age-dependent)	1:50	yes (amniocentesis)	chromosomal
Hemophilia	1:3000	1:4 (50% of all males)	yes (amniocentesis)	single gene (sex-linked)
Pyloric stenosis (obstructed opening from stomach into intestine)	1:1000	1:30	no	multifactorial
Sickle-cell anemia	1:500*	1:4	yes (amniocentesis)	single gene
Spina bifida	1:1000	1:20	usually (amniocentesis)	multifactorial
Tay-Sachs disease	1:3000**	1:4	yes (amniocentesis)	single gene

* Frequency among blacks
** Frequency among Jews of eastern European ancestry

ration may become more available for couples who choose to preselect the sex of their child.

Where to Get Help

If you need more information about birth defects and genetics (see Table 23), start with your family physician or obstetrician, who may make the appropriate local referral if he or she cannot do the counseling. There are counseling centers located in most major cities throughout the United States.

For further information on genetic counseling, contact:

March of Dimes Birth Defects Foundation
1275 Mamaroneck Avenue
White Plains, New York 10605
(914) 428-7100

CHAPTER 12

Pregnancy After Thirty-Five

Many women are choosing to wait until their thirties or even their early forties to have a child. From 1980 to 1986 the rate of first births to U.S. women between the ages of thirty-five and thirty-nine increased 81%. For women over thirty-nine, this rate doubled. The trends toward establishing one's career and completing one's education before having children, marrying later, having smaller families, having children in second and third marriages, and spending fewer years at home as a full-time homemaker have paralleled one another. The increased longevity and better health of women have also been factors. The impetus of the women's movement, changing life-styles, modern methods of birth control, and availability of child-care facilities have also contributed toward the shift in the timing of childbearing.

There is probably no "perfect" time to have a baby. There can be advantages and disadvantages at every age of childbearing when all the factors—social, financial, psychological, and medical—are considered. Your marital happiness, financial security, and, when you have the opportunity, the satisfaction that comes from planning a child when the time is right for you are important considerations which you must weigh against strictly medical factors. A recent study found that parents who consciously chose to start families in their twenties saw their forties as the time to be child-free. Parents who chose their thirties and forties were unanimous in their conviction that their twenties were the time to be free and unencumbered by parenthood. Midlife parents cited only one age-related drawback: energy level.

Let's consider here first the medical concerns of pregnancy and childbirth after the age of thirty-five. Evidence suggests that pregnancy poses few significant risks to maternal health after age thirty-five unless the woman has diabetes, hypertension, or gynecological complications such as large uterine fibroids (see Chapter 35). Actually the likelihood of medical complications increases gradually, without sudden escalation, starting at about the age of thirty. For example, the risk of pregnancy-related deaths per 100,000 births increases from 11 in the late twenties to 18 in the early thirties, rising to 46 in the late thirties, and so on; but keep in mind that this rate is still a very small percentage.

Although it is true that certain birth defects increase with maternal age, many of these abnormalities are detectable in early pregnancy and they affect a very small percentage of women over the age of thirty-five. The most well-known and frequent risk of pregnancy after age thirty-five is the birth of an infant with a chromosomal abnormality, such as Down syndrome (see Chapter 11). The incidence of Down syndrome rises from less than one per thousand before age thirty to one per hundred by age forty. Women over thirty-five have a 2% chance of having a child with a chromosomal birth defect. For some women, the emotional stress of genetic testing is so great that they choose not to have the testing done, especially if abortion is not an option. Others choose to have the tests because they feel it is better to be prepared in advance to deal with the birth defect. The more immediate results of chorionic villus sampling and "early" amniocentesis, which can detect genetic abnormalities one to two months earlier than traditional methods, may make these tests preferable.

Infertility increases with age and has become more common at all ages, especially infertility due to pelvic infections resulting from sexually transmitted diseases. Human reproductive capacity peaks for both sexes in the midtwenties and then appears to decline steadily in women over thirty and in men over forty. Tubal infections, endometriosis, and fibroid tumors occur more often in older women and are among the common causes of infertility in this age group.

Other pregnancy complications which are at least twice as frequent in mothers over the age of thirty-five compared to those in their twenties include miscarriage, stillbirths, placenta previa, diabetes, and high blood pressure. (See index for more information.) Multiple births also occur more often with increasing age, so that women in their thirties have a 30% greater chance of having twins than they did in their twenties. The risk of premature births and infant deaths is only *slightly* greater in older mothers, even up to age forty-four; and it is not nearly so great as in pregnant teen-agers.

With adequate rest, diet, and prenatal care, some of these risks can be minimized. Amniocentesis (see Chapter 20) and sonography (see Chapter 16) identify possible pregnancies at risk and make early intervention—sometimes by cesarean section—possible, if needed.

Psychologically, there are special concerns and advantages for the woman who delays pregnancy until after age thirty-five. If a pregnancy complication, such as miscarriage, does occur, the disappointment may be much greater as she waited longer to have her family. Or she may be concerned about potential problems with sibling rivalry because of the need to have her children spaced closer together in age than she ideally would like. Keep in mind, however, that sibling rivalry occurs no matter what the age spacing of children, and planning for spending individual time with each child will help to minimize it. If you are a mother with older chil-

dren, you may feel excited or depressed, or both, initially at the thought of giving birth to and rearing another child. When the baby arrives, depending on your circumstances, you may find you react either more or less enthusiastically toward caring for this newborn and observing his or her development compared to your initial feelings with your earlier children.

You may feel isolated from your friends who are close to your age and who are freer from child care responsibilities and involved with other things. You may long to have your neat and tidy house back after the arrival of a new baby and envy the free time your contemporaries with grown children have. On the other hand, some new mothers report that they enjoy motherhood more fully with this later child. In either case, getting more help with child care is important. You may decide to go back to work and spend less time at home with this child than you did with your previous children. Or you may feel more relaxed and want to spend more time to "enjoy" this child than you did with your others.

More and more today when both parents work, couples are electing to wait until their

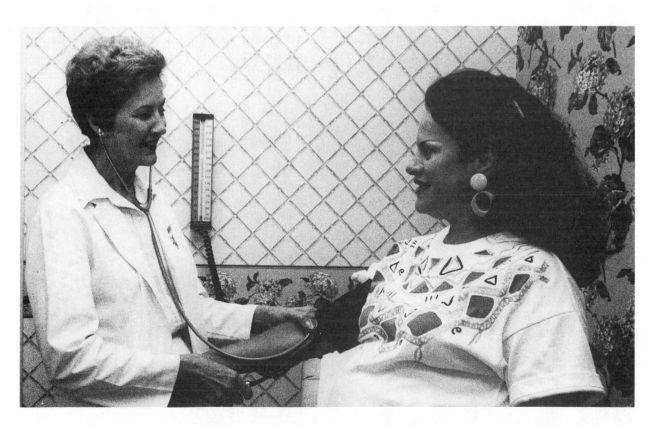

thirties to start a family. One advantage of this delay is often that both parents are more mature and more likely to have had time to establish their marriage as well as to consider their desire for parenthood. Parenthood is an adjustment regardless of age; and a couple's past experience, separately and together, in coping with stress and change may help smooth their transition into parenthood.

Having a clear idea of career goals is particularly helpful to the older woman just starting a family. A woman who is comfortable and secure with her own career plans may find it easier to maintain her identity as an individual with her own needs as separate from those of her developing family. She has had more practice balancing personal needs at home and at work and may have developed better management skills in adapting to motherhood than the less experienced young woman. Women who choose late childbearing tend to have more years of schooling and may be in better health than those who have given birth in their earlier decades.

Financial concerns connected with raising children are often a matter of major importance. Having a child today represents a substantial economic commitment, and a couple may feel more financially secure at this later point in their lives. If both parents work, it may be possible for either or both of them to arrange a leave of absence or to work part-time during the baby's first years.

In this chapter, we have dealt with some of the special concerns, medical and otherwise, you may have if you are, or plan to be, pregnant and are over the age of thirty-five. As a result of later marriage, infertility problems, or other reasons, you may suddenly be faced with the fact that if you are to have children, you will be an older-than-average mother. But the dangers are not nearly so great as is often believed. What is "ideal" for your body biologically may not suit your personal, social, or emotional needs, and, on balance, the advantages to delaying pregnancy until later in life often outweigh the disadvantages. For the woman in good general health, the medical risks of childbearing after thirty-five are indeed relatively low. Although childbearing complications for mother and baby do increase with age, this factor cannot be isolated from other aspects of your life. Increasingly, midlife women are electing to have children. Some single women decide to have children as they approach their forties, sometimes through use of a sperm bank. Adoption of older children has also increased, with many midlife women choosing older children whom they can more easily care for within the demands of their work schedules. Some couples are trying foster parenthood, adopting children from underdeveloped nations or of different racial groups, or adopting children who have special medical problems and needs and who have been hard to place.

CHAPTER 13

Infertility—Causes and Treatment

Despite apparent dwindling social pressures to have children, pregnancy and childbirth remain major milestones in the lives of many women. Psychiatrists report that even women who choose to remain childless often experience depression during their thirties related to unfulfilled motherhood. The psychological impact of an inability to bear children that are desired can be even more devastating.

A predictable and nearly universal sequence of feelings accompanies the infertility experience. The sequence resembles the pattern of coping that people go through during other crises, such as serious illness or the loss of a loved one. Some couples entering infertility evaluation are already in a state of crisis. The evaluation itself can produce further stress in the form of embarrassing questions, physical discomfort, costly tests, and the emotional anguish of having to wait several months for results. Even though a couple undergoes evaluation because they suspect they are infertile, a diagnosis suspecting or confirming infertility shocks them. They may even initially deny this diagnosis.

As the investigation proceeds, feelings of isolation and anger often develop. During this time, many couples experience marital discord or sexual difficulties, such as impotence or a decrease in sex drive. Sex, misguidedly planned around temperature charting, often becomes work instead of play. A cycle may develop with increasing emotional tension after ovulation, followed by depression when menses ensues. At this point, guilt feelings add to an already lowered sense of self-esteem. Many women may ask themselves why they have been singled out not to achieve what the rest of the world takes for granted. They may attribute infertility to some past deed, such as abortion or infrequent medical checkups. Such factors rarely account for infertility but may explain the severe depression and guilt that infertile couples so often experience.

Grief normally becomes a prominent emotional feature of an infertility evaluation. Since infertility is rarely absolute, the process of grieving may be prolonged by uncertainty surrounding the outcome of the evaluation and the potential treatment. Grieving involves acknowledging many losses in addition to the loss of potential children. There is also the loss of genetic continuity, the loss of all that fertility means to one's sexuality, and the loss of the pregnancy itself. When these feelings are dealt with openly, couples can begin to accept infertility. This acceptance allows couples to consider their remaining alternatives.

Counseling may be helpful at this point. Counseling is sometimes available through local support groups consisting of couples who have also experienced infertility problems. Many of these groups have been established through RESOLVE, Inc., a national organization offering infertile couples a variety of services, including telephone counseling and referrals for medical help. For further information, write to: RESOLVE, Inc., 1310 Broadway, Somerville, Massachusetts 02144.

What Is Infertility?

Infertility is the inability to become pregnant after one year of unprotected intercourse. Sixty percent of couples achieve conception after six months and 85% by one year. On this basis, an estimated 15% of all married couples are infertile. After the age of thirty, when a woman's fertility begins to decline somewhat, most authorities recommend an infertility evaluation if pregnancy is unsuccessfully attempted for more than six months. Infertility currently affects at least three million couples. An increasing trend to put off childbearing until after age thirty, or to stop having babies and not start again until after thirty, may increase the number of couples seeking infertility evaluation in the 1990s.

This infertility evaluation is usually done by a primary care physician such as an obstetrician-gynecologist. OB-GYNs can handle most infertility problems. Frequently gynecologists list themselves in the yellow pages of the phone book as infertility specialists. However, fewer than 5% of gynecologists have received additional subspecialty training required for treating the more uncommon infertility problems.

About half of all couples seeking infertility evaluation and treatment will ultimately be able to have children. Sometimes pregnancy occurs fortuitously during the evaluation, which takes several months or more to complete. Over 80% of the time a specific diagnosis is made. Among known causes of infertility, about one-third are attributed to a problem in the male, one-third to a problem in the female, and a final third to factors that involve both male and female partners.

Ideally the infertility evaluation is a mutually shared investigation that begins with a medical history and physical examination; the history taking includes some questions that could be directly related to the infertility (see Table 24). A sequence of laboratory tests follows the examination. In practice, this evaluation often starts with the woman who seeks advice from her gynecologist during a regular office visit. Most infertility experts recommend having both partners present at least initially to explain the upcoming tests and to lessen misplaced guilt that either one may experience by feeling responsible for the infertility.

The Causes and Treatment of Infertility

Problems found in the four areas investigated in an infertility evaluation account for more than 90% of known causes of infertility. The next part of this chapter covers these four areas and discusses causes, tests, and traditional treatment. At the end of the chapter, we will also look at some newer "high-tech" treatments, such as in vitro fertilization, which have become increasingly available in the past decade.

Tubal factors

Tubal problems contribute to infertility nearly 30% of the time and are now the leading cause of female-related infertility. Tubal blockage often occurs as a result of scarring of the Fallopian tubes due to previous infection. Although such infection is usually transmitted sexually (venereal infection), previous surgery or the prior use of an IUD could be responsible. Other tubal problems associated with infertility include endometriosis (see Chapter 36) and tubal (ectopic) pregnancy, which may require surgical removal of the involved tube.

Common tests to evaluate the Fallopian tubes: There are three basic tests to evaluate whether the Fallopian tubes are open.

The *Rubin test*, an office procedure, involves injecting carbon dioxide gas through the cervix and into the uterus and tubes. When the tubes are open, the test produces slight shoulder pain. This is due to an irritating effect of the gas, which refers pain from the abdomen to the shoulder area.

A somewhat more elaborate test, a *hysterosalpingogram* (see Figure 16), is an X-ray performed in the radiology department. The radiologist injects a special dye into the uterus and tubes, allowing an outline of the inside of the uterus and tubes to be seen on the X-ray. Both the Rubin test and hysterosalpingogram (HSG) involve some discomfort, and both are subject to about a 25% error. An apparently blocked tube, for example, may only be in spasm.

The Rubin test is not used widely today because the test results are often unclear or misleading. For example, a woman with damaged Fallopian tubes may have an apparently normal Rubin test (indicated by shoulder pain) unless her tubes are completely blocked. The HSG is a much more complete test, however, which identifies certain uterine abnormalities, pinpoints the location of tubal blockage, and provides a permanent record.

Laparoscopy, the third method of tubal evaluation, is the most definitive method. In an infertility evaluation, laparoscopy should be one of the last procedures since it is also the costliest and most hazardous. Laparoscopy, usually done on an outpatient basis under general anesthesia, involves inserting a long, thin, telescopelike instrument into the abdominal cavity through a small incision in the navel. This allows direct visualization of the pelvic organs. During this procedure, an assistant injects dye through the cervix while the clinician observes the dye as it comes out the tubes into the abdominal cavity. The location of any tubal blockage can be determined, and sometimes adhesions around the tubes can be cut apart by the clinician as a part of this procedure. Approximately 40% of women with infertility will have some unsuspected ab-

Figure 16   *Diagram of an X-ray of uterus and tubes (hysterosalpingogram).*

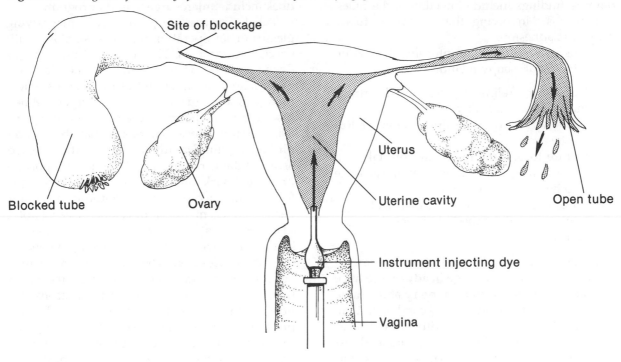

Table 24   QUESTIONS COMMONLY ASKED BY THE DOCTOR DURING THE INFERTILITY HISTORY

Question	Significance	Treatment
Are your periods regular?	infrequent periods often associated with faulty ovulation	fertility drug (e.g., Clomid) to stimulate ovulation
Do you have painful intercourse?	may be associated with certain causes of infertility affecting the tubes—infection, adhesions, or endometriosis	laparoscopy; possible tubal microsurgery
Do you have an irritating vaginal discharge?	may be associated with cervical infection	antibiotics or vaginal creams
Do you have very painful periods?	may be associated with cervical stenosis from previous surgery involving the cervix (cone biopsy) or with endometriosis	D & C (for cervical stenosis); laparoscopy (to evaluate for endometriosis)
How often do you have intercourse?	too frequently—decreases sperm count; too infrequently—decreases sperm activity	ideally, have intercourse every other day during midportion of the cycle
Have you had previous abdominal surgery?	may have caused adhesions	laparoscopy; release of adhesions if present
Have you had several miscarriages?	may be due to a uterine abnormality	diagnosis by hysterosalpingogram; may require uterine surgery
Have you noticed dry skin, sudden weight gain, and intolerance to cold?	may be due to low thyroid	thyroid pills

normality at the time of laparoscopy. The most common findings include infection of the tubes, endometriosis involving the ovaries or tubes, and pelvic adhesions.

The usual reasons in an infertility evaluation for having laparoscopy include:

1. Failure of preliminary tests to determine the cause of infertility.
2. An abnormal hysterosalpingogram or Rubin test.
3. Failure to become pregnant after taking a fertility drug for six months in the absence of other identifiable causes.
4. To determine whether a tubal ligation (a tying off of the tubes) that was done can be reversed.

If blocked tubes are discovered at the time of laparoscopy, you can arrange in advance to have your surgeon perform tubal surgery at the same time to prevent the need for a second operation. Because the extent of disease with blocked tubes varies widely, many physicians recommend discussing the findings of the laparoscopy first and planning definite tubal surgery later. Another reason to wait is that following any of the diagnostic procedures—Rubin test, hysterosalpingogram, or laparoscopy—your chances of pregnancy increase slightly. This may be due to the procedure itself, which can open up small adhesions inside the tubes.

Treatment: Tubal infections are treated with antibiotics. As noted, minor adhesions can be cut apart at the time of laparoscopy without making a regular abdominal incision. (Tubal adhesions occur when tissue surfaces stick together during the healing process after surgery, from infections involving the internal pelvic organs, or from diseases such as endometriosis.) More serious adhesions, either surrounding or within the tube, require special surgery; using techniques like microsurgery and laser surgery, up to 50% of women with blocked tubes may be helped by an experienced reproductive surgeon.

Today, many OB-GYNs take courses to acquire skills in microsurgery and laser therapy. Individual expertise varies greatly. Only recently have these areas become a standard part of most OB-GYN residency training programs. If you need tubal surgery, it may be an advantage to have it done at a hospital affiliated with an infertility center or with a medical school that does include microsurgery in its program.

Tubal microsurgery requires magnifying glasses or an operating microscope, along with special instruments. The success of this surgery depends partly on the location of the blockage. Obstructions at either end of the tube have less than a 50% pregnancy rate after surgery. When blockage is at the uterine end of the tube, the least common location, repair may be accomplished by implantation. That is, the blocked area of tube is removed and the healthy portion implanted back into the uterus. A new technique for treating such blockages—without major surgery—has recently been developed (see Chapter 41). Blockage at the far end of the tube may result from venereal infection, causing the end of the tube to close off. The scar tissue must then be cut away and a new opening created. A higher success rate is achieved with reconstruction of the midportion of the tube. In this procedure, known as *anastomosis*, the blocked segment of the tube is cut out and the cut ends are sewn together. This procedure is most often done to reverse previous elective tubal sterilization. In this instance, the best results are obtained when the sterilizing technique involved a nonburning surgical procedure to mechanically block the tube, using a "clip" or "band." (See Chapter 43.)

The laser (see Chapters 37 and 41) represents another, newer development in the field of tubal surgery. The laser cuts tissue very precisely and can be used alone or in combination with microsurgery. When used alone, the laser can be hand-held if the tubal surgery is performed through a regular abdominal incision, or it can be attached to a laparoscope (see page 78). In appropriately selected patients, *laser laparoscopy* avoids the need for a long abdominal incision and is used to remove adhesions around the tube or to open the ends of blocked tubes (an operation known as *fimbrioplasty*). These techniques are currently gaining wide popularity. However, laser surgery, including laser laparoscopy, has definite risks, such as injury to the bowel or other organs if the laser beam is accidently misdirected.

For some women with tubal diseases, who do not choose to have or cannot be helped by tubal surgery, another option is in vitro fertilization or related technologies (see page 83).

Ovarian factors

Absent or infrequent ovulation accounts for 15% to 20% of infertility problems. Women who menstruate every two to four months ovulate infrequently. Among the causes of infrequent periods and ovulation are polycystic ovaries (see Chapter 78), serious illness, and emotional stress. Thyroid problems, especially hypothyroidism (see glossary), occasionally cause infrequent ovulation.

Common tests to evaluate the ovaries: The basal body temperature (BBT) chart is the simplest test to determine if you are ovulating, although drugstore ovulation test-kits that are now available may be more convenient. The sex hormone produced in the second half of the menstrual cycle causes a slight (half a degree) but abrupt rise in temperature twenty-four hours after ovulation. This rise can be documented on a chart by taking your temperature every morning. (The correct method for this procedure is described in Chapter 6, Natural Family Planning.) If the results of the BBT test are unclear, the clinician may determine if ovulation has occurred by performing an endometrial biopsy or by obtaining a blood hormone (progesterone) level approximately ten days after ovulation. The biopsy, an office procedure, involves removal of a tiny amount of uterine tissue by means of a small instrument inserted into the uterine cavity. The appearance of the tissue under microscope indicates whether ovulation has occurred.

Additional tests measuring the level of various hormones are rarely necessary and add considerable cost to the infertility evaluation. However, women who have never had a period (see Chapter 78) or who have experienced other hormonal problems such as hair growth (see Chapter 66) or breast discharge (see Chapter 57) may need to have further diagnostic testing.

Treatment: Fertility drugs effectively induce ovulation within three months in more than 90% of women with infrequent or absent ovulation. Clomiphene (Clomid, Serophene), the principal fertility drug, acts on the brain, causing release of the hormones which stimulate ovulation. Clomiphene is indicated only in women who do not ovulate or ovulate infrequently. For the woman who produces an egg each month, fertility pills are of no value. Further, pregnancy rates average only about 40% with clomiphene, since not all women who ovulate as a result of taking this drug conceive. Eight percent of women who conceive while taking clomiphene experience multiple births; this rate is ten times more often than multiple births in the general population.

Clomiphene is usually taken for five consecutive days starting from the fifth day of your menstrual period. To increase chances of conception, you should have intercourse every other night starting five days after you take the last pill. More frequent intercourse may actually decrease the sperm count slightly. Women who do not have regular periods may need to have a period induced each month with a drug containing progesterone, such as Provera, before starting clomiphene. Clinicians evaluate clomiphene therapy by using the BBT chart to detect the presence of ovulation. If your temperature does not rise, ovulation has not occurred and subsequently the dose of clomiphene may need to be increased.

Contraindications to the use of clomiphene may include the presence of ovarian cysts, liver disease, or abnormal vaginal bleeding. Clomiphene is not known to cause congenital abnormalities, but, like any other drug, its use is best avoided in pregnancy. Relatively common side effects of clomiphene include hot flashes, nausea, headaches, and breast tenderness. Blurred vision is an uncommon side effect and indicates that clomiphene should be discontinued. Approximately 14% of women taking clomiphene develop ovarian cysts. For this reason, you need a pelvic exam at least every two months when you are taking this drug, to check for ovarian enlargement. Such cysts shrink on their own after the drug is discontinued.

If ovulation does not occur after adjustments in clomiphene dosage, the clinician may prescribe other fertility drugs including human chorionic gonadotropin (HCG) and Pergonal. Compared to clomiphene, Pergonal has more serious side effects, is more costly (presently $400 per menstrual cycle), and requires constant monitoring by a fertility expert.

Other, newer drugs used in the stimulation of ovulation include bromocriptine (Parlodel) and the still-experimental gonadotropin-releasing hormone (GnRH). Bromocriptine is a specialized drug used to treat some disorders of the pituitary gland that cause breast discharge (galactorrhea) in addition to lack of ovulation.

Fertility drugs such as clomiphene (Clomid) have been used widely in the past because of their apparent safety and effectiveness. However, in 1993 the Collaborative Ovarian Cancer Group reported three studies that suggested a possible link between fertility drugs and ovarian cancer. While this connection is by no means proven, the National Cancer Institute is currently studying the issue and groups like the American Society for Reproductive Medicine currently recommend treatment with clomiphene be limited to no more than six months.

Uterine factors

Approximately 20% of infertility results from a problem within the uterus, often involving the cervix. For a few days before ovulation, the cervical glands secrete a watery mucus that supports sperm migration from the vagina into the uterus. Most of the time no one knows what causes impairment of the quantity and quality of cervical mucus. Cervical stenosis, a narrowing of the cervical canal, may block the passage of sperm into the uterus or diminish mucus quantity. The scarring associated with this condition can result from overzealous cautery (see glossary) of the cervix or from previous dilation and curettage (D & C) or cone biopsy (see Chapter 37). DES syndrome (see Chapter 38) causes various abnormalities in the shape of the uterine cavity and of the cervix, which may result in infertility. One of the least frequent uterine factors responsible for infertility is the presence of sperm antibodies in the cervical mucus. Such antibodies prevent conception by destroying sperm just as other types of antibodies in the body destroy bacteria.

Common tests to evaluate the uterus: The postcoital, or *Sims-Huhner*, test involves microscopic examination of sperm and cervical mucus a few hours after intercourse. The clinician performs this painless test near the time of ovulation when the mucus is most copious. A normal test, showing copious clear mucus within the cervix and active sperm, would indicate that a tubal or an ovarian factor more likely accounts for the infertility.

Hysteroscopy, a new and increasingly used office procedure, allows visualization of the cervical canal and inside of the uterus. Hysteroscopy requires the use of a thin, telescopelike instrument similar to the laparoscope. The clinician can utilize the hysteroscope to visualize and often release adhesions and remove cervical polyps and other growths inside the uterus. The tubes, ovaries, and outer side of the uterus cannot be seen. The HSG, described above, also allows evaluation of the inside of the uterus.

Treatment: Antibiotics, vaginal creams, and occasionally cryosurgery (see glossary) are used to treat cervical infections that may contribute to abnormal cervical mucus. Women with inadequate cervical mucus production sometimes respond well to treatment with low doses of estrogen. Those with stenosis of the cervix may need a D & C to widen the canal or artificial insemination to bypass the narrowed cervix. Recently, a new procedure called *intrauterine insemination* (IUI) has been gaining steady popularity as a means of helping couples with cervix-factor infertility (see page 85).

Male factors

Approximately 40% of infertility problems are due to male factors, initially evaluated by sperm count or semen analysis. Normal counts range from 20 million to over 100 million sperm per cubic centimeter. Counts below 20 million are often associated with some degree of infertility. Azospermia, a very uncommon finding, refers to complete absence of sperm. A small and often temporary decrease in the sperm count may be due to a variety of factors such as fatigue, poor diet, excessive alcohol or other drug abuse, smoking, occupational exposure to chemicals, or prostate gland infection. A common and surgically correctable form of male infertility is due to varicose veins in the scrotum (varicocele). This condition raises the temperature near the sperm, thus impairing their development.

The common test to evaluate male infertility is called a *semen analysis*. In addition to measuring volume and acidity of the ejaculate, the semen analysis test involves microscopic evaluation of sperm activity, appearance, and number. For the semen analysis test, the man should abstain from sexual activity for three days before producing a sperm sample, and the sample should be collected by masturbation into a clean, dry container. To get the most accurate evaluation, he should bring the sample to the lab at once since sperm activity decreases with time.

Treatment: An abnormal semen analysis requires referral to a urologist or another infertility specialist. Men with low sperm counts occasionally respond to Clomid or other hormonal therapy. Artificial insemination represents an alternative to raising the sperm count by medical means. This may be conducted with sperm from the husband or from a donor. In either case, the technique involves introduction of semen into the upper vagina or cervix. To enhance the chances for pregnancy, several inseminations are performed during a single cycle near the time of ovulation as calculated by use of the BBT chart (see above under the paragraphs on *Ovarian factors*).

A newer and sometimes more successful method of artificial insemination is called *intrauterine insemination* (IUI—see page 85). With IUI, the physician, using a small tube (catheter), places the semen sample directly into the uterus and bypasses the cervix. Other, more involved, treatments like IVF and the GIFT procedure may ultimately be necessary to help some couples with male-factor infertility. A very recent breakthrough in the field of male infertility is microinsemination, a technique in which the sperm is directly injected into the egg cytoplasm. This new procedure, called direct intracytoplasmic sperm injection (ICSI), potentially enables a male who produces any sperm to father a child. This expensive technique requires in vitro fertilization and is too new to have produced any data on the risk of birth defects or other complications.

Results of artificial insemination using the husband's sperm (AIH) have been disappointing. The low pregnancy rate of 25% reflects the fact that the usual indication for AIH is low sperm count. When performed for reasons such as impotence, the success rate of AIH increases.

Artificial insemination from a donor (AID) may be indicated if the husband is sterile, is impotent, has a very low sperm count, or carries a genetic disease likely to be transmitted to the child. Donors are carefully selected by the physician, who searches the donor's background to rule out hereditary diseases, chronic conditions, or current infection. Pregnancy rates with AID run between 50% and 80%.

The legal status of AID is complicated. Most states do not have laws establishing legitimacy of children conceived by artificial insemination from donors.

The psychological implications of AID are enormous. Some couples or religious groups find AID immoral. Many couples experience guilt feelings resulting from the secrecy that often surrounds the procedure, owing to the anonymity of the donor. Men may feel left out when their wives conceive by AID, and women may feel there is something improper about being fertilized by another man's sperm. The long-term psychological effects of AID upon husband, wife, child, and donor remain unclear. Certainly artificial insemination, particularly by a donor, aggravates the emotional stress normally associated with infertility.

Information concerning physicians who perform artificial insemination may be obtained by contacting: The American Fertility Society, 2140 Eleventh Avenue South, Suite 200, Birmingham, Alabama 35205.

The New Technologies

The work of British researchers Patrick Steptoe and Robert Edwards culminated in 1978 with the birth of the first baby conceived by fertilization outside the body, a process known as *in vitro fertilization* (IVF). IVF was just the first of several new "assisted reproductive technologies" that have since offered a wide range of options to infertile couples and have permitted nearly 5,000 "miracle births" worldwide. Prior to IVF, those infertile couples who could not be helped by traditional means could only look to adoption or artificial insemination. During the 1980s and 1990s the new infertility technologies, led by IVF, developed rapidly, and infertility specialists, spurred on by both medical and monetary reasons, soon set up more than 300 IVF centers throughout the United States. But there have also been problems: high costs, long waiting lists, unresolved ethical and legal questions, and more importantly, only a one-in-three chance—or less—of bringing home a baby.

In Vitro Fertilization (IVF)

IVF involves removing an egg (ovum) from the mother's ovary and then fertilizing the egg in a laboratory dish using the father's sperm. The resulting embryo is then transferred to the mother's uterus, where it develops as a normal pregnancy. The term *in vitro*—Latin for "in glass"—refers to the glass dish or test tube where the egg is fertilized. IVF was first designed to help women with infertility due to blocked Fallopian tubes. Today, IVF is used to aid couples with various other infertility problems, including endometriosis, male infertility, and unexplained infertility. (Unexplained infertility is sometimes defined as infertility lasting at least two years with all the usual infertility tests showing no abnormalities.) Some IVF candidates have a combination of infertility factors—for example, a low sperm count and damaged Fallopian tubes. Overall, a couple's chances of a clinical pregnancy during one IVF cycle is about 15% to 20%. The rate goes up to 60% to 70% after six cycles. (*Clinical pregnancies* are those in which some physical evidence of pregnancy, such as fetal heart tones, is present, as distinguished from *chemical pregnancies*, which are very early and are detected only by a blood test that measures the presence of the pregnancy hormone, human chorionic gonadotropin. Since some of these early pregnancies miscarry before a pregnancy becomes clinically evident, only true clinical pregnancies are included in the statistics.) In the United States, data are collected annually by the American Fertility Society in cooperation with the Society for Assisted Reproductive Technology (SART) on the approximately 250 participating IVF programs nationwide. In 1992, these programs reported to the SART Registry that among 29,404 IVF cycles a total of 5,279 or about 18% resulted in clinical pregnancies. The chance of having a baby is a little less, however, due to miscarriages. For couples who don't succeed in their first cycle, additional cycles may be necessary. After three or four unsuccessful cycles, the pregnancy rate falls off rapidly.

A single cycle of IVF consists of four basic steps, which are carried out by a team including an OB-GYN, nurse specialists, lab technicians, and (usually) a reproductive endocrinologist. Most centers are hospital-based to allow access to specialized laboratory services as well as an operating room and ultrasound equipment. The four steps are:

1. Follicle stimulation

    During the first week of an IVF cycle, potent drugs such as clomiphene (Clomid, Serophene) and HMG (Pergonal) are given to stimulate the growth of follicles within the ovary. Each follicle is a tiny fluid-filled structure containing an egg. Unlike a spontaneous, natural cycle, in which usually only one egg will be released, an IVF cycle enables many egg-containing follicles to develop. While this enhances the pregnancy rate of a given IVF cycle, its drawback is that multiple pregnancies occur relatively often. The chance of twins or higher-order births is 15% to 20% among IVF births, compared to 1% to 2% in fertile women.

    Follicle growth is monitored by hormone tests and ultrasound (sonography), which track the number and size of the follicles to determine when they are "ripe." With these methods, eggs ready for ovulation can be predicted quite accurately to within 24 hours.

2. Egg recovery

    Egg recovery is accomplished by ultrasound, which produces an image of the follicles on a viewing screen. Then the physician passes a needle through the vagina to collect the eggs from the follicles. Nearly 90% of the time one egg and often two or more may be recovered.

3. Fertilization

    The egg (or eggs) are placed in a special culture dish and fertilized with approximately 100,000 sperm per egg. Additional steps may be taken to separate out the most active, healthy sperm for fertilization, especially if male-factor infertility is present. This step usually results in successful fertilization of one or more eggs following an approximate forty-eight-hour incubation period.

    An important ethical question for couples using IVF arises at this point: what should be done with any "extra" embryos if more than one egg is fertilized? Some programs transfer all the embryos into the woman's uterus. Other centers transfer a maximum of four to avoid increasing chances for twins or higher-order pregnancies and freeze the other embryos for later use. But what happens if the couple conceive and do not want additional children later? Suppose they divorce or die? Embryo donation to other infertile couples is, of course, a possibility, but medical and legal questions make this option controversial. Another sensitive issue concerns the possible use of these early embryos for research. Currently, a number of other countries permit fetal research on such "pre-embryos" for up to fourteen days of life. In the United States, federally funded fetal research was banned in the 1980s. This ban was lifted by Congress in 1993 and in 1994 a directive by President Clinton opened the way for potential but limited research on "spare" human embryos left over from IVF attempts. Several national organizations, including the American Society for Reproductive Medicine and the American College of Obstetricians and Gynecologists, have recently issued ethical guidelines concerning the many complex and difficult social issues surrounding IVF techniques.

4. Embryo transfer

In this step, the fertilized egg, which has begun the process of cell division in the laboratory, is transferred to the woman's uterus using a small catheter. The transfer of the tiny embryo, which usually consists of about 4-8 cells at this stage, is the rate-limiting step in IVF. Only 10% of embryos successfully attach to the wall of the uterus and go on to develop as a normal pregnancy. Since the chance of a pregnancy is related to the number of embryos transferred, when multiple eggs are retrieved and fertilized successfully, pregnancy rates go up. Following embryo transfer, the rest of the pregnancy occurs as it normally would.

The main risk of IVF relates to the increased rate of multiple births, which are often accompanied by prematurity, high blood pressure, and other problems. Twins often require cesarean birth, and higher-order pregnancies nearly always do. The rate of miscarriage among IVF couples is slightly higher due to the earlier, more frequent, diagnosis of pregnancy. Birth defects in babies born by IVF are not greater compared to the rate in the fertile population.

Intrauterine Insemination (IUI)

IUI is the least-known, simplest, and least expensive of the new infertility technologies, costing less than one-third of IVF. This technique is performed much like artificial insemination except that the physician, using a tiny catheter, places the semen inside the uterus instead of within the upper vagina or cervix. There may be two other differences from artificial insemination: the use of hormones to stimulate follicle growth, as in IVF, and the use of special methods to prepare the sperm to facilitate fertilization. IUI is performed as close as possible to the time of ovulation as judged by the BBT method, ultrasound, or home test kits. IUI may be particularly useful for some couples with cervix-factor infertility, male-factor infertility or unexplained infertility and should be considered before turning to more costly options like IVF or GIFT. In a recent study, 85 couples who underwent a total of 148 cycles of IUI achieved a 27% pregnancy rate per couple—comparable to IVF. Like IVF, the rate of twins and higher-order pregnancies is increased with the use of potent hormones that stimulate more than one follicle to develop. IUI does not require anesthesia or surgery and can be done in a doctor's office if lab facilities for special sperm preparation are present.

The GIFT procedure (Gamete Intra-Fallopian Transfer)

This procedure with its catchy acronym represents the main alternative to IVF. First reported in 1984, the GIFT procedure involves a variation of IVF that allows fertilization to occur in a woman's Fallopian tube rather than in the lab. Here's how it works: the surgeon first removes one or more eggs stimulated by ovulation-inducing drugs from the woman's ovary, usually by laparoscopy. Then the eggs are visualized with a microscope, and the most mature eggs (usually 2-4) are tranferred to a tiny catheter along with a sperm sample (sperm and eggs are separated by an air bubble). The surgeon then introduces the catheter, again by laparoscopy, into the open end of one or both of the woman's Fallopian tubes and injects the sperm and eggs. This way, fertilization occurs where it naturally would in a normal cycle. To

Table 25   HOW A DOCTOR EVALUATES INFERTILITY

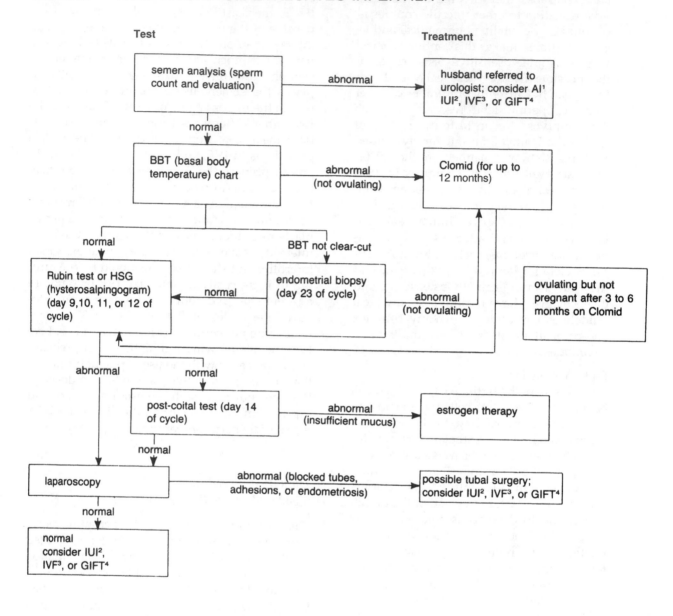

1. Artificial insemination
2. Intrauterine insemination
3. In vitro fertilization
4. Gamete Intra-Fallopian Transfer

qualify for the GIFT procedure, the couple must meet the same criteria as for IVF, and in addition, the woman must have at least one healthy Fallopian tube. If both tubes are healthy, the GIFT procedure is usually performed on both tubes. The procedure takes approximately one hour and can be performed on an outpatient basis. Another technique, known as ZIFT (the Z stands for *zygote*), calls for transfer of the just-fertilized egg, or zygote, into the Fallopian tube. A simpler variation of GIFT and ZIFT calls for transfer of sperm and eggs by ultrasound guided catheters placed through the uterus into the Fallopian tubes. Like IVF, the GIFT procedure may be appropriate when traditional infertility therapy doesn't work and is especially suitable in cases of endometriosis, male-factor infertility (with sperm counts as low as 5 million), or unexplained infertility.

According to the IVF Registry, the number of patients having the GIFT procedure increased nearly tenfold—from 47 to 419—between 1985 and 1986. By 1992, nearly 6,000 GIFT cycles per year were being reported. In that year the overall clinical pregnancy rate for GIFT was 28% while the rate for IVF was 18%. Even higher rates—up to 42%—have been reported, especially among couples with unexplained infertility. However, GIFT's apparent superiority over IVF remains unexplained at this time, and the procedure's main risk—higher rates of multiple pregnancies—is similar to that reported for IVF. Advocates of GIFT correctly point out that the procedure is somewhat less expensive than IVF and requires less extensive laboratory facilities (since fertilization occurs in the body rather than in a lab). In fact, the relative ease with which the GIFT procedure could be performed by most OB-GYNs in an office and with minimal lab facilities makes quality control for this procedure a potential problem. For this reason, the American Fertility Society has established minimal standards for the GIFT procedure as it has for IVF: the couple should first have completed basic infertility tests to qualify, and the facility must have equipment and personnel that meet AFS minimal standards for IVF programs.

Donor sperm or eggs

A woman may require donor sperm or eggs because of infertility, due to genetic factors or for other reasons. Sperm donation or artificial insemination from a donor other than her husband or partner is a well-established procedure. Donor sperm may be used if the husband is sterile, has a very low sperm count, or carries a genetic disease. And the procedure may be performed in association with IUI, IVF, or GIFT. Guidelines by the Centers for Disease Control now call for freezing of donor sperm for a minimum of six months so that the donor may be screened for AIDS and retested six months later. Although most sperm are unaffected, it is known that a small percentage of stored frozen sperm will lose their activity as a result of cold shock. How long sperm can survive freezing remains unclear, although some pregnancies have occurred

after several years of sperm storage. No one knows how the freezing of semen affects the rate of mutations or other abnormalities, since relatively few babies have been conceived through the use of stored sperm. Fertility experts report somewhat lower conception rates with stored semen (compared to fresh semen). For more information on sperm banks, write to the American Fertility Society (see Appendix D).

Egg donation, combined with IVF or GIFT, allows a woman with an intact uterus to have her own pregnancy using her husband's sperm to fertilize the donor eggs. Egg donation may be necessary if the woman's ovaries are inactive (e.g., due to premature menopause), inaccessible due to disease such as endometriosis, or absent due to surgery. Inherited disease may be another reason for using an egg donor in connection with IVF or the GIFT procedure.

IVF technology has made donor eggs more available than ever before. With improved cryopreservation (freezing) methods, egg banks may become more of an option in the future. However, concern about AIDS will mean freezing and storage for six months as is done for sperm banks.

To avoid using frozen eggs, another option is to obtain donor eggs at the same time as IVF or GIFT is done. For example, donor eggs may be supplied by relatives or friends who are willing to go through the egg-retrieval process. In these instances, the hormonal cycle of the donor must be coordinated with that of the recipient. This carefully timed "egg harvesting" is accomplished by giving the donor hormones for a few days to stimulate follicle growth before the egg is retrieved. And, of course, the donor is screened for medical and genetic conditions.

Until recently, ovum donation has not been widely performed. As of 1990, however, 37% of clinics reporting to the IVF Registry were using donor eggs in some cycles. Among a total of 498 patients receiving donor eggs, 160, or 29%, had clinical pregnancies. These resulted in a total of 122 live births including 36 sets of twins and three sets of triplets.

In actual practice, the use of donor gametes in IVF and GIFT represents a relatively small percentage of cases. However, these cases often involve special ethical and legal considerations. Issues such as confidentiality and the method of selecting donors must be carefully worked out by each program. The American College of Obstetricians and Gynecologists as well as the American Fertility Society find gamete (sperm or egg) donation ethically acceptable provided the physician is properly trained and experienced in the techniques involved. These organizations also recommend a nonprofit system for sperm and egg banks to avoid the potential abuses of a commercial system.

Cryopreservation of eggs and embryos

Cryopreservation is a technique used to freeze eggs or early-stage embryos (fertilized in the lab, but not yet transferred) for use in later IVF cycles. Cryopreservation for IVF was first performed successfully in Australia in 1984. In the United States, the first IVF birth using a frozen embryo occurred in 1986, and relatively few of such cryopreservation births have been achieved subsequently. Worldwide, several hundred cryopreservation infants have been born, mainly in Australia, the United Kingdom, and Europe. The IVF Registry reported that in 1992 among 5,354 cycles using frozen embryos, a total of 820 pregnancies resulted for a clinical pregnancy rate of 15%. This rate is somewhat lower than for traditional IVF. Ethical concerns include questions about how long an embryo should be preserved and what steps to take if the parents die, or don't want the extra embryos. The question of what a cryopreserved embryo's legal rights are remains unresolved as well.

Egg freezing, while less controversial than embryo freezing, has not yet been used widely in IVF or GIFT procedures. Technically, egg freezing is similar to sperm banking, which has been available for a number of years, but is not as successful. Now, with IVF technology, a ready supply of extra eggs may become available. At least three children have been born from cryopreservation of eggs, in Australia, West Germany, and in the United States. The potential for genetic damage resulting from either egg or embryo freezing, as well as the possibility of sexually transmitted disease, including AIDS, remain concerns with these techniques.

Surrogate Mothers

Typically when people speak of surrogate mothers, they are referring to a woman who is artificially inseminated with the sperm of a man who is not her husband. This surrogate "biological mother"—selected, usually, because the man's wife is infertile—then gives up the child to the biological father and his wife to rear. The procedure, which only involves the technology of artificial insemination, is done in order to allow the man to have a child with a genetic link to him. But IVF allows another type of surrogacy—the surrogate "gestational mother." In this variation, the surrogate mother provides the uterus for the child but not the egg, which is supplied by the infertile woman herself. This option can be considered by women with medical conditions contraindicating pregnancy (for example, high blood pressure) or who have had a hysterectomy early in life but retained their ovaries. The process starts out just like IVF, using the sperm and egg of the infertile couple. The resulting embryo is then transferred into the surrogate's uterus. The surrogate mother by written agreement relinquishes any claim to rear the resulting child. The first reported U.S. birth by a surrogate gestational mother occurred in 1986. Since then seventy-five programs have evolved offering gestational surrogacy. Both types of surrogate motherhood raise a number of important legal and ethical concerns. The ethics committee of the American Fertility Society presently recognizes a limited role for this still-experimental alternative and has "serious ethical reservations about surrogacy . . . until appropriate data are available for assessment of the risks and virtues of this alternative."

Selecting an IVF program

According to a 1988 congressional report, a number of U.S. IVF centers had, at that time, never had a birth. In Canada, in a recent survey involving 3,500 women attempting IVF at twelve separate clinics, only 10% successfully conceived and took home a baby. Such statistics have caught the attention of government officials and consumers and produced mixed reviews of the IVF concept in the media.

As of 1995, there are more than 300 IVF centers in the United States, twice the number that were in operation a decade earlier. Despite an overall increase in the number of programs reporting to the SART Registry in 1992, success rates were only slightly increased compared to those of 1990 and 1991. The larger programs tend to be more successful. Many U.S. programs are modeled after the first U.S. clinic, the Jones Institute for Reproductive Medicine in Norfolk, Virginia. This center delivers approximately 100 babies per year. Another large, well-run program is IVF America, which opened in 1986 and has facilities in Long Island, Port Chester, New York, Boston, and Philadelphia. Such clinics are run as franchise operations using the expertise of one of the world's leading IVF centers in Melbourne, Australia. Smaller programs, however, have also done well. For example, Tampa's Humana Women's Hospital, a 200-bed private facility, reports a 20% live-birth rate among couples entering their program since 1986—certainly within the national norm. Regardless of size or locale, successful programs all seem to have three basic ingredients: the programs have a full-time director (usually a reproductive endocrinologist); IVF staff privileges are limited to M.D.s with special training in this procedure; and the programs follow specific protocols that follow previously established successful guidelines.

Couples considering IVF and related technologies have to be smart consumers. IVF programs use a variety of statistics to back up—and market—their program's successes. Pregnancy rates can be confusing because they can be quoted as per cycle of treatment, per laparoscopy, per patient, or per year. These rates may not take into account canceled cycles—cycles which in every program must be dropped—and egg retrieval not attempted because of failure to develop adequate follicles. Success rates vary from program to program and even at the same facility since there is normal cyclic variation, with higher pregnancy rates reported in some periods and lower rates in others. Also, the patient population is a critical determinant of success rates. Higher pregnancy rates are expected in centers treating less difficult infertility cases. The American Fertility Society lists recognized IVF programs and may serve as a valuable resource in locating one. In addition to calling the AFS, here are some questions to consider before selecting an IVF or GIFT program:

1. Have all the standard infertility treatments, including microsurgery, been considered?
2. Does the program try intrauterine insemination, if applicable, before going on to more expensive options like IVF and GIFT?
3. How many of the program's couples have actually had babies?
4. What are the total costs per cycle?
5. Which method of egg retrieval is used, laparoscopy or ultrasound? (The latter is less expensive and has been used increasingly by larger centers.)
6. Is a full-time reproductive endocrinologist present to oversee the program?
7. Is the IVF lab on site and adjacent to the operating suite (as opposed to an outside lab)?
8. Does the program provide references from patients who have used the facility previously?

Before selecting an IVF or GIFT program, emotional and financial costs must also be considered. Any infertility evaluation, but especially IVF, with its elaborate testing and the tension associated with high expectations, is likely to be stressful. There may be financial strains as most insurance companies may exclude IVF and GIFT in their coverage. Not having insurance can be a real burden; the cost is approximately $8,000 per cycle of IVF or GIFT. But couples who do have financial coverage and who accept the medical limitations of this new technology may find it offers a new hope, other than adoption, for having a child when traditional methods have been unsuccessful.

References for Section Three

Chapter 11—Identifying Birth Defects

American College of Obstetricians and Gynecologists *Technical Bulletin* 208. Genetic technologies, July 1995.

American College of Obstetricians and Gynecologists *Technical Bulletin* 108. Antenatal diagnosis of genetic disorders, Sep 1987.

Simpson, J. Genetics: the future is here. *Contemporary OB/GYN* 31(1):116–118, Jan 1988.

American College of Obstetricians and Gynecologists. *Guidelines for Perinatal Care*, 2d ed., Antenatal detection of genetic disorders, 235–242, 1988.

Orris, L. Fetal sex preselection: technology/prospects/issues. *OB/GYN Topics* 2(5): Sep/Oct 1987.

Research Reports from the National Institute for Child Health and Human Development, Results of first major CVS study announced. Sep 1989.

Lilford, R. Transabdominal chorionvillus biopsy, 100 consecutive cases. *Lancet* 1:1415–1416, 1987.

Kardon, N. Genetic abnormalities—their role in amenorrhea and infertility. *The Female Patient* 14(19):17–26, Sep 1989.

Feinn, D. Funicentesis: a review of sonographically-guided unbilical cord sampling. *The Female Patient* 14:10–86, June 1989.

Muggah, H. Difficulties encountered in a randomization trial of CVS vs. amniocentesis for prenatal diagnosis. *Clinical Genetics* 32:235–239, 1987.

Klein, V. Genetics for the obstetrician. *Williams Obstetrics* Supplement 17: Apr/May 1988.

Chapter 12—Pregnancy After Thirty-five

Daniels, P. *Sooner or Later: The Timing of Parenting in Adult Lives.* New York: W.W. Norton, 1988.

Redwine, F. Pregnancy in women over 35. *The Female Patient* 13:30–36, May 1988.

Winslow, W. First pregnancy after 35: what is the experience? *Maternal and child health nursing* 12:92–96, Mar/Apr 1987.

Kirz, D. Advanced maternal age: The mature gravida. *American Journal of Obstetrics and Gynecology* 152:7–12, 1985.

Hansen, J. Older maternal age and pregnancy outcome: a review of the literature. *Obstetrical and Gynecological Survey* 41:726–742, 1986.

Spellacy, W. Pregnancy after 40 years of age. *Obstetrics and Gynecology* 68:452–454, 1986.

Chapter 13—Infertility: Causes and Treatment

American Fertility Society. *Guideline for Practice,* Intrauterine insemination. 1991.

American Society for Reproductive Medicine. *Guideline for Practice,* Induction of ovulation with clomiphene citrate. 1991.

Gray, R. Infertility epidemiology: current scene. *Contemporary OB/GYN* 70–81, May 1994.

American Fertility Society. *Fertility and Sterility* 62(6):1121–1128. Assisted Reproductive Technology in the United States and Canada: 1992. Results Generated from the American Fertility Society/Society for Assisted Reproductive Technology Registry, Dec 1994.

The Ethics Committee of the American Fertility Society. *Ethical Considerations of Assisted Reproductive Technologies* 62(5):895–925, Nov 1994.

American College of Obstetricians and Gynecologists *Technical Bulletin* 142. Male infertility, June 1990.

American College of Obstetricians and Gynecologists *Technical Bulletin* 140. New reproductive technologies, Mar 1990.

American College of Obstetricians and Gynecologists *Technical Bulletin* 125. Infertility, Feb 1989.

American College of Obstetricians and Gynecologists, Committee on gynecologic practice, *Committee Opinion* 119. Zygote intrafallopian transfer, Feb 1993.

American College of Obstetricians and Gynecologists, Committee on ethics, *Committee Opinion* 47. Ethical issues in human in vitro fertilization and embryo placement, July 1956.

Shephard, B. New hope for infertile couples. *Encyclopaedia Britannica, Health Annual*: 455–458, 1988.

Hammond, M. Monitoring ovulation. *Contemporary OB/GYN* Special Issue: 59–68, Feb 1987.

ACOG Committee provides information on at-home ovulation predictor kits. *ACOG Newsletter.* Aug 1988.

Azziz, R. Reproductive loss: the role of congenital uterine anomalies. *The Female Patient* 12:20–34, Aug 1987.

Goldfarb, A. Ovulation induction: state of the art. *The Journal of Reproductive Medicine* 34(1):65–115, Jan 1989.

Ory, S. Keeping up to date on donor insemination. *Contemporary OB/GYN* 33(3):88–112, Mar 1989.

Marik, J. Oocyte donation. *The Female Patient* 14(4):39–46, Apr 1989.

Sarafini, P. Diagnosis of female infertility: the comprehensive approach. *The Journal of Reproductive Medicine* 34(1):29–40, Jan 1989.

American Fertility Society. Minimum standards for programs in in-vitro fertilization. *Fertility and Sterility* 41(1):13, Jan 1984.

Russell, J. Helping patients choose an IVF program. *Contemporary OB/GYN* Special Issue: Feb 1987.

Horvath, P. In-vitro fertilization: a review of the last decade. *The Female Patient* 13:93–107, May 1988.

Speroff, L. Exploring super ovulation for infertile patients. *Contemporary OB/GYN* 33(3):128–162, Mar 1989.

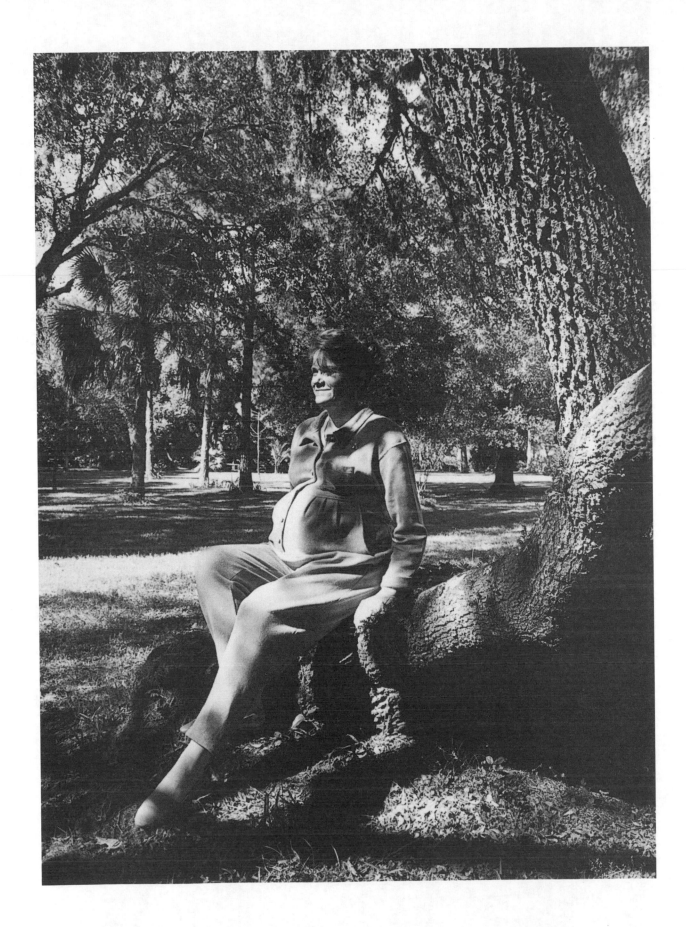

PREGNANCY AND CHILDBIRTH

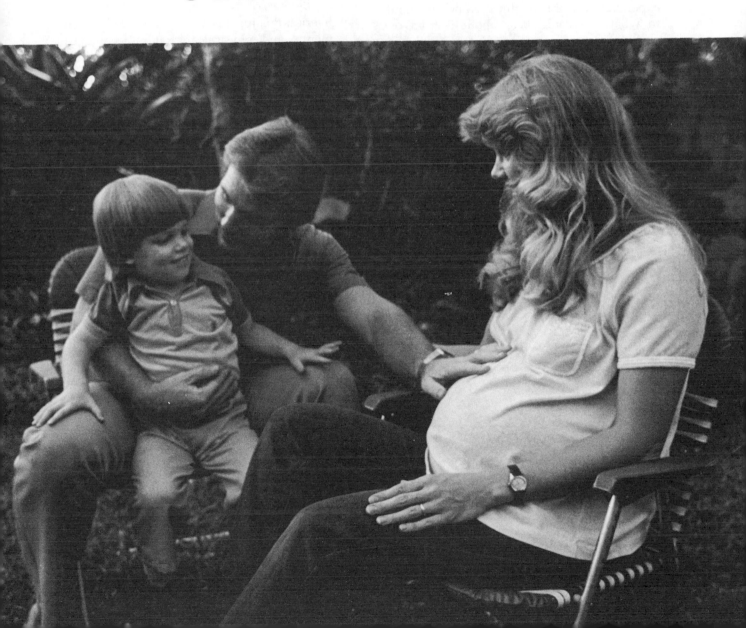

CHAPTER 14

Childbirth Education

During the late nineteenth century, attempts to reduce maternal and infant infections and to provide relief from pain brought childbirth from the home setting into the hospital. As the hospital began to take responsibility for the birthing experience, childbirth education became limited to what one could hear about it from one's mother or among peers. But because many women of this era were put to sleep under general anesthesia during childbirth, even they were not sure what happened. Pregnant women thus found themselves unprepared for childbirth and dependent on their physicians to "deliver" them. Before long, women grew dissatisfied with their passive role in childbearing.

Today's pregnant woman wants to be more fully informed and involved in decisions that affect her pregnancy and delivery. For this reason, you'll find classes for expectant parents in almost every community in the United States. Hospitals, community colleges, the American Red Cross, private organizations, and some physicians now provide courses to meet the increasing demand for childbirth preparation. Some goals of prepared childbirth are to minimize the discomfort of labor and delivery, to decrease potential risks to you and your newborn, and to help you and your family have the best experience possible for your unique situation.

Most childbirth preparation classes provide nutrition counseling and information about labor and delivery, as well as the opportunity for you to share experiences with other mothers-to-be. Because of the increased rate of cesarean deliveries, this topic is usually included. Teaching mental and physical relaxation techniques to deal with contraction discomfort is an important part of the classes. Childbirth education emphasizes minimal use of pain medication during labor and more active participation of the father or significant other. With such preparation, a mother is likely to be less anxious and fearful and she may feel greater satisfaction by actively participating in the birth process.

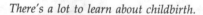

There's a lot to learn about childbirth.

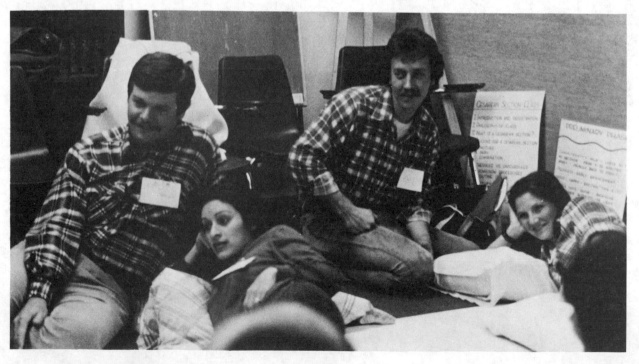

Choosing prepared childbirth, which requires an active decision on the parents' part, means that you elect to become more aware of what will happen to you so that you can make informed choices throughout your labor, delivery, and postpartum period. *Choosing* to be prepared for childbirth is more important, we feel, than the particular method you select. The types of prepared childbirth classes are discussed below. Ask your clinician or a nurse which methods are available in your community, or write for more information to the organizations that interest you; you'll find a list of addresses at the end of this chapter, in Table 26.

The Dick-Read Method

About 1914, Dr. Grantly Dick-Read, a British obstetrician, pioneered the concept of childbirth as a normal, natural process, as opposed to a medical condition. Women, he believed, had been unnecessarily conditioned to fear the pain of labor. Dr. Dick-Read believed that this fear produced muscle tension that led to much of the experienced "pain of childbirth." The Dick-Read method attempts to break the fear-tension-pain cycle by making the woman more knowledge-

able about childbirth and by teaching muscle relaxation exercises ("passive relaxation"). Some of the techniques used resemble yoga in that the mother learns to develop an attitude of passivity and acceptance toward childbirth. She becomes conditioned to focus inward, concentrating on herself and meeting each contraction as it comes. This method relies heavily upon close communication between the laboring woman and the hospital staff, who help to reduce childbirth fears by answering questions about what to expect each step of the way. An outgrowth of this work, sometimes called the *modified Read method*, has developed, teaching more specific techniques of relaxing and submitting to the body's demands during labor, such as breathing more rapidly and deeply as the strength of the contractions increase, to ensure adequate respiratory exchanges.

Many other childbirth preparation techniques have been developed from the Dick-Read method, the oldest type of childbirth preparation in the United States. Classes, which begin in the seventh month, last eight weeks. The father, or labor coach, also attends class to learn how to provide support during labor and delivery. Classes are loosely structured, with emphasis on meeting the unique needs of each group.

Discussing the three stages of labor.

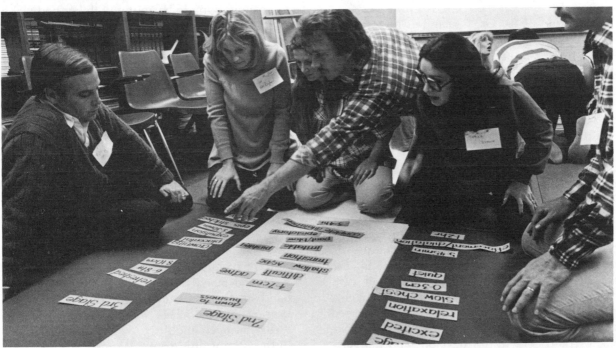

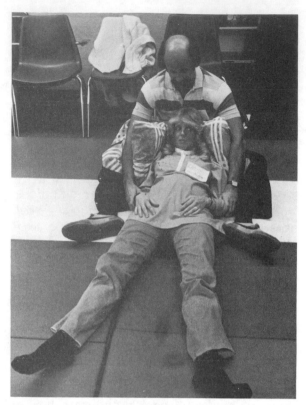

Practicing breathing techniques in preparation for labor and delivery.

Lamaze (Psychoprophylaxis)

In the early 1950s, Dr. Fernand Lamaze developed a method of childbirth preparation to minimize the pain and discomfort of labor and delivery. This method teaches specific breathing techniques for dealing with painful contractions. Proper exercise and a thorough knowledge of the labor and delivery process are also stressed. Essential to the Lamaze technique is the use of a coach (usually but not necessarily the father), who attends the classes and helps the mother-to-be practice her relaxation and breathing skills. The coach accompanies her during labor and delivery, to provide support, to time contractions, and to help her relax. Its highly structured approach teaches specific breathing techniques in response to contractions. The woman is also taught to focus all of her concentration on these breathing techniques and thus away from any pain. Discipline and commitment are required for the practice that will make this method useful for pain control during labor and delivery.

Lamaze is currently the most popular method of childbirth preparation in the United States. Classes are usually six weeks in length and begin about the seventh month of pregnancy. Elisabeth Bing, R.P.T., a prominent authority on the Lamaze method, has written *Six Practical Lessons for an Easier Childbirth*, which has become the standard text for many Lamaze classes.

Psychosexual Preparation

This approach was developed by Sheila Kitzinger, a British social anthropologist, as she taught childbirth education classes in the late 1950s. Although Kitzinger has not developed a specific method, her ideas have been incorporated in various childbirth education classes. Kitzinger is concerned with the social context of birth, how women communicate with their care givers, and especially with the psychological aspects of pregnancy. Birth is seen as a sexual experience. Sex in pregnancy and how sexual adjustment relates to acceptance of labor and delivery are seen as important. Pregnancy is seen as a developmental crisis in a woman's life, with renewed focus on common feminine concerns as well as the importance of the early mother-child relationship. The physical exercises are similar to those of Dick-Read, with the emphasis on the woman working in harmony with her body. She uses imagery, the recollection of past experiences, and tactile cues to aid in relaxation. The woman's ability to control the muscles of the perineum and birth canal are given special attention. Because Kitzinger views pregnancy as part of the whole psychosexual cycle, including the woman's relationship with her husband, parents, and children, marriage counseling and private sessions may be included as part of this method.

Bradley Husband-Coached Childbirth

In 1947, Dr. Robert A. Bradley developed the concept of husband-coached natural childbirth, a method heavily emphasizing the use of husband support and supervision during the childbearing process. This method also advocates "true natural childbirth," which means giving birth without any drugs. Women are prepared to experience the "intensity and pleasure" of birth by using deep relaxation and "tuning in" to the body's sensations during labor, rather than "distracting breathing techniques." The husband/coach is taught to observe his wife in sleep and note her natural sleep position and her deep breathing, as these will be used in labor. He is taught to praise, encourage, and assure his wife of her progress during labor. Breast-feeding immediately after birth and early, frequent contact between mother and baby are encouraged.

Bradley classes differ from others in that the first class, which covers nutrition and exercise, is held early in the third month. Eight more classes follow, beginning during the sixth or seventh month of pregnancy, followed by review classes every two weeks in the final months. Breathing exercises and pushing techniques differ from the other methods. Because Bradley stresses nonmedicated participation during childbirth, this method has become popular for some home births and birth centers.

Hypnosis

Interest in self-hypnosis to control pain and anxiety during pregnancy and childbirth is increasing. Hypnosis training for childbirth means reeducating women about childbirth pain, with the message that pain is not always the overriding experience of childbirth. Self-hypnosis techniques enable a woman to forget the pain associated with childbirth and to relax with contractions. One learns to experience the contractions as "pressure," rather than "pain." The woman is taught to relax and focus her concentration so that she can direct her mind somewhere else when experiencing a contraction, thereby increasing her feeling of control.

Successful hypnosis requires both motivation and practice. Obstetricians who use hypnosis prefer the father or support person to attend classes and to help the expectant mother practice at home. Classes usually take place over a twelve-week period and involve education about what to expect during labor and delivery. Hypnosis aims to produce total amnesia or to selectively dull the perception of pain. It also offers the advantage of posthypnotic suggestion— for example, in some individuals episiotomy

pain can be reduced at the suggestion of the hypnotist. There are no drug dangers or discomfort to being hypnotized; however, it requires considerable time and commitment from both the hypnotist and the patient.

Prenatal Yoga

Prenatal hatha yoga classes, a helpful way to psychologically approach pregnancy through exercise and breathing techniques, can be used during your entire pregnancy. The focus is to integrate pregnancy with the yogic way of life. Specific yoga positions that have been adapted for pregnancy are used to help the woman become calm and flexible. The practice of daily yoga exercises is seen as helpful in preparing for the actual labor, delivery, and postpartum periods. These classes focus on teaching relaxation techniques but they seldom include the physiology of labor and delivery and other practical aspects of childbirth. For this reason, if you use prenatal yoga, we recommend that you attend another form of prepared childbirth classes as well.

Early Parenting Classes

Some "prenatal" classes that are taught by private organizations last twelve months. After delivery, the classes cover the needs and activities of the infant during the first year of life as well as those of the parents. You'll be able to "practice" taking care of your baby because parents bring their babies to class where they can also observe normal variations in growth and development. These classes provide an opportunity to share ideas and support for those first difficult months of adjustment to parenthood. Infant massage classes have also been helpful in promoting bonding in early parent-child relationships.

Prenatal Classes for Repeat Parents

Pregnancy, birth, and parenting are not necessarily easier for experienced parents. Many repeat parents feel that they need more than a simple review of the labor-and-delivery

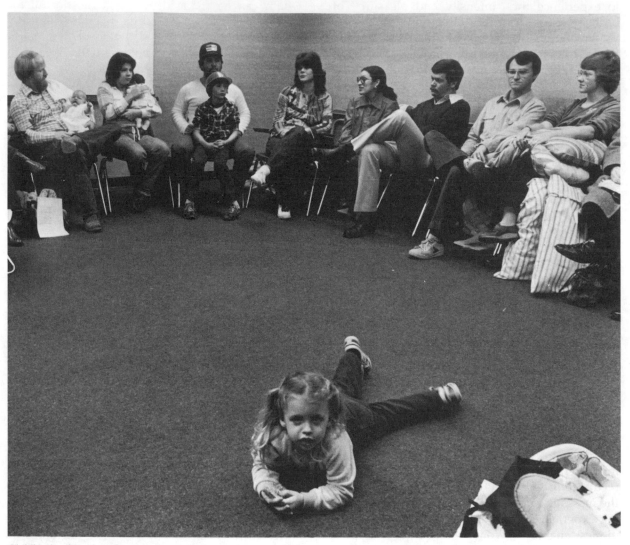

Childbirth education class.

breathing techniques. Some communities offer classes to meet the special needs of repeat parents. Subject matter usually includes preparation of siblings for the baby and new ideas on how to fit the proper rest and nutrition into a busy mother's schedule. Many women worry about differences in fetal movement between this pregnancy and their previous pregnancies. Some are concerned as to whether they can love another child as much as they loved their older child or children. Often mothers feel more uncomfortable or tired with a second or subsequent pregnancy than with the first pregnancy. Getting support from mothers in similar situations helps to make up for the usually less enthusiastic reactions of

friends and relatives to a second pregnancy. A repeat mother knows what it is like to be responsible for a child's care twenty-four hours a day and is realistically concerned about the demands of this additional child. She is in some ways more aware of the realistic stresses that she will face with a new child than is the mother who is pregnant for the first time.

If no such classes exist in your community, you might approach your local chapter of the International Childbirth Education Association or child-birth educator. Or organize your own group of second- and third-time mothers to share ideas about adjusting to the second or third baby.

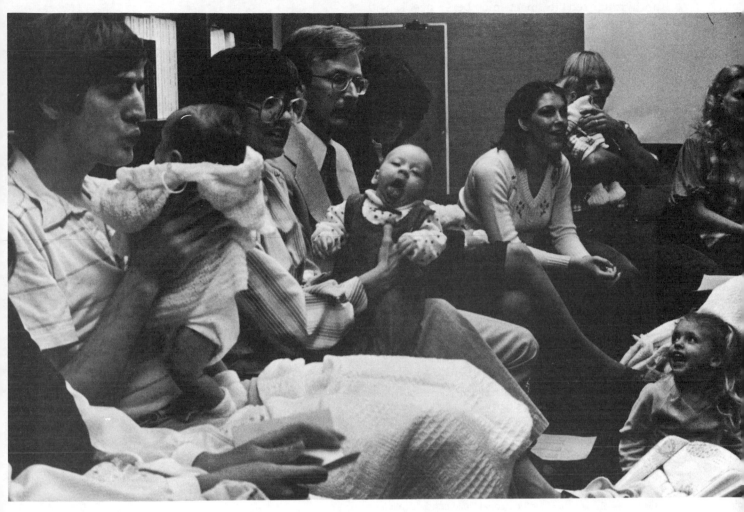

Parents share delivery experiences and show off their newborns at a prenatal class reunion.

Prenatal fitness classes

Increasingly, these classes are being offered by local health clubs and organizations. Exercise is healthful and usually recommended but may need to be tailored to meet your individual needs (see Chapter 16). You should, therefore, check with your clinician prior to attending any class.

Family preparation classes

Many hospitals offer sibling classes that vary according to the age of the sibling. Topics usually include care and appearance of the newborn, a practice period with dolls, and discussion about the feelings of the older sibling. Some programs

offer films about labor and delivery for children who will attend the birth (see Chapter 15). "Grandparent" classes are also offered in order to acquaint expectant grandparents with the new theories of child care and options during childbirth. These classes are helpful in facilitating optimal contributions of grandparents to the expanding family.

Childbirth Education for High-Risk Mothers

Increasingly, hospitals are forming groups for emotional support and education for those mothers who must remain hospitalized or on bed rest due to complications. These groups are individualized to meet members' needs and have been found to be quite helpful in dealing with all aspects of the upcoming birth. Ask your hospital for a list of classes available to help you with specific problems of high risk pregnancies.

Table 26 CHILDBIRTH EDUCATION ORGANIZATIONS

Type of Childbirth Education	Where You Can Get Information
Dick-Read	Read Natural Childbirth Foundation, Inc. P.O. Box 5442 Sherman Oaks, California 91413
Lamaze	ASPO/Lamaze 1200 19th Street, N.W., Suite 300 Washington, D.C. 20036-2401
Bradley Husband-Coached Childbirth	American Academy of Husband-Coached Childbirth P.O. Box 5224 Sherman Oaks, California 91413 800-4-ABIRTH
Hypnosis	To request information about a physician near you who practices hypnosis, write or call: The American Society of Clinical Hypnosis 2200 East Devon Avenue, Des Plaines, Illinois 60018-4534 (708) 297-3317
General Information	International Childbirth Education Association P.O. Box 20048 Minneapolis, Minnesota 55420 (612) 854-8660
	NAPSAC International The International Association of Parents & Professionals for Safe Alternatives in Childbirth Route 1, Box 646 Marble Hill, Missouri 63764-9725 (314) 238-2010

CHAPTER 15

Hospital Birth and Its Alternatives

More than in any other area of women's health, people have been urgently challenging the way care is provided during pregnancy, labor, and delivery. The feminist movement and consumer activism have much to do with new options that are now available for the pregnant mother and her family. Birthing alternatives vary greatly from community to community and often reflect the differing reference points from which physicians and pregnant women view pregnancy and childbirth. Physicians tend to think of potential *medical* risks to both mother and baby and how they can best anticipate and treat emergencies that might occur. The obstetrician clearly prefers to deliver the baby in the hospital, where equipment and personnel are available to meet any emergency. More and more women, on the other hand, view pregnancy as a natural biological process involving the whole family and needing minimal medical attention. They aren't sick—they're just pregnant! These women sometimes prefer to share the childbearing experience with their family in the warmer, more intimate surroundings of their home or a birth center. They reason that they can always go to a hospital should an emergency occur.

Because the birth rate has decreased and the number of home deliveries has increased in the last decade or so, hospitals now have an economic incentive to provide birthing alternatives in order to attract prospective parents to their institution. Many hospitals have therefore developed the concept of *family-centered maternity care*. The meaning of family-centered maternity care varies among hospitals, but it may include classes for expectant parents, a tour of the hospital before delivery, and birthing alternatives such as fathers being present in the delivery room, rooming-in, bonding periods, and sibling visitation (see Chapter 19).

A recent trend in birth-setting alternatives is the designation of regional centers for high-risk mothers. These facilities, often located at university medical centers, employ special staff round-the-clock to care for mothers with complicated pregnancies. If your pregnancy is identified as being high risk (see Chapter 20), you may be referred to one of these centers.

Physicians, nurses, and other people who are concerned about the availability of alternative birth settings have formed their own organizations to which you can write for further information:

NAPSAC International
The International Association of Parents & Professionals for Safe Alternatives in Childbirth
Route 1, Box 646
Marble Hill, Missouri 63764-9725

How Do I Choose Where to Have My Baby?

There is no *one* right way to have your baby. You won't be a better mother just by choosing a birthing center, for instance, over a traditional hospital setting. Some parents feel guilty about not selecting a new, trendy alternative. What may be most suitable for another couple may not be the best choice for you. It's a good idea to investigate the alternatives your community has to offer and to see what meets your personal goals. Here is a preview of the birth-setting alternatives you may find during your investigation.

Alternatives Within the Hospital

Traditional childbirth

Hospitals vary widely in their labor-and-delivery policies, but many hospitals do provide childbirth preparation classes. If you are having your baby in the hospital, insist on a tour of the labor and delivery area beforehand. This will help you feel more comfortable when you enter the hospital for childbirth. Under traditional hospital care, the laboring woman is admitted

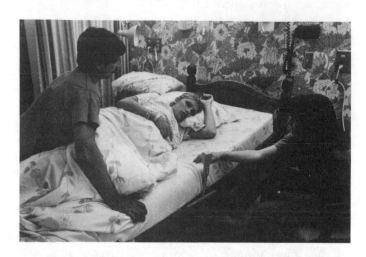

Labor and midwife-attended delivery in a birthing room.

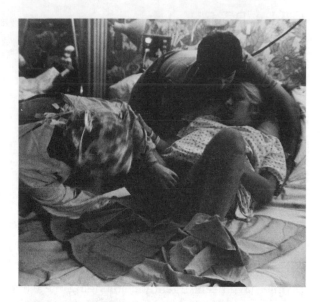

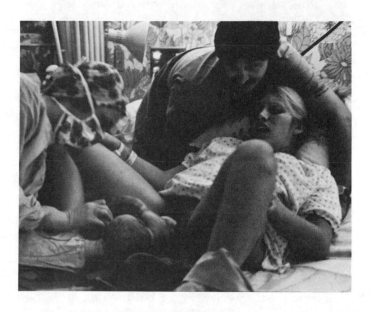

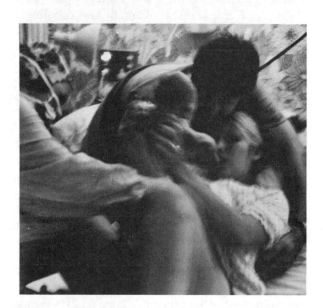

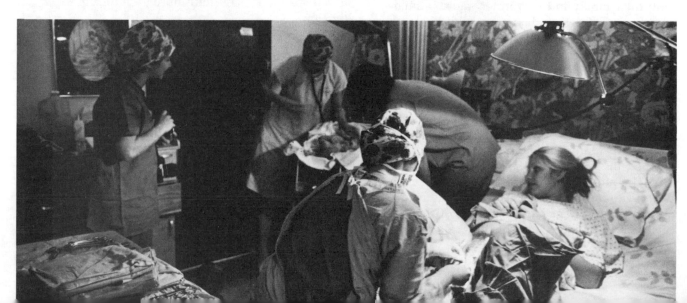

into a small, so-called labor room, either private or shared, and is usually permitted a limited number of visitors. The physician may order an enema, some form of perineal shave, and an IV (intravenous solution). Electronic monitoring of the unborn fetus and pain medication or anesthesia may be prescribed routinely unless you specifically request otherwise at the time of hospital admission.

When completely dilated, the woman is transferred by stretcher to the sterile delivery room; her support person might accompany her, if the hospital permits. Following delivery, she may stay in the delivery room or go to a recovery room for several hours. Here, nurses evaluate uterine bleeding and then transfer the stable patient to a hospital room. The baby may stay with the mother during this period or may be immediately taken to a newborn nursery. The mother may see her baby only at feeding time, or the baby may be with her constantly if rooming-in is available.

The average length of stay in the hospital is now twenty-four to forty-eight hours for a routine delivery. Early discharge planning has become routine and may include home visitation by a nurse. Most hospitals offer classes on breast-feeding and newborn care.

Birthing Rooms and LDRs

Birthing rooms and labor-and-delivery rooms (LDRs) offer alternatives to home births in providing a more intimate, personal experience within the hospital setting. A birthing room is cheerfully decorated and informal, with a couch, magazines, and often a television available to both the mother-to-be and her visitors. A labor bed easily transforms to a delivery bed as the mother stays in one room for both labor and delivery and remains there until discharged. LDRs are similar to birthing rooms in look and design. The difference is that after delivery in an LDR, the woman is usually transferred to a postpartum area or floor for the remainder of her stay.

Hospitals vary in their rules and procedures. Smaller facilities may be a bit more flexible. Some hospitals limit visitors while others let the parents decide who may be present during labor and delivery. Certain procedures such as enemas, episiotomies, and fetal monitoring, once considered routine, may be optional unless you want or need them. Occasionally, fathers are al-

lowed to participate in the actual delivery. Immediate breast-feeding and sibling participation are typical options in birthing room and LDR settings, as are the use of video cameras to record the event and cassette tapes to provide preselected background music.

In hospitals where very early discharge is possible, mother and baby may stay in the birthing room for six to eight hours after delivery and then leave for home if all has progressed normally. This markedly reduces hospital costs. However, many experts question the wisdom of sending patients home before they are ready—and for many women having a vaginal birth, this means staying in the hospital for up to forty-eight hours.

Increasingly, hospitals are utilizing certified nurse-midwives (CNMs). The percentage of CNM-attended hospital births in the United States grew from less than 1% in 1975 to 4.4% in 1992. These midwives are usually supervised by an OB/GYN who may or may not be "in-house" during midwife deliveries. Among the 185,000 CNM-attended births in the United States in 1992, 95% occurred in hospitals.

Alternatives Outside the Hospital

Birth centers

Of 4,065,000 total births in the United States in 1992, 43,000 were out-of-hospital births, according to the National Center for Health Statistics. Out-of-hospital births include deliveries at birth centers, home deliveries (usually attended by midwives), and unattended births. About 0.3% of all births in 1992—13,255—were reported as occurring in birth centers.

These centers provide for a labor-and-delivery experience in a low-cost, homelike setting. Use of birthing centers is an economic and personal alternative to private-physician care and hospitalization. A mother-to-be and her family usually stay in one room for labor, delivery, and the immediate recovery period under the supervision of a nurse-midwife. Bonding, gentle birth, breast-feeding, sibling participation, and early discharge are readily available. Should an emergency occur, these centers usually have arrangements for immediate transfer to a hospital or back-up service by a physician. Extensive parent education classes are usually part of the center's prenatal program.

Because requirements for licensure differ from state to state, birth centers vary greatly both in the quality of professional care and emergency provisions. If you select this option, make sure the birth center has an arrangement with a nearby hospital to accept patients from the center should an emergency arise that requires hospitalization during labor.

Home births

In 1950, only half of all births took place in hospitals; by 1975, that figure had climbed to 99% and has remained essentially unchanged since. In 1992, the National Center for Health Statistics reported that out of 4,065,000 total births in the United States, 26,000 (less than 1%) were home births. The issue of home birth appears to have become somewhat less visible in the past few years, with more emphasis being placed on the birth attendant than on the place of birth. The number of physician-attended out-of-hospital births is definitely declining, while those attended by midwives is increasing.

Although a good deal has been written about the outcome of home births, little statistical data has actually been collected. This lack of data arises partly from the fact that in some states the birth setting may not be recorded on the birth certificate. The American College of Obstetricians and Gynecologists compiled statistics on out-of-hospital births from twelve states that showed a two- to five-times-higher stillbirth or newborn death rate for births outside hospitals. Although there is no consensus among the various reports available as to the safety of home birth, the response of physicians to home birth generally has been negative. Many physicians view home birth as an irresponsible risk to mother and child and hence refuse to support or attend home delivery.

A number of couples continue to select home birth. A few studies indicate that such couples tend to be white, middle-class, and often college-educated. Women often choose to have their babies at home because the home is seen as the most natural place to have a baby, to celebrate the miracle of a new member of the family. Home birth is much less costly and gives the mother much greater control of her birth experience. For some women the experience of a previous hospital childbirth, including the subtle pressure to take drugs for pain relief, is their main reason for wanting a home birth. The parents' desire for early and unlimited contact with the newborn, photographing and recording the childbirth, and flexibility of delivery position are other reasons often given for the choice of home birth delivery, especially when these options are unavailable in a nearby hospital.

The types of home birth services that are available vary widely. The delivery may be done by a physician or by a certified or lay midwife with or without a back-up physician available. Home birth services usually include medical screening by a physician, nutrition counseling, preparation for childbirth, and a postpartum checkup. Enemas, IVs, and episiotomies are usually not performed at home. Some home birth services teach couples to recognize the signs of hemorrhage and to learn newborn resuscitation should it be needed. Self-birthing, where the parents actually do the delivery with supervision, is now part of some home birth classes. Comprehensive health insurance often pays for maternity hospitalization and prenatal care but may not pay for costs of a home delivery.

For information about midwives, write to:

American College of Nurse-Midwives
818 Connecticut Avenue, N.W., Suite 900
Washington, D.C. 20006

Midwives' Alliance of North America
P.O. Box 175
Newton, Kansas 67114

For information about birth centers, write to:

National Association of Childbearing Centers
3123 Gottschall Road
Perkiomenville, Pennsylvania 18074

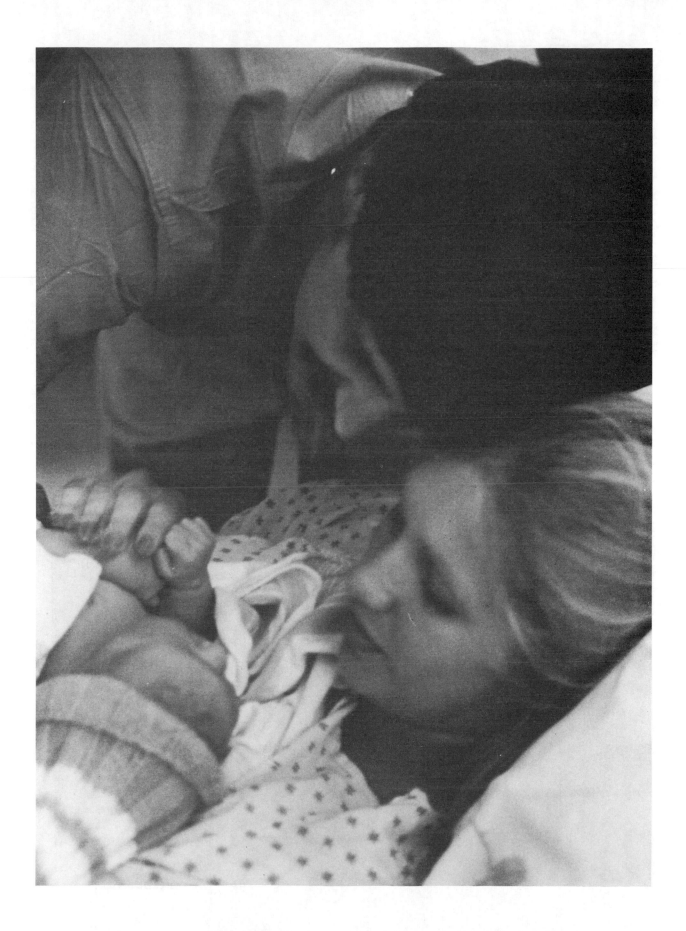

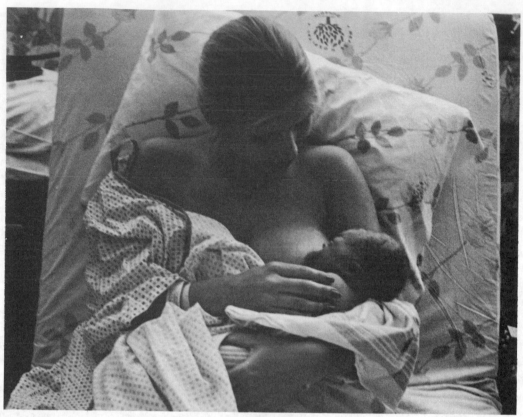

Bonding (below) and breast-feeding (above) immediately following delivery.

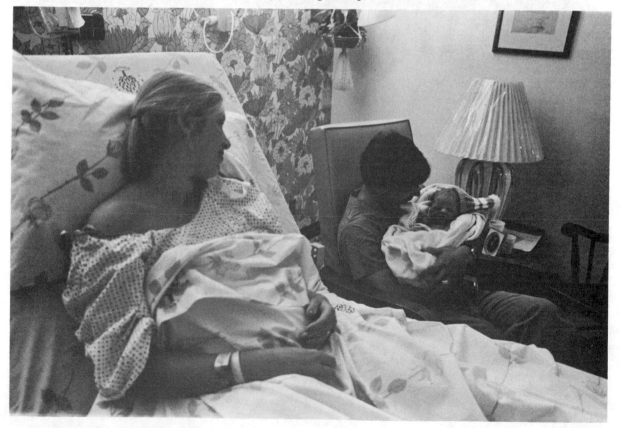

CHAPTER 16

Pregnancy

In your mother's childbearing era, a woman whose period was two weeks late made an appointment that was scheduled for 2 to 4 weeks later, at which time a pregnancy test and a pelvic exam would confirm this now 6-to-8 week pregnancy. Thus, prenatal care really began six weeks or more after conception. Today, we know that this sequence of events is not optimal, that planning for pregnancy should begin much earlier. Ideally, a couple should start planning for a pregnancy several months in advance. During this time, they can schedule a visit with the physician for "preconception counseling" to discuss personal risk factors and other matters that may affect a pregnancy and to arrange for any tests that might need to be completed before trying to conceive.

Preconception Counseling

Typically, preconception counseling focuses on four areas: dos, don'ts, possible tests, and the question of early prenatal vitamins. Topping the list of "dos" are proper nutrition and frequent, regular exercise (see Chapters 48 and 49). Pregnancy is not a time to diet and neither are the weeks that precede it. Adequate calories and a balanced, healthy diet are important to correct nutritional deficiencies and to maintain the nutritional stores needed in pregnancy. Regular, preferably aerobic, exercise in the months before pregnancy helps promote cardiovascular fitness, control weight, and improve muscle tone. Such conditioning also may help with the fatigue and general physical stress that accompany pregnancy. One of the most important "don'ts" is taking medicines (either prescription or nonprescription) not ordered by your doctor—from the moment you start trying to become pregnant. This is because the baby is especially at risk for birth defects during the first eight weeks—when a woman may not yet know she has conceived. Birth control pills should be discontinued two to three months before you become pregnant (see page 53).

It is important to stop smoking or taking drugs even before you conceive. Cigarette smoking, in addition to being a risk to the fetus (see Chapters 31 and 61), can reduce a man's sperm count and increase the number of abnormal sperm. Smoking should be stopped for at least three months before conceiving as it may take this long for cancer-causing ingredients in cigarettes to be cleared from the body. Smoking marijuana may inhibit ovulation in the woman and sperm production in the man. Excessive alcohol consumption should be avoided, as current research shows that consumption of ten drinks per week (five per week if you smoke) during the weeks prior to conception is linked to low birth weight (below the tenth percentile). Possible risks from consuming alcohol during pregnancy are discussed in Chapter 31. It is also important to cut down on caffeine during the preconception time, drinking no more than three cups of coffee or its equivalent per day, as excessive caffeine may pose a slight risk of miscarriage. Also to be avoided are soft drinks containing caffeine. Use of cocaine has been shown in recent studies to lead to addicted babies with later development of irritability and frustration in performing simple tasks and more difficulty in establishing personal relationships in early childhood.

In the months before pregnancy, too, a woman must also consider potential risks in the work place, including chemicals and X-rays. It is important to discuss any possible job-related risks with your doctor. For example, women working in day-care centers or in other occupations that involve contact with small children may want to take special precautions to minimize the risk of exposure to CMV infections (see Chapter 20). For couples with cats, other precautions apply (see Chapter 20).

Certain tests may be desirable prior to pregnancy. For example, if you are unsure of your immunity to German measles (rubella), you should have a rubella antibody test (see Chapter 20). Couples belonging to racial or ethnic groups that are at risk for certain inherited diseases may want to have appropriate genetic screening tests (see Chapter 11).

Finally, obstetricians now routinely prescribe prenatal vitamins for women planning a pregnancy. Typical examples of prenatal vitamins include Materna Tablets, Niferex-P N Tablets, PreCare Caplets, Stuartnatal Plus Tablets, and ZENATE Tablets. Recent studies indicate that some neural tube defects may be prevented by taking prenatal vitamins very early in pregnancy (during the first six weeks). Prenatal vitamins are particularly advisable if you smoke, as smoking decreases levels of vitamins B_1 and C as well as levels of calcium and zinc. Vitamins are especially important if a women has a history of giving birth to a child with a neural tube defect (see Chapter 11). Recent research has found that starting such women on folic acid during the month before they conceived again caused a decrease in the recurrence risk of this birth defect from 5% to less than 1%. Other women for whom multivitamins should be prescribed include those formerly on weight-loss diets or special diets (e.g., vegetarians), endurance runners, and women taking birth control pills, which may cause minor deficiencies in certain vitamins. Vitamins taken prior to as well as during pregnancy should not contain more than 100% of the recommended daily allowance (RDA), as high doses of vitamins, especially megadosages (dosages greater than 1000% of RDA) have been shown to cause birth defects in animals. Particular caution must be used with vitamin A, since dosages of just 25,000 IU have been associated with birth defects.

Ovulation Test Kits

New ovulation test kits have become available in recent years and have changed the process of determining when you are most likely to conceive. Using the chemistry of *monoclonal antibodies* (see Glossary), these test kits measure a hormone (luteinizing hormone, or LH) in the woman's urine. This hormone surges—suddenly increases in concentration—about twenty-four hours before ovulation each month. The woman performs the test each day, beginning on about the tenth day of her cycle. Once the test detects the LH surge (by a distinct color change on test paper), intercourse should be planned for approximately twenty-four to thirty-six hours later. Ovulation kits are available through physicians' offices or over the counter under brand names such as OvuQuick, OvuKit, First Response Ovulation Predictor Test, Q-Test, ClearPlan Easy,

and Answer, and cost about $25 per kit. These tests predict ovulation very accurately and can help you time intercourse so that you are more likely to deliver in the month desired.

Confirmation of Pregnancy

You may have some or none of the early signs of pregnancy listed in Table 27. If you have been taking your basal body temperature (see Figure 9 in Chapter 6) and it stays elevated for sixteen days with no menstruation, you can be reasonably sure you are pregnant. If you haven't been taking your temperature, then confirmation of pregnancy requires a test and an examination.

Both a pregnancy test and a pelvic exam are necessary to confirm pregnancy because either procedure alone may be misleading. The test may be inaccurate, or uterine enlargement detected during pelvic examination may be due to some cause other than pregnancy. For most women, the simplest approach is to have a pregnancy test two weeks after a missed period—or earlier (see below)—followed by an appointment with her clinician if the test is positive. If the test is negative, you can repeat the test in one to two weeks and put off the examination until after the second test report. If you have unexpected pain or unusual vaginal bleeding, however, see your clinician immediately even if your pregnancy test is negative.

The main purpose of the pelvic exam in early pregnancy is to evaluate the size of the uterus. The clinician determines how many weeks you have been pregnant by evaluating uterine enlargement, initially detectable about four weeks after conception (that is, two weeks after your period was due). Besides uterine enlargement, the clinician looks for two other findings indicative of pregnancy: uterine softening and a slight bluish coloration of the cervix.

Urine pregnancy tests

All pregnancy tests are based upon the detection of pregnancy hormone (see Chapter 3) found in the urine or blood. Newer over-the-counter home pregnancy tests diagnose pregnancy earlier and with greater accuracy than ever before.

Table 27   EARLY SIGNS OF PREGNANCY

1. Missed period(s)
2. Breast changes (enlargement, tenderness)
3. Nausea, vomiting (morning sickness)
4. Increased frequency of urination
5. Fatigue
6. Slight weight gain
7. Abdominal enlargement

Since these tests depend upon the concentration of pregnancy hormone in the urine, always use your first urine specimen of the day because it is most concentrated. Office pregnancy tests may be performed in a matter of a few minutes and accurately diagnose pregnancy as early as four to five days *before* a missed period. Home pregnancy tests typically are capable of diagnosing pregnancy as early as the first day of an anticipated period. Typical home tests include First Response Pregnancy Test, Advance, E.P.T., Answer, Fact Plus, Clearblue Easy, Confirm, and Conceive.

False-positive and false-negative urine pregnancy tests do sometimes occur. The greatest number of incorrect tests are false negatives, occurring in up to 20% of women using home tests and in a smaller percentage when tests are performed in a hospital lab or in the doctor's office. Most false negatives occur because the test was performed too soon or with a diluted urine specimen. Very occasionally, a false-negative test may also result if an ectopic pregnancy (see Chapter 54) has developed. For this reason, a woman should consult her clinician if she has skipped a period or has symptoms of pregnancy after a negative reading.

Blood pregnancy tests: Blood pregnancy tests are the costliest as well as the most sensitive and reliable of pregnancy tests. The basic type is called the *radioimmunoassay* (RIA) or beta-subunit HCG. This test is often reserved for pregnancy complications such as a suspected tubal pregnancy, but it can also be used to determine if a woman is pregnant *before* the missed period. Essentially 100% accurate, test results usually take about one hour. This test can also establish approximately how far your pregnancy has progressed in weeks.

How Is My Due Date Determined?

The clinician calculates your due date from the first day of your last known period (since the date of conception is usually unknown) using Nägele's Rule: count back three months from the first day of your last menstrual period and add seven days. For example, if your last menstrual period began May 1, your due date would be February 8. Fewer than 10% of women deliver exactly on their due date, and it's normal to have your baby as much as two weeks early or two weeks late. Because of the inaccuracies of calendar calculations, a number of fetal maturity tests have been developed to determine the age of the fetus. *Sonography* is one type of fetal maturity test.

Uses of Sonography During Pregnancy

During pregnancy sonography may be used to evaluate the fetus, amniotic fluid, and placenta. It works like this: sound waves are sent out by an instrument called a *scanner*, and the reflected waves (the echo) are displayed on a screen, appearing as a black-and-white image that looks similar to an X-ray. The sonography procedure is painless except for the discomfort of lying on your back and temporarily having a full bladder. You will be asked to drink fluids and not urinate until after your sonogram, because the clinician can read the pattern better when your bladder is full. The clinician coats your abdomen with mineral oil or aqua gel to improve the quality of sound waves from the hand-held scanner. Many physicians have begun using a newer technique in which a specialized scanner is inserted into the vagina in early pregnancy. This scanner, called the *vaginal probe*, can usually assess the health of an early pregnancy much better than the abdominal technique. As you watch the screen, you can see the outline of the fetus and see movement. Your clinician can point out the head and other parts of the body.

Sonography performed in early pregnancy can diagnose the cause of bleeding complications, including ectopic pregnancies (see Chapter 54). Later in pregnancy, abdominal sonography may be used to diagnose birth defects or accompany chorionic villus sampling or genetic amniocentesis for accurate needle placement (see

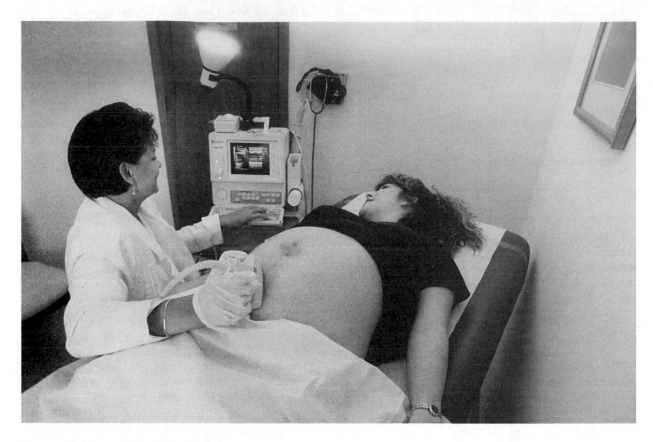

Sonography helps evaluate the baby's growth, position, and well-being.

Chapter 11). When performed prior to twenty-five weeks, sonography is one of the best methods for determining gestational age, which may be especially helpful if the date of your last menstrual period is uncertain. The calculation of gestational age is based on certain measurements, including head circumference and another measurement called the *biparietal diameter* (BPD). After twenty-six weeks, the BPD and other measurements that are taken are less reliable in detecting gestational age because of the greater variability in fetal head growth during the latter part of pregnancy. Sonography is also the most reliable technique for assessing potential growth problems (see Chapter 20). The newest use of sonography in pregnancy has been in the development of a very sophisticated test of fetal well-being called the *biophysical profile* (see Chapter 20). This test is often performed every week or so in the last few weeks of high-risk pregnancies. Other uses of sonography include assessment of the position of the fetus (head-first or breech) and detection of twins. Localization of the placenta by sonography allows the physician to identify when certain placental complications may occur (see Chapter 55).

With sonography, your body is exposed to sound waves only for a fraction of a second. There are no known harmful effects. The technique has been studied for many years and is generally considered extremely safe, both for you and your baby. While still not recommended for routine use in pregnancy (as it is in some European countries), in many pregnancies there will be an appropriate indication for this procedure. Table 28 summarizes some of the reasons for the use of sonography during pregnancy.

Table 28 POSSIBLE REASONS FOR A SONOGRAM (ULTRASOUND) DURING PREGNANCY

When Performed*	Reason or Indication	What Sonogram Shows
6–12 weeks	Bleeding in early pregnancy.	Fetal movement is detectable (using vaginal probe) by 6–7 weeks: absence of movement indicates possible miscarriage; fetal movement is reassuring sign.
6–12 weeks	Pelvic pain in early pregnancy.	Can detect some causes of pain—e.g., ovarian cyst and ectopic pregnancy.
9–11 weeks	Chorionic villus sampling for genetic screening.	Identifies site of placenta where tissue sample is obtained.
11–18 weeks	Amniocentesis is planned to screen for genetic defects.	Identifies "pocket" of amniotic fluid as well as placenta and fetus, both of which must be avoided by amniocentesis needle.
14–25 weeks	History of previous child with anencephaly, spina bifida, or hydrocephaly.	These abnormalities are detectable.
16–25 weeks	High-risk pregnancies in which labor may be induced (e.g., high blood pressure, diabetes) or repeat cesarean section planned.	Measurement of fetal head size allows calculation of gestational age and due date.
16–25 weeks	Maternal family history of twins or suspected twins because of apparent large size of fetus.	Shows presence of one fetus or more (may be detected as early as 10 weeks).
32–40 weeks	High-risk pregnancy.	Detection of fetal motion and breathing and amount of amniotic fluid (biophysical profile test—see Chapter 20).

* Counting from the first day of your last menstrual period.

Physical and Emotional Changes During Pregnancy

Pregnancy lasts about nine months and averages 38 weeks from the date of conception, or about 40 weeks from the first day of your last menstrual period, depending on the usual length of your cycle. After your initial visit to your clinician, you will usually have a check-up once a month until your seventh or eighth month when visits become more frequent. During these visits, your clinician measures fetal growth by recording the expansion of your uterus (see Figure 23). Your weight and blood pressure are checked and urine samples are taken to check for albumin (indicator of toxemia) and sugar (indicator of diabetes). You and your clinician should use these visits to get to know and feel comfortable with each other. It is important to thoroughly discuss attitudes and decisions about your childbirth experience so your plans and expectations coincide.

The events of pregnancy fall naturally into three equal time periods, called *trimesters* of pregnancy. The physical and emotional changes in the mother, which are discussed below, vary predictably within each trimester. It is important to remember, however, that each pregnancy is unique and that this discussion is only a general outline of what you might experience. If you notice symptoms that worry you, look them up in the symptoms section of this book (Section Eleven) for their possible causes and treatment. Diet and nutrition in pregnancy are discussed below (see also Chapter 48).

Warning signs in pregnancy—that is, indications that your pregnancy may be threatened—are shown in Table 29.

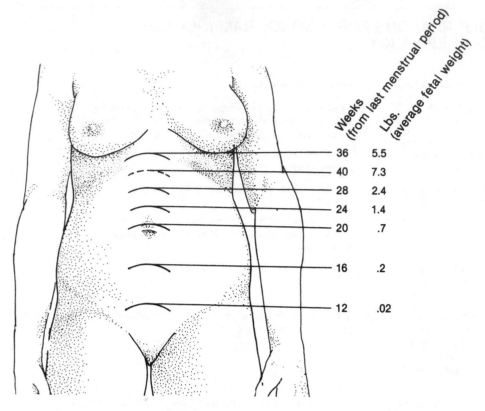

Weeks (from last menstrual period)	Lbs. (average fetal weight)
36	5.5
40	7.3
28	2.4
24	1.4
20	.7
16	.2
12	.02

Figure 17   *Curved marks indicate the location of the top of the uterus (fundus) at various weeks of pregnancy. The approximate weight of the fetus at each of these weeks is shown. Note that by 40 weeks, the fundus has become slightly lower than at 36 weeks because the fetus "drops" in the last month of pregnancy. Most of the fetal weight is gained in the last 12 weeks.*

Figure 18
Pregnancy at 12 weeks. At 12 weeks you are beginning to "show." Morning sickness is subsiding. The heartbeat can easily be heard using a Doppler device. Length: 3 inches. Weight: 1 ounce.

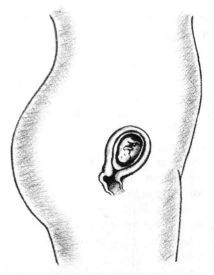

The first trimester (1 to 3 months)

During the first trimester (the first three months), the fetus makes its greatest developmental strides. The head, brain, heart, body, and limbs begin to form. Fingers and toes are recognizable. Sex organs begin to develop but cannot yet be observed. Except for the first week after conception, all drugs and chemicals to which you are exposed may cross the placenta and possibly influence the development of the fetus.

Your physical changes: You may experience some or none of the early signs of pregnancy listed in Table 27. The most common symptoms of early pregnancy are a missed period, morning sickness, fatigue, decreased appetite, breast tenderness, and frequent urination.

Your emotional changes: Most women have conflicting feelings about pregnancy throughout the first trimester. Even women who have had difficulty conceiving go through mood swings that pass from exuberance to despair. Both parents-to-be often worry about the financial and psychological responsibility of parenthood. You may wonder if you want to be a mother after all, or if you can be a good mother. Sometimes a father finds himself feeling just as worried and torn about the pregnancy as the expectant mother is. It often helps to share your feelings with each other.

During the first trimester, many women are preoccupied with the changes in their bodies and what seems to be happening to them. They frequently feel at this time more dependent upon others. The need to share the frustrations and pleasures of pregnancy is likely to continue through the entire nine months. It's best to depend on someone besides your clinician since he or she may not always be available. Ideally, the person you select should also be the one who will be with you in labor and delivery. If you have a close friend who is pregnant at the same time, you can offer each other mutual support and understanding.

The second trimester (4 to 6 months)

The heart and circulatory system of the fetus develops during this time; and by the fifth or sixth month the clinician, using an instrument called a *doptone* (see glossary), can hear the heartbeat. By the end of the sixth month, the fetus will have grown to about twelve inches in length. The clinician continues to measure uterine growth in centimeters during your monthly checkups. This is the time to start preparing for breast-feeding if that is what you wish to do. You may want to contact your local La Leche League office for group support and instruction. See Chapter 19 for more information about breast-feeding.

Your physical changes: If you felt some discomfort during the first trimester, you are likely to feel better the second trimester. If you felt well during the first trimester, you may feel even better during this time.

As the fetus increases in size, so does your waist. You gain weight more rapidly in the second trimester and find that your clothes become uncomfortably tight. By the twentieth week or so of your pregnancy, the fetus becomes large enough for *you* to feel its movements, called *quickening*. Repeat pregnant mothers usually no-

tice it earlier in their second pregnancy since they are familiar with the fluttering movement. Be sure to tell your clinician the date on which you first felt fetal movement.

Indigestion problems such as heartburn, gas, and constipation may appear. Your heart is working harder because your blood volume has increased, and this circumstance may lead to greater fatigue and some fluid retention. You may find that some discomfort can be relieved by continued regular exercise (see Chapter 49). Other conditions which may begin to occur in midpregnancy include varicose veins, hemorrhoids, and skin changes, including the appearance of stretch marks, called *striae*. Pregnancy support hose are often helpful in preventing worsening of varicose veins and decreasing fluid retention. Braxton-Hicks contractions (false labor pains) may occur and often continue through the third trimester. If they seem to become regular, as often as every fifteen to twenty minutes, or become painful, you should contact your doctor as they may be a sign of premature labor. Now is the time to assess your activities and eliminate the nonessentials. You may find you'll need to gradually slow down work activities and allow

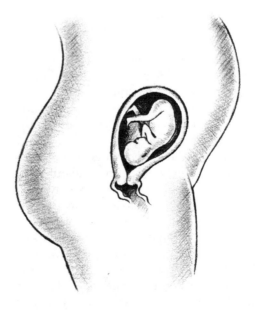

Figure 19
Pregnancy at 20 weeks. You're a little more than halfway there. The middle trimester is perhaps the most enjoyable one, as digestive problems are usually manageable and you're still not dealing with the discomforts of the third trimester. The baby's organs have developed and are maturing. Fetal movement can now be felt. Length: 10 to 12 inches. Weight: ½ to 1 pound.

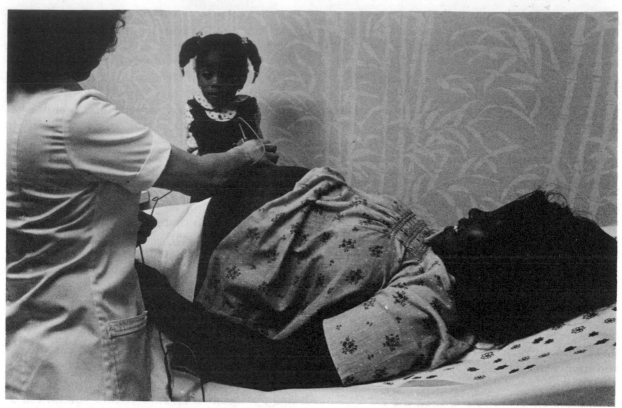

The fetal heartbeat can be heard through an instrument called a doptone.

for more frequent rest periods during the day.
Your emotional changes: Many women feel very well during this time, partly as a result of the disappearance of the unpleasant symptoms of early pregnancy. You are obviously pregnant yet not too big to move around comfortably. The reality of the pregnancy is obvious to everyone, and you will probably get more immediate support and recognition from others.

The feelings of the movements of the fetus can be thrilling. If you are upset about your pregnancy, however, the movements may seem to focus your anger and make you feel less in control of your body. Repeat mothers often compare their current pregnancy with their previous pregnancies and the amount of fetal movement, wondering how the differences between this pregnancy and earlier pregnancies will be reflected in this newborn's personality. If you have a sonogram during this period, you may form a clear picture in your mind of what your baby looks like. You may be surprised at how much affection you feel from this early "bonding" as you hold your child's first, blurred photograph after the sonogram. A previous experience of a miscarriage or stillbirth may elicit unresolved

feelings and cause you to be more anxious about the outcome of this pregnancy.

As you begin to wear maternity clothes and lose your figure, you may still experience conflicting feelings toward this pregnancy. A change in your image—in the way you see yourself physically—normally occurs by the second trimester. You may experience many different emotions as you watch the growth of your abdomen and realize you have been sharing your body with a growing fetus. You may feel protective and maternal toward what is inside your abdomen. It is common to continue to wonder if your newborn will be normal.

Even in the most wanted and planned pregnancies, feelings of confusion, anxiety, or depression may lurk below the surface. It is normal to turn your thoughts more to yourself, to look more into your own mind and feelings, and to spend time thinking about your own mother and your childhood. If you have a close relationship with your mother, and she is nearby, you may find her support comforting. If your mother is far away or you have conflicts in your relationship, you may use a great deal of energy in trying to develop your own separate, distinct style of maternal role and identity. Second and subsequent pregnancies may be harder at this point because of the demands of older children. Every pregnant woman needs some time to think about becoming a mother and to identify her feelings about it.

The third trimester (7 to 9 months)

The fetus grows rapidly during the last three months, multiplying its weight about three to four times. You may note the hands or feet of the fetus poking out in a lump in your abdomen or appearing as a wave when it changes position. You are constantly aware of its movements, from kicking to hiccuping. The last trimester is usually the time to begin preparation classes for childbirth (see Chapter 14). Sonograms at this time present a more realistic picture of your child.

Your physical changes: Your abdomen is very large, and you can see the movements of the fetus clearly. Your abdomen feels very firm and big; your navel may be pushed out flat. The fetus moves into the position for delivery, usually head down. Your awareness of these movements may wake you, and sleeping may be difficult. Finding a comfortable sleeping position isn't easy. Sometimes slight contractions, called *Braxton-Hicks,* cause your uterus to tighten. These contractions seem like menstrual cramps and usually go away quickly. Shortness of breath is a common symptom during this period; this condition is due to the fact that the uterus is pushing up other abdominal organs and thus restricting movement of the diaphragm. At the end of the eighth month, the top of the uterus may be felt just below the lower edge of the ribs. This may cause an uncomfortable feeling of stretching below your lower ribs. Pressure from the fetus may be felt in many ways: aches and pains in the legs, thighs, or perineum; frequent urinating; constipation; and occasional lightheadedness or dizziness. You may experience indigestion because the uterus presses against your stomach. Nausea and vomiting may return. Fatigue usually increases because of sleep difficulties and the added body weight. It is important to plan for short, frequent rest periods and to sit with your legs and feet up when possible. Red spots or spider vein

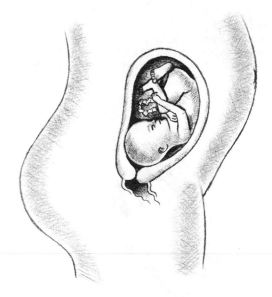

Figure 20
Pregnancy at 28 weeks. You're now beginning your last trimester of pregnancy. You may notice occasional contractions from time to time. The baby's lungs, while still immature, have developed to the point at which, if you were to deliver now, the baby's chance of intact survival would be very good in many hospitals. Fetal weight is rapidly increasing. Length: 13 to 15 inches. Weight: 1½ to 3 pounds.

Table 29   TEN WARNING SIGNS IN PREGNANCY

Report any of these symptoms to your clinician immediately:

1. Any vaginal bleeding or spotting
2. Severe, persistent headaches
3. Prolonged vomiting (over one to two days, preventing adequate intake of liquids)
4. Blurring of vision; spots before the eyes
5. Fever (over 100°F.) and chills not accompanied by symptoms of a cold
6. Sudden intense or continual abdominal pains
7. Sudden gush of fluid from the vagina
8. Sudden swelling of hands, feet, and ankles
9. Frequent, burning urination
10. Pronounced decrease in fetal movement

Figure 21
Pregnancy at 36 weeks. You've got one month to go! Discomforts in the lower abdomen and upper legs and vagina increase now. The baby is probably in the head-first position in preparation for birth. Length: 17 to 20 inches. Weight: 4½ to 6½ pounds.

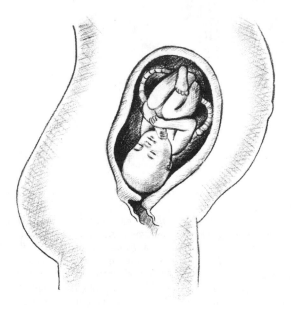

The illustrations for figures 18–21 were provided courtesy of Wyeth-Ayerst Laboratories.

marks may form on your skin as a result of circulation changes. Yeast infections may become a problem and should be reported to your physician. Backache, too, is common because you tend to lean backward to compensate for your heavy abdomen. *Lightening* refers to the slight descent of the uterus that occurs when the head of the fetus drops into the birth canal; it usually occurs two to four weeks before delivery. This process is more pronounced in first-time mothers and may not occur until labor in repeat mothers. Lightening relieves the pressure on your stomach and diaphragm, making it easier to breathe. Lightening means that your body is getting ready for delivery.

Your emotional changes: Now is a time of expectancy, of waiting for labor to begin. Many women experience a feeling of wanting the delivery soon but at the same time fear the experience of labor and delivery. Taking childbirth preparation classes helps you to lessen your anxiety as well as to share your excitement with other pregnant women. Anxiety about birth defects may increase. You may feel a deep sense of

oneness and at the same time be ready to give up this oneness in order to see and hear and touch what you have anticipated for nine months.

You begin to picture your newborn's appearance. You may dream or fantasize about what he or she looks like. It is normal to imagine how this child will fit into your family and its future. It is also common to imagine what activities you would like your child to be involved in and how you and the child will share them together. Knowing the sex of your child may lead to specific fantasies or expectations for the future. The baby's increasing activity won't let you forget him or her or the fact that you are soon to be a mother. The last month may drag by as you eagerly await the arrival of the baby. People constantly ask you how you feel and when you expect to have the baby. These comments can be upsetting as you have no answer for what you want to know most, and no one can tell when "labor day" will arrive. The last few weeks of pregnancy are a hard time during which to plan anything, and most women stay close to home. Each day you wonder if this will be "the day," though you know the waiting is well worth it.

Feelings of dependency on friends and relatives increase. This is the time, it is hoped, when you should be getting some extra help. Your husband or an older son or daughter can help with the heavier chores, and perhaps one of them can spend more time with your other children. If you are alone, stay close to a friend who will be available for help.

Nutrition in Pregnancy and Breast-feeding

Adequate fetal growth and development depends upon a constant supply of nutrients from the mother. Inadequate nutrition, in fact, is considered a major risk factor in pregnancy and can lead to fetal malnutrition and low birth weight babies, which have more than their share of difficulties after birth. (See also Chapter 89 on weight gain and weight loss.) If you are a teenager, you need to increase your caloric intake to meet both the baby's and your "growth" needs.

During pregnancy, your diet should consist of a variety of foods selected from the five basic food groups shown in Table 87 in Chapter 48.

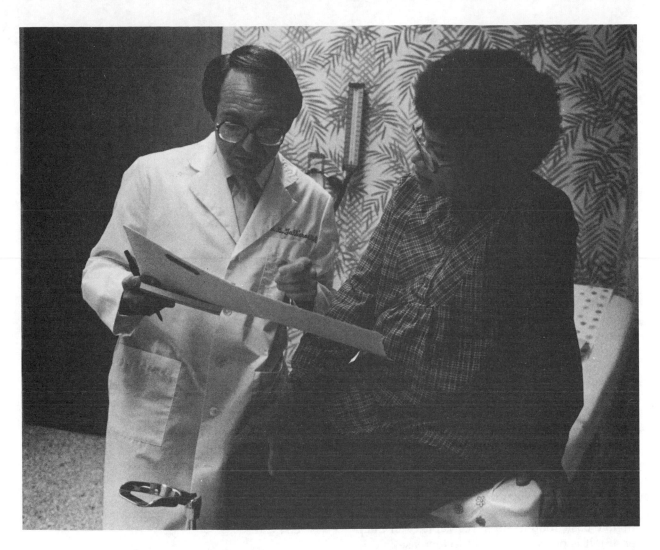

Emphasize fresh fruits, vegetables, meat, and milk. Eat as few canned and processed foods as possible. The effects on the fetus of food additives such as monosodium glutamate (MSG) and nitrates are unknown.

The recommended vitamin requirements for pregnant and breast-feeding women are given in Table 79 (Chapter 48). Fresh fruits, vegetables, and whole grain products provide a dietary source for these vitamins although prenatal vitamins are often prescribed routinely, as noted earlier in this chapter.

The recommended daily amount of calcium during pregnancy and breast-feeding increases significantly from 800 to 1200 mg (an increase of approximately two 8-oz. glasses of milk). Eggs and fortified milk are nutritious sources of calcium and protein as well as vitamins A and D for pregnant and breast-feeding women. If you dislike drinking milk, try getting some of your

calcium in creamed foods, yogurt, puddings, or cheese or ask your doctor for a calcium supplement. In addition to being an excellent source of calcium and protein, yogurt containing active cultures helps digest the milk sugar lactose, which may be of particular benefit to women who are lactose-intolerant.

Salt does not have to be restricted in pregnancy in healthy women. Research in recent years has shown that salt intake has little or no relationship to the development of toxemia (see Chapter 20).

When you are breast-feeding, you need to eat slightly more of most nutrients than you did during your pregnancy, especially as your baby grows. This is because your body requires more energy to produce the milk, and the milk itself requires substantial calories. In order to produce about one quart of milk per day when breast-feeding, you need to consume about 900 extra calories daily. This is not the time to start a weight-loss diet. There are no nourishing foods that need to be eliminated from your diet. Chocolate sometimes has been found to have a laxative effect on some babies; and broccoli, Brussels sprouts, cabbage, dried beans, and cauliflower sometimes create gas. Spicy foods may flavor the milk or cause gas pains in your baby. Moderation is a helpful rule, as most foods eaten by a breast-feeding mother in small amounts are well-tolerated by newborns.

If you don't breast-feed and you want to lose weight, you can begin a weight-loss diet at once after your baby is born. You may, however, want to wait several weeks before beginning any strenuous diet to lose weight because the process of childbirth is stressful and nutritionally demanding as are the first weeks at home. Refer to Chapter 89, on weight gain and weight loss, for healthy approaches to dieting and for a suggested diet plan to lose weight.

Normal Weight Gain During Pregnancy

Many scientific studies have shown the advantages of good nutrition before and during pregnancy. In general, fewer complications of pregnancy occur in women rated as having well-balanced diets consisting of foods from each of the five basic food groups (see Table 87 in Chapter 48). It is not so important to increase calories in pregnancy as it is to improve the quality of the diet. In the second half of pregnancy, however, caloric intake does need to be increased by approximately 10%, and this increase should continue through breast-feeding.

The subject of weight gain during pregnancy has been controversial for many years. Obstetricians now impose less severe restrictions on weight gain than in the past in an effort to decrease the number of babies with low birth weights. According to the National Academy of Scientists, weight gain in pregnancy should reflect the woman's prepregnancy weight. Women who are underweight should gain twenty-eight to forty pounds; overweight women should gain fifteen to twenty-five pounds. For most women —those neither significantly overweight nor underweight—total weight gain in pregnancy should average between twenty-five and thirty-five pounds.

There are several reasons for weight gain during pregnancy: the growing fetus and its surrounding amniotic fluid, the growth of specific organs such as the uterus and breasts, the increase in your blood volume, and fluid retention. The pattern of weight gain is more important than the total amount gained. You should gain weight gradually and primarily during the second two-thirds of your pregnancy. In the first third of pregnancy, weight gain averages three pounds but may be less if nausea and vomiting are severe.

Table 30 WEIGHT GAIN IN PREGNANCY

Weight	Pounds
Baby	7–8
Placenta	1½
Amniotic fluid	2
Uterus	2
Breasts	1–1½
Blood	3–4
Fluid (retained in body tissues)	2–3
Maternal stores (fat, protein not in nutrients)	3½–6
Total	22–28

Exercise During and After Pregnancy

More women than ever before are interested in maintaining fitness during pregnancy. Benefits include a feeling of well-being and a reduction in minor physical complaints, such as constipation, backache, edema, and poor posture. If you haven't exercised before becoming pregnant, this is not the time to start a rigorous program. Ideally, if you plan to become pregnant and want to begin exercising, give yourself a good six months to begin working out before you try to become pregnant.

Exercise helps prepare a woman's body for labor and delivery, and in moderation, it usually poses no danger to mother or baby. Check with your doctor if you have a medical problem such as high blood pressure, however. Concern about exercise in pregnancy is centered around exces-

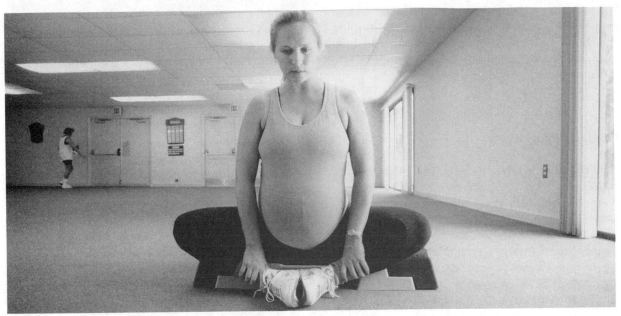

Stretching and exercise help prepare a woman's body for giving birth.

sively strenuous or risky activity or activity that could decrease oxygen to the fetus. Scuba diving, sprinting, competitive exercises, high-altitude training, and contact sports are off-limits. So are activities where water could be forced into the vagina during a fall, as may happen in water-skiing and surfing. Exercises that emphasize stretching and relaxation are appropriate during pregnancy. Jerky, bouncy movements as well as jumping and jarring motions should be avoided because of increased joint instability. For added protection, exercise on a carpeted floor to reduce shock and provide safe footing, and avoid overstretching.

It is especially important to drink plenty of fluid before, during, and after exercise during pregnancy. Dehydration can be a potential problem if the mother becomes overheated. Avoid exercise if you have a fever and try not to work out in hot, humid weather. High body temperatures have been linked to birth defects. Women at risk for premature labor should not exercise unless their doctor approves. Regular exercise (i.e., several times a week) can be continued during most of pregnancy.

Women who haven't been participating in endurance sports such as running, cycling, and aerobic dancing probably shouldn't take them up during pregnancy, although many women can continue with their previous nonpregnant level of aerobic exercise during pregnancy. Some

may find exercising in water helpful, especially during the latter part of the pregnancy. The American College of Obstetricians and Gynecologists (ACOG) has helped develop a highly acclaimed videocassette for home use called "Pregnancy Exercise Program," designed for expectant mothers. Another video, "Postnatal Exercise Program," covers safe exercises especially designed for the first few months after delivery. Instructional booklets accompany these programs and can be ordered by calling 1-800-428-4488. Helpful exercises for pregnancy and postpartum are also described in *Essential Exercises for the Childbearing Year*, by physical therapist Elizabeth Noble.

Getting up and walking around is the first exercise you'll do after childbirth. With your physician's approval, exercises can be started twenty-four hours after a normal delivery. Mild, regular exercising helps to strengthen the muscles and get you back into shape.

In about six weeks, your uterus should be back to its normal size and position, and your weight should have dropped near to what it was before you became pregnant. You may notice that certain parts of your body appear heavier. This is due to stretching of tissues and sometimes to increased fat deposits that accumulate during pregnancy. During this time, do exercises that tone your thighs, stomach, waist and hips. You can exercise if you've chosen to breast-feed, but be sure to drink plenty of fluids to remain well hydrated. Your general body conditioning and how you are feeling will determine how soon you can participate in active sports. Use common sense and discuss your exercise plans with your clinician.

Teenage Pregnancy

Teen pregnancy rates in the United States are the highest of any Western country. One out of every ten women aged fifteen to nineteen becomes pregnant in the United States each year. Approximately 50% of these pregnancies are aborted, the same percentage as found in other Western countries. American women do not start sexual activity at an earlier age than their European counterparts, but they are less likely to use or have access to birth control. American teens also are likely to have had less extensive sex education than European adolescents. School problems, crime, and drug and alcohol abuse are high-risk behaviors that are associated with teenage pregnancy. The presence of self-esteem, a knowledge of health, sex, and contraceptives, and communication skills to delay the initiation of sexual activity are all found to decrease the incidence of teen pregnancy.

The social and emotional consequences of teenage pregnancy can be devastating to a young girl and her family. Unintended pregnancy at this age is likely to have an adverse effect upon her education, independence, and later opportunities. Informative sex education provided by the parents and acceptable community resources are the first steps toward making the responsibility of pregnancy and parenthood realistic for teenagers (see Chapter 3).

If you are a teenager, and find yourself pregnant, seek medical help immediately. As you are still physically growing yourself, your body has special nutritional needs that must be met. Plan to continue your education, if at all possible.

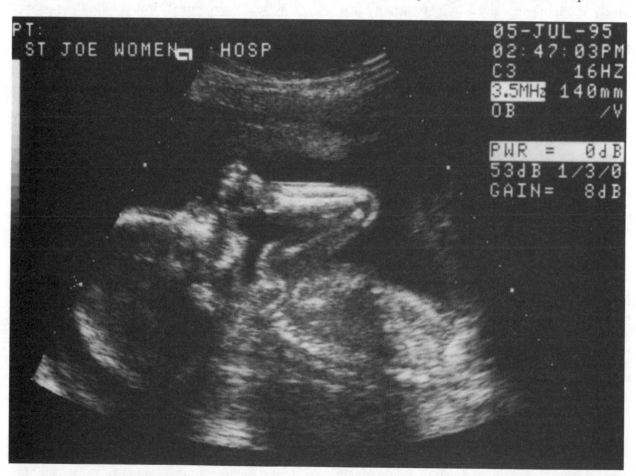

The outline of the baby as viewed on a sonogram.

Table 31 COMMON CONCERNS DURING PREGNANCY

Trips by car . . .	Wear a seat belt and shoulder strap at all times, fitting the belt loosely over your thighs as opposed to tightly around your abdomen. Take frequent (hourly) breaks for exercise and nourishment. Stay close to home during your ninth month in case the baby decides to make an early appearance.
Air travel . . .	Fly only in a pressurized aircraft. It is recommended that you move about every 45 minutes to promote circulation.
Sex . . .	During a normal pregnancy, sexual intercourse is in no way harmful. Some women experience increased sexual desire during pregnancy. Avoid intercourse if you have vaginal bleeding or ruptured membranes, or in the last six weeks of pregnancy if you are pregnant with twins or have a history of premature labor. (See Chapter 23.)
Pets—like cats . . .	Cats may carry a rare microorganism that causes a disease called toxoplasmosis and that is excreted in their stools. An ample precaution is to have someone else change the kitty litter and to wash your hands after you have handled a cat.
Exercise . . .	A safe rule to follow is to continue whatever exercise you were doing before pregnancy as long as you feel comfortable. Jogging, horseback riding, swimming, and skiing have all been done safely by pregnant women. Use your common sense and if you find you are uncomfortable and tired, stop. Walking and prenatal exercises are particularly helpful. Check with your clinician about your exercise program. (See Chapter 49.)
Work . . .	In most uncomplicated pregnancies the woman can work throughout the pregnancy, including the ninth month. In general, avoid strenuous activity, extreme temperatures, smoking areas, and excessive stair climbing. Take frequent breaks, stop working when fatigued, elevate your legs periodically, and wear support hose. Prolonged standing (greater than four hours), repetitive heavy lifting (greater than twenty-five pounds), and frequent stooping and bending below knee level should be avoided in the last three months. Women with previous preterm babies or other high-risk factors such as high blood pressure, diabetes, or inadequate fetal growth should seriously consider only light duties throughout pregnancy. Exposure to environmental toxic substances (that is, chemicals) may be hazardous to the fetus, especially in early pregnancy.
Video display terminals . . .	VDTs have not been found to be a hazard to the fetus, but you may experience neck pains or headaches from sitting in a fixed position for prolonged periods.
Hot tubs . . .	Animal experiments suggest that high maternal temperatures result in a reduction of blood flow to the fetus. In uncomplicated pregnancies, short stretches in a sauna or hot tub are probably not harmful if the temperature is less than 102° F and exposure does not exceed ten minutes.

Take care of yourself, especially now, and seek out the support of a trusted adult to help you plan to deal with your pregnancy.

Common Concerns During Pregnancy

There are many concerns that women may have during pregnancy. Table 31 discusses some of the more common ones.

Further Information

For more information about what to expect during pregnancy, you can send a self-addressed stamped envelope to the American College of Obstetricians and Gynecologists and they will provide a single copy of the following pamphlets free of charge:

Nutrition During Pregnancy
Car Safety for You and Your Baby
Especially for Fathers
Working During Your Pregnancy
Travel During Pregnancy
Special Needs for Pregnant Teens

The address is:
Resource Center
American College of Obstetricians and
   Gynecologists
409 Twelfth Street, S.W.
Washington, D.C. 20024
(202) 638–5577

Table 32   HOW LONG CAN WOMEN WORK DURING PREGNANCY?

Job Function	When You Should Stop Working (weeks of pregnancy from last menstrual period)
Secretarial, light clerical, professional, managerial	40 weeks
Seated: light tasks (prolonged or intermittent)	40 weeks
Standing	
Prolonged (>4 hrs)	24 weeks
Intermittent (>30 mins/hr)	32 weeks
(<30 mins/hr)	40 weeks
Stooping and bending below knee level	
Repetitive (>10 times/hr)	20 weeks
Intermittent (<10>2 times/hr)	28 weeks
(<2 times/hr)	40 weeks
Climbing vertical ladders and poles	
Repetitive (>4 times/8-hr shift)	20 weeks
Intermittent (<4 times/8-hr shift)	28 weeks
Climbing stairs	
Repetitive (>4 times/8-hr shift)	28 weeks
Intermittent (<4 times/8-hr shift)	40 weeks
Lifting	
Repetitive >50 lbs	20 weeks
<50>25 lbs	24 weeks
<25 lbs	40 weeks
Intermittent >50 lbs	30 weeks
<50>25 lbs	40 weeks
<25 lbs	40 weeks

Source: American Medical Association, Council on Scientific Affairs: Effects of pregnancy on work performance, 1983.

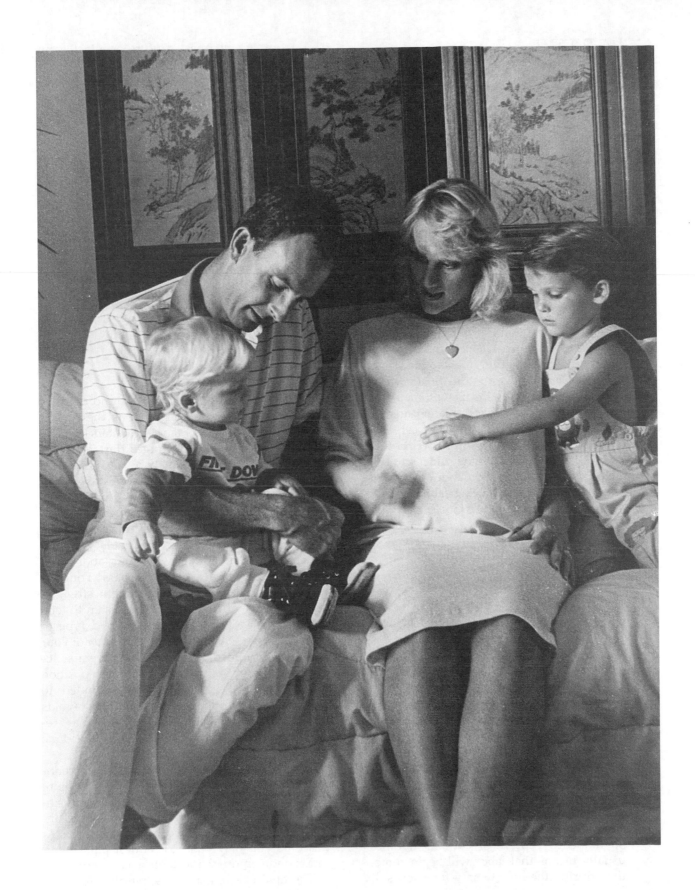

CHAPTER 17

Labor and Delivery

Labor is the process by which uterine contractions cause the cervix to dilate (become widened), allowing delivery of the baby. No one knows what causes these involuntary contractions to begin. Prior to labor the cervix undergoes a process (sometimes called *ripening*) in which it becomes thinner (*effaced*), more pliable, and slightly dilated. Dilation refers to the size of the cervical *opening*. During the final two or three prenatal visits, the clinician estimates by pelvic examination how much dilation and effacement have occurred. Even if your cervix is closed, labor can begin within twenty-four hours. Once the cervical opening widens to two to three centimeters, however, labor often starts within one or two days. During labor, uterine contractions will complete the process of cervical dilation, which must reach ten centimeters (about four inches) for vaginal delivery to occur.

How Do I Know When Labor Begins?

There are three signs that labor may soon begin:

1. You may notice a blood-tinged mucous discharge known as *bloody show*. This discharge means that the mucus plug sealing the bottom of the uterus has been dislodged. Labor often begins within twenty-four hours following bloody show.
2. Leakage of fluid from the vagina, in a constant trickle or a sudden gush, usually indicates rupture of the bag of waters. ("Waters" means simply the amniotic fluid surrounding the fetus during pregnancy.) Spontaneous rupture of your membranes usually means that labor will begin sometime during the next twenty-four hours. If your membranes rupture, contact your clinician.
3. Frequently, backache or painless abdominal tightening (*false labor*) indicates that labor will soon begin. These Braxton-Hicks contractions help prepare your uterus for real labor, which is characterized by regular, often painful contractions which occur initially at ten- to fifteen-minute intervals. As a general rule you should contact your clinician and prepare to leave for the hospital (or other birth setting) once these contractions become regular, occurring at least every ten minutes and lasting thirty seconds or longer. Table 110 in Chapter 83 explains differences between real labor and false labor.

Stages of Labor

There are three stages in the labor and delivery process. The first stage of labor is the time it takes the cervix to dilate ten centimeters (see Figure 22). The first stage averages thirteen hours in a woman having her first baby; in subsequent childbirths, this period is shorter, averaging about eight hours. This stage is divided into three phases: *early*, *active*, and *transition*. Often the *early* phase (up to three to four centimeters dilation) will not be too uncomfortable. Walking, watching TV, and talking with your labor coach (if you have one) help the time pass. Your clinician or a nurse will record the length, strength, and frequency of contractions and listen to fetal heart tones. Decisions on enemas and type of perineal shave will be made. The *position* of your baby is determined, and you may have a sonogram if the baby seems to be in a breech position (see Chapter 21). You may be reminded to empty your bladder frequently. This avoids bladder distention (stretching) which may require catheterization. Vaginal exams are done periodically between contractions.

During the *active* phase (four to seven centimeters), when contractions become more intense, you will rely more on breathing techniques to help relieve discomfort and need increased emotional support from your coach. At this time you may want to request pain medication or an epidural anesthetic (see Chapter 19).

The final phase, known as *transition* (eight to

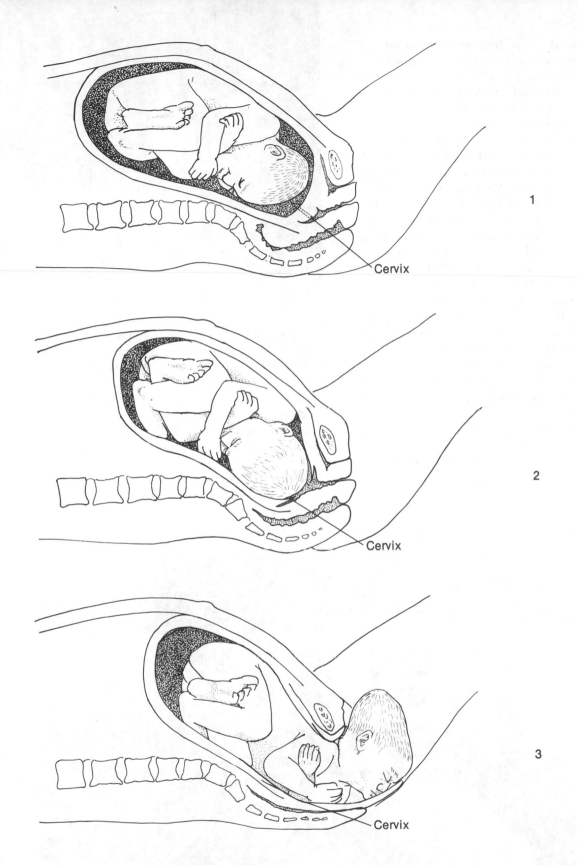

Figure 22 *Prior to labor the cervix is closed or slightly dilated (1). As labor begins, the cervix begins to dilate (2). For delivery to occur the cervix must be completely dilated (3).*

ten centimeters), is the time when most intense pressure and pain occur during contractions. This phase is the hardest but also the shortest part of labor; maintaining your breathing patterns may become difficult. You may want to "push" or bear down before you reach complete dilation (ten centimeters). You need the most support and encouragement from your coach at this time to help you stay in control. Once you are fully dilated, the hardest part is finished.

The second stage of labor begins when the cervix is completely dilated. The second stage usually lasts no more than an hour in a woman having her first baby and averages less than thirty minutes in subsequent childbirths. It ends when the baby is born. During this stage, you feel a tremendous urge to bear down and push the baby out. It can be a very satisfying experience to push with each of your contractions. Pushing lessens the contraction pains. If the birth setting and situation allow for it, you can observe your baby's head in a mirror as you push. If you have an epidural anesthetic, your coach or the nurse can feel your abdomen for the start of your next contraction and tell you when to push. If you have had no other anesthesia, either a local anesthetic or a pudendal block (see Chapter 19) is almost always used just prior to delivery.

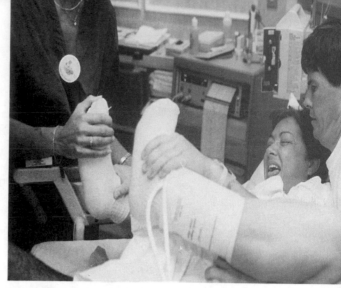

"Pushing" during the second stage of labor.

After the baby's head is pushed out, the baby may cry before being completely delivered. The baby's shoulders come next, followed quickly by the rest of the body. Your baby can be placed on your abdomen, where the cord is cut. Or the cord may be cut while the baby is still in the hands of the clinician. Mucus from the baby's mouth is quickly removed by a small suction bulb.

When you first see your newborn, don't be

Footprinting the newborn in the delivery room.

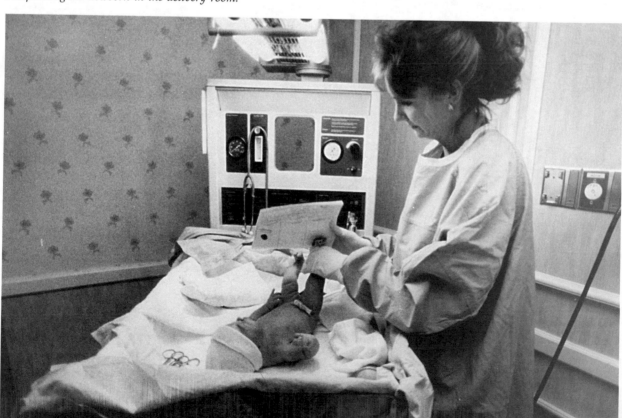

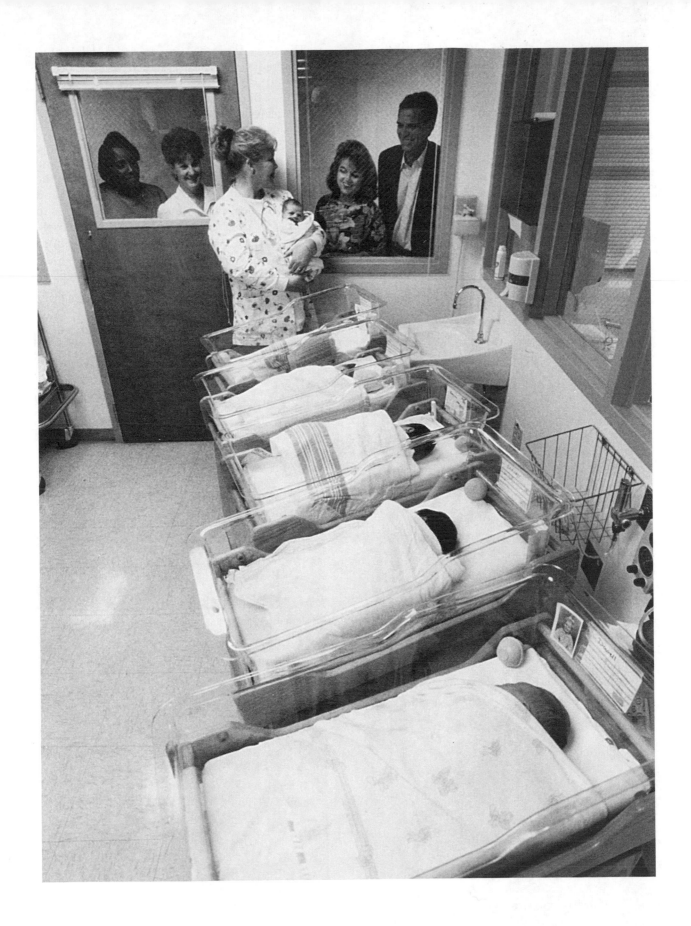

surprised if your baby doesn't look like the pictures you've seen in magazines. He or she may appear smaller and is usually wet looking and covered with a white, creamy substance called vernix. Normally a newborn's hands and feet may look blue. The baby's head may look strange—often swollen or elongated—a result of passing through the birth canal. This temporary condition is known as *molding*. Newborns seems so tiny and fragile; even the most experienced parents feel awkward in holding them. It's natural for you and the father or support coach to want to hold and touch your baby, to fully realize the reality of your having given birth. Childbirth is such an amazing process that it takes a while to absorb the experience.

The third stage of labor includes delivery of the placenta (afterbirth), which usually occurs within fifteen minutes after birth. The clinician examines the expelled placenta to make sure it is complete because any part left in the uterus may cause subsequent bleeding or infection. After delivery of the placenta and repair of any tears and the episiotomy, if performed, you are usually taken to a recovery area. There the nurses observe you closely for bleeding and other complications and massage your uterus to minimize blood loss. Your baby is also closely observed in the recovery area or in the newborn nursery. When you and your baby appear to be progressing without complications, you will be transferred to a room or allowed to go home, depending on your birth setting.

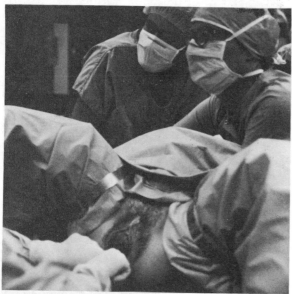

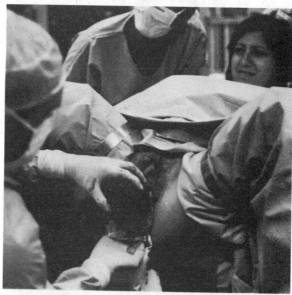

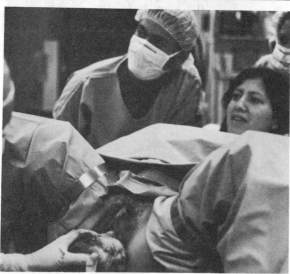

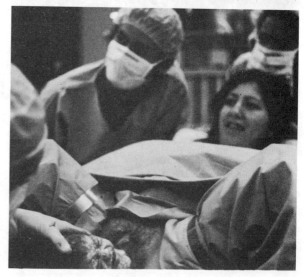

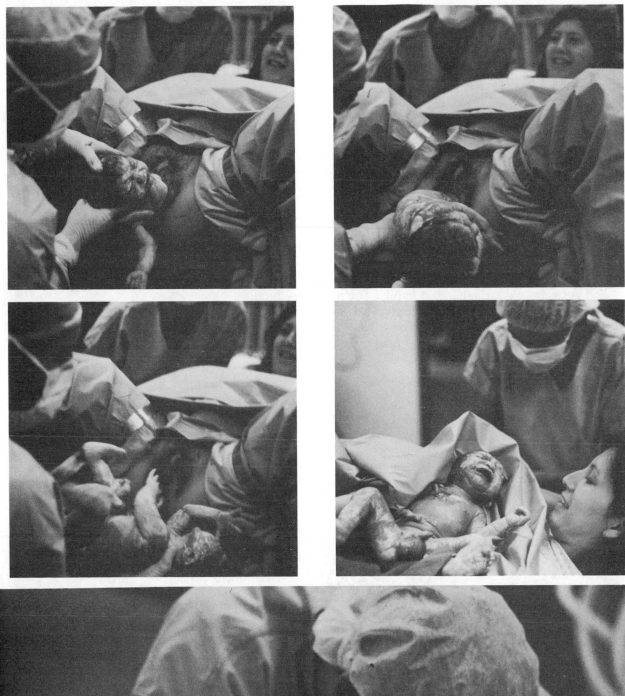
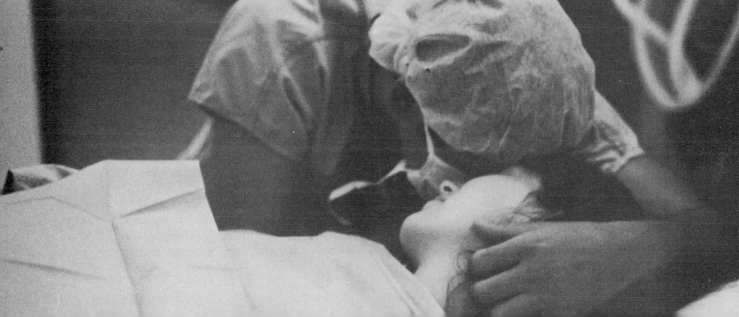

CHAPTER 18

Your First Weeks as a Mother

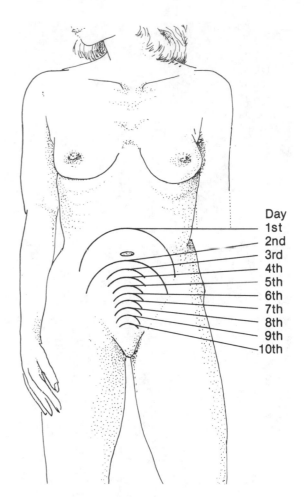

Birth climaxes months of waiting. With the birth of a first child, it transforms spouses into parents and converts a marriage into a family. The new mother undergoes changes in her physical state, feelings, and style of living. These first few weeks after your baby's birth are known as the

Figure 23
The location of the top of the uterus (fundus) during the first ten days after childbirth. After about a week the fundus can no longer be felt by pressing on the abdomen.

postpartum period. It may take several days after childbirth for a woman to feel she has regained control over the physical changes affecting her body. This chapter talks about what to expect physically and emotionally in the postpartum period.

Physiologic Changes

The uterus gradually returns to its nonpregnant size in a process called *involution,* which takes about six weeks (see Figure 23). The uterus continues to contract mildly following delivery, thereby controlling possible bleeding. Immediately after delivery, you can feel the top of the

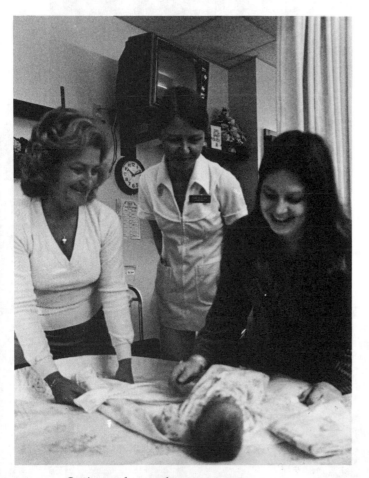

Getting ready to go home.

uterus (fundus) above your umbilicus (bellybutton). The fundus feels round and solid, somewhat like a grapefruit, for the first few days after you deliver. The nurse will press on your abdomen to check for the firmness of your uterus, and she may massage it to keep it firm in the first few hours after childbirth. You may be encouraged to massage the fundus, as well, to help prevent bleeding. The periodic cramping some women experience for a few days after having a baby is called *afterpains*. These uterine contractions are less common in women having their first baby and thus may come as a surprise to a woman having a subsequent child. These contractions after childbirth may feel especially strong during breast-feeding, which stimulates them.

If you have a cesarean birth, your body will undergo the usual changes that occur after a vaginal birth, plus the additional alterations required to recover from a major surgical operation. Recovery after a cesarean birth means that some added discomforts will accompany those associated with vaginal birth. While you won't have the perineal pain that goes with having an episiotomy, the incisional pain from stitches located under your abdominal scar is likely to be uncomfortable. Sometimes, especially with a midline incision, it is difficult to hold the baby and uncomfortable to breast-feed. Using supportive pillows or lying on one side may help. Talk to your physician about what physical exercises you can do in the postpartum period. It is a good idea to arrange for some help at home during the first few weeks, especially in running errands and doing the physical tasks that will be most difficult.

The abdominal wall muscles remain stretched following childbirth. When you first stand up after your delivery, the abdominal muscles will fall forward, pushed out somewhat by the uterus, giving you a slight still-pregnant appearance. This is very disappointing, especially if you had expected to be flat right away! In the next few days, your abdomen will begin to firm up; and with frequent postpartum exercise (see Chapter 49), you can be zipping up and buttoning your pants in about six weeks. Most women require a few months to return to their prepregnancy weight. You may want to wear a sup-

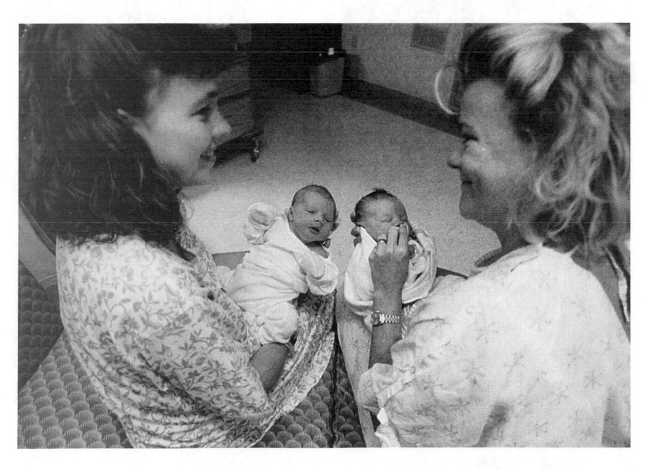

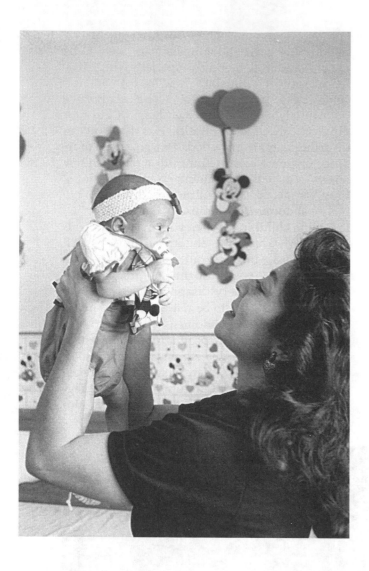

and in four months or so in women who do. Remember, it is possible to get pregnant before you menstruate, so use contraception as soon as you resume sexual intercourse. Couples vary as to when they resume sexual intercourse. Vaginal discomfort, physical fatigue, and lack of sexual interest due to demands of new parenthood are all factors. For help regarding breast engorgement or tenderness, see Chapters 57 and 59.

Many women worry about the discomfort of having their first bowel movement, which normally does not occur until a few days after delivery. This delay is usually a result of the lack of recent food intake or if you had an enema during labor. Stool softeners are frequently given after delivery; a laxative will also help. A nutritious diet of vegetables and fruit as well as plenty of fluids is also beneficial (see Chapters 16 and 48).

Your stitches may cause discomfort or itching for several weeks. Sitting on an inflatable cushion that is shaped like a doughnut or on a pillow helps to relieve direct pressure on your incision. Heat from a tub bath or heat lamp and a Tucks pad, a pre-moistened gauze pad (available in your drugstore), held in place by your sanitary napkin also help relieve the pain from stitches. When you go home, you may want to ask for pain medication; but remember, if you are breast-feeding, that the drug will pass into your milk (see Chapter 31). Ask your clinician for examples of postpartum exercises that will help to reduce your discomfort.

Adequate Rest and Sleep

A few hours after delivery, you will feel very tired, though excited from the delivery. It is important to continue to force yourself to rest so you won't become frustrated and irritated in taking care of your new baby. If you are breast-feeding but really exhausted, you might want to let the nurses feed the baby water through the night so that you can get some sleep. The baby mainly needs fluids at this time.

With the first baby it is easy to nap; but when older children are at home, it is very difficult. If possible, ask friends or relatives to help during the first few weeks so that you can rest. Involve the other family members in housekeeping chores by delegating some day-to-day tasks. Limit your visitors during the first few weeks. It

porting girdle initially to hold these muscles in, although it really isn't necessary.

Some women worry that if they begin walking too soon after delivery "everything will fall out." This isn't true; nor is the belief that walking increases vaginal bleeding true. Vaginal bleeding continues for three to six weeks after delivery. All women experience vaginal drainage called *lochia* for the first few days after childbirth. Normally this vaginal discharge changes in a few days from red or pink to brown or yellow. It is important to wash the vaginal area with warm water (usually from a squeeze bottle or pitcher) when you change your sanitary napkin or urinate. This helps to keep the area clean and reduces the chance of infection.

Women who breast-feed may not menstruate while they are nursing. Menstruation usually begins in two months in women who do not nurse

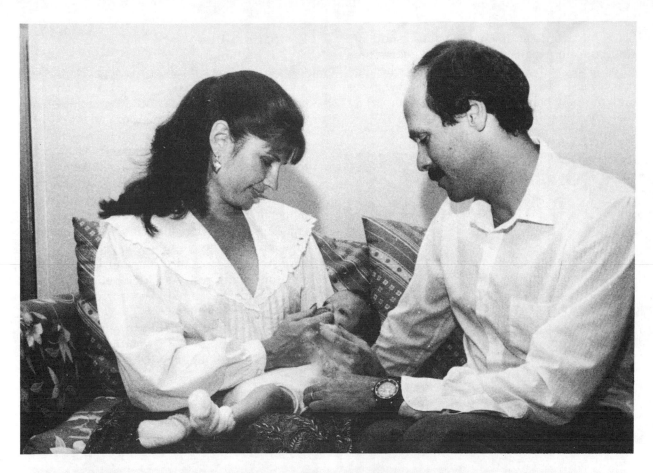

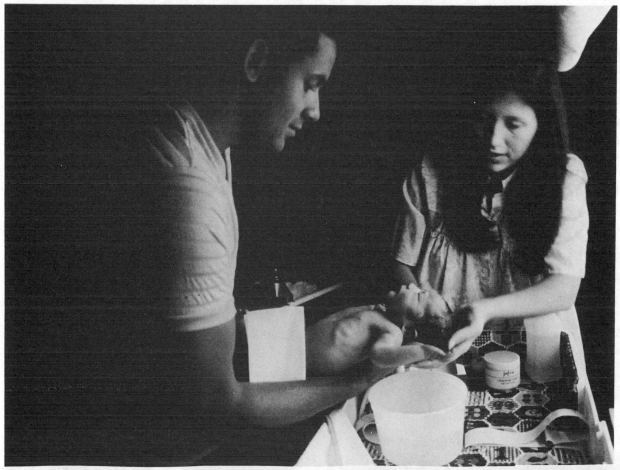

is easy to overdo at first, and you may suddenly find yourself exhausted. Arrange for some time to be alone with your husband. Remember that chronic sleep loss will make you less able to enjoy your new baby, and *you* are more important than the chores to be done.

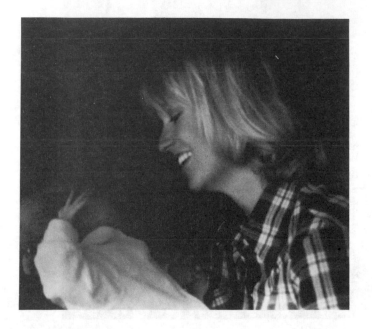

Postpartum Blues

Postpartum blues refers to the slight depression normally experienced by most woman after childbirth. The blues may occur as a letdown following the initial excitement of childbirth, or it may come three to six weeks later. These feelings may reflect changes in hormone levels after delivery or may be due to the realization of the reality of motherhood. Some women never acknowledge or experience any depression, while others find themselves crying frequently for several days. Most often, all that's needed is a little time for you and your family to get used to your new schedule, a chance for your body to heal, and some extra rest. Ask for emotional support from friends and family, and express your feelings and needs to them.

A new mother is often unprepared for how the baby will upset her former life style. She often finds herself juggling baby's needs, possibly older children's needs, and husband's needs while her own needs go unmet—no wonder she may get upset!

Ten to fifteen percent of women experience postpartum depression; it could occur with your

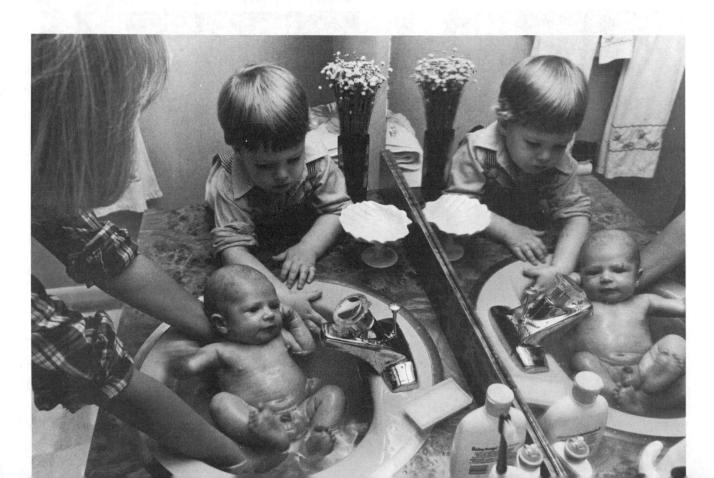

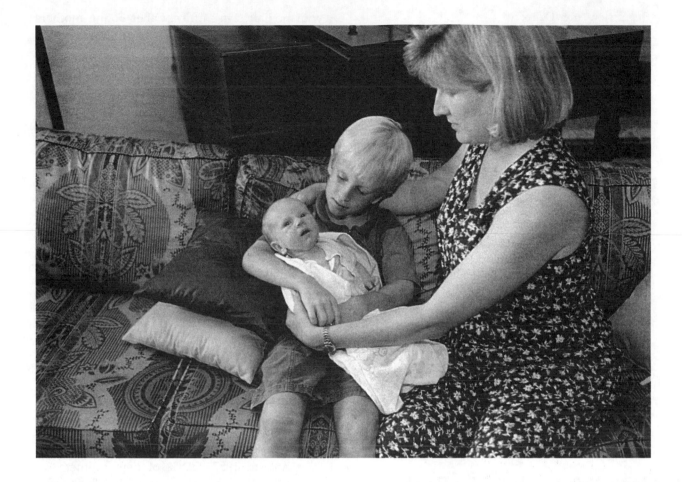

first child or your fifth. Women report guilt, crying, worry, changes in sleep patterns, or feeling they cannot care for their baby in the "right way." If extra rest and being with friends does not help, and you feel worse each day, talk to your physician. If you continue to feel depressed, unmotivated, and tired for no special reason, you may be suffering from postpartum depression. You may need emotional support through counseling. Women who have had a previous postpartum depression, or manic-depressive illness, are more at risk for developing postpartum depression. Having a difficult or prolonged birth, an unwanted pregnancy, or premature or ill infant also are risk factors. Call your clinician to ask for special help (see Chapter 62).

Table 33   HELPFUL ACTIVITIES FOR POSTPARTUM ADJUSTMENT

1. Obtaining experienced help for baby care
2. De-emphasizing tidiness in the home
3. Continued couple socializing outside the home, but on a less frequent basis
4. Increased availability of husband at home
5. No moving soon after the baby is born
6. Getting plenty of rest and sleep
7. Maintaining outside interests but at a reduced rate
8. Limiting outside responsibilities
9. Making friends with other couples who are experienced with young children
10. Planning and arranging for babysitters in advance
11. Avoiding people who make you feel drained or uncomfortable

---

Resources

Postpartum Support International
927 N. Kellogg Avenue
Santa Barbara, California 93111
(805) 967-7636

Depression After Delivery
P.O. Box 1282
Morrisville, Pennsylvania 19067
800-944-4773

Adjusting to the New Baby

Most women have unrealistic expectations for themselves and their behavior as mothers. Parenting behavior is learned—not instinctive—and our society provides few personal opportunities to learn about infant care until parenthood. It may take as long as a year to "feel like a mother" and adjust to your new role in life. And it also takes time for you to understand your newborn's needs. Each baby is so different! Baby-care classes are offered at most hospitals with obstetrical services, and the hospital nurses can help you with specific questions about caring for your baby. The American Red Cross offers parenting classes for parents of newborns. When you are at home, call your clinician's office if you need help or have questions. Your physician can refer you to a public health nurse if you need one. You could also call the nursery nurses if you have a question and, of course,

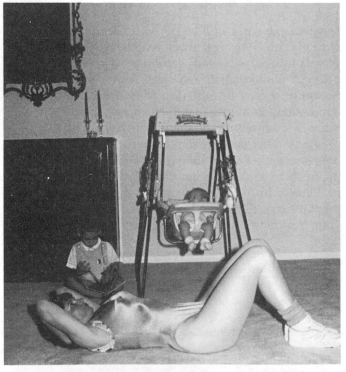

Finding time to exercise at home isn't always easy.

your pediatrician's office. Other young mothers or relatives with whom you are comfortable may be among your best resources.

Each family member has his or her own period of readjustment when the new baby arrives. New parenthood necessarily involves reduction of some nonfamily needs and interests, but don't let them all go. It is important to return after a few weeks to some outside activity that interests you. If you have stopped working, you may miss the loss of income as well as the social contacts involved in your job. The additional laundry and caretaking activities may seem overwhelming. You may find your husband or your other children, or both, more demanding, and this relationship may worry you. Your husband may feel an increased financial pressure now that he is a family man or now that there is an additional family member. Siblings, too, usually have mixed feelings about the attention paid to the new baby—although they may outwardly act otherwise. It is important to acknowledge these normal feelings in your other children. In time, with support and understanding, these stresses will resolve and your family will stabilize once again.

According to the Census Bureau, children today are more likely to have a working mother than not. In 1987, 50.8% of new mothers remained on the job, compared with 31% in 1976. Those mothers most likely to continue to work are college-educated women, those who have their first child after age thirty, black women, and widowed, separated, or divorced women. More than 40% of all married couples of childbearing age are "two-worker" families. Planning for child care after returning to work has now become a part of the childbirth experience. Women are asking for better-regulated childcare facilities and encourage planning for child care within the workplace. But many mothers, especially those living far from close relatives, find arrangements for child care are a constant cause of stress. High cost, insufficient government regulation, and lack of federal support for daycare have contributed to infant daycare problems. Live-in help, especially for young children, in the form of au pairs or college students, has become popular. Professional nannies and housekeepers are also in demand.

Some communities have organized parent discussion groups, baby classes, or support groups. Ask your physician or nurse what is available in your community. Parent-arranged baby-sitting co-ops or play groups are also helpful.

Pregnancy Loss

The loss of a baby through miscarriage, stillbirth, or illness has always been a devastating experience for both parents. Strong attachment to the baby begins early in pregnancy and is intensified by hearing the fetal heartbeat, observing the fetus through ultrasound, and feeling the unborn baby move. The grief following such a loss can be as great as that when a parent or older child dies.

Studies of grief and mourning indicate that a normal period of grieving is a necessary response to the loss and that the absence of such mourning is not a healthy sign but a cause for alarm. Couples who experience abortion, whether induced or spontaneous, often grieve as well. Following pregnancy loss, the initial response is usually one of shock and numbness. It is common to feel that it's a nightmare and really not happening. Disbelief, denial, loss of appetite, fatigue, heart flutters, and shortness of breath all are common reactions. Feelings of anger, loneliness, and emptiness are normal. Mothers particularly feel the loss as a physical one. As expressed by one mother, "I feel as if my arm has been cut off—as though a part of me has died." The authors experienced the loss of an infant daughter at ten days of age and were surprised at the acute pain and intensity of their feelings. Parental support groups, allowing for the sharing of common feelings with each other, help to ease the pain of such a loss. Parents need to realize their feelings are normal and that it's all right to express them to their family and friends. The grieving process may last anywhere from six months to two years or more.

The next stage of grief, the searching stage, encompasses feelings of guilt, hostility, anger, and emptiness. Self-examination for something the parents did to cause or could have done to prevent the death is common. Parental anger and disappointment expressed toward the hospital staff, toward religious beliefs, or to each other may occur. At this time it is important that parents recognize that they each grieve individually and that both may be feeling the same emotion expressed differently. As a consequence, they may not always be able to help each other. The disorientation phase is characterized by increased acceptance, leading toward the acknowledgment of the death. Depression and difficulty in returning to normal living patterns are commonly felt. Peer support groups are helpful at this time as well. The last stage, reorganization, is characterized by adaptation to the loss, an increase in energy, and a reinvestment in the normal activities and relationships of daily living. Though the pain is never completely gone, the loss has been integrated into the parents' lives and is no longer immobilizing. If you find you continue to feel depressed and unable to function, it is advisable to get professional help (see Chapter 62).

It has been found that involvement in the planning of the labor and delivery is helpful if you know in advance you are having a stillbirth.

Table 34   NORMAL GRIEF REACTIONS FOLLOWING THE LOSS OF A CHILD

1. Periods of crying for no apparent reason
2. Mood changes over the slightest things
3. Feeling guilty at times and angry at others
4. Wandering aimlessly around the house; forgetting and not finishing tasks
5. Feeling the loss isn't real, that it didn't actually happen
6. Experiencing difficulty in sleeping; dreaming of the baby
7. Wishing to have your baby back and searching for things you could have done to prevent the loss
8. Finding solace in a special attachment to something of the baby's, such as a blanket or the hat worn in the hospital
9. A feeling that part of you has been cut off—the part of you that was involved with your baby
10. Needing to tell and retell things about the baby and the experience of his or her death
11. Feeling the need to be protective of others who are uncomfortable by politely not talking about feelings of grief
12. Feeling heaviness in your chest or a tightness in your throat
13. Having an empty, aching feeling in the pit of your stomach and a loss of appetite
14. Decreased interest in sex
15. Later, feeling guilty when you forget about it and find you are enjoying an activity
16. Wanting to remember or include your baby's memory in family occasions or holidays

---

Seeing and holding your baby after its birth acknowledges the baby's reality. Ask for a private room after delivery. Pictures of the baby and hospital remembrances are usually treasured. You may wish to consider an autopsy to uncover the cause of death or ascertain that there are no congenital malformations. Planning a funeral for the baby helps parents to formally acknowledge the importance of their baby's life, however brief, and gives friends and family an opportunity to grieve and provide support. Telling siblings about the baby's death as soon as possible and arranging for them to see and hold the baby is also helpful.

Pregnancy loss is a difficult subject in our society where normal, healthy, successful pregnancies have become the expected results rather than hoped-for blessings; an unsuccessful outcome of pregnancy is a shock to everyone. If you have a friend who loses a baby, encourage her to talk about her feelings as much as possible rather than to deny the event. Only when feelings of grief have been dealt with can your friend become mobilized to reinvest in old activities and relationships. It is not helpful to return all the baby's things while the mother is in the hospital—let her do it when she is ready. Being there for emotional support and acceptance is what counts. In cases of multiple births, it is also important to recognize that having one healthy baby does not make up for the loss of the other(s). This situation is particularly difficult for mothers who are trying to bond and take care of one infant while mourning the loss of their other(s).

Many parents feel that they want to become pregnant again soon after a pregnancy loss. It has been found that it is most helpful to wait at least several months before trying to conceive again. Grief cannot be rushed; one baby cannot make up for the loss of another. Having another baby too soon can make it hard to appreciate the new child as a separate and special individual, and overprotectiveness of the second child may be the result if you do not allow yourself to recover from the first loss. Giving yourself time to grieve, planning for frequent exercise and physical activity, and maintaining important relationships all help in overcoming grief.

Resources

SHARE
St. Joseph's Health Center
300 First Capital Drive
St. Charles, Missouri 63301
800-821-6819

Pregnancy and Infant Loss Center
1421 E. Wayzata Boulevard, Suite 30
Wayzata, Minnesota 55391
(612) 473–9372

The Compassionate Friends, Inc.
National Headquarters
P.O. Box 3696
Oak Brook, Illinois 60522-3696
(708) 990–0010

Amend
c/o Maureen Connelly
4324 Berrywick Terrace
St. Louis, Missouri 63128
(314) 487–7582

CHAPTER 19

Options During and After Childbirth

This chapter discusses the possible options you can select from during and after your childbirth experience. As you read about these options, decide which are important to you, and ask your clinician which ones are permitted and encouraged in your birth setting. If there are procedures you wish to avoid—such as an IV (intravenous fluid) in early labor—you may need to sign a statement releasing the birthing facility from medical liability should complications arise. It is important that both you and whoever delivers your baby feel comfortable with the options you choose or eliminate.

After you have read this chapter, look over Table 36. If any of these questions concern you or you want to know more about these topics, be sure to discuss them with your clinician.

Optional Procedures During Early Labor

An enema, IV, and perineal shaving are not always performed automatically. Some of the pros and cons of these procedures are discussed below.

Enema

Routine enemas for women in labor began in an effort to decrease the chance of maternal and infant infection during delivery. If the rectum is not emptied prior to childbirth, feces may be un-controllably expelled at delivery. Some women feel more comfortable pushing at delivery if they know their rectum is empty.

An enema consists of a warm sudsy solution that is inserted into the rectum through a tube. The presence of this fluid stimulates a bowel movement. As the enema is administered, you may notice some mild discomfort from rectal pressure. You will use either the bedpan or the bathroom for expelling the solution. If you want to avoid an enema, ask your clinician during a prenatal visit about omitting this procedure. For many if not most women, this procedure is unnecessary.

IV (intravenous fluid)

Most physicians advise women, once labor has begun, not to eat, in order to prevent nausea. An IV may be inserted into a vein in your hand or arm to provide the fluid replacement you and your baby require during labor. A most important advantage of the IV is that it provides immediate access for drugs, fluid, or blood should an emergency occur.

The main disadvantage of an IV is that it limits your movement to some extent and may be uncomfortable during the insertion of the needle. If you are in early labor and want to write or walk around, you could ask the staff to delay IV insertion. Suggest placing the IV in the arm you are less likely to use, that is, your left arm if you are right-handed.

The prep (perineal shaving)

Although most physicians consider this procedure completely unnecessary, shaving the perineal area theoretically lessens the chance of infection stemming from contamination of the birth canal during childbirth. Its main practical advantage, however, is in allowing better visualization of the area for the clinician during repair of the episiotomy. There are some disadvantages to perineal shaving—itching may occur as the hair begins to grow back and razor nicks or abrasions may themselves be a source of infection. Where routine perineal shaving continues, its use may be a result of convenience or even ignorance of research concerning this practice. Discuss this with your clinician during a prenatal visit.

Drugs for Pain Relief in Labor and Delivery

Pain relief through drugs during labor are generally of two types: direct administration of painkillers (narcotics) or sedatives, and regional anesthesia in which a local anesthetic blocks pain sensation in a particular area of the body. For the relief of pain during delivery, there are five types of anesthetic available. These methods are summarized in Table 35.

Drugs used during labor

There are two types of pain relief used during labor. Both are described here.

Narcotics and sedatives: Sedatives, such as Seconal, may be used in early labor to decrease anxiety. Narcotics, such as Demerol, relieve pain in more advanced labor; these drugs decrease the perception of pain by acting on the central nervous system. Other effects may include euphoria, sleepiness, or restlessness. Sedatives and narcotics readily cross the placenta and, while having no apparent ill effects in usual dosages, can delay the newborn's ability to breathe fully. This occurs most often if the baby is born prematurely or has experienced *fetal distress* (see Chapter 21) during labor. Other possible short-term effects on newborns include decreased interest in breast-feeding, decreased temperature or muscle tone after delivery, and decreased responsiveness to visual and auditory stimuli. Research continues to focus on possible long-term problems in infants exposed to these and other anesthetic drugs during labor and delivery. These drugs appear to be safe, however, when used in recommended dosages and when pregnancy is not complicated by premature labor or signs of fetal distress.

Regional anesthetics: The two types of regional anesthetics used in labor are known as the *paracervical block* and *epidural anesthesia*. Both allow you to remain awake and be aware of your labor while experiencing little or no pain. Only minimal amounts of the drug reach the baby.

Paracervical block involves injection of a local anesthetic into the vaginal tissue around the cervix to block the nerves to the uterus. The physician performs paracervical block during the pelvic exam usually when you are dilated four or more centimeters. This method provides good pain relief for an hour or two and may be repeated. A separate anesthetic is needed at delivery since the paracervical block does not anesthetize the vagina. Fetal monitoring is recommended when the paracervical block is used since heart rate abnormalities occasionally occur briefly following this procedure. Because of this risk to the fetus and due to the need for repeated injections during labor, this technique is used for pain relief in only 5% of vaginal births.

Epidural anesthesia, one of the safest and most effective methods of pain relief, is usually performed by an anesthesiologist and thus may be available only at medical centers and large hospitals. Epidural anesthesia requires placement of a small tube into the outer covering of the spinal cord through which travel nerves that sense pain from the uterus. Local anesthetic medication injected through the tube relieves pain during both labor and delivery.

Like paracervical block, epidural anesthesia is considered good reason for electronic fetal monitoring since this procedure is occasionally associated with brief drops in the baby's heart rate during contractions. The epidural is usually administered when you reach four or more centimeters of cervical dilation. When properly performed, an epidural does not slow your contractions; but if administered too early, an epidural sometimes prolongs labor. Also, a high dose of an epidural in late labor may decrease the urge to push, increasing the need for a forceps delivery.

Drugs used during delivery

Anesthesia for delivery may be one of five different types, including the epidural already described. The other four are described below.

Spinal anesthesia, a form of regional anesthetic performed by the obstetrician or anesthesiologist, involves injection of a local anesthetic into the spinal canal that surrounds the spinal column. Anesthesia in the lower half of the body is thereby provided. With "saddle block" spinal anesthesia, the procedure produces anesthesia in that area of the body that would be in contact with a saddle during horseback riding. In other words with a saddle block, the anesthesia is restricted to the vulva and vagina and does not extend to the lower abdomen and legs. Compared to an epidural, spinal anesthesia is more likely to cause headaches and a drop in blood

Table 35   DRUG METHODS OF PAIN RELIEF IN LABOR AND DELIVERY

Method	When Given	Advantages	Disadvantages	Possible Effects on Baby
Sedative drugs (e.g., Seconal, Valium)	Early labor (1 to 3 cm. dilated)	Decreases anxiety	May cause drowsiness	Decreased initial responsiveness; respiratory problems (especially if premature)
Narcotic drugs (e.g., Demerol)	Active labor (after 3 cm. dilation usually)	Decreases pain at start of active labor without slowing contractions	Drowsiness during labor; may cause nausea and vomiting; pain relief using lower dosages may be minimal	Decreased initial responsiveness; respiratory problems (especially if premature)
Paracervical block	Active labor (after 3 cm. dilation usually)	Does not cause maternal or fetal sedation	Lasts only 1 to 2 hrs; not always effective	Occasional severe drop in fetal heart rate follows procedure (fetal monitoring recommended)
Epidural	Active labor (after 5 cm. dilation usually) or for cesarean section	Effective, safe anesthesia during labor and delivery	Requires trained personnel (usually anesthesiologist) so more expensive and less available than other methods; increased chance of forceps delivery	Occasional dips in fetal heart rate (fetal monitoring recommended)
Spinal	After completely dilated or at delivery	Effective, safe anesthesia for delivery	Risk of headaches (5%); increased chance of forceps delivery; increased chance of temporary drop in blood pressure	Drop in fetal heart rate may occur (especially in high-risk pregnancies)
Pudendal or local anesthesia	At delivery	Safe; provides relief of pain for episiotomy and from vaginal stretching at time of delivery; may be used with nitrous oxide (inhalation anesthetic)	No relief of uterine pain (from contractions)	Rare
General anesthesia	Rarely, except for cesarean section	Complete pain relief; fast anesthetic for an emergency delivery	Possible aspiration (vomiting into the lungs); no participation in delivery	Decreased initial responsiveness; respiratory problems (especially if premature)

pressure. This problem is usually solved by simply increasing your IV fluids. Despite disadvantages when compared to the epidural, the spinal remains a popular, rapid, and effective method of childbirth anesthesia. Since minimal amounts of drug reach the baby, fetal well-being can be assured by close monitoring of fetal heart rate and the mother's blood pressure.

A *pudendal anesthetic block*, administered by the clinician just prior to delivery, involves injecting a local anesthetic around the pudendal nerve, which supplies sensation to the lower vagina. This procedure, performed much like a paracervical block, anesthetizes the lower birth canal but does not eliminate the pain of contractions. Some clinicians combine a pudendal block with inhalation of nitrous oxide (so-called laughing gas). Brief exposure to this inhalation anesthetic is considered safe since low concentrations are used. Along with pain relief, nitrous oxide may produce temporary euphoria or confusion. This is why most women prefer to use breathing techniques rather than nitrous oxide to supplement the pudendal block during delivery.

Local anesthesia involves injecting a small amount of local anesthetic directly into the vaginal opening. The anesthetic effect is only slightly less than a pudendal block. Except for rare instances of allergy to local anesthetics, local and pudendal techniques provide safe methods of delivery anesthesia for both mother and baby.

General anesthesia is rarely used for vaginal deliveries today because of the greater risk of breathing difficulties in the newborn and the high maternal risks associated with aspiration (vomiting into the lungs). In emergency situations, however, general anesthesia is often the method of choice especially when immediate delivery is needed. In this situation, the mother can be put to sleep in a matter of seconds, allowing prompt intervention which may be lifesaving to the baby.

Over the last several decades, epidural anesthesia and lower drug dosages have made childbirth pain relief much safer than previously. As a result, the view that natural childbirth should exclude all medication is questioned by some childbirth educators. While some educators in the women's health movement feel that doctors are still too quick to use medications in labor and women are too quick to ask for them, others support the administration of some pain relievers, like epidural anesthesia, that allow a woman to participate actively in her labor. Most hospitals with family-centered policies offer both medical and nonmedical approaches toward childbirth pain relief. According to this view, Lamaze-prepared childbirth and epidural anesthesia, for example, can, and should be, complementary rather than competing techniques. In our experience, a combination of the two offers an optimal way of providing safe, effective childbirth pain relief for many patients.

Fetal Monitoring

Electronic fetal monitoring (EFM), once considered one of the most important advances in modern obstetrics, is currently undergoing reevaluation. While most obstetricians have been taught that fetal monitoring contributes greatly to fetal safety during labor, the use of routine monitoring has been controversial for a number of years. As early as 1979, a National Institutes of Health task force concluded that routine electronic fetal monitoring is not justified in low-risk pregnancies. Subsequently, medical professionals and consumers alike have pointed to EFM as one (although not a major) cause of higher C-section rates. In 1989, the American College of Obstetricians and Gynecologists (ACOG) concluded that routine EFM was not always necessary—even in high-risk pregnancies—as long as the physician or nurse listened to the fetal heart at appropriate intervals, using a fetoscope (a stethoscope for listening to the baby's heart) or doptone (see glossary). In arriving at this conclusion, ACOG reviewed eight major studies, including data on more than 50,000 deliveries. In six of the studies, the outcome was no different whether monitoring or auscultation (the use of either a fetoscope or doptone) was used. In the other two studies, blood oxygen levels were slightly better in the monitored group in one, while in the other, the monitored group had a slightly lower rate of seizures. How ACOG's new position on fetal monitoring will affect the use of EFM in actual practice is hard to say. While most physicians and many patients are very comfortable with the procedure, electronic monitoring appears to be an option over which couples soon will have greater control.

EFM continuously records the infant's heart activity as well as the frequency and duration of uterine contractions. There are two types of fetal monitoring: external and internal. One or the other may be used.

During *internal* fetal monitoring, a small wire electrode is attached to the fetal scalp to record fetal heart activity (see Figure 24). A second device, a thin, plastic tube, is passed into the uterine cavity to measure uterine contractions.

The *external* monitor consists of two straps placed around the woman's abdomen. The upper belt holds a device which measures the frequency and length of uterine contractions; the lower strap monitors the fetal heart rate. The two belts may have to be adjusted frequently during labor and may be slightly uncomfortable. External monitoring has the advantage of avoiding uterine or fetal scalp infections which occasionally occur with internal monitoring. The external monitor, however, may not record the fetal heart tracing clearly when mother or baby moves. For this reason, internal monitoring is preferred if there is any question of fetal heart abnormality.

Whether the internal or external monitor is used, it is attached to a machine next to your bed. This machine prints out a recording of fetal heart rate and uterine contractions. By looking at this paper, you can see when a contraction begins before you even feel it. The normal fetal heart rate ranges between 120 and 160 beats per minute. A heart rate slightly below or above these rates does not necessarily indicate fetal distress. The condition of the fetus is better judged by other aspects of the tracing, especially patterns in which the heart rate rises or falls during contractions. Both physicians and nurses recognize which patterns may indicate fetal distress. Figure 25 shows a typical "normal" or reassuring fetal heart and uterine contraction pattern. Figure 26 depicts an "abnormal" or nonreassuring tracing in which the fetal heart rate drops (decelerates) briefly during and after each contraction. This pattern, known as *late decelerations*, indicates that the fetus may not be getting enough oxygen. There are no known dangers in using external monitoring and only minimal risks with the internal monitor (mainly fetal and uterine infection).

Some women feel that the monitor distracts their clinician or labor coach away from more

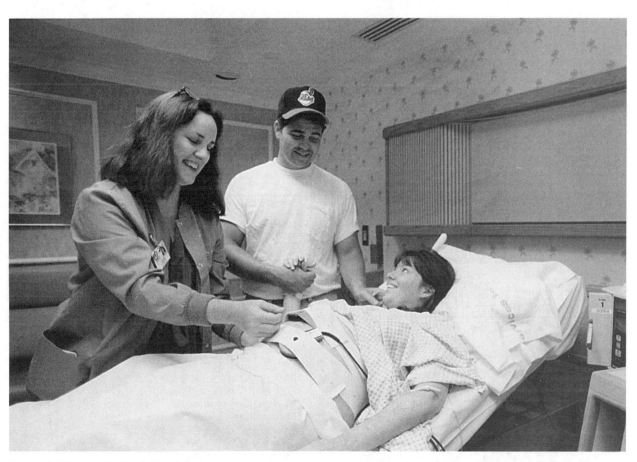

External fetal monitoring during labor.

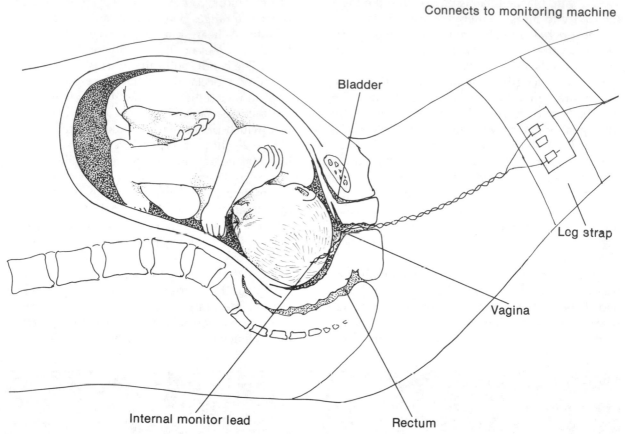

Figure 24 *Fetal monitoring. The internal fetal monitor attaches to the fetal head. The other end of the lead attaches to the monitoring machine, which records the fetal heartbeat.*

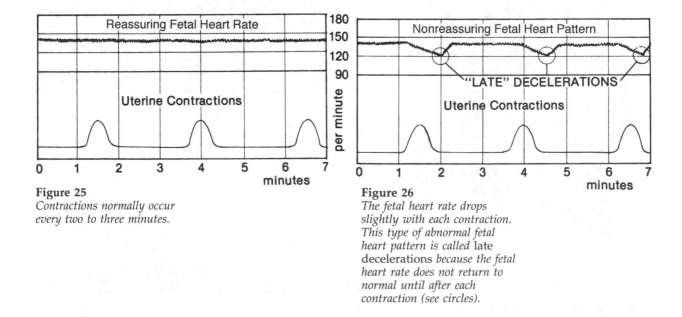

Figure 25
Contractions normally occur every two to three minutes.

Figure 26
The fetal heart rate drops slightly with each contraction. This type of abnormal fetal heart pattern is called late decelerations *because the fetal heart rate does not return to normal until after each contraction (see circles).*

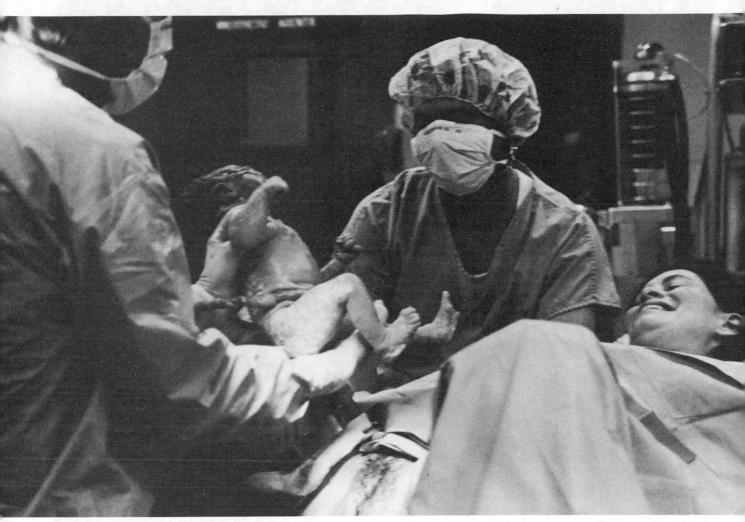

Father-attended birth.

Father-attended cesarean birth.

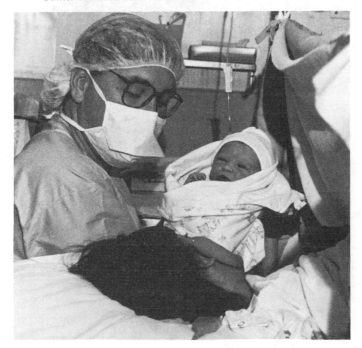

direct participation in her care. Some see the monitor as highly restrictive (because of interference with movement) and an infringement on their control of the labor situation. Others view monitoring as beneficial in lessening anxiety about the baby's condition. Some couples participating in prepared childbirth use the monitor as a second "coach" which helps in timing breathing techniques.

Positions for Labor and Delivery

From the viewpoint of a woman's body structure, the squatting position offers the least resistance to the baby about to be born. Women delivering in many primitive cultures naturally assume a vertical squatting position. Hospitals approximate this position by having the woman

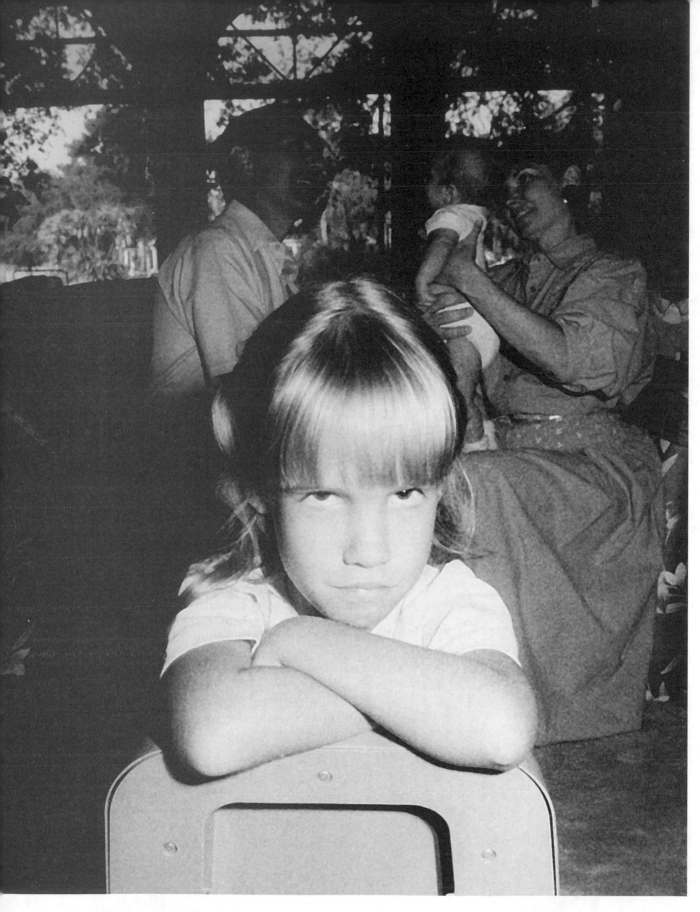

lie on her back with her legs resting in stirrups. While convenient for physicians and nurses to examine the woman in labor, this position is not the most beneficial physiologically. A woman lying on her back is more likely to experience hypotension (low blood pressure) as the pregnant uterus compresses the large blood vessels near the heart, and even a small drop in blood pressure may mean that less blood (and oxygen) reaches the baby. In many delivery rooms, the nurses encourage the mother to sit up and pull back on her knees while pushing. Most hospital labor beds can be cranked into the sitting position so you can assume a near squatting position during labor.

Despite widespread discussion of different labor positions, the fact that there is not much data makes it difficult to conclude which position will be best for you and safest for your baby. You should find the position which is most comfortable whether it is sitting, squatting, or lying flat. Obviously certain limitations may be imposed by such factors as fetal monitoring, blood pressure cuffs, and so on. As a general rule, avoid lying on your back for long periods (although it can't be helped when pushing during delivery). If the baby has any difficulties such as fetal distress, many authorities recommend lying on your left side to maximize good circulation to the fetus.

Father-attended Birth

Childbirth educators stress the importance of having the baby's father present during labor and immediately after birth when father-child attachment (see Bonding, discussed later in this chapter) should begin. Hospitals now routinely allow the father in the delivery room with childbirth education classes as a prerequisite. The father can offer special support to the laboring mother; still, some women feel more comfortable not having their husband present.

Fathers now also attend most cesarean births. The mother has an epidural anesthetic so that she and her husband may share the first moments after delivery. Most hospitals don't allow fathers to be present if a general anesthetic is used. Support groups have become popular throughout the United States to promote father attendance at cesareans. Special classes for prep-

aration for cesarean childbirth are now available in most communities.

When circumstances prevent the father from being present at childbirth, often another "significant other," such as a good friend or mother, can act as your labor support person. Recently, the concept of a "Doula," a labor support person specifically trained for this task, has developed across the United States. At times Doulas may help both mother and father maximize the labor and delivery experience.

Inclusion of Siblings in the Birth Experience

With increasing emphasis on birth as a family event, more parents want their children to share in the labor and delivery experience. This may be an important reason for couples to choose a home or birth center setting over a hospital for childbirth. The response of children witnessing childbirth depends upon their age, family attitudes toward childbearing, and the manner of preparing the child for what will happen. The few studies that have been done on sibling-attended birth have stressed adequate preparation as the key to making this a positive experience. Studies indicate that most children react positively and with varying degrees of interest to

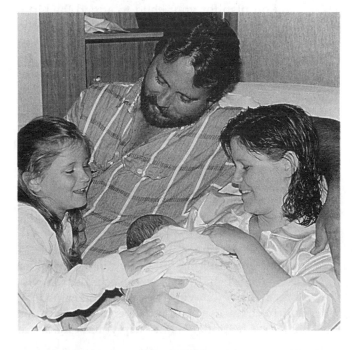

the experience. Children should not be forced to attend a birth if they do not wish it. Anderson (see reference list at the end of this section) feels that all children need to participate as much as possible in the birth of a sibling. Other researchers stress the importance of allowing children to see their mother promptly *after* delivery. If your child or children aren't allowed to visit you, be certain to talk with them on the phone and reassure them that you are all right.

Whether or not you choose to have siblings at the actual birth, their preparation for the arrival of a new baby is important. Tell a child as soon as possible about the anticipated sibling. Explore his feelings, especially the negative ones, often. Accept his feeling that it will be difficult for him to share his parents and his home with the new child and reassure him that you will be there to listen and help him handle the situation. Visit the library for books about new babies and older brothers and sisters to help your child anticipate these feelings. Take your child to at least one prenatal visit where he can hear the heart beat. If you have a sonogram, bring your other children along. Older children, especially, enjoy watching the sonogram and having their own "picture" of their baby. If possible, visit a family with a new baby so your child can see how tiny a newborn will be. Tell about how all babies cry and need to sleep and eat often; explain that the newborn won't be an ideal playmate immediately!

If you plan for your child to attend the birth, show him movies, books, or slides (preferably, in color) about childbirth. Pay particular attention to the blood that will be noticed on both the mother and baby and to the working sounds of childbirth, which could be frightening to your child if he is not prepared. Explain how the umbilical cord will be cut and that it won't hurt mother or baby. Show your child pictures of you when you were pregnant with him and pictures of his birth if available. Have a caretaker at the birth whose job it is to explain what is happening to the child and to meet his needs.

Many parents buy a special toy for the older sibling and give it to him as a gift from the new baby. Some parents stock small items such as crayons and coloring books to give to the older child when the new baby receives gifts from visitors at home. Buying the preschooler a baby doll to dress, wash, and diaper along with his mother is helpful. Let him help you fix the space

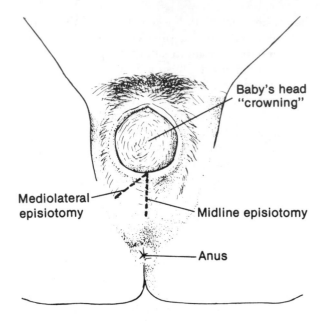

Figure 27
Types of episiotomy.

for the newborn, and make certain he still has his own private area at home.

Even the most careful preparation can still not be enough for the young child to understand what is about to happen. One three-year-old told us, "Yes, my mother's going to get a baby. They're on sale at the hospital. I saw them in the window there."

Episiotomy

An episiotomy is an incision that enlarges the vaginal opening for the delivery of the baby. This incision is made when the baby's head is visible at the vaginal opening and the perineum is well distended or stretched. When it appears that the lower part of the vagina is not stretching adequately and a large peritoneal tear may result, an episiotomy is done. Sometimes a laceration (tearing) occurs during childbirth at the place where an episiotomy would be made, especially if the baby is large. The need for an episiotomy may be lessened by patience (on the physician's part) and by performing regular exercises during pregnancy to stretch the perineum. Some physicians recommend having your husband insert two fingers about an inch inside the vagina and, with the help of a lubricant, exert firm downward pressure while making a sweeping motion from side to side. When done several times a week during the last few weeks of pregnancy, such stretching may prevent the need for an episiotomy or make a smaller one possible.

Many childbirth educators and an increasing number of physicians question the practice of performing episiotomies routinely for childbirth.

Some physicians routinely use an episiotomy in a woman having her first baby because of the greater chance of tearing. This is unnecessary as a routine procedure, and it is difficult to prove whether this approach actually prevents such problems as a "dropped" uterus (uterine prolapse) later. You may want to ask your physician to perform an episiotomy only if he or she feels a tear is inevitable.

There are two types of episiotomy: *midline* and *mediolateral* (see Figure 27). If you do have to have an episiotomy, ask your physician to use the midline type because it heals more easily and causes much less discomfort.

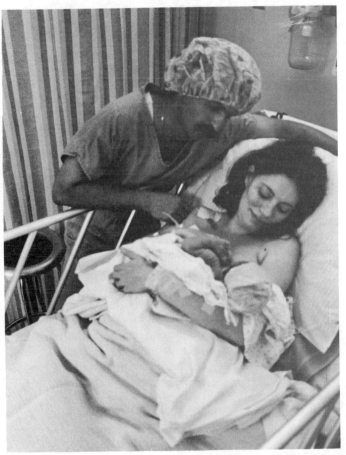

Parents and newborn share the first moments after childbirth as part of the bonding process.

Infant Massage

Infant massage has become an increasingly popular technique to enhance the parent-baby bond. The International Association of Infant Massage was founded in 1981. Vimala Schneider McClure observed the daily massage of infants while traveling in India and began massaging her own babies upon her return to the United States. She recorded her personal observations and wrote *Infant Massage*, a handbook for loving parents, in 1977. Currently there are 1,000 Certified Infant Massage Instructors (CIMIs) in the United States.

Infant massage can be taught as part of a childbirth education class or separately. This practice can begin immediately after birth, and the technique emphasizes that babies are aware human beings who deserve tenderness, warmth, respect, and compassion through touch and a nurturing attitude. Although infant massage was originally designed for healthy babies and their care givers, instructors are branching out to special-needs populations as well. Currently some licensed massage therapists have become interested in utilizing massage through both pregnancy and labor. For information regarding a trainer or an instructor near you contact:

The International Association of Infant Massage Resource Center
2350 Bowen Road, P.O. Box 438
Elma, New York 14059-0438
1-800-248-5432

Bonding

Bonding refers to the internal process by which a mother or father forms a loving relationship with her or his offspring. It may begin when a mother first feels her baby move or the first time a father-to-be hears the fetal heartbeat. Or bonding may begin during or after childbirth. Although parents want to love their new baby right away, he or she is a little stranger to them, and it takes a while for each to get to know the other, to feel comfortable, and to develop love. "Mother's instinct" refers to a woman's natural desire to nurture and care for her baby. It is often through caring for the newborn that bonding, or feeling love toward the child, develops.

The first hour after birth is an especially critical time for bonding. Klaus and Kennell (see ref-

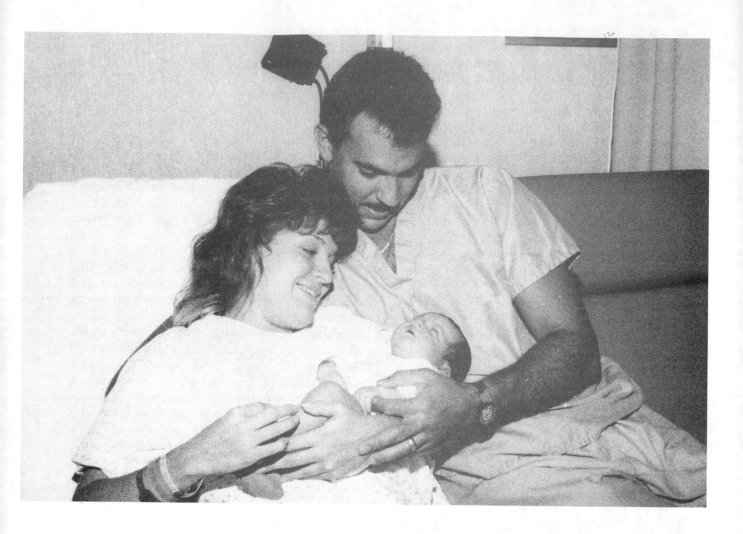

erence list at the end of this section) call this time the "early sensitive period" when mother and infant are mutually receptive to each other. At this time most babies are active and able to focus well on their surroundings. The mother is feeling happy with completion of childbirth and anxious to get to know her newborn. As the mother and father touch, kiss, hold, and care for their baby, they begin to become attached to the infant. Watching the child respond to caresses and having eye-to-eye contact with the baby evokes the stirrings of parental love. Though no one knows what a newborn feels, the baby seems to look closely at his or her parents and to enjoy close contact with them.

The idea of bonding is as old as childbirth itself. In years past, when home births were common, the bonding experience between parents and child occurred naturally and often encompassed the entire family. Today many hospitals encourage parents to spend the first

hour or two after delivery with their newborn. In fact, the American Medical Association endorses the concept of providing a bonding experience for the new mother and her newborn baby.

Awareness of the possible significance of bonding began in the intensive care nursery. Through various follow-up studies, researchers discovered that a higher rate of child abuse existed among parents of prematurely born infants with prolonged hospitalization (and decreased maternal contact) than among parents of healthy newborns. Whether or not a postpartum bonding experience has permanent beneficial effects on the newborn or on the parents is still debated. Nevertheless, an early bonding experience between parents and child is becoming more and more popular and is an important element in a more humanistic, family-centered approach to childbirth.

Siblings are encouraged to begin the bonding

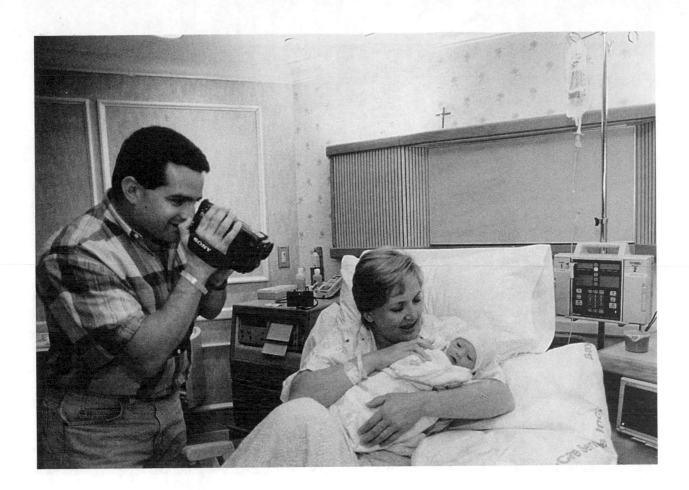

process as soon after childbirth as possible, through seeing or touching the newborn. This is important for premature infants as well; siblings can see the infant in the nursery. Bonding in multiple births is more difficult and requires more time from the parents. Klaus and Kennell have found that parents of multiple births usually bond first to one child and need to be encouraged to spend bonding time with each of the other infants as well. When one infant is seriously ill and demands more attention from the parents, they will more quickly bond to that child.

Bonding is an option to discuss with your clinician prior to labor. For the maximum effect of bonding, the child should receive antibiotic eye ointment *after* the bonding experience, because the ointment clouds the baby's vision and his or her ability to see the parents. When there is no evidence of maternal venereal disease, this delay will not harm the infant. For more information about bonding read *Parent-Infant Bonding* by M. H. Klaus and J. H. Kennell.

Breast-feeding

The American Academy of Pediatrics strongly recommends breast-feeding for all infants during the first four to six months of life. More and more women have been breast-feeding in the last decade probably because numerous studies indicate that breast milk is nutritionally superior to manufactured formulas or cow's milk. Breast-feeding is especially important for the premature or low-birth-weight infant who has special nutritional needs. In addition, breast milk has antibodies that help protect your infant against infection until he or she can produce his or her own antibodies (at about six months of age).

If you decide to breast-feed your baby, there are several things you can do in preparation. You'll need several supportive nursing bras to wear during the latter part of pregnancy and for nursing, because your breasts will be increased in size as long as you nurse. Once you stop nursing, your breasts will return to normal size or

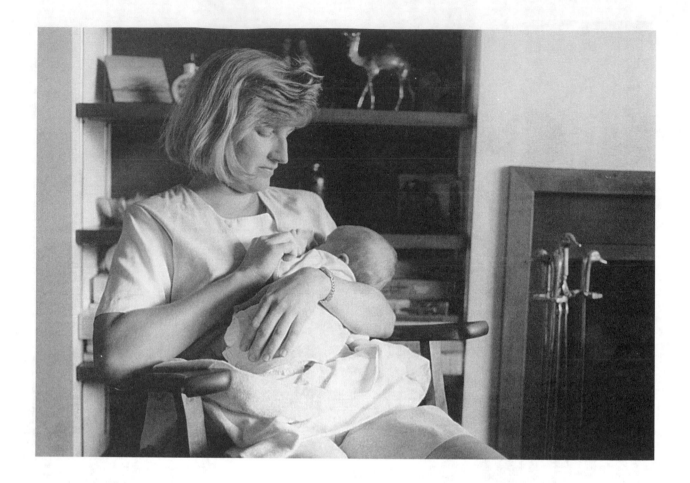

only slightly larger than before pregnancy. During the last two months of pregnancy, rub your nipples with a rough towel after bathing, and periodically massage your nipples between your thumb and forefinger to help toughen them for breast-feeding. Breast cream or A and D Ointment applied daily will help to prevent dryness around the nipple. Even before childbirth, your breasts may leak enough fluid to require the use of breast pads.

When you begin nursing, you can continue eating the same well-balanced diet as you did throughout pregnancy, although you need to increase your fluid intake to a total of two or three quarts per day. At least one quart (four 8-oz. glasses) of these fluids should consist of whole or low-fat milk or skim milk for extra protein and calcium (see Chapter 16, Pregnancy). If you don't like milk, substitute another dairy product, such as yogurt, cheese, or ice cream. Producing milk takes extra energy, so make an effort to get enough rest. Emotional tension may temporarily decrease your milk flow but will not affect its

quality. See Chapter 31 for discussion of drugs and breast-feeding.

Begin nursing gradually to prevent sore nipples. Feed your baby on demand, but no more often than every two hours. Don't be surprised if it takes a few days to establish a regular breast-feeding schedule. Relax. It *will* happen. A newborn takes three or four hours to empty his or her stomach and will naturally regulate himself or herself to a schedule. Fortunately, infants eat more frequently during the day and less often at night. Alternate breasts and gradually build up to nursing no longer than ten minutes on the first breast and twenty minutes on the other. If your baby does not want to nurse twenty minutes on the second side, don't worry, because the baby sucks harder on the first side, getting about ninety percent of the milk in that breast in five to ten minutes. A pacifier may be helpful for babies who want to suck longer than twenty minutes. Release the baby from your breast by inserting your forefinger between the baby's mouth and your breast. Remember that

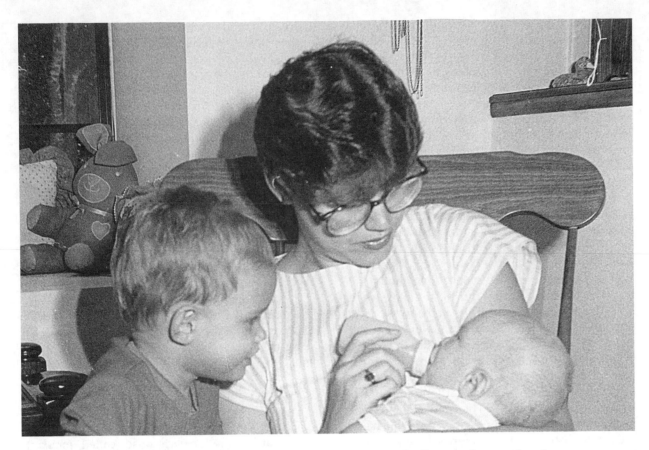

your baby will get enough milk because whenever your infant sucks more, your breasts produce more milk.

Some working mothers breast-feed by using a breast pump or hand-expressing their milk during lunch hour to provide milk for the child's feedings when they are away from home. Breast milk can be safely stored in a refrigerator for forty-eight hours. Other mothers use formula milk when they are not at home to breast-feed their babies themselves. The working mother and other mothers often find total breast-feeding very demanding, and it is important to work out an arrangement that is comfortable for you. Some mothers have their babies fed jello-water (ungelled gelatin and water mixture), sugar water, or Gatorade rather than formula for the feeding when they are not with the babies. Some mothers use these liquids when they feel their baby is thirsty as opposed to hungry. Discuss this situation with your pediatrician and decide what best meets your family's needs. There are many resources, such as the La Leche League, that help breast-feeding mothers. For information about the La Leche League consult your telephone directory or write to:

La Leche League International
1400 N. Meacham Road
Schaumburg, Illinois 60173

International Lactation Consultants Association (ILCA)
200 N. Michigan Avenue
Chicago, Illinois 60101
(312) 541-1710

Bottle Feeding

Despite the current popularity and benefits of breast-feeding, bottle feeding is preferred by many mothers. The advent of disposable bottles, bottle liners, and nipples have made bottle feeding easier now than ever before. Today's manufactured formulas are safe and, if used properly, will keep your baby strong and healthy. A particular advantage of bottle feeding is that anyone can feed the baby, thereby freeing the mother for other activities. The mother who bottle feeds often feels satisfied that her child is getting adequate nutrition because she knows exactly how much formula the baby takes.

Pediatricians differ in their approach toward bottle sterilization, tending more toward "clean" as opposed to "sterile." Cleaning and rinsing the bottles thoroughly and washing or perhaps boiling the nipples is adequate for formula preparation. Some pediatricians still insist that bottles be sterilized for the first three months of the baby's life. You can buy formula as powdered milk formula (the cheapest), concentrated formula, or ready-to-use formula. All of these are easy to prepare for individual bottles.

It is better to avoid propping up a bottle because the infant may choke on the formula while lying on his or her back. Besides, the comfort the baby feels from being held close to you while you feed him or her is also very important.

It is a demanding experience for a mother to feed her new baby often during the day. As in breast-feeding, try to keep the baby awake long enough to complete the feeding. Newborns fall asleep easily after feeding. Make sure the nipple is not clogged. Feed your baby no more often than every two hours and preferably every three or four hours since it takes that long for the baby's stomach to empty. The baby will let you know when he or she is hungry and will naturally establish his or her own schedule. Newborns should be fed formula for the first four to six months of age, as this is the nutrient best absorbed in the intestinal tract. After six months, you can start your baby on solids, but be sure to keep the baby on formula (rather than whole cow's milk) throughout the first year.

Rooming-in

Rooming-in, now available in most hospitals, means that the baby stays in the mother's room where she can provide care and feeding on demand. The baby's crib may be at the mother's bedside or in a nursery nearby. With rooming-in, the father usually has unrestricted visiting privileges, and some institutions allow grandparents and siblings to hold and feed the baby as well. Ideally, rooming-in is available twenty-four hours a day though the mother may return the baby to the nursery whenever she needs to rest or wants to see visitors (called partial rooming-in).

Rooming-in programs stress parent education. A nurse usually works closely with the family, offering advice and support in newborn care. The mother practices bathing her baby and other skills, such as taking the baby's temperature, in this reassuring environment. Rooming-in promotes bonding and prepares the mother for what to expect at home. The experience is often more popular with first-time mothers who are anxious to learn all they can, although some second-time mothers eagerly approach rooming-in as the only time they will have alone with their new child unhampered by older children at home.

Opponents of rooming-in say it is hard on mothers who are already exhausted after labor and delivery. They feel the mother needs the time now to rest and will have plenty of time to learn to care for the baby at home. New parents sometimes resent paying the high cost of hospitalization and then doing all of the baby care themselves. Mothers who already have one child may welcome their hospital stay as a chance to rest and take a break from child care.

Circumcision

Circumcision (a "cutting around") is the surgical removal of the *prepuce* (also called *foreskin*), which is the loose skin around the head of the male newborn's penis. The prepuce protects the meatus, which is the opening into the urethra, the tube through which urine passes from the bladder. When the prepuce is removed through circumcision, the glans is exposed and is therefore easier to clean. As the uncircumcised male grows and the penis develops, the foreskin eventually separates naturally from the glans. At this time the skin can be gently pulled back and effective hygiene accomplished.

While not a routine procedure, circumcision is still widely performed, largely due to tradition: about 70% of American male newborns are circumcised. In early 1989, a task force of the American Academy of Pediatrics issued a new statement on circumcision, suggesting possible medical benefits from the procedure. This report represents a dramatic change for the Academy, which for the past eighteen years has deemed circumcision medically unnecessary. However, current research indicates that uncircumcised newborns are more than ten times as likely as circumcised newborns to get urinary tract infections. The report also confirmed previous studies that showed that cancer of the penis, which affects one in 100,000 males, occurs almost entirely among uncircumcised men.

While these medical findings appear well documented, the role of circumcision in protecting against sexually transmitted diseases is less certain. Although some reports have found that various sexually transmitted diseases, including syphilis, human papilloma virus, genital herpes, and AIDS, are more frequent in uncircumcised males, these reports have statistical problems that make them inconclusive.

The relationship between circumcision and cervical cancer in women is also unclear. Previously, the theory that circumcision protects against cancer of the cervix has been firmly disputed. However, recent studies suggesting higher rates of precancerous conditions, like genital herpes and papilloma virus infections, in uncircumcised men have again raised the question of whether sexual contact with an uncircumcised male is a risk factor for this form of cancer.

Aside from medical and hygienic considerations, there are also social and religious reasons that some parents choose infant circumcision. Sometimes a father feels that since he was circumcised, his son should be, too. Parents may feel that it is the "proper" thing to do, or simply that it "looks" better.

When circumcision is performed by a skilled practitioner several hours or more after birth, the risks of complications are minimal, although hemorrhage or infection can occur. Removal of too much tissue may be uncomfortable during later life; and narrowing of the end of the urethra may occur, requiring surgery to widen the urethral opening. The procedure is painful, but a local anesthetic is generally not used because of the small but added risk of a drug reaction.

The long-term psychological effects of circumcision on the newborn, if any, are unknown. Delaying circumcision until later preschool years or adolescence, when a child is more acutely aware of his penis, could be seen by him as threatening. If circumcision is to be done, any psychological effects of this procedure would probably be less during the first few months of life.

If you have your baby circumcised, be certain to request that it be done at least a day after birth to make certain the baby is healthy. After circumcision the penis may be cleansed with mild soap and water. In the first few days after

---

Table 36   QUESTIONS TO CONSIDER WHEN YOU BECOME PREGNANT*

As your pregnancy progresses, you will probably have many questions about what to expect during childbirth. This may be particularly true if you're having your first baby. Listed below are questions about some aspects of labor and delivery which women are often curious about. Some of these questions may have been answered by the information in this chapter, and others you may want to ask your clinician.

1. Do I want to attend childbirth education classes for a so-called prepared childbirth?
2. If I've prepared for natural childbirth, can I change my mind during labor and receive anesthetics and/or other drugs?
3. What types of anesthetic does my doctor usually use during delivery, and what effect might they have on me or the baby?
4. How much does my husband or partner want to participate during labor and childbirth? Is he willing to be my "coach" if I decide on a prepared labor and delivery? If not, can someone else coach?
5. What kinds of alternative birth settings are available to me? What are the risks and benefits of each?
6. How do I know if I'm having a normal, low-risk pregnancy? What are the chances that I'll have a cesarean birth?
7. Are enemas and prepping—or shaving of the pubic area—always necessary?
8. Will I automatically be given an IV during labor?
9. When is it necessary for labor to be induced artificially?
10. Is fetal monitoring used routinely?
11. Are forceps likely to be used during delivery?
12. Is an episiotomy performed routinely? How will my doctor decide on whether to give me one?
13. Do I want to know more about so-called gentle birth, with dim lights, music, a quiet delivery room, and a warm bath for the baby?
14. Is a parent-infant bonding experience available? Do I have to prepare for this? How soon can I breastfeed?
15. Will I get to see my baby as often as I like, for as long as I like, while I'm still in the hospital?
16. How long does my health plan allow me to stay in the hospital?

---

* Modified with permission of Syntex Laboratories, Inc. (Effective Communication Series #8, 1978).

circumcision diapers should be changed often to avoid irritation to the glans. If your baby is not circumcised, gently retract the foreskin and clean the glans when you give him his bath.

CHAPTER 20

Complicated Pregnancies

Sometimes doctors talk about *high-risk pregnancies* when factors related to such things as age, smoking, or chronic illness are present. This labeling only serves as a warning to be especially careful about your pregnancy because you have a higher chance of developing complications. A high-risk pregnancy does *not* mean you won't have a normal pregnancy, labor, and delivery.

Certain "life-style" risk factors can be minimized or avoided by identifying potential problems *before* you conceive. This is one of the reasons why preconception counseling is important (see Chapter 11). For example, a woman who smokes may cut down or quit when she realizes that smoking more than a pack of cigarettes daily increases her baby's risk of fetal or infant death by more than 50%. Other "life-style" risks include alcohol use, drug use, and exposure to toxins or chemicals in the workplace (see Chapters 16, 30, and 31). Chapter 12 deals with the risks associated with pregnancy over the age of thirty-five.

This chapter discusses some of the common high-risk conditions that develop during pregnancy as a result of a medical or obstetrical problem. We also included discussion of tests that the high-risk mother may undergo to evaluate the fetus. Risk evaluation by the obstetrician is a continuing process, as some complications do not develop until late in pregnancy or in labor. Fortunately, most conditions, if recognized quickly, can be managed safely.

Miscarriage

Miscarriage (known medically as *spontaneous abortion*) refers to loss of the pregnancy during the first twenty weeks. In about 10% to 15% of pregnancies, miscarriage occurs with obvious

cramping and bleeding, usually in the first two or three months (see Chapter 54 for causes and treatment of bleeding in early pregnancy, including ectopic pregnancy). But the true rate of miscarriage is about 40%, since many occur earlier and may be confused with a "heavy" or "late" period and go unrecognized.

About 50% to 60% of miscarriages are due to random chromosome abnormalities in the sperm or egg that are not inherited from the parents. Maternal factors associated with an increased risk of miscarriage include being over the age of thirty-five, smoking, alcohol consumption, exposure to X-rays or toxic chemicals, and some medical conditions, such as insulin diabetes. The age of either the sperm or the egg also may influence miscarriage, which is slightly more likely if fertilization occurs as much as four days after intercourse. Conditions that do *not* appear to add to the risk of miscarriage include cancer, high blood pressure, use of birth control pills or spermicides, morning sickness, and emotional stress. Chlamydia infections rarely result in miscarriage, nor do most uterine fibroids (see Chapter 35), except, sometimes, for those located inside the uterine cavity.

Recurrent abortion has been defined as having three or more consecutive spontaneous miscarriages. Certain uncommon infections (caused by the mycoplasma or ureaplasma organisms) and poorly understood immunological conditions may cause this to occur. More often the cause is an anatomical defect within the uterus that may require surgical repair. Such abnormalities are more common among DES daughters (see Chapter 38), about 25% of whom experience repeated miscarriages. Such women may have a smaller-than-average, T-shaped uterus or an abnormality known as *incompetent cervix*. In this condition, a weakness within the cervix leads to painless dilation of the cervix, and miscarriage becomes inevitable. If diagnosed early enough, the condition can be effectively treated by a surgical procedure called *cerclage*, in which the widened cervix is sewn shut. The cerclage operation may be performed after the third month in a subsequent pregnancy to prevent this condition from recurring. Another uncommon finding in women with recurrent abortion is *luteal phase defect* (LPD), in which inadequate progesterone is produced by the corpus luteum of the ovary (see page 15). The condition is diagnosed by endometrial biopsy (see glossary) and treated with progesterone vaginal suppositories in the early weeks of pregnancy.

A woman with a history of recurrent miscarriage still has at least a 60% chance of a successful pregnancy, even if no specific cause for the miscarriages is found. Such patients may not need as many tests as previously thought. The basics usually include blood tests for unusual conditions (e.g., lupus anticoagulant test), an endometrial biopsy to rule out LPD, and an X-ray called a *hysterogram* to look for abnormalities of the uterus. If the results of these tests are normal, chromosome analysis, or *karyotyping*, is done to see if either parent is a carrier of abnormal chromosomes that may be inherited. When chromosomal abnormalities are identified, the couple may elect to have chromosome studies of the fetus performed in a subsequent pregnancy (see Chapter 11).

Having a miscarriage may create considerable emotional stress and produce many grief reactions similar to those after the loss of a newborn. Depression, guilt, anger, disbelief, and insomnia all are commonly seen. For the sake of one's emotional and physical health, it is advisable to wait two to three months after a miscarriage before trying to conceive once again. Fortunately, most miscarriages are random events that don't recur or threaten the woman's future ability to bear children.

High Blood Pressure in Pregnancy

High blood pressure in pregnancy, sometimes known as pre-eclampsia or *toxemia*,[1] occurs in about 7% of all pregnancies. This condition, while more common during a first pregnancy, can also affect a woman who has previously given birth, especially if she has a prior history of high blood pressure.

The first sign of toxemia may be a weight gain of five to ten pounds within a week, as a result of fluid retention. Although leg swelling in pregnancy is normal, prominent swelling of the hands and face is not. Report these or other possible symptoms of excessive water retention, such as severe headaches or blurred vision, to your doctor.

Fetal complications of high blood pressure include inadequate fetal growth (see Chapter 16) and premature labor as well as possible fetal distress during labor (see Chapter 21 for both). Because of these complications, the physician often starts fetal testing as early as 32 to 34 weeks when toxemia is present. Abnormal tests sometimes indicate the need for early delivery. In most pregnancies associated with high blood pressure, however, the fetus is not in serious danger and can be delivered at about 37 weeks of pregnancy, or as soon as fetal maturity is confirmed.

A woman with severe toxemia may be hospitalized to control high blood pressure or for fetal testing. More often, these tests are done on an outpatient basis. Extra rest, especially done lying on your left side, improves circulation and is one of the most beneficial measures for a woman with high blood pressure. The use of a salt-free diet and so-called water pills have possible fetal hazards and are infrequently used today.

Rh Disease

The Rh factor is a substance in the blood of approximately 85% of white people and 95% of blacks. These individuals are known as *Rh positive*. The people who have no Rh factor in their blood are called *Rh negative*. Having Rh negative blood in no way affects your general health. However, a condition called Rh disease (hemolytic disease of the newborn) can occur in babies born to Rh negative women when the father and the baby are both Rh positive. A few cells of the fetus's Rh positive blood (inherited from the father) may "leak" into the mother's circulation during pregnancy, usually at delivery. The mother's system, because it is Rh negative, acts on the Rh positive cells as a foreign substance and produces antibodies (see glossary). These antibodies can cross the placenta and destroy some of the fetal red blood cells, producing anemia, which can lead to serious or even fatal brain damage. This condition rarely occurs in a first pregnancy.

Rh disease is uncommon today even in subsequent pregnancies because a drug called Rho-GAM, developed in 1968, prevents the formation of antibodies when given to Rh negative women within seventy-two hours after delivering an Rh

---

[1] Newer terminology refers to *pregnancy-induced hypertension* when high blood pressure in pregnancy develops in a woman whose blood pressure has been normal before.

positive baby. Rh negative women should also receive a "mini-dose" RhoGAM injection after a miscarriage, therapeutic abortion, or ectopic pregnancy. In 1983, the American College of Obstetricians and Gynecologists began recommending RhoGAM for all susceptible Rh negative women *during* pregnancy as well as postpartum. The drug is also given near the twenty-eighth week of pregnancy to benefit a few women who will otherwise develop Rh antibodies in late pregnancy. Despite the availability of RhoGAM, nearly one out of ten women for whom the drug is indicated do not receive it for one reason or another. Once developed, Rh antibodies are permanent and RhoGAM is of no benefit. Such antibodies represent a continuing risk of Rh disease in subsequent pregnancies if the fetus is Rh positive.

Rh blood typing and antibody testing are routinely done at the initial office visit. If you are Rh positive, you need not worry about Rh disease even if the father is Rh negative. If you are Rh negative, however, the father's blood type should be checked. If both you and he are Rh negative, your baby will also be negative and, therefore, unaffected by Rh disease. If the father, however, is Rh positive and you are Rh negative, then you are susceptible to Rh disease. In such susceptible Rh negative women, the clinician repeats the blood test, to check for antibodies, in the sixth and eighth months of pregnancy as well as at delivery.

If antibodies are detected in your blood during pregnancy, the physician may perform an amniocentesis (see later in this chapter and also Chapter 11) to assess the condition of the fetus by analyzing the amniotic fluid. When fetal blood cells are broken down by maternal Rh antibodies, the cells release bilirubin, a substance which shows up in the amniotic fluid. High bilirubin levels may indicate the need for early delivery to protect the fetus from further antibody damage. This approach is usually lifesaving to the fetus. Rarely, blood transfusions need to be given to the fetus in severe disease.

Infections in Pregnancy

Rubella (German measles)

Birth defects, including mental retardation, heart disease, hearing loss, and blindness, occur up to 50% of the time when rubella is contracted by the mother in the first eight to twelve weeks of pregnancy. Symptoms of rubella may mimic the common cold and include skin rash, swollen neck glands, and a slight fever. Blood tests can detect if you have had recent or past rubella infection, based on the presence in the blood of antibodies. Typically a high level of antibodies (or a rising level based on successive blood tests two weeks apart) indicates recent infection. A low antibody level indicates past infection and thus present immunity to (protection against) rubella. Absence of antibodies means you have not had rubella. Fortunately, a vaccine can be given *prior to* pregnancy to prevent the disease in such women. Nearly 20% of women entering childbearing age have not acquired immunity either from having had the disease or from the vaccination and are therefore susceptible to rubella. It's best to have your blood tested for rubella antibodies three months before you plan to get pregnant. This way, if your antibody level is too low (less than 1 to 20), you can get the rubella vaccine for complete protection. Although physicians routinely screen pregnant women for rubella, you cannot be vaccinated once you are pregnant or within three months before you become pregnant, because the vaccine itself could be harmful to the fetus. This is why you should avoid pregnancy for three months following vaccination. Vaccination is recommended *following* pregnancy in women found not to have immunity.

Herpes infections (herpes genitalis, genital herpes)

Herpes genitalis, a sexually transmitted disease (see Chapter 24), causes painful sores around the vaginal opening. The newborn may acquire this virus by direct contact with the sores at the time of vaginal delivery.

A first-time herpes infection during pregnancy involves greater risk to the baby than a recurring infection. About 50% of infants born vaginally to mothers during a first-time infection will contract herpes, compared with only 4% of infants born to mothers experiencing repeat infections. Testing for herpes (performed like a Pap smear) can detect the presence of the virus in the vagina and cervix; the virus may be present even without a previous history of herpes infection. However, a positive culture during pregnancy does *not* mean that infection will occur subsequently in the newborn. Some large-scale studies to test pregnant patients selected randomly (including those with, as well as without, a history of herpes) have shown that the frequency of positive herpes cultures during delivery is about 1 per 250 deliveries (or even less). Yet the frequency of actual newborn herpes infection in random populations is no greater than 1 per 2,500 deliveries. Why so many infants exposed to this virus escape infection is unclear, but it may result from the presence of protective maternal antibodies. If infection in the newborn does occur, herpes can be fatal or produce serious damage to the nervous system, including mental retardation and seizures. Fortunately, such serious infection is rare unless the baby's exposure follows a first-time outbreak in the mother at or just before delivery.

The management of patients with a history of herpes has changed in recent years. The practice of performing weekly herpes cultures in such patients in the last month of pregnancy and of allowing patients to deliver vaginally (if cultures remain negative) has not reduced the frequency of newborn herpes. This is partly due to the fact that even in the presence of a positive herpes culture, the chance of serious infection in the newborn is small. In fact, most cases of newborn herpes occur *without* a prior history of maternal herpes or evidence of an outbreak at the time of delivery. In addition, it has been shown that even performing a prompt cesarean section does not always prevent herpes infections from developing in the newborn. At present, the American College of Obstetricians and Gynecologists does not recommend routine cultures for patients with a history of herpes. A herpes culture is recommended when and if an outbreak of herpes occurs during pregnancy. If the outbreak develops at the start of labor or in the presence of ruptured membranes at term, a cesarean section is performed—otherwise, vaginal birth is allowed. Some obstetricians still turn to cesarean birth if a woman goes into labor and has not had a negative culture subsequent to a recent herpes outbreak.

Cytomegalovirus infections (CMV)

Cytomegalovirus (CMV) infections are an uncommon cause of birth defects in newborns whose mothers have been infected with this virus. CMV infections in adults are very mild and usually go unnoticed. In adults, transmission occurs by saliva or sexual contact; in pregnancy the virus can cross the placenta, affecting the baby. Newborn problems can include various neurological problems, from hearing loss to mental retardation.

Approximately 50% to 85% of mothers have antibodies to CMV, indicating prior infection. These mothers have some immunity to CMV and are at low risk for having a baby with CMV-related birth defects (1 out of 10,000). Mothers without antibodies are at slightly higher risk of having an impaired infant as a result of acquiring this symptomless infection for the first time in pregnancy (about 1 in 1,000). At this time, there is no treatment for CMV in adults and no test to identify infection or disease in the fetus. Fortunately, the risk of neurologic damage in the newborn as a result of exposure to this disease in pregnancy is relatively rare, and affects only about 2,500 newborns annually. Since mothers who have not had a primary infection with CMV are at greatest risk, those whose jobs place them in frequent contact with babies may want to be tested and, if antibodies are not present, take special precautions, since exposure to infants who shed the CMV virus in sputum or urine may be a source of infection.

Hepatitis-B infections

This form of viral hepatitis, also known as *serum hepatitis* or *HBV infection*, may cause serious or chronic liver damage in the mother and chronic infection in the newborn. While an acute case produces symptoms of fatigue and yellow coloring of the skin and the whites of the eyes (jaundice), many cases of HBV infection are chronic and symptomless. HBV infections may be contracted in several ways: from contaminated blood; sexually; through IV drug abuse with contaminated needles; or it may cross the placenta during pregnancy. Women who are chronic, symptomless carriers of HBV infection may belong to certain risk groups—for example, Pacific Islanders or Alaskan Natives, among whom HBV infection is highly endemic. Another risk group includes individuals working in medical or dental settings, where frequent occupational exposure to blood is likely. Since many chronic carriers do not belong to risk groups, uniform screening through a blood test (called the *hepatitis B surface antigen*) is now recommended for all pregnant women. While no specific treatment is available in the mother, prevention of infection in the newborn is possible by treating exposed newborns with hepatitis-B immune globulin and hepatitis-B vaccine immediately after birth.

Toxoplasmosis

About 30% of the U.S. population has previously had toxoplasmosis, an infection caused by the protozoan *Toxoplasma gondii*. Symptoms may include a flulike syndrome, with a sore throat and fever, but usually the disease in adults is symptomless. Maternal infection may cause varied complications in the baby, including permanent eye damage and mental retardation. Birth defects are most likely when infection occurs in the first three months of pregnancy; maternal infection in later pregnancy is much less likely to be associated with serious fetal problems.

Toxoplasmosis in humans is acquired by eating uncooked meat or by ingesting *Toxoplasma* as a result of contact with cat feces containing the organism. Contrary to popular belief, it is fairly difficult to catch this infection just by caring for a cat. However, it is advisable to have someone else change the kitty litter and to minimize contact with the cat during pregnancy. Changing the litter box daily helps prevent this infection, since *Toxoplasma* is not infective during the first twenty-four hours after the cat's stool is passed. Also, if you have outdoor cats, it is best to avoid gardening or yard work in areas that may be contaminated with cat feces.

Screening tests for this disease have not been successful, since they do not clearly distinguish between a recent infection, which can affect the fetus, and a prior infection, which generally does not. Treatment of toxoplasmosis involves antibiotics that may be toxic to the fetus and are usually given after the first trimester of pregnancy. Because of the risks of birth defects, women who acquire an active case of this disease in the first three months of pregnancy may consider terminating the pregnancy. In some countries in Europe, testing for toxoplasmosis in pregnancy has become routine. In France, screening for *Toxoplasma* and the use of new drugs not yet approved in the United States, as well as the practice of starting antibiotics in early pregnancy, have decreased the rate of congenital toxoplasmosis to babies born to infected mothers to only 3% to 4%.

AIDS (Acquired Immune Deficiency Syndrome)

This disease is now the leading cause of death in women twenty-five to thirty-four years old, the age when most childbearing in women occurs. (For a complete discussion of AIDS see Chapter 24). A pregnant woman who has AIDS may experience a worsening of her disease. For this reason, health professionals recommend that patients with AIDS avoid pregnancy. Transmission of the AIDS virus to the newborn is estimated to occur in 40% to 50% of cases and can occur at any stage of pregnancy, during delivery, and during breast-feeding. When the mother is HIV positive, her newborn will have HIV-positive blood that may stay positive for twelve to fifteen months. The virus can then disappear permanently, remain, or reappear later.

It is estimated that about 7,000 infants are born to HIV-infected mothers each year. Most likely this number will increase for several years to come based on increasing rates of HIV infection in women. Recent research by the National Institute of Allergy and Infectious Diseases indicates that HIV-positive pregnant women who take zidovudine (AZT) can dramatically lower the risk of maternal-child transmission of HIV. For this reason, the CDC has drafted recommendations pertaining to voluntary HIV testing for all pregnant women and treatment with AZT for most of those who are confirmed as HIV positive. AZT can both improve the woman's health as well as prevent transmission of the virus to her fetus.

Childhood mortality among HIV-infected children is about 45%, and many die before the age of two. The low survival rate as well as quality of life concerns place HIV-positive women in a contraception vs. conception dilemma. For women who become too ill to function during their early motherhood, there are also legal, moral, social, and political issues regarding the care of their infected infants. Ideally, prescreening for HIV in high-risk population groups (e.g., IV drug users and women with multiple sexual relationships), accompanied by sensitive counseling prior to conception, would help women to make decisions about pregnancy. Even with counseling, some HIV-positive women choose to try to "beat the odds" and have a child. Others elect not to use contraception because to do so may risk the loss of financial or emotional support for themselves and their children if their disease becomes known to others.

Premature Rupture of Membranes (PROM)

Spontaneous leakage of amniotic fluid (usually in a gush) before the onset of labor occurs in 10% of pregnancies. Such leakage, called *premature rupture of membranes* (PROM), is usually not a problem unless it occurs several weeks before your due date, when premature labor and early delivery could occur. A specific cause of PROM is usually not identified, although infection, including sexually transmitted disease, is sometimes a suspected factor. PROM is more common among teens, single women, and women who smoke. If you are "leaking water" or you think your membranes have ruptured, call your physician or go to the hospital.

When PROM occurs at thirty-six weeks or after, labor is likely to begin within twenty-four hours. If it does not, the physician usually induces labor, if your cervix is "favorable"—i.e., has become softer, shorter (effaced), or begun to dilate. If your cervix is unfavorable, the physician may wait for your cervix to "ripen" before inducing labor. This conservative approach in the face of an unfavorable cervix requires frequent fetal testing, but it is less likely to result in a cesarean birth.

When PROM occurs before thirty-six weeks, the risk of prematurity from early delivery is usually the single greatest concern. In such instances, the obstetrician often elects not to induce labor unless you show signs of infection.

Diabetes

Two forms of diabetes may complicate pregnancy: diabetes first discovered during pregnancy, called *gestational diabetes*, and preexisting diabetes. By far the more common form in pregnancy is gestational diabetes. It is diagnosed when a woman has higher-than-normal blood sugar (glucose) levels after drinking a sugar so-

lution, a test called a *glucose tolerance test* (GTT). While there are various types of GTTs, today, many obstetricians first screen patients for gestational diabetes by using a one-hour test in which a single blood-glucose sample is obtained exactly one hour after drinking the sugar solution. If this test is abnormal, a more exact three-hour GTT is then performed to confirm the diagnosis of gestational diabetes. This condition is found in 1% to 3% of pregnant women in the United States and is more common among overweight women, those over thirty-five, and among women with a history of large babies (more than 8½ pounds) or stillbirths. Although gestational diabetes usually subsides within six weeks of delivery, some women with this diagnosis will ultimately develop permanent diabetes and require either oral medication or insulin.

While either form of diabetes can make a pregnancy "high risk," the risks—both maternal and fetal—are much greater with preexisting diabetes. Preexisting diabetes is associated with significantly higher-than-average rates of birth defects, stillbirth, preterm labor, and various problems in the newborn, such as low blood sugar. Insulin diabetes also presents significant risks to the mother, including increased rates of high blood pressure and difficulty in controlling blood-sugar levels.

Gestational diabetics may be assessed using "non-stress" tests (see page 164) in the last few weeks of pregnancy. In insulin diabetics, a blood test for alpha-fetoprotein at sixteen to eighteen weeks of pregnancy and a sonogram at eighteen to twenty weeks may be useful in ruling out birth defects. In the last eight weeks these patients require weekly "non-stress" tests until delivery. Serial sonograms, to assess growth and to test fetal health (see below), are also performed regularly in insulin diabetics. In both forms of diabetes, the sugar level in the blood is measured periodically by blood tests. Calorie intake should be maintained at between 2,000 and 2,500 calories a day, and simple sugars should be avoided. The number-one goal in both forms of diabetes is to maintain a normal blood-sugar level, which protects the fetus in many ways. Pregnancy complications, such as stillbirth, occur with much greater frequency when blood-sugar levels are too high.

Planned early delivery at about thirty-eight weeks is customary in insulin diabetics, while gestational diabetics usually can expect to de-

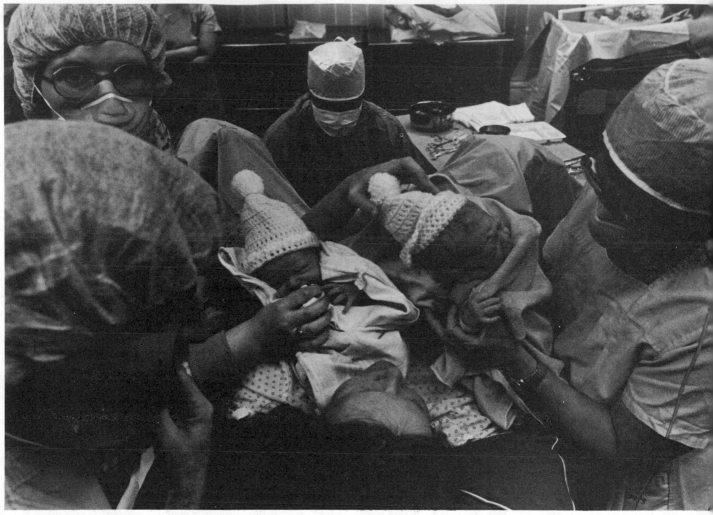

Parents greeting their newborn twins.

liver close to their "due" date. Cesarean birth rates are significantly higher among insulin-dependent women (due, partly, to having larger babies), and the rate is slightly increased among patients with gestational diabetes.

Multiple Pregnancies

Twins are delivered in about 1 out of 90 pregnancies and triplets in 1 out of every 9,000. The use of fertility drugs and procedures like in-vitro fertilization (see Chapter 13) have increased the rate of multiple pregnancies in recent years. Today, with the frequent use of sonography, most twins are diagnosed within the first five months of pregnancy.

Having twins, triplets, and other multiple pregnancies is most stressful on your body, and you will need to be watched closely by your physician. Frequent problems include greater physical discomforts due to the added fetal weight and increased amniotic fluid. Later in pregnancy you might find yourself tiring more easily and having difficulty keeping up with normal activities. Bedrest is often recommended for the last trimester.

You will be more closely monitored than in an ordinary pregnancy to prevent such maternal complications as high blood pressure and anemia, and more frequent prenatal visits will be important. Multiple births present the added risk of possible premature labor and fetal growth problems. Sonograms are done to screen for birth defects and to monitor fetal growth. "Non-stress tests" and biophysical profiles (see pages 164–165) may be performed weekly in the last three months. This extra medical attention may seem demanding while you are pregnant, but the added precautions are worth it. Having a multiple birth can be very exciting, overwhelming, and frightening all at the same time. Cesarean birth is more common in multiple pregnancies, due most often to breech presentation at the time of labor, difficult labor, or prematurity.

Resource

Twins Magazine
P.O. Box 12045
Overland Park, Kansas 66282
(913) 722–1090

Intrauterine Growth Retardation (IUGR)

Abnormal fetal growth, sometimes referred to as *intrauterine growth retardation* (IUGR), occurs in 3% to 5% of all pregnancies. There are various causes of IUGR, including heavy smoking, poor nutrition, and alcohol or drug abuse. These conditions often lead to a decrease in blood flow through the placenta, the baby's nutrition pipeline. IUGR can also result from medical problems, such as high blood pressure, or obstetrical conditions causing bleeding. And, rarely, a birth defect (such as a chromosome disorder) or a viral condition, like herpes, cytomegalovirus, or rubella, can cause IUGR.

The physician may suspect a growth problem if the baby's size seems small or the fundal height (see page 112) does not seem to increase appropriately during successive prenatal visits. The best test for this condition is the sonogram. Usually two or more sonograms at least three weeks apart are needed to give a precise indication of the baby's growth. The measurements are compared to a normal range (to allow for individual differences) for that gestational age. If the measured growth is below the tenth percentile (i.e., the baby is smaller than 90% of ba-

bies in a similar population for that stage of pregnancy), IUGR is said to occur.

In addition to inadequate growth, repeat sonography often reveals another finding common to IUGR: decreased amniotic fluid. This is a warning sign in this condition, often associated with chronic "stress" in the fetus. Frequent "non-stress" tests are performed once IUGR is diagnosed. Abnormal fetal testing or decreased fluid may require delivery before your due date if the tests indicate that the risk to the baby of continuing pregnancy exceeds that of prematurity.

Bleeding Problems

In the first few weeks of pregnancy, spotting or vaginal bleeding may be associated with miscarriage or ectopic pregnancy (see Chapter 54). In the second half of pregnancy, vaginal bleeding is commonly associated with placental problems, like placenta previa and abruptio placenta (see Chapter 55). Whenever it occurs, vaginal bleeding is an important symptom to promptly report to your doctor.

Post Maturity—When Your Baby Is Overdue

The newborn is considered overdue, or *post mature*, when delivery occurs two weeks or more after your due date. No one knows why this occurs in 10% of all pregnancies. In late pregnancy, as the placenta ages, transfer of oxygen and other nutrients to the baby normally diminishes. Post-mature babies, especially those three or more weeks overdue, have an increased risk of fetal distress (see Chapter 21) in labor. This risk is further compounded when the woman is over the age of thirty-four or is having her first baby. Post maturity also imposes greater likelihood of a difficult delivery as a result of large fetal size since over 70% of overdue newborns weigh more than 8½ pounds. In the nursery, post-mature infants have a slightly higher rate of low blood sugar, jaundice (see glossary), and respiratory problems.

Today, obstetricians usually begin fetal testing at forty-one weeks, starting with a non-stress test once each week. When a pregnancy is truly post-date—i.e., forty-two weeks or more—other tests, such as the biophysical profile, may be performed as well, and labor may be induced if the cervix is favorable. If the cervix is unfavorable, induction may be delayed for a time as long as the fetal testing remains normal. Most physicians will attempt to deliver their patient once she has reached forty-three weeks. One of the most important considerations in a post-date pregnancy is knowing the exact due date. When this is in doubt due to irregular periods or because the date predicted by a sonogram does not agree with the date predicted by your last menstrual period, the physician may move more cautiously. Sometimes a fetal maturity test, such as amniocentesis, is performed to confirm that the baby's lungs are mature before inducing labor.

High-risk Pregnancy Testing

The kinds of tests performed in the first twenty weeks of high-risk pregnancies are aimed at identifying birth defects or the cause of bleeding problems. As early as the fifth week after a missed period, an ultrasound exam using the newer vaginal probe technique can help diagnose whether unexplained vaginal bleeding is due to a miscarriage or ectopic pregnancy (see Chapter 54). At sixteen weeks some women who are at risk for having a baby with a birth defect or who are over age thirty-five may elect to have an amniocentesis, a test to screen for chromosomal abnormalities (see Chapter 11). At about the seventeenth week, many women choose to have the alpha-fetoprotein blood test performed. This is a screening test for certain birth defects like open spine (see Chapter 11). If there has been exposure to drugs or excessive alcohol in early pregnancy, a "level II" sonogram, which looks at the baby's organ development at about eighteen to twenty weeks, may be done to check for various abnormalities.

In the second half of a high-risk pregnancy, testing often seeks to identify the fetus in distress, who needs prompt delivery. Prior to fetal monitoring and sonography, assessing the baby's health was more subjective—e.g., by counting the number of times the baby moved within a certain period of time. While still used today, few randomized studies have demonstrated the benefits of "kick counts," although maternal perception of a general decrease in fetal activity may indicate fetal distress. Currently, the nonstress test, contraction stress test, and biophysical profile are the three main tests used for diagnosing fetal distress—i.e., whether the fetus is healthy or becoming "sick" due to reduced blood flow or for other reasons. Normal test results—which are usually the case—allow the obstetrician to take a "wait and see" approach and avoid premature delivery. Complementing these tests of fetal health is amniocentesis, a widely used test to evaluate the baby's lung maturity. The amniocentesis tells the obstetrician whether or not premature delivery will itself be a significant risk to the baby. Occasionally fetal blood samples need to be tested and a needle inserted into the umbilical cord for this (see Chapter 11 for more information on umbilical cord sampling). Managing many high-risk pregnancies often comes down to one important decision: when to deliver the baby. This process amounts to a balancing act between the need to deliver the baby as early as possible (because of the threat of the high-risk condition itself) and the need for delaying delivery as long as possible to prevent newborn complications of prematurity.

The Non-stress Test (NST)

The NST is the most basic and widely used screening test in high-risk pregnancies. This test looks for and evaluates brief increases or "accelerations" of the fetal heart rate. These often occur during fetal movement or with spontaneous (Braxton-Hicks) uterine contractions. During this test, you are connected to a fetal monitor (see Chapter 19) and push a button that makes a mark on the monitor strip when you feel the fetus move. A normal, or *reactive*, test shows two or more fetal heart-rate accelerations of at least ten to fifteen beats per minute and lasting ten to fifteen seconds within a set time period usually lasting not more than forty minutes. A reactive test almost always means the fetus is in healthy condition and will probably remain so for the next several days. An abnormal, or *nonreactive*, test is one without fetal heart-rate accelerations that meet the above criteria during the test period. A nonreactive test indicates the need for additional testing, such as a contraction stress test or biophysical profile. While there are very few false-negative NSTs, a major drawback of the test is the high number of false-positive tests: that is, tests that appear to show a fetal problem when in fact the fetus is healthy. Thus, an abnormal test does not necessarily mean the fetus is in danger. A newer technique, *acoustic stimulation*, has been used to reduce the number of false-positive NSTs. Using acoustic stimulation such as a doorbell buzzer, researchers have been able to evoke fetal heart responses (accelerations) like those used in the NST test. In one study, incorporating acoustic stimulation into the NST procedure reduced the number of nonreactive NSTs by 36% and cut testing time significantly.

Contraction Stress Test (CST)

This test evaluates the fetal heart rate during contractions that are stimulated through the use of the drug oxytocin. In a normal, or negative, test, the fetal heart rate will remain unchanged or may increase slightly during contractions. A negative CST requires at least three contractions within a ten-minute period without decelerations of the fetal heart rate. In definitely abnormal, or positive, tests, the fetal heart rate drops slightly (decelerates) during and after each contraction (see Figure 26). Most CSTs are negative. In fact, there are even fewer false negatives among CSTs than among NSTs, which makes the CST an extremely reliable test if it is negative. In that case, it is usually safe to wait a week, at which time the CST will be repeated. A suspicious test (neither positive nor negative) is usually repeated in twenty-four hours. A positive test, found in 5% to 10% of high-risk pregnancies, may indicate the need for immediate delivery, often by cesarean section.

The CST is a backup test to the NST and is usually not the first test performed in evaluating the fetus in a high-risk pregnancy. Compared to the NST, the CST is costlier and usually requires the use of an IV to administer the oxytocin. To avoid the need for oxytocin and an IV, a variation of the CST uses breast stimulation to induce uterine contractions. Through gentle self-stimulation of one nipple, a pregnant woman can produce enough of a surge of her own natural oxytocin to cause a few contractions and successfully complete the test at least 50% of the time. A slight risk of the CST is that preterm labor may be started. For this reason the CST is usually avoided in women with twins or threatened preterm labor.

Biophysical Profile (BPP)

This test uses ultrasound (see page 109), usually combined with the NST, to perform a fetal "physical exam." In this test the physician evaluates and scores five separate activities: fetal breathing movements; movement of fetal limbs; fetal tone (extension and flexion of the spinal column); the amount of amniotic fluid; and fetal heart rate. The first four activities are evaluated by ultrasound and the last by NST. Each activity receives a score of 2 (if normal) or 0 (if abnormal). In general, a score of 8 to 10 is considered normal and is associated with fetal well-being for one week, after which the test is usually repeated. In pregnancies two weeks or more overdue or complicated by insulin diabetes, however, more frequent testing is occasionally performed.

Unlike the NST or CST, which are performed by the obstetrician, the more technically complex biophysical profile (BPP) may require the services of a radiologist or perinatologist (high-risk specialist). In addition, the biophysical profile may cost $300 or more—about three times the cost of an NST or CST. For this reason, the BPP is usually reserved for the more severe high-risk pregnancies or in situations where the NST is unreactive and further evaluation is needed. The biophysical profile has some advantages over the other "second line" test, the CST, in being a noninvasive test and also in providing information about the baby's size and position. Lower scores require individual interpretation and may require repeat testing in twenty-four hours or in preparation for delivery. With a score of 6, for example, the physician may simply repeat the test in twenty-four hours in a thirty-four-week pregnancy; in a full-term pregnancy, he may opt for inducing labor. Scores of 4 or less are ominous and may require prompt delivery.

The frequency of high-risk testing depends on the nature of the risk factors involved. Following a normal NST, CST, or biophysical profile, the usual interval is one week for many moderate-risk conditions, such as gestational diabetes. Depending on the maternal and fetal condition, more frequent testing may be performed, especially as the pregnancy progresses toward the fortieth week. Such testing provides a wide margin of safety in most circumstances. But even with persistently normal tests a baby is occasionally lost due to unpredictable catastrophes, such as a prolapsed umbilical cord or cord "accident," in which the cord becomes compressed without actual prolapse. Fortunately, such things are very infrequent.

Amniocentesis

This procedure is widely used in the second half of pregnancy to diagnose fetal maturity—that is, confirmation that the fetal lungs are sufficiently developed to function normally after birth. In this procedure, a sample of amniotic fluid is removed, as shown in Figure 28. Analysis of the fluid provides a measure of fetal lung maturity. If the lungs are not yet fully developed, the new-

Figure 28   *Amniocentesis. Amniotic fluid is withdrawn from the "bag of waters" surrounding the fetus and sent to a laboratory for various tests. Modified with permission of G. D. Searle and Co. (The Female Reproductive System. San Juan, Puerto Rico, 1976).*

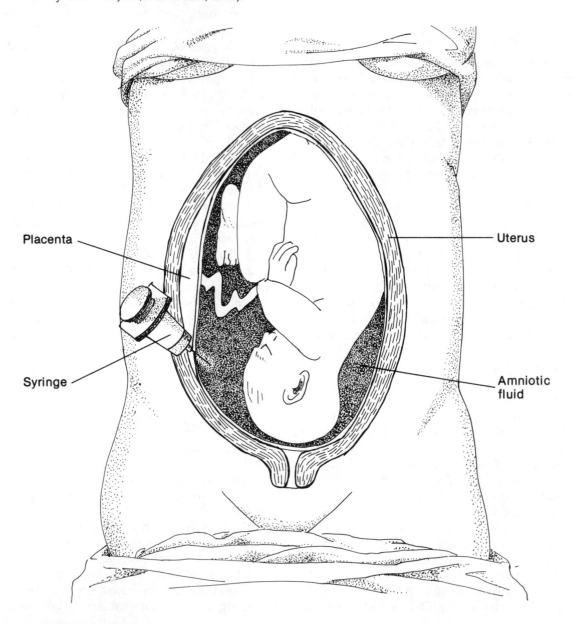

Placenta

Syringe

Uterus

Amniotic fluid

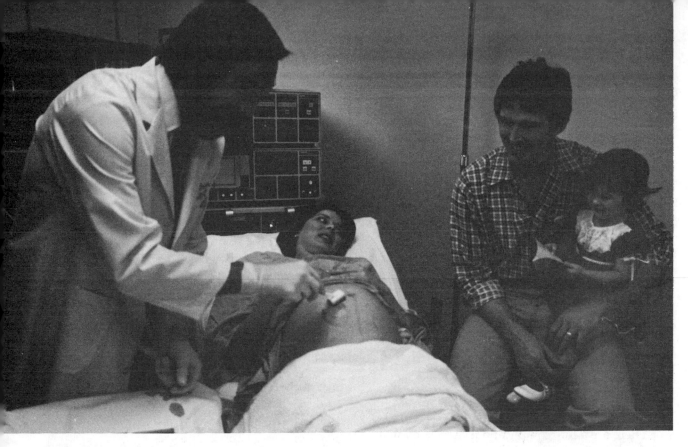

The mother's abdomen is cleaned with antiseptic solution prior to amniocentesis.

Performing an amniocentesis.

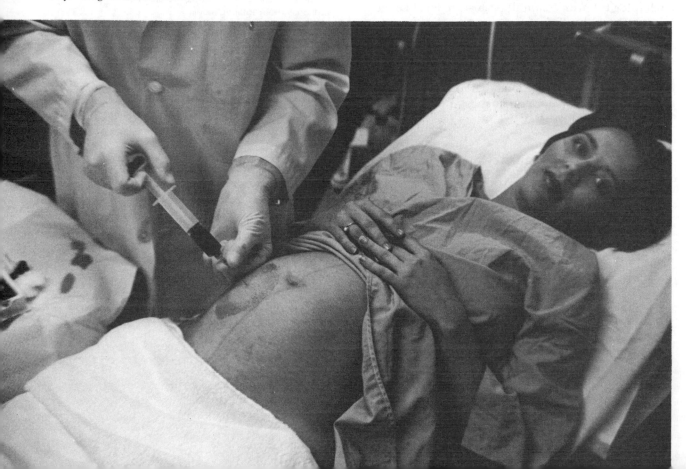

Table 37 POSSIBLE REASONS FOR AMNIOCENTESIS

Reason	When Usually Performed*
Evaluation for certain specific birth defects	16 to 18 weeks
Evaluation for fetal maturity when repeat cesarean section is planned	38 to 39 weeks
Evaluation for fetal maturity in high-risk pregnancies (e.g., high blood pressure, diabetes, Rh disease, overdue more than two weeks, inadequate fetal growth)	34 to 39 weeks

* Weeks of pregnancy counting from the first day of the last menstrual period (term pregnancy is 40 weeks).

born may have respiratory problems, a serious complication in the premature newborn.

There are a few complications associated with amniocentesis, the most common of which is failure to obtain fluid. This situation usually can be prevented by the use of sonography (see Chapter 16) prior to amniocentesis to localize the fluid. Fetal bleeding, infection and premature labor can also occur but they are rare. Amniocentesis is not painful because a local anesthetic is administered. Perhaps the hardest part of the procedure is waiting several hours for the results, whether or not you suspect a problem.

Risk Factors in Pregnancy

In order to help predict whether problems may develop during labor, scoring systems have been developed to identify high-risk mothers such as shown in Table 38. It identifies high-risk pregnancies according to risk factors, with a point score assigned to each risk factor according to its potential for causing problems. Women with ten points or more total score can be considered high risk. A score of less than ten points total indicates low risk. Unfortunately, high-risk scoring systems do not identify all women who will develop complications during labor. Some women who are low risk during pregnancy may develop risk factors during labor, such as a pro-

Table 38 IDENTIFYING HIGH-RISK PREGNANCIES ACCORDING TO RISK FACTORS*

Risk Factor	Point Score**
High blood pressure (moderate or severe, often requiring hospitalization in pregnancy)	10
Severe kidney or heart disease	10
Diabetes (requiring insulin)	10
Previous stillbirth, premature or low birth weight infant, or newborn death that occurred within one month of birth	10
Overdue three or more weeks	10
Twins	10
Baby in breech position (in the last six weeks of pregnancy)	10
Previous multiple miscarriages (three or more)	10
Age older than 35 or younger than 15	10
Excessive drug use, including alcohol	10
Moderate alcohol intake	10
Previous kidney (not bladder) infection	5
High blood pressure (mild, not requiring hospitalization in pregnancy)	5
Pregnancy diabetes (diabetes developing in pregnancy, not requiring insulin)	5
Previous cesarean section	5
Previous delivery of baby weighing more than 10 pounds	5
Have been pregnant five times or more	5
Severe flu, bronchitis, or viral illness	5
Severe anemia (hemoglobin less than 9 grams)	5
Weight less than 100 or more than 200 pounds	5
Height less than five feet	5
Previous child with a birth defect	5
Vaginal spotting	5
Smoking more than one pack of cigarettes a day	5
Emotional problems	5
Bladder infection	1
Previous high blood pressure in an earlier pregnancy	1
Family history of diabetes	1

* Adapted from Hobel, C. J., Prenatal and Intrapartum High-Risk Screening, *American Journal of Obstetrics and Gynecology*, 117(1): 1–9, 1973.
** Score of 10 points or more = high risk
Score of less than 10 points = low risk

lapsed cord (in which the umbilical cord "drops" into the vagina where it may become dangerously compressed by the baby's head), bleeding, or prolonged labor. Your clinician will evaluate these factors throughout your pregnancy.

Resources

March of Dimes
1275 Mamaroneck Avenue
White Plains, New York 10605
(914) 428-7100

Center for Study of Multiple Births
333 East Superior Street
Chicago, Illinois 60611
(312) 266–9093

CHAPTER 21

Complications of Labor and Delivery

At any time during labor, complications may arise and lead to inadequate oxygen supply to the fetus. This problem is particularly prevalent in women whose pregnancies have been complicated by such factors as high blood pressure or diabetes. Unexpected events, such as a prolapsed cord or severe bleeding in a previously normal pregnancy, may also complicate labor and delivery. For these reasons, close observation of your condition and that of your baby is very important throughout labor and delivery.

The fetus normally experiences mild oxygen deprivation during birth due to the stress of labor. When oxygen deprivation is moderate to severe in labor—a condition called *fetal distress*—the newborn is likely to be less responsive at birth as measured by what is called Apgar scores. These scores measure the general condition of the newborn at one minute and five minutes after birth by evaluating muscle tone, color, cry, respiration, and heart rate. Most healthy newborns score seven to ten. Low Apgar scores are not necessarily cause for alarm—most of these babies grow up to be perfectly healthy, too. Early detection and treatment of fetal distress can increase the newborn's chances for a healthy outcome.

Determining Fetal Distress

Except for a crisis such as a prolapsed umbilical cord (in which the cord "drops" into the vagina where it may become dangerously compressed by the baby's head), fetal distress in labor usually develops gradually and can be evaluated in three ways:

1. *Amniotic fluid*, normally clear, may become brown or green-colored from fetal stool, which is called *meconium*. This demands careful observation of the condition of the fetus.
2. *Fetal heart rate* is evaluated intermittently with a stethoscope or continually with electronic fetal monitoring (EFM) (see Chapter 19). With a stethoscope, the clinician can recognize a sustained drop in heart rate. But with the electronic fetal monitor the clinician is aware of brief, less severe drops in heart rate as well as more subtle patterns of fetal heart irregularity related to decreased oxygen flow to the baby. Thus, EFM may lead to earlier detection of fetal distress.
3. *Fetal blood oxygen levels* are obtained through fetal scalp sampling, which means the doctor obtains a tiny drop of blood from the fetal scalp during labor and analyzes the oxygen content. Fetal scalp sampling seeks to confirm or prove false the apparent fetal stress indicated by fetal monitoring. The use of this procedure, which is somewhat cumbersome technically, has declined in recent years.

Premature (Preterm) Labor

Premature labor, one of the most common serious complications of pregnancy, occurs in approximately 10% of all pregnancies. Nearly three-fourths of all newborn deaths are associated with prematurity. Although prematurity is often associated with vaginal bleeding in late pregnancy, high blood pressure, and other medical complications, the cause is unknown over half the time. An increase in prematurity has been associated with a previous history of premature labors, with twins, and in pregnancies occurring before age seventeen or after age thirty-five. There is a slightly increased chance of prematurity in individuals who smoke, use drugs, are poorly nourished, or have a previous history of two or more therapeutic abortions.

Premature labor used to be defined as labor resulting in either the delivery of an infant weighing less than 5½ pounds at birth or an infant being delivered before 37 weeks of pregnancy. This definition failed to differentiate between babies born before 40 weeks (*premature*)

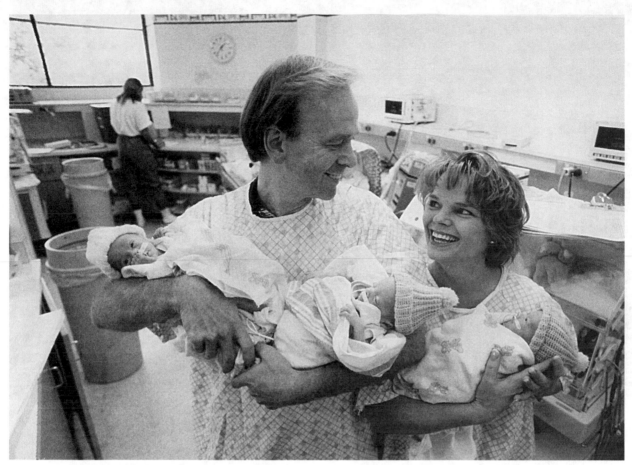

TRIPLETS! Alex, Harrison, and Spencer.

and those born at 40 weeks but with low birth weight (*growth retarded*). Low-birth-weight babies born on schedule have fewer newborn complications than premature infants. When growth retardation coexists with prematurity, the risk to the newborn is greater than that for premature babies.

Treatment of premature labor

Premature, or preterm, labor is usually treated with strict bed rest and increased fluids as dehydration may promote contractions. The success of this treatment by itself has been about 50%. Traditional labor-stopping drugs include magnesium sulfate, indomethacin, and a group known as beta-adrenergics (ritodrine, terbutaline), which mimic the adrenalin-releasing sympathetic nervous system. "Mag" is often the first choice because of its relative lack of side effects compared to the nervousness and palpitations that may accompany the beta-adrenergic group.

None of these drugs has been particularly successful at stopping labor for more than a few days, however. A new category under study called calcium channel blockers (e.g., nifedipine) shows promise.

Drug therapy may be used whenever preterm labor begins after twenty weeks of pregnancy and is usually continued as long as possible until about thirty-six weeks. The physician initially will hospitalize you to evaluate the contractions. If started, drug therapy is initiated in its most potent form by IV (intravenously). Once your cervix dilates more than 5 centimeters or your membranes rupture, drug therapy probably will not work. More often than not, however, preterm labor can be stopped, and after several days, you can usually go home. Some physicians also prescribe a home monitor, which allows you to monitor yourself periodically for contractions during the day, but its value is unproven at this time. Most home monitor systems allow you to telephone a recording of your monitor

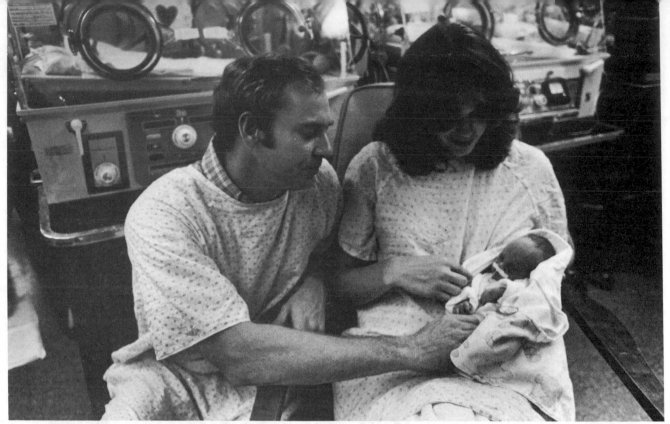

Parents holding their premature baby in the newborn intensive care unit.

Feeding a premature infant may require the help of both parents. In this photo, mother feeds while father holds the oxygen supply close by.

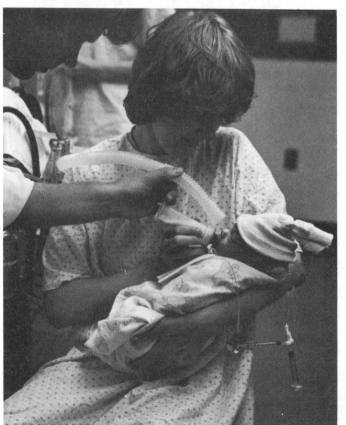

strip back to the monitoring service, where the strip is read by an obstetrical nurse.

Also complementing drugs to stop labor are other medicines known as corticosteroids (steroids). Newer studies report that steroids such as betamethasone help speed up lung maturation in some preterm fetuses. Steroids are given by weekly injection between the twenty-fourth and thirty-fourth week of pregnancy when preterm labor threatens early delivery. Steroids are given at the same time as labor-stopping drugs.

Drug therapy to stop labor, while promising in select individual circumstances, is not by itself likely to change the overall picture of prematurity. Recognition of early signs of preterm labor is important. These signs may include an increase in backache, cramping in the lower abdomen, or irregular contractions. When in doubt, see your physician promptly. A pelvic exam can tell whether you have started labor, and external monitoring can help in the evaluation of persistent contractions even before your cervix is dilated too far.

Table 39   POSSIBLE MEDICAL REASONS FOR INDUCING LABOR

Reason	Comment
High blood pressure (toxemia or "pregnancy-induced hypertension")	Timing of induction depends on severity of disease. Labor is induced near term (40 weeks) if pre-eclampsia is mild but earlier if severe or if fetal tests are abnormal.
Diabetes (requiring insulin)	If you take insulin, labor may be induced two or more weeks early.
Rh disease (you are Rh negative and have had a blood test showing the presence of Rh antibodies—see Chapter 20)	Rare today; timing of induction depends on amniocentesis, which tells how severely fetus is affected.
Overdue (more than two weeks past your due date if this date is definitely established)	Amniocentesis may be done first to confirm fetal maturity if there is uncertainty about your due date.
Inadequate fetal growth	Depends on severity of growth problem as determined by successive sonograms and fetal tests.
Ruptured bag of waters (amniotic fluid leaking)	Labor is often induced within 24 hours of rupture if 36 weeks or more or if signs of infection are present (see Chapter 20) regardless of gestational age.

Induction of Labor

There are several medical reasons for inducing labor. Your physician can induce labor by rupturing the fluid-filled sac which surrounds the fetus (this procedure is called an *amniotomy)* or by giving synthetic *oxytocin*, a hormonal drug which stimulates contractions. Rupturing these membranes initiates labor within twenty-four hours in over 75% of women. When both methods of inducing labor are combined, 98% of women deliver within twenty-four hours. Some clinicians start oxytocin at the same time as amniotomy, while others wait for contractions to start on their own after the membranes have been ruptured. At other times, oxytocin may be started without breaking your waters when your cervix is so-called unfavorable—that is, when your cervix is hard, thick, and completely closed—and delivery is unexpected for at least twelve hours.

The obstetrician may have patients with an "unfavorable" cervix come into the hospital the night before their induction for "cervical ripening." This added step to increase chances for a successful induction of labor involves the use of a vaginal gel containing the hormone prostaglandin. These gels help to soften the cervix to make the induction shorter and easier. Because prostaglandin has oxytocin-like effects (may cause contractions) you must be monitored for a few hours after the gel is inserted and you will usually stay overnight in the hospital.

Amniotomy, the safer and simpler of the two techniques, also allows assessment of the baby's amniotic fluid as noted earlier in this chapter. Once performed, amniotomy commits the clinician to delivery within twenty-four hours because of the increasing chance of infection after this time.

Oxytocin is a powerful drug, a synthesized form of the same hormone found in the brain, which works by stimulating the uterus to contract. It is given intravenously. The flow of oxytocin is increased very slowly to prevent overstimulation of the uterus since too frequent contractions may reduce the baby's oxygen supply. The major maternal risk of oxytocin, uterine rupture, is a rare occurrence. Although uterine contractions induced by oxytocin are identical to the contractions of normal labor, it is theoretically possible that improper use of the drug could cause fetal distress or uterine rupture. Some mothers who have experienced both types of contraction have felt that the induced labor is more painful.

Elective induction of labor, for the convenience of choosing your labor day, may subject the fetus as well as the mother to unnecessary risks during labor and delivery. Some studies associate elective induction of labor with a slightly increased incidence of prematurity (due to miscalculation of the baby's gestational age) and of cesarean births.

Medical reasons for inducing labor are listed in Table 39. In high-risk pregnancies, medically indicated inductions improve the chances of a healthy outcome for both mother and baby. The success of an induction depends upon the readiness of the cervix. A cervix that is soft, thin, and already dilated two to three centimeters responds more readily to oxytocin than an unfavorable cervix, which is undilated, thick, and firm.

Augmentation of Labor

Stimulation, or augmentation, of labor means that the doctor attempts to enhance uterine contractions that have already begun, either by amniotomy or by administering oxytocin, or by a combination of both methods. The oxytocin method is used only if labor is not progressing properly. Amniotomy, however, is often performed routinely whether contractions are normal or not. This is because, in addition to facilitating regular contractions, the procedure enables the clinician to evaluate the condition of the fetus by noting whether the amniotic fluid is clear or stained with meconium (see glossary). Amniotomy is usually performed after you reach about four centimeters of cervical dilation.

Oxytocin is generally indicated when labor contractions are weak or irregular. When contractions are strong and regular, yet labor does not progress, oxytocin is of no benefit and cesarean section may be a more appropriate intervention.

Once the active phase of labor begins (usually after four centimeters dilation), prolonged labor may be of three types:

1. stoppage of labor (there is no change in cervical dilation for two hours or more);
2. slow labor (cervical dilation occurs at a rate slower than one centimeter an hour); and
3. failure of descent (the baby's head does not drop progressively deeper into the birth canal).

All types of prolonged labor are abnormal and may indicate a small pelvis, a large or abnormally positioned baby, or inadequate uterine contractions. When oxytocin is used to stimulate labor which is not progressing normally, delivery usually occurs within two to six hours. If

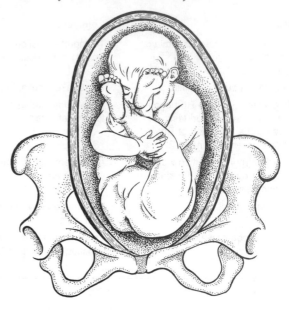

Figure 29
Breech presentation. In the breech position, the baby's bottom or feet enter the birth canal first.

labor does not progress normally with oxytocin, then cesarean birth may be unavoidable.

Breech Birth

In approximately 3% of all deliveries, the baby is in the *breech* position, with the baby's bottom or feet entering the birth canal first rather than the head. Breech presentation is a high-risk condition because of the greater likelihood of prematurity, a prolapsed cord, or fetal injury at the time of delivery.

Because of the high risk associated with breech delivery, many physicians automatically perform a cesarean section when it is the woman's first baby or the baby's feet are entering the birth canal (*footling breech)*, as opposed to the baby's buttocks alone (*frank breech*). In a breech, particularly a premature breech, the head is relatively large compared to the buttocks and may become dangerously trapped within the cervix during vaginal delivery. If delivery is thereby delayed for several minutes, the supply of oxygen to the baby can be threatened. Efforts to release the head when it becomes entrapped during delivery may result in damage to the baby's brain, spinal column, or soft internal organs. Many physicians believe that if vaginal breech delivery is to occur successfully, it is most

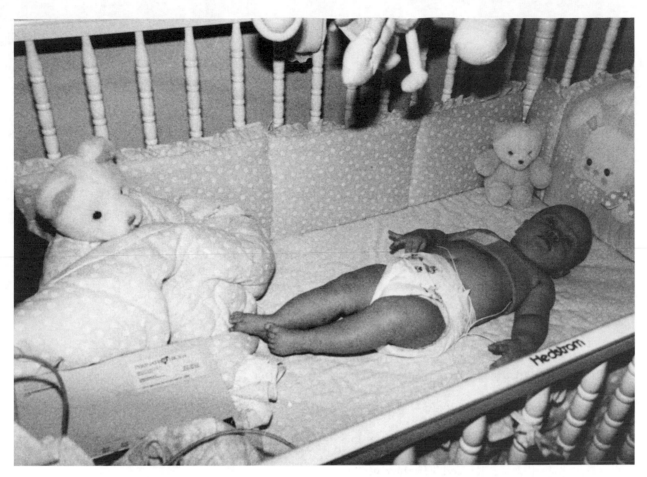

Sometimes after complicated pregnancies, the baby must continue to be monitored at home by the parents.

likely to be accomplished safely in a woman who has previously given birth and who has an average-size baby positioned as a frank breech where the buttocks alone enter the birth canal.

To prevent breech births, some obstetricians are returning to external version, a once-popular procedure in which the baby is manually "turned" from the breech to the normal head-first position. To aid in performing this maneuver, the doctor first gives an intravenous medication to the mother which temporarily relaxes the uterus. The procedure is done before labor begins, around the thirty-seventh week, and most often in a hospital where fetal monitoring is available.

Cesarean Section

A cesarean section, performed if the health of the mother or baby is threatened by vaginal deliv-

ery, is an operation to deliver a baby through an incision in the abdomen. Two types of abdominal incision can be used. The horizontal Pfannenstiel incision, which may be preferred for cosmetic reasons, is made at or just above the pubic hairline. This incision may require several additional minutes to make and thus is not used in an emergency. The other type of incision, called *midline* or *vertical*, starts just below the bellybutton and extends downward. (These two types of incision are shown in Figure 45, in Chapter 43.) The usual time from initial skin incision to delivery ordinarily takes only a few minutes. After the baby is removed from the uterus, the baby breathes normally and cries just like babies born vaginally.

The incision in the *uterus*, unlike the abdominal incision, is almost always one that runs horizontally across the lower part of the uterus, the so-called *low-transverse* incision. Although there are exceptions, this incision is preferred if possible because of its minimal association with infection, bleeding, and subsequent uterine rupture.

Cesarean births are more painful, more disabling, and more expensive than vaginal deliveries. Hospital stays for cesareans now average 2–3 days as opposed to 1–2 days or less for normal deliveries. The most common complication of cesarean births, uterine infection, occurs 15 to 20% of the time, ten times the rate for vaginal deliveries. Although mortality associated with cesarean delivery is extremely low, approximately 4 per 10,000, this risk is 4 times that of normal deliveries. Cesareans have also been linked to prematurity and an increased risk of breathing problems in the newborn, especially when the operation is carried out early without a medical reason.

Why the increase in cesarean births?

One of the most dramatic trends in modern obstetrics has been the rise in cesarean birth rates, which have quadrupled in less than twenty years, in the United States. In 1970 the overall cesarean rate was 6%, rising to 16% in 1980 and to 24% by 1987. Of 3.7 million births in that year, nearly one in four was by cesarean. Several factors help to explain this trend, although the rate of cesarean births has leveled off through the mid-1990s. Opponents of high cesarean rates cite fear of lawsuits as a cause and argue that the cesarean is easier for the doctor than waiting or performing a complicated delivery with the use of forceps. Yet many obstetricians have abandoned some forceps operations like the *midforceps delivery* (see Figure 31), which can be more dangerous to the baby than delivery by cesarean. The safer, gentler, *low-forceps delivery* is still performed by most obstetricians, but in general, less frequent use of forceps in cases of prolonged labor or fetal distress has meant that the obstetrician more often turns to cesarean when these situations arise.

The real culprit in the latest statistics is not first-time cesareans but repeat cesarean births, which contributed one-third of the 966,000 cesarean sections done in 1990. The high number of repeats results in part from an ingrained U.S. tradition that says "once a cesarean, always a cesarean"—a practice not followed in other countries. This dictum originated in 1914, when most obstetricians performed cesareans by making a vertical incision in the upper part of the

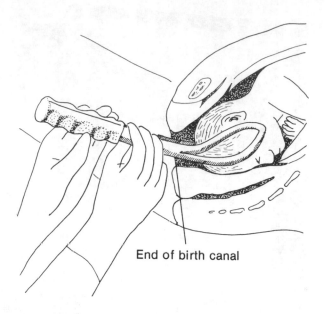

Figure 30
Low-forceps delivery. The baby's head has reached the lower end of the birth canal before the forceps are applied.

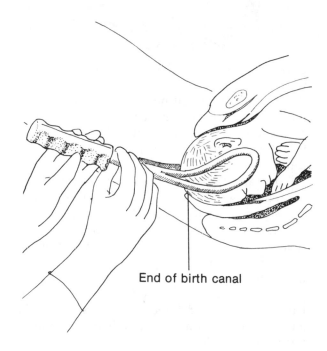

Figure 31
Mid-forceps delivery. The baby's head still has not reached the lower end of the birth canal when the forceps are applied. In this situation considerably more traction may be required to deliver the baby vaginally compared to a low-forceps procedure.

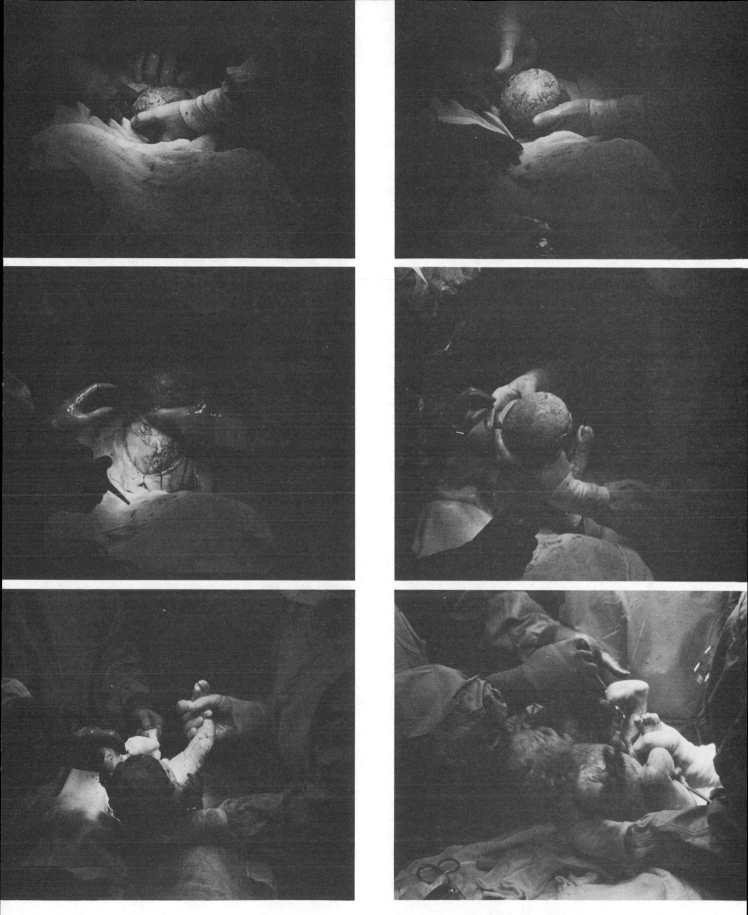

uterus, the so-called classical cesarean operation. Classical cesareans *do* represent a significant risk for uterine rupture when labor begins. Today, however, the classical operation is rarely performed; instead, doctors use a low horizontal incision (called *low-transverse* or *low-segment* cesarean section) most of the time. The low-transverse incision minimizes the risk of uterine rupture and is generally a safe incision for subsequent vaginal birth.

In an attempt to encourage physicians to change their practice patterns (and to lower the cesarean birth rate in the United States), the American College of Obstetricians and Gynecologists issued guidelines in 1988 and then again in 1994 on the subject of vaginal birth after cesarean (VBAC). The guidelines currently suggest hospitals and obstetricians routinely give their patients a trial of labor and vaginal birth after most cesarean sections. The guidelines note that the hospital should be able to perform an emergency cesarean and that the prior cesarean should have utilized a lower uterine incision (not the "classical" type). Previous studies show that vaginal deliveries will be successful in 60% to 80% of women with previous cesarean births and can also be attempted by those with two previous cesareans. Women in whom a prior cesarean was performed for failure to progress also have an excellent chance of successful vaginal birth subsequently.

The extent to which the increased use of VBAC births can reduce cesarean rates is not clear. For some patients and physicians, having a repeat cesarean appears to be a simpler, easier solution. Hospital staffs will have to take an active role if VBAC rather than a cesarean section is to become the norm. A few practitioners still have mixed feelings about VBAC. However, the number of VBAC births is growing. In 1993, 25% of the women who had a previous cesarean birth delivered their infants vaginally compared to only 12.6% of such mothers in 1988.

Other ways to lower cesarean section rates can be found and have been urged by various consumer groups as well as an expert NIH panel that convened on the subject over a decade ago. The panel recommended, for example, that some babies in breech position be allowed to deliver vaginally if the mother's pelvis is normal and the baby is of average size. But the greatest reduction in C-section rates must come from altering management of patients with difficult or prolonged labors. These patients account for more first-time cesarean births than any other group. Prolonged labor may be due to any combination of weak contractions, a small pelvis, or a large baby. Allowing patients with difficult labors to labor longer, especially when the baby's size isn't excessive, is another important way to further lower the cesarean section rate.

Options with cesarean birth

Even if you have your baby by cesarean, you can still experience a number of birth options in most hospitals. Fathers are usually allowed in the operating room, and, in a few institutions, you can observe the birth procedure by means of a mirror. Also, you can usually hold your baby and sometimes breast-feed right after delivery while the physician is closing your incision.

Resources

Some communities have cesarean support groups or special classes for repeat cesarean mothers. Find out what is available in your area from the local childbirth education association.

International Cesarean Awareness Network (ICAN)
1304 Kingsdale Avenue
Redondo Beach, California 90278
(310) 542-6400

C/SEC
c/o Norma Shulman
22 Forrest Road
Framington, Massachusetts 01701

References for Section Four

Chapter 14—Childbirth Education

MacDonald, J. Prenatal review classes . . . expectant couples who aready have children. *Canadian Nurse* 83(9):26–29, Oct 1987.

Lindell, S. Education for childbirth: a time for change. *Journal of Obstetric, Gynecologic and Neonatal Nursing* 17(2):108–112, Mar/Apr 1988.

Nunnerly, R. Parent education. *Nursing Times* 84 (29): July 1988.

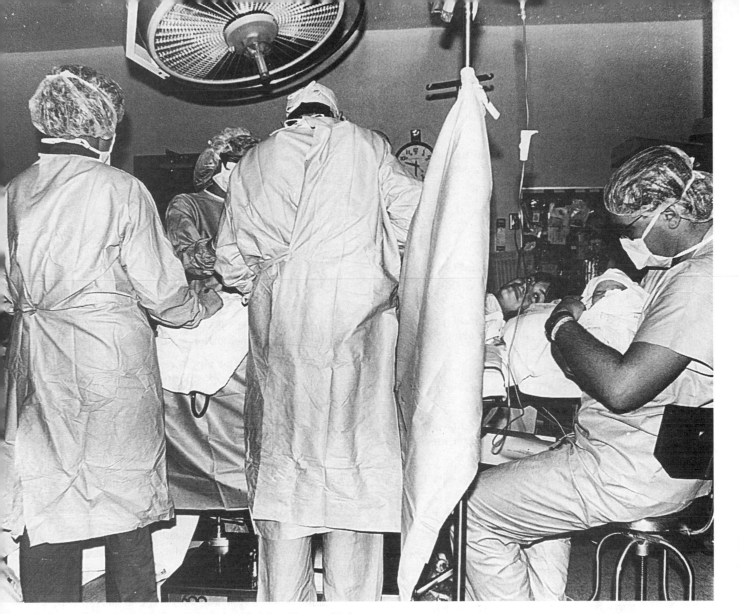

A father holds his new baby moments after cesarean birth.

Avery, P. Expanding the scope for childbirth education to meet the needs of hospitalized, high-risk clients. *Journal of Obstetric, Gynecologic and Neonatal Nursing* 16(6):418–421, Nov/Dec 1987.

Aaronson, L. Seeking information: where do pregnant women go? *Health Education Quarterly* 15(3):335–345, Fall 1988.

Jimenez, S. Education for the childbearing years—comprehensive application of psychoprophylaxis. *Journal of Obstetric, Gynecologic and Neonatal Nursing* 9:97–99, Mar/Apr 1980.

Dick-Read, G. *Childbirth Without Fear.* New York: Harper & Row, 1979.

Kitzinger, S. *Six Practical Lessons for Easier Childbirth.* New York: Bantam Books, 1981.

Chapter 15—Hospital Birth and Its Alternatives

Flint, C. Know your midwife . . . one who would tend to mother's birth at home and in hospital. *Nursing Times* 84(38):28–32, Sep 1988.

Flint, C. Home services. *Nursing Times* 83(24): 22–24, June 1987.

Faison, J. B. The childbearing center: an alternative birth setting. *Obstetrics and Gynecology* 54(4):527–532, 1979.

Anderson, J. Alternative birth center gives parents a new option. *Hospital Forum* 19:4–5, July 1976.

Wertz, R. W., and Wertz, D. C. *Lying-In: A History of Childbirth in America.* New York: Free Press, 1977.

Devitt, N. The transition from home to hospital birth in the U.S. 1930–1960. *Birth and the Family Journal* 4:47–58, Summer 1977.

Dobbs, K. B., et al. Alternative birth rooms and birth options. *Obstetrics and Gynecology* 58(5):626–630, 1981.

Chapter 16—Pregnancy
Chapter 17—Labor and Delivery

American College of Obstetricians and Gynecologists *Technical Bulletin* 187. Ultrasonography in pregnancy, Dec 1993.

American College of Obstetricians and Gynecologists *Technical Bulletin* 179. Nutrition during pregnancy, Apr 1993.

American College of Obstetricians and Gynecologists *Technical Bulletin* 205. Preconceptional care, May 1995.

American College of Obstetricians and Gynecologists *Practice Patterns* 1. Vaginal birth after previous cesarean birth, Aug 1995.

Williams Obstetrics, Supplement 13: Obesity in pregnancy, June/July 1995.

Sciscione, A. Update on fetal assessment. *The Female Patient* 19: 75–88, Sep 1994.

Artal, R. Exercise during pregnancy and postpartum. *Contemporary OB/GYN* 62–90, May 1995.

American College of Obstetricians and Gynecologists *Technical Bulletin* 207. Fetal heart patterns: monitoring, interpretation, and management, July 1995.

American College of Obstetricians and Gynecologists *Technical Bulletin* 189. Exercise during pregnancy and the postpartum period, Feb 1994.

American College of Obstetricians and Gynecologists *Technical Bulletin* 154. Alpha-fetoprotein, Apr 1991.

American College of Obstetricians and Gynecologists *Technical Bulletin* 151. Automobile passenger restraints for children and pregnant women, Jan 1991.

American College of Obstetricians and Gynecologists, Committee on obstetrics, maternal and fetal medicine (ACOG) and committee on fetus and newborn (AAP), *Committee Opinion* 49. Use and misuse of apgar score, Nov 1986.

Leveno, K. Forecasting fetal health. *Williams Obstetrics*, Supplement 19:1–11, Aug/Sep 1988.

Sabbagaha, R. Recent trends in ultrasound. *The Female Patient* 13:77–93, Apr 1988.

Coppel, J. Doppler ultrasound in obstetrics. *Williams Obstetrics*, Supplement 16: Feb/Mar 1988.

Rebar, R. Early home detection of pregnancy. *Journal of Reproductive Medicine* 32(9):710–716, Sep 1987.

Charles, D. How colostrum and milk protect the newborn. *Contemporary OB/GYN* 24(1):143–166, July 1984.

Cunningham, F. *Williams Obstetrics*, 18th ed. Norwalk, Conn: Appleton and Lange, 1989.

Chapter 18—Your First Weeks as a Mother

American College of Obstetricians and Gynecologists *Technical Bulletin* 148. Diagnosis and management of postpartum hemorrhage, July 1990.

Storr, G. Prevention of nipple tenderness and breast engorgement in the postpartum period. *Journal of Obstetric, Gynecologic and Neonatal Nursing* 17(3): 203–209, May/June 1988.

Affonso, D. D. Missing pieces—a study of postpartum feelings. *Birth and the Family Journal* 4:159–164, Winter 1977.

Jones, F., et al. Maternal responsiveness of primiparous mothers during the postpartum period—age differences. *Pediatrics* 65:579–584, Mar 1980.

Johannsen, L. As birth and death coincide. *Maternal Child Nursing* 14(2):89–92, Mar/Apr 1989.

Brewer, M. Postpartum changes in maternal weight and body fat deposits in lactating versus nonlactating women. *American Journal of Clinical Nutrition* 49(2):259–265, Feb 1989.

Broderick, E. Baby bottle tooth decay in Native American children in Head-Start centers. *Public Health Reports* 104(1):50–54, Jan/Feb 1989.

Chapter 19—Options During and After Childbirth

Goldstein, S. Early pregnancy scanning with the endovaginal probe. *Contemporary OB/GYN* 31(6):54–64, June 1988.

Eisenach, J. Patient-controlled analgesia following caesarian section: a comparison with epidural and intramuscular narcotics. *Anesthesiology* 68:444–448, 1988.

Harrison, D. Epidural narcotic and patient-controlled analgesia for post-caesarian section pain relief. *Anesthesiology* 68:454–457, 1988.

American Academy of Pediatrics. *Report of the task force on circumcision*, 1989.

Mahan, C. Preps and enemas—keep or discard? *Contemporary OB/GYN* 22(5):241–248, Nov 1983.

McKay, S. Laboring patients need more freedom to move. *Contemporary OB/GYN* 24(1):90–119, July 1984.

Klaus, M., and Kennel, J. *Maternal-infant Bonding*. St. Louis: C. V. Mosby Co., 1976.

Is circumcision medically justified? *Patient Care* 23 (2): 86–89, Jan 1989.

Hill, P. Effects of heat and cold on the perineum after episiotomy—laceration. *Journal of Obstetric, Gynecologic and Neonatal Nursing* 18(2):124–129, Mar/Apr 1989.

Rockner, G. Episiotomy and perinatal trauma during childbirth. *Journal of Advanced Nursing* 14(4):264–268, Apr 1989.

Liu, Y. The effects of the upright position during childbirth. *Journal of Nursing Scholarship* 21(1):14–18, Spring 1989.

Chapter 20—Complicated Pregnancies

American College of Obstetricians and Gynecologists *Technical Bulletin* 91. Management of preeclampsia, Feb 1986.

American College of Obstetricians and Gynecologists *Technical Bulletin* 117. Antimicrobial therapy for obstetric patients, June 1988.

American College of Obstetricians and Gynecologists *Technical Bulletin* 115. Premature rupture of membranes, Apr 1988.

American College of Obstetricians and Gynecologists *Technical Bulletin* 122. Perinatal herpes simplex virus infections, Nov 1988.

American College of Obstetricians and Gynecologists *Technical Bulletin* 131. Multiple gestation, Aug 1989.

American College of Obstetricians and Gynecologists *Technical Bulletin* 130. Diagnosis and management of postterm pregnancy, July 1989.

American College of Obstetricians and Gynecologists *Technical Bulletin* 148. Management of isoimmunization in pregnancy, Oct 1990.

American College of Obstetricians and Gynecologists *Technical Bulletin* 161. Trauma during pregnancy, Nov 1991.

American College of Obstetricians and Gynecologists *Technical Bulletin* 168. Cardiac disease in pregnancy, June 1992.

American College of Obstetricians and Gynecologists *Technical Bulletin* 170. Group B streptococcal infections, July 1992.

American College of Obstetricians and Gynecologists *Technical Bulletin* 171. Rubella and pregnancy, Aug 1992.

American College of Obstetricians and Gynecologists *Technical Bulletin* 174. Hepatitis in pregnancy, Nov 1992.

American College of Obstetricians and Gynecologists *Technical Bulletin* 188. Antepartum fetal surveillance, Jan 1994.

American College of Obstetricians and Gynecologists *Technical Bulletin* 200. Diabetes and pregnancy, Dec 1994.

Dorfman, S. AIDS and pregnancy. *The Female Patient* 14:86–90, Feb 1989.

Sachs, B. Acquired immunodeficiency syndrome: suggested protocol for counseling and screening in pregnancy, *Obstetrics and Gynecology* 70:408–411, 1987.

Phelan, J. Antepartum fetal assessment: newer techniques. *Seminars in Perinatology* 12(1):57–65, 1988.

Shephard, B. Problem pregnancies. *Encyclopaedia Britannica Health Annual:* 433–436, 1987.

Romero, R. A critical appraisal of fetal acoustic stimulation as an antenatal test for fetal well-being. *Obstetrics and Gynecology* 71:781–786, 1988.

Stabile, I. Ultrasonic assessment of complications during first trimester pregnancy. *Lancet* 2:1237–1240, 1987.

Chervenak, F. Multiple gestation: diagnosis and management. *The Female Patient* 14(3):38–53, Mar 1989.

Chez, R. Meeting the challenge of gestational diabetes. *Contemporary OB/GYN* 34(3):120–140, Sep 1989.

Research Reports from the National Institute of Child Health and Human Development. Diabetes in early pregnancy study yields important results, June 1988.

Leveno, K. Gestational diabetes: evolving concepts and misconceptions. *Williams Obstetrics*, Supplement 9: Nov/Dec 1986.

Maslow, A. Herpes in pregnancy: exploring clinical options. *Contemporary OB/GYN* 32(4):44–61, Oct 1988.

Amstey, M. High risk pregnancy: confining herpes infection. *Contemporary OB/GYN* 34(3):73–81, Sep 1989.

Friedman, S. Hepatitis B screening in a New York City obstetrics service. *American Journal of Public Health* 78:308–310, 1988.

Centers For Disease Control, Immunization practices advisory committee. Prevention of perinatal transmission of hepatitis B virus: prenatal screening of all pregnant patients for hepatitis B surface antigen. *Morbidity and Mortality Weekly Report* 37(22): 341–345, June 1988.

Garite, T. Premature rupture of membranes—exploring management strategies. *Contemporary OB/GYN* 30(4):153–168, Oct 1987.

Gant, N. Inappropriate fetal growth: diagnosis and management of fetal growth retardation. *Williams Obstetrics*, Supplement 14: Sep/Oct 1987.

Carlan, S. Post dates pregnancy—a new look at management. *The Female Patient* 14(3):87–99, Mar 1989.

Resarias, F. Postdatism and the law—the minimum standards. *The Female Patient* 14:28–37, May 1989.

Stear, L. Understanding acquired immune deficiency syndrome: implications for pregnancy. *Journal of Perinatal Neonatal Nursing* 4:33–46, Apr 1988.

Kemp, V. Maternal self-esteem and prenatal attachment in high risk pregnancy. *Maternal Child Nursing Journal* 16(3):195–206, Fall, 1987.

Chapter 21—Complications of Labor and Delivery

American College of Obstetricians and Gynecologists *Technical Bulletin* 206. Preterm labor, June 1995.

American College of Obstetricians and Gynecologists *Technical Bulletin* 95. Management of the breech presentation, Aug 1986.

American College of Obstetricians and Gynecologists *Technical Bulletin* 86. Grief related to perinatal death, Apr 1985.

American College of Obstetricians and Gynecologists, Committee on obstetrics: maternal and fetal medicine, *Committee Opinion* 115. Home uterine activity monitoring, Sep 1992.

Flamm, B. Vaginal birth after caesarian section: results of a multicenter study. *American Journal of Obstetrics and Gynecology* 158:1079–1084, 1988.

Vaginal birth after caesarian revisited—does it work in rural areas? *ACOG Newsletter* 33(9):1, Sep 1989.

Phelan, J. Twice a caesarian, always a caesarian? *Obstetrics and Gynecology* 73:161–165, 1989.

Queenan, J. Today's high c/s rate: can we reduce it? *Contemporary OB/GYN* 32(1):154–166, July 1988.

Phelan, J. Finding alternatives to caesarian section. *Contemporary OB/GYN* 31(1):191–210, Jan 1988.

Beguin, E. Vaginal birth after caesarian section: what are the risks? *The Female Patient* 13:16–29, Aug 1988.

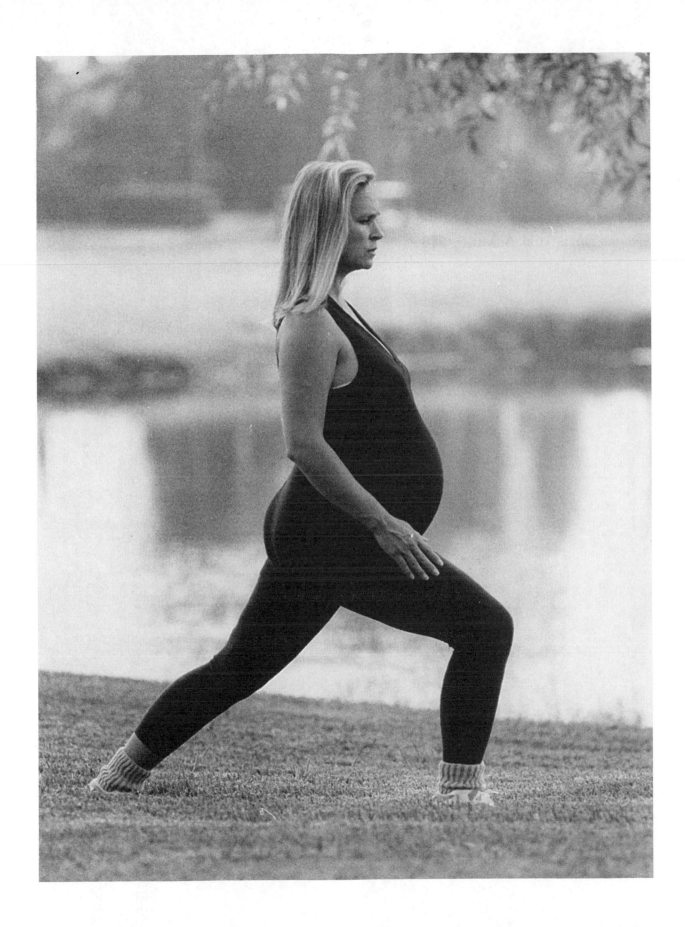

F·I·V·E

SEXUAL ISSUES FOR TODAY'S WOMAN

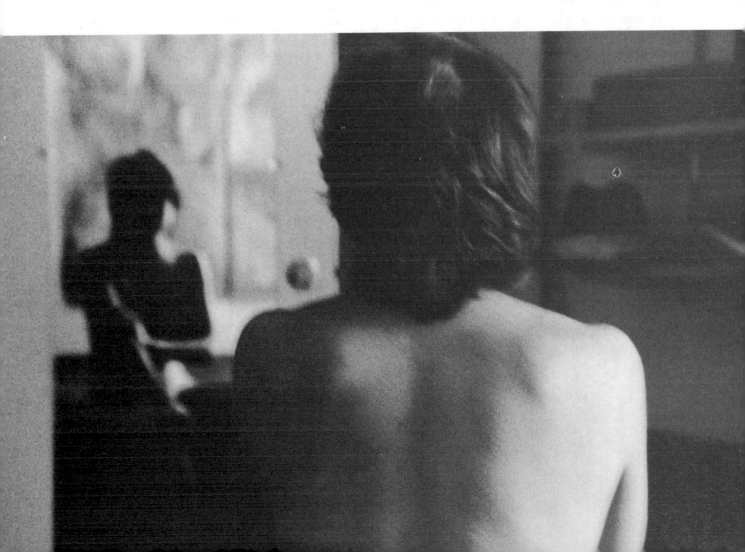

CHAPTER 22

Female Sexuality

A woman's attitude toward her own sexuality is greatly influenced by the information and "messages" she received about sex while she was growing up. In spite of today's greater sexual freedom, sex still remains a hidden, secret, or even taboo subject much of the time.

Formal sex education in school, for example, fails to offer enough information to answer the questions young people may be too embarrassed to ask. In addition, parents often do not provide adequate sex information, either because they do not have enough information themselves or because they, perhaps like their own parents, feel uncomfortable discussing sex with their children. The message we may receive from all this is that sex is not a proper topic for open or easy conversation, and, hence, sex itself is to be suppressed.

The words people use to talk about sex and sexual parts of the body also give us clues about sexual attitudes. Terms that mean sexual intercourse are often vague ("doing it") or technical ("coitus") or evasive ("sleeping together"). Our sexual vocabulary seldom includes words that are plain and simple and human. No wonder people often feel embarrassed or nervous talking about sex!

So-called double messages are also abundant in our everyday lives, and it is easy to understand why many women (and men) feel confused about their sexuality. Your family or your religion may tell you to "be a virgin until you are married," while the media, through sexually explicit movies, and more recently through the television, encourages sexual casualness. We may be torn between peer pressure for sexual freedom and our own determination of what is "right" and "wrong," "healthy" and "unhealthy," or "moral" and "immoral." Such conflicts may interfere with a person's ability to clarify his or her *own* values and needs.

If you feel uncertain about your own sexual

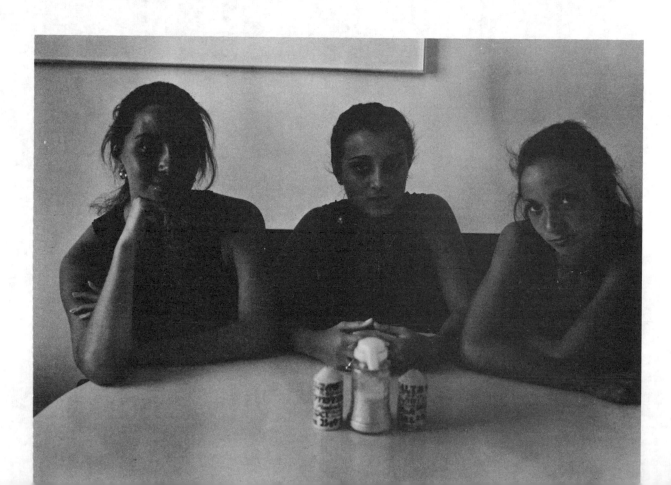

beliefs, you might try to review what you learned about sex from family, school, religion, peers, and society in general. Are there many conflicting messages? Try to decide which values are meaningful for you right now. You might find you have grown up with some sexual attitudes or beliefs you don't care to live with. Changing longstanding attitudes is not easy, but just being aware of them may help you substitute more desirable ones. Some people find that talking with partners, friends, or even a therapist may help them clarify or redefine their sexual goals.

Sexual Response Cycle

Our society often equates sex with intercourse. Though it is helpful to know about the sexual response cycle, there is nothing mandatory about having to go through the whole cycle each time. Kissing, hugging, and other acts of physical affection can be just as sexually satisfying as intercourse at times.

A woman responds to sexual excitement emotionally and physically. While the emotional response varies widely depending on several factors (your sexual attitudes, your relationship with your partner, the physical setting, and so on), the physical changes that the body goes through are similar in all situations. The *sexual response cycle* is the name given to these natural physical changes that a person experiences from initial sexual stimulation through orgasm and back to the original state. Although this cycle is divided into four basic stages—*excitement, plateau, orgasm,* and *resolution*—there isn't always a sharp line between the end of one stage and the beginning of the next. These changes result from two physiologic processes: engorgement (increased circulation of blood to certain parts of the body) and increased muscle tension.

When a woman becomes sexually aroused, whether from sexual fantasy, masturbation, or a sexual partner, the *excitement* state begins. The first response is vaginal lubrication; that is, the woman's vagina gets wet because vaginal blood vessels become engorged during excitement and force a mucuslike fluid into the vaginal canal. The amount of lubricant in the vagina can be affected by a number of different factors, including a woman's past sexual experience. When anxiety or pain is associated with previous in-tercourse, vaginal lubrication may decrease. The older woman, too, usually finds that vaginal fluid naturally decreases. If you need additional lubrication, simply use a water-soluble lubricant, such as K-Y or Transi-Lube, which you can find in most drugstores. Contraceptive creams, jellies, and foams also provide extra lubrication, as does the new vaginal moisturizer, Replens. Avoid using a petroleum jelly (such as Vaseline) as a vaginal lubricant, however; a greasy jelly (that is, one that is not water soluble) does not wash out of the vagina by itself and can thus become a breeding place for bacteria.

During the excitement stage, increased blood circulation to the genital area deepens the color of the vulva to deep pink or reddish and makes the labia puffy and thicker. (You may want to refer at this point to Chapter 3, on female anatomy.) The clitoris also swells. Meanwhile, muscles in the woman's uterus begin to tense.

As sexual stimulation continues, the woman moves into the *plateau* stage of the sexual response cycle when the vaginal lips become even more engorged and puffy. The clitoris moves closer to the body and tucks itself up under its hood. Directly stimulating the sensitive clitoris at this time might be painful, but touching the hood with the clitoris underneath it only heightens the pleasurable sensations. During plateau, muscles all over your body tense up. Your heartbeat, blood pressure, and breathing rate increase with continued stimulation. The breast nipples become erect, and the breasts themselves become somewhat larger.

Women need continued sexual stimulation to reach the *orgasm* phase, the third stage in the response cycle. Orgasm, physiologically a reflex, occurs when the engorgement and muscle tension reach a peak and then release. Fewer than half of American women have orgasm during intercourse. Different women need different kinds of stimulation to produce an orgasm. Some women prefer breast stimulation or whole-body contact, while others like frequent touching of the clitoral area, and still others enjoy some other form of stimulation. Most women require at least some clitoral stimulation to achieve orgasm.

How women react to orgasm depends on the specific situation: whether or not you are alone or with a partner, the physical setting, the intensity of the orgasm, and so on. Some women tremble, some thrash a bit, others remain still.

Some people are quiet, others may moan or weep or cry out. The important thing is to recognize that there is no "right" pattern to follow, and the amount of noise or movement a person makes does not necessarily show how much pleasure she is experiencing.

During the *resolution* stage of the sexual response cycle, engorgement subsides, the muscles relax, and you may perspire as your body returns to its pre-excitement stage. The swollen clitoris and other parts of the body return to their normal state, as does your heart rate and blood pressure. A woman's body goes through the resolution stage whether or not she reaches orgasm. If she did not have an orgasm, the resolution stage lasts a bit longer.

Sexual Responsiveness

You probably find that you enjoy various approaches to sexual experiences. Sometimes, while becoming very excited, you may want to alter the pace of activity, slowing down and then building up to intense excitement once or several times to prolong the warm, tingly sensations. Or you might enjoy moving rapidly and directly into a state of higher excitement and orgasm. At other times, you may prefer the warmth of hugging without the goal of intercourse in mind.

Cultural beliefs about female sexual responsiveness have changed over the years. During the early part of this century many people did not believe that women had sexual urges and satisfactions comparable to a man's, so no one expected women to have orgasms. When researchers found that women did indeed experience orgasms, they believed orgasms were possible only during intercourse. Later, it was believed that women had two distinct kinds of orgasm: the "clitoral" type from clitoral stimulation and the "vaginal" type, which was believed to occur in the vagina during sexual intercourse. It is now known, however, that there is only one kind of orgasm, in which the clitoris and vagina each play a part: the clitoris *receives* the stimulation, and the vagina *reacts* to this stimulation with muscular contractions during orgasm. Although this physical reflex always happens in the same way, women may experience the feelings of orgasm in different places. Sometimes a woman may be more aware of the orgasmic feeling in her vagina, sometimes around the clitoris, sometimes in the entire genital area, with these feelings sometimes "spreading" to other parts of the body. Some women experience several orgasms at a time; others have one orgasm. Having multiple orgasms, however, does not necessarily make the experience any more enjoyable. Only you can measure your own sexual satisfaction and thereby determine what is personally satisfying.

Sexual Expression

The variety of activities we take part in as we respond to our sexual needs is limited only by the imagination. This part of the chapter discusses common forms of sexual expression.

Although it is one of the most common and frequent sexual practices, masturbation, or self-stimulation, is a subject surrounded by ignorance and shame. Masturbation is in no way harmful, and some sex therapists even suggest masturbating techniques to increase body awareness, which often helps overcome certain sexual problems. Many individuals continue to masturbate even when involved in long-term sexual relationships.

When women masturbate, they generally stimulate the area of the clitoris, moving their fingers in small circles or using a pressing motion. These strokes gradually become more intense as a woman reaches orgasm, and most women continue to stimulate themselves through the orgasm. Some women find that tensing the muscles in their thighs or in their genitals increases sexual stimulation. Others use electric or battery-operated vibrators for stimulation. Many people have sexual fantasies while they are masturbating. The content of these fantasies, which may include, say, having sex with someone not available as a partner in reality, is limited only by the imagination.

When women are involved in sexual relationships with men, there are any number of sexual activities in which the two partners may engage, depending upon their shared interests, desires, and values.

Some women prefer to have sexual relationships with other women. Although our society has a history of prejudice against relationships between two people of the same sex, such relationships are becoming more commonly accepted as valid expressions of the individual's sexual and emotional needs. Some lesbian couples have established families through artificial insemination, adoption, or in cooperation with gay men.

Some people in our society are bisexual; that is, they have relationships with partners of both sexes. Many bisexuals choose a partner on the basis of personality rather than on gender. That is, the woman is attracted to others on the basis of their personal qualities, and, for her, such relationships with either a man or a woman might become sexual. Other women feel they can have different kinds of experiences with a woman from what they can have with a man, and they like to experience both of these relationships.

Another sexual option is celibacy: the voluntary decision not to have sexual partners for a given period of time. A person might choose to be celibate for many different reasons—to take time to heal after a relationship has ended, or to concentrate one's time and energy on other things.

Sexual Problems

The natural bodily responses to sexual stimulation do not always occur exactly as you might think they should or just in the way that you want. This brings up a sensitive question: when, if ever, does failure to achieve a desired response mean you have a sexual problem? There are times in everyone's life when they just are not feeling sensual or sexual. Illness, financial worry, and stressful work demands are only a few of life's crises that naturally decrease sexual interest and responsiveness.

There may also be times when you feel ready for a sexual experience but your body does not respond as expected—you just don't feel aroused. Such events happen to everyone from time to time and are not problems unless they begin to interfere with your relationship or occur with increasing frequency. In this sense, you are the one to decide whether or not there is a problem. This part of the chapter discusses the causes of some sexual difficulties.

Anxiety causes many sexual problems. The kind of anxiety that interferes with a person's ability to function sexually is very common and has many sources. Conflicting or inadequate information about sex is an important factor.

Women are often brought up to repress or ignore their sexuality. They may, for example, be discouraged from the natural childhood activity of exploring their genitals, and they may not even be taught about their anatomy. If a woman does not understand how her body functions sexually, she may experience difficulty or simply may not know what to do in a sexual situation. Sometimes uncertainties about sexual values underlie nervousness about sex if your partner wants to engage in a certain sexual activity but you do not. Other things that may make us anxious include unrealistic expectations about ourselves or our partners or too much emphasis on technique. Guilt feelings about sexuality, possibly because of what we have been taught about sex as children, can easily cause anxiety. Or a woman may be afraid that she is not a "good lover," or that her partner will reject her. If you have a sexual problem related to anxiety, it's important to explore the roots of your sexual attitudes and values on your own or with your partner or a therapist, so you will be able to clarify your own sexual needs, values, and goals. This self-exploration alone may relieve the anxiety and therefore the problem.

Anxiety about a sexual situation can make you do "sex-watching." That is, you begin watching yourself as if you were watching an actress in a movie. You may look at yourself and say, "I look too fat," or "What am I doing here?" and so on. Watching the "movie" as it plays in your head reduces your anxiety, because you are so preoccupied with the "movie" that you do not experience your feelings of anxiety. However, this means that you do not allow yourself the full benefits of your pleasurable feelings either. A person cannot completely enjoy the sexual experience while sex-watching; your energy cannot go both ways. It is fairly common to engage in sex-watching; and, if you find yourself doing it, try to refocus your attention and get into the experience, or maybe take time out to talk with your partner about how you are feeling.

Sex-watching is not the same as having a sexual fantasy. In a fantasy, you think sexual thoughts and imagine sexual activities. Sex-watching takes you and your feelings out of the sexual situation, while fantasy can be a way to get even more deeply involved.

Another major source of sexual difficulties is poor communication between sexual partners.

Some people will not talk to their partners about sexuality, fearing, for example, that talking during sex will "spoil the mood." Or sometimes sexual preferences go unexpressed because one partner assumes that the other already knows which manner of touching, for example, gives the greatest pleasure. At other times you may feel shy or nervous about telling your partner what you like because you are afraid that he may think you are criticizing him. In all of these situations, the partners need to talk with each other. It may help to begin by acknowledging feelings such as fear, shyness, or embarrassment. Such open communication may make it less threatening to discuss sexual problems.

Sexual problem areas

There are three basic areas in which a person might experience sexual problems: sexual desire, sexual arousal (excitement), and orgasm.

Lack of desire is a very common sexual problem. While everyone experiences variation in sexual interest from time to time, a problem may arise when lack of desire persists. People who experience a lack of desire do not initiate sexual activities and may have few sexual fantasies. Such individuals may participate in sex but do not find the experience very satisfying.

Occasionally, lack of sexual desire has a physical cause, such as chronic illness or drugs, like sedatives or alcohol. More often this problem results from psychological factors. Anxiety, depression, and guilt, and any of the situations which produce these symptoms, may contribute to a lack of sexual desire. The problem may be a relationship conflict, especially where differences in attitudes or values exist or where an underlying power struggle between partners leads to resentment or hostility. Other relationship problems such as unresolved anger or fear of intimacy can lower an individual's sexual desire.

Some therapists use what might be called relearning methods to treat lack of sexual desire. The therapist may, for example, help the client learn positive attitudes about sexuality. However, the underlying causes of this problem are usually more complicated than other sexual problems. Thus, treatment for lack of sexual desire often requires the use of more traditional counseling methods to explore relevant individual and/or relationship conflicts.

In the second problem area—sexual arousal—a woman has sexual desires and wants to be sexual, but her vagina will not lubricate. The woman and her partner may not know how to trigger stimuli for lubrication, or the woman may have that information but not know how to share it with her partner. Sometimes even when a woman wants to be sexual, her anxiety about sex prevents her body from functioning normally. This situation might occur in a woman who was told as a child that sex is "bad" and has not unlearned this message as an adult.

Related to lack of sexual arousal is the problem of painful intercourse, called *dyspareunia*. Sometimes a woman has intercourse when she has not had enough time to become aroused or when she is not getting aroused because of psychological reasons. In such cases, her vagina may not lubricate, and intercourse will be painful or uncomfortable. But most of the time, dyspareunia is due to a physical problem. A vaginal irritation or infection is a very common cause. Quite simply, if there is an infection in the vagina, movement of the penis inside will hurt. An allergic reaction to a douche or a contraceptive product may also cause painful intercourse. There is a difference between vaginal discomfort during intercourse caused by vaginal infections or allergic symptoms, and deep dyspareunia which is felt as pain or discomfort in the lower abdomen during intercourse. Deep dyspareunia is sometimes caused by a pelvic infection, endometriosis, or scarring after previous surgery (see Chapter 83 on pelvic pain). Once the symptoms of the physical problem are treated, dyspareunia typically disappears. As long as painful intercourse continues, however, anticipation of discomfort may lead to decreased vaginal lubrication and further contribute to the pain.

One of the most common sexual complaints of American women is the third sexual problem area—difficulty in reaching orgasm. As discussed earlier, a majority of women do not reach orgasm during intercourse. Sometimes a woman may have orgasms through masturbation but never with her partner. Or she may be able to experience orgasm with one partner but not with another. If a woman can have orgasms by, for example, self-stimulation or when a partner touches her, lack of orgasm during intercourse need not be defined as a sexual problem. If, however, a woman does not reach orgasm by means of any type of sexual stimulation, and if failure to have an orgasm disturbs her or her relationship, then she and her partner may want to consider sex therapy (see below).

In general, the causes of difficulties with orgasm are similar to the reasons for other sexual problems. Frequently, a woman simply does not receive either enough stimulation or the kind of stimulation she needs. Sometimes a woman is so eager to have an orgasm that she tries too hard, and she is so busy being anxious about this orgasm that her body cannot respond.

Treatment for failure to experience orgasm involves dealing with any anxiety that may be present and having the couple learn the appropriate and adequate stimulation needed. This often involves exercises to learn how the female body responds, along with an understanding that this process takes some time to unlearn old responses and learn new ones.

Sex Therapy

What are your options if you decide you have a sexual problem? You might begin by getting more information. There are a number of useful books available that focus on specific topics, for example, offering women information with which they can teach themselves how to have orgasms. Sometimes, especially if self-help does not work, you might want to seek professional help from a person who has been specially trained in the field of sex therapy.

Barring physical causes, most sexual problems are not "individual" problems but are problems of the couple. Most sex therapists approach sexual problems with this view and work only with the couple. In other words, contrary to what may be expressed by a woman's partner (implicitly or explicitly), he is part of the problem.

Sex therapy today approaches sexual problems as learned behavior patterns. We are born with the ability to be sexual, but such factors as ignorance, guilt, cultural attitudes, and other contributing factors may place roadblocks in the way of normal sexual responsiveness. In this approach, the therapist helps the couple identify and remove these roadblocks by a process of relearning while also helping them to explore any problem areas in their relationship that might have a bearing on the sexual difficulty.

Sex therapists often give couples exercises in

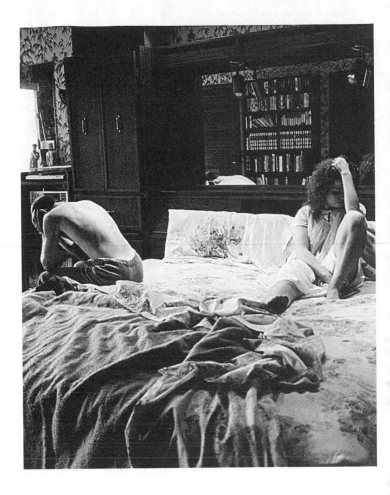

what is called *sensate focus* to practice at home between sessions. Sensate focus refers to a massage technique that teaches you to focus on the pleasurable sensations you feel when your body is being touched. The first set of exercises involves your partner massaging your body but without touching your breasts or genitals. Only later is direct genital stimulation permitted. In this way, you can experience pleasurable feelings without worrying about either sexual performance or having an orgasm.

What constitutes a qualified sex therapist? Unfortunately, many people call themselves sex therapists but are not qualified as such. Moreover, authorities within the profession do not agree on the qualifications for a competent sex therapist. There is some consensus, however, as to certain base lines that should be used to evaluate a sex therapist. These base lines include the following:

1. The therapist should have a terminal (or advanced) degree in his or her profession:

for example, M.D. (psychiatrist), Ph.D. (psychologist), M.S.W. (social worker), M.A. or M.S. (Marital and Family therapist), M.S. (nurse).

2. He or she should be competent in doing marital therapy or marital counseling—that is, working with couples who have marriage problems.

3. The therapist should be trained both in human sexuality (including the physiology of the sexual organs) and in the treatment of sexual dysfunctions. This training should include supervised experience in sex therapy.

State licensure is not always a good measure of competence: not all states have licensing programs for certain professions, like social workers. Affiliation with a professional association may or may not be a good indicator of competence in this area. There are, throughout the country, organizations that certify sex therapists according to certain standards. One such group is the American Association of Sex Educators, Counselors, and Therapists (AASECT). AASECT demands, for certification, 100 hours of individual supervised experience or 150 hours of group supervision. Such certification alone may not ensure competence, but that in combination with the base lines described above may be a good indicator of qualification.

How do you find a qualified sex therapist?

1. Look for a clinic that is sponsored by a university, medical school, or social agency. Such clinics are geared to education and training and often charge lower fees.

2. Call the nearest university department of psychology or social work or medical school department of psychiatry for a referral.

3. Check the list of sex therapists certified by AASECT (see Resources below).

4. Do not simply accept a referral from a doctor, clergyman, friend, etc. Check out the person's qualifications as suggested above.

Before you make an appointment with a prospective therapist, don't be afraid to ask questions about his or her qualifications as a sex therapist. The following questions are appropriate to ask: Do you have special training in sex therapy techniques? Where did you receive your training? How long was the training? Did you have supervised experience? If the person is qualified, he or she will not mind answering your questions.

Resources

This organization will provide information about qualified sex therapists in your area:

American Association of Sex Educators, Counselors, and Therapists
435 N. Michigan Avenue, Suite 1717
Chicago, Illinois 60611

Write for a list of publications available from this organization:

Sexuality Information and Education Council of the U.S.
130 W. 42nd Street, Suite 350
New York, New York 10036

CHAPTER 23

Sexuality and Pregnancy

A woman's sexual feelings during pregnancy can be affected by previous sexual attitudes, her relationship with her partner, and how she feels about the pregnancy itself. Some women feel markedly more sensual and free, and they even experience more intense orgasms than when they are not pregnant. It is natural for a pregnant woman to have more vaginal secretions, and the added lubrication may enhance the sexual pleasure of both partners. Other women feel more inhibited by feelings of unattractiveness or by a sense of protectiveness toward their unborn. Changes in hormones, too, may increase or decrease sexual drive as can your partner's response to your new appearance.

It is helpful to realize that some fluctuation in sexual appetite normally accompanies pregnancy. Fatigue and nausea may dampen one's ardor during early pregnancy. From most accounts, sex appears most satisfactory during the second trimester when a woman is generally feeling very well. Many couples find that pregnancy encourages sexual experimentation at this time. Positions with the woman on top or entry from the side or rear are often more comfortable. During the last few months of pregnancy, sexual activity often declines as a result of increasing physical discomfort.

Many pregnant women experience a greater need for affectionate body touching as opposed to sexual intercourse. During pregnancy, as at any other time of lovemaking, it is important to communicate your concerns and needs to your partner. Otherwise, expression of a need to be touched, for example, may confuse your partner, who may infer that your behavior indicates a desire for intercourse. Satisfying sexual activity can be an experience of mutual pleasuring through a variety of means, not just genital stimulation.

Despite misconceptions that the penis can rupture the membranes or hurt the fetus, sexual activity may continue up to the time of labor in a normal pregnancy. In a woman with a history of premature labor, however, many physicians recommend abstinence during the last few months of pregnancy. Conditions causing bleeding (see Chapters 54 and 55) may also require sexual abstinence. If you have questions pertaining to sexual activity, discuss them with your clinician. If your clinician recommends abstinence, find out exactly what that means—in most situations, sexual activity outside of intercourse can continue. Mutual fondling or masturbation may relieve tension in the event that sexual intercourse is limited.

Following childbirth, it is wise to abstain for two to three weeks since the cervix remains partially open during this time, thus increasing susceptibility to infection. Episiotomy stitches vary in the degree of discomfort they produce. Many women are understandably apprehensive about experiencing painful intercourse after childbirth, and this fear alone creates tension that may cause some discomfort. Exercising extra gentleness, sometimes with the aid of lubricants such as K-Y Jelly or Astroglide, makes intercourse more comfortable. Sometimes pain persists even though nothing is wrong. That is a signal to relax, slow down, and concentrate on enjoying pleasurable sensations that accompany each step along the way to intercourse. The postpartum period is a time of stress in general, and it is often hard for a new parent to find time to relax and enjoy sex.

If you are breast-feeding, you may find that you are more sexually stimulated. Your breasts and genitalia are apt to be more sensitive, requiring more gentleness in sexual play. Nursing also tends to decrease vaginal secretions so you may need added lubrication. Some women find the fullness of their breasts increases their sexual self-image, making them feel more erotic and sensual. A husband's sexual response to his wife's breast-feeding varies, and it is important to share these feelings with each other.

Some couples find that childbirth changes the vaginal size, resulting in decreased sexual feeling. This may result from stretching or tearing of vaginal muscles during childbirth. Special exercises can help (see Chapter 28).

CHAPTER 24

Sexually Transmitted Diseases

Sexually transmitted diseases (STDs) or venereal diseases—infections transmitted from one person to another during intercourse or other intimate contact—are the second most common type of infection in the United States today, surpassed only by the common cold. Since 1981, when the first cases of Acquired Immune Deficiency Syndrome (AIDS) were diagnosed, most women have become more aware of venereal diseases generally.

The continuing high rates of sexually transmitted infections of all types cannot be explained by any single cause. This trend continues to reflect a lack of awareness and education about STDs, especially among teens. Another factor includes an increase in numbers of single adults due to divorce and population growth. A disconcerting factor in the growth of STDs is the continuing unwillingness of many couples to use barrier methods like the latex condom and diaphragm, which help protect against many sexually transmitted diseases.

In addition to classical forms of VD such as gonorrhea and syphilis, new forms have appeared. These include human papilloma virus (HPV) infections, hepatitis-B, and, of course, AIDS. Finally, the growth in the rate of STDs has occurred because the viral infections, such as herpes, HPV, hepatitis-B, and AIDS, cannot be cured, while others such as chlamydia and gonorrhea (which can be cured) display few if any symptoms. Hepatitis-B virus, in particular, has emerged as a growing sexually transmitted disease both in the United States and worldwide and can be transmitted to the newborn (see also Chapter 20). In women, especially, the lack of

symptoms with many forms of VD may cause a delay in or lack of treatment. For this reason women are especially susceptible to the complications that follow these infections.

The shame, fear, and embarrassment that have surrounded STDs for centuries are still present today, although some women are better informed about symptoms, newer treatments, and support groups. The fear of death from contracting AIDS has moved some women to become more open and direct in asking potential sexual partners about their possible risks. Race, religion, and social or economic conditions offer no protection from this frightening disease.

There are some ways you can minimize the risk of getting a sexually transmitted infection. These ways—commonly called practicing "safe sex," more accurately described as "safer sex"—include the following:

- Avoid sexual activity and seek medical care if you or your partner show signs of VD, including discharge from the vagina or penis, painful urination, the presence of sores, blisters, and bumps on or itching of the genitals or rectal area, or pain during intercourse.
- Limit sexual partners. Your chances for acquiring VD increase if your partner has more than one partner. Ideally, sexual contact should be limited to a monogamous partner. Avoid high-risk partners, such as drug abusers and those who have multiple sexual partners.
- Use barrier methods of contraception, preferably a latex condom in combination with a spermicide (see Chapter 7). Use these methods even if you are on the pill, have an IUD, or have had an operation for sterilization.
- Talk to your partner about your concerns prior to intercourse. Avoid intercouse if you or your partner suspect that you may have VD. Avoid sex during treatment until medical tests confirm you are both cured.
- Avoid anal intercourse.
- Urinate immediately after intercourse.

In this chapter we discuss the symptoms, diagnosis, and treatment of the major sexually transmitted infections. Vaginal infections and skin infestations, such as lice and scabies, both of which may be transmitted sexually, are included in Chapter 87. Also, hepatitis-B, a less frequent but important form of VD, is discussed separately in Chapter 20.

Table 42, which appears at the end of this chapter, lists some things you should and should not do if you have been exposed to a sexually transmitted disease. For information on all aspects of VD, write to the following address for a list of current pamphlets:

Centers for Disease Control
1600 Cliffon Road, N.E.
Atlanta, Georgia 30333

or call the CDC at 1-800-227-8922.

For another excellent resource write to:

American Social Health Association
Post Office Box 13827
Research Triangle Park, North Carolina 27709

AIDS

AIDS (Acquired Immune Deficiency Syndrome) is now the leading cause of death in women aged twenty to thirty-four years. Women account for 13% of all U.S. AIDS cases, an increase of more than twentyfold since 1981. As of 1993, 40,000 women and thousands of children with perinatal infections have been diagnosed with AIDS. Among U.S. women with AIDS, 74% are women of color with many living in large, urban areas in the Northeast or South. Fifty-one percent of women with AIDS have a history of intravenous drug use, while 33% contract the disease heterosexually (62% of the time from a partner who is a drug user). Although presently only 6% of AIDS cases have been acquired through heterosexual contact, heterosexual transmission represents the fastest growing segment of AIDS cases, with a 130% increase from 1992 to 1993 in the United States. And worldwide among women with AIDS, an estimated 75% acquire the disease through sexual intercourse. Recent studies indicate women are two to five times more likely than men to acquire HIV from heterosexual sex. Researchers believe one explanation for this is that the semen of an HIV-infected man may be more infectious than the vaginal secretions of an HIV-infected woman.

As of 1993, an estimated one million persons in the United States have been infected with the HIV virus, including approximately 140,000 women. Such worrisome statistics strongly indicate the need for education, preventive measures, and awareness of risk factors. Women at particularly increased risk include those who received a blood transfusion prior to 1985, IV drug abusers, prostitutes, or those who have had contact with an infected partner. Cocaine abusers are particularly at risk. Because of the short highs associated with cocaine use, more frequent injections and shared-needle experiences have been found among users. AIDS is commonly transmitted through anal sex; this form of sexual intercourse is particularly dangerous because the anal tissues are fragile and tear easily, allowing the AIDS virus to enter the bloodstream.

AIDS is the end stage of infection with HIV (Human Immune Deficiency Virus), also known as Human T-Lymphotropic Virus Type III (HTLV-III) or Lymphadenopathy Associated Virus (LAV). This virus invades the body and attacks the T-4 lymphocyte, which ordinarily aids the body in combating infection. Once the body is infected, the disease is chronic and lasts for the lifetime of the infected person. AIDS by itself usually doesn't kill, but the virus slowly damages the brain and central nervous system of the person infected. It also weakens the body's lymphatic "disease prevention" system (immune system) so that other life-threatening diseases (such as cancer or pneumonia) invade the body. HIV lives only in infected humans and is relatively hard to catch. It can only be transmitted in three ways: by sexual contact (heterosexual and male homosexual); by intravenous injection of the virus through sharing of contaminated needles; and perinatally, from an infected woman to her fetus or newborn.

Prior to mid-1985, some AIDS cases were transmitted through infected blood transfusions, an occurrence that caused a high prevalence of HIV infections among hemophiliacs. Today, however, all donated blood and blood components (e.g., plasma) are screened for HIV. People who received transfusions or treatment with clotting-factor concentrates before 1985 could be infected. When infected, the virus is present in several body fluids, including blood, semen, and vaginal and cervical secretions. The virus has also been isolated from saliva, tears, and urine, but in such low concentrations that the appearance of the virus in these fluids is not considered contagious. You cannot contact AIDS by casual social contact, in a swimming pool, or by contact with inanimate objects.

Symptoms

Women infected with HIV may experience no symptoms or may initially have a mononucleosislike syndrome including fatigue, weight loss, swollen glands, diarrhea, night sweats, dry cough, and fever. One of the frustrations faced by researchers is that no one knows how many people carry this virus, as it can exist in the body for years before any symptoms appear. Many researchers believe that there are people who have been infected who may never develop the symptoms of AIDS. Researchers disagree about the length of time it takes for HIV antibodies to appear in the blood after initial infection, but in general, antibodies appear within six months of contact with an infected person.

Some studies show that nervous-system dysfunction is often the first manifestation; this can be seen as recent memory loss, poor concentration, decreased spontaneity, and poor cognitive flexibility. Later on, symptoms may include coordination problems, unsteady gait, mental confusion, blindness, delirium, and seizures. Estimates of people experiencing neuropsychiatric symptoms range from 30% to 70% of the AIDS population.

The major psychological reactions to diagnosis—disbelief, numbness, and denial, followed by feelings of anger, acute stress, and anxiety—result from the stress of the patient being aware that he or she has a fatal disease. Depression and even suicidal thoughts are common. For this reason it is important to seek out as much emotional support as possible, including counseling. Fears of debilitation and the stress of living with a chronic, probably fatal disease can be overwhelming. These fears and anxieties lead to an increased sense of social isolation and dependence on health professionals for maintenance of life. Fears of possible abandonment by friends and relatives continue to be a concern.

Persons with AIDS are subject to a number of internal conflicts regarding the transmission of this disease, including thoughts about who gave it to them and to whom it might have been transmitted. Many experience guilt over their previous life-style and experience fears of abandonment after informing sexual partners. Persons who have treated their drug use or sexual preference as a private matter are now at risk of possible exposure to and subsequent rejection by

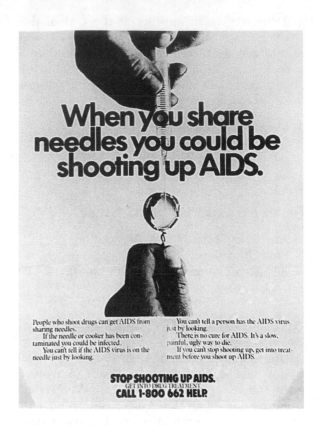

When you share needles you could be shooting up AIDS.

People who shoot drugs can get AIDS from sharing needles.
If the needle or cooker has been contaminated you could be infected.
You can't tell if the AIDS virus is on the needle just by looking.

You can't tell a person has the AIDS virus just by looking.
There is no cure for AIDS. It's a slow, painful, ugly way to die.
If you can't stop shooting up, get into treatment before you shoot up AIDS.

STOP SHOOTING UP AIDS.
GET INTO DRUG TREATMENT
CALL 1-800 662 HELP.

family and friends. Persons with AIDS are faced with the need to make changes in their sexual behavior that can leave them feeling bereft of physical expressions of affection and comfort, even in stable relationships. Financial and health resources may be exhausted due to the prolonged nature of this illness.

Diagnosis

The clinician cannot tell by physical examination that you have AIDS. The only way a diagnosis can be made is through voluntary blood testing for the antibody to the AIDS virus. All the screening tests for HIV antibodies now licensed in the United States are based upon an enzyme-linked immunoassay (EIA). The sensitivity of these initial screening tests for AIDS has varied from one laboratory kit to another. False-positive tests, in which a patient tests positive but doesn't in fact have the AIDS virus, have decreased since the tests were first introduced. All initial reactive or positive tests are repeated. If the second test is also reactive, the sample is interpreted as *repeatedly reactive*, and the results are validated by more definitive tests. The Western Blot test is more specific than EIA tests and is widely used as a confirming test; it identifies antibodies to specific viral proteins. The concentration of antibodies to HIV generally rises after their first appearance, and indeterminate Western Blot tests should be repeated every three to six weeks over a period of several months.

Physicians and health clinic staffs have been encouraged to provide pre- and post-test counseling to assess possible exposure to AIDS due to high-risk behaviors. If an initial test is positive, the clinician assesses the client's understanding of the result, including the possibility of a false positive. The client then will be encouraged to tell his or her previous sexual partners and to recommend that they be tested. Psychological referral is recommended to help plan for the effects of a chronic illness. Results of the test are confidential, and some states—California, for one—separate the results from the rest of the medical record. If you have tested positive, however, it is recommended that you tell your physician and dentist before receiving treatments, as this knowledge could affect your medical treatment.

An HIV-positive test result is not synonymous with a diagnosis of AIDS; it just shows that you are infected with the virus. Your body fluids are considered to be infected for life. A person who tests positive for the AIDS virus has a 20% to 30% chance of developing AIDS over a five-year period. The results of a Walter Reed study in 1987 showed that HIV-infected women who had chronic yeast infections were at increased risk for developing AIDS. Some diseases have been defined as warning indicators that a person may have AIDS; these include Kaposi's sarcoma (a skin disorder), certain types of persistent pneumonia, and some cancers, such as lymphoma.

Effect in pregnancy

Health officials estimate that HIV infection is passed from an infected mother to her newborn in approximately 40% to 50% of all cases. Transmission of the AIDS virus may occur at any stage of pregnancy, during delivery, or during breast-feeding. Pregnancy may accelerate the progression of AIDS in some cases. The American College of Obstetricians and Gynecologists recommends that pregnancy be avoided in women who have AIDS (see also Chapter 20).

Treatment

Disclosure to the patient of positive HIV test results is usually so upsetting that not much else is done in an initial medical visit. The physician will usually schedule a follow-up visit for a few days later, and the client is encouraged to bring all her questions and concerns. At this later visit, the client is advised to practice "safe sex" (see page 194); further exposure to the virus should be avoided. Local phone numbers for AIDS support groups should be shared. Clients are advised to tell their other physicians and dentist about the test results. The patient may request that the physician do so for her. Positive things that a client can do to strengthen her health include obtaining good nutrition, adequate rest, and exercise, and avoiding stress, drugs, and alcohol.

Zidovudine (Retrovir) or AZT is the most widely used antiviral drug approved for AIDS treatment. AZT suppresses the AIDS virus but doesn't eradicate it. Other approved antiviral drugs to treat HIV infection include didanosine and zalcitabine. Much of the effort in finding and studying new drugs to treat AIDS is being coordinated by the National Institute of Allergy and Infectious Diseases through its AIDS Clinical Trials Program. In addition, dozens of drugs are being studied and developed in clinical trials around the world. Development of a vaccine against AIDS offers the best hope for an ultimate cure for this disease and is the subject of continuing extensive research. So far, such a vaccine has been unsuccessful because of the virus's high rate of mutation.

Resources

A toll-free number has been established by the Public Health Service for information about AIDS trials being conducted by the National Institute of Allergy and Infectious Diseases. All calls are confidential. Call 800–HIV-0440, Monday through Friday, 9 A.M. to 7 P.M. Eastern Time.

National AIDS Information Hotline (verbal information): 800-342-2437.

National AIDS Information Clearing House (printed information): 800-458-5231.

Common Questions Asked About AIDS

Question: Answer:

1. What is AIDS?

Acquired (i.e., not innate or arising naturally; the virus is passed from one person to another) Immune (body's defense system) Deficiency (lack of something) Syndrome (presence of signs and symptoms that indicate the existence of a particular condition).

2. What is HIV?

Human (men and women) Immuno-(body's defense system is involved) Virus (a particular organism that involves the human body and attacks the T-4 lymphocyte cell).

3. What is HIV positive (HIV+)?

An individual so described has been infected with the HIV. She or he may remain without symptoms for a very long time.

4. How can I keep myself from getting AIDS?

First, recognize that you alone are responsible for protecting yourself. Get to know your sexual partner prior to intercourse. Limit your sexual activity to one continuous monogamous partner. Use a latex condom and diaphragm with a spermicide. Avoid anal sex. Don't share IV needles with anyone.

5. How can I tell if I have AIDS?

The only way to tell for certain is by having the HIV blood test. You can have the virus and not be aware of it, thus transmitting it to others. You may also carry the virus without it being converted to the infective stage.

6. What should I do if I think I have AIDS?

Talk to your physician or local health clinician about being tested. Testing is voluntary and can be done anonymously or confidentially.

7. Can't I tell if someone else has AIDS?

No. Most people who are infected look and feel fine. You can be infected by anyone who has the virus even though they show no symptoms of disease.

8. What are some signs of AIDS?

In the early stages of the infection, there may not be any symptoms. Swollen glands, diarrhea, night sweats, ongoing fever, loss of ten pounds or more without dieting, unexplained dry cough, white patching in the mouth, fatigue, pink or purplish raised spots on the skin, and bruising and bleeding easily can all be symptoms of AIDS.

9. Is there a cure for AIDS?

No. Not yet.

10. Does the presence of other STDs increase my chances of contracting AIDS?

An increased risk of HIV infection is associated with genital ulcers, including herpes and syphilis.

11. Why does my dentist wear gloves?

It has been recommended that dental workers wear gloves because of the common contamination of saliva with blood during dental procedures. Blood spattering and hand trauma may also occur.

12. Can I catch AIDS from kissing?

Kissing a person who has AIDS on the cheek is safe. No cases have been reported from kissing on the mouth. Experts advise against prolonged, deep "French" kissing with an infected individual.

13. Can I get AIDS from one sexual encounter?

Yes, one sexual contact is all that is needed. Your risk of infection increases with multiple sexual contacts.

14. Can I get AIDS from my pets or from an insect bite?

No. The AIDS virus is only found in humans.

15. Can I get AIDS from a blood transfusion?

Very rarely today. All the blood and blood components used in transfusions are tested for AIDS. If you are concerned and know you're going to have surgery, you might want to pre-donate your blood to be given back to you should you need it (autologous transfusion).

16. Can I get AIDS from donating blood?

No. New equipment is used for each donor when blood is donated.

17. Can I get AIDS from a toilet seat?

No.

18. Can AIDS be transmitted by breast milk?

Yes. The newborn nursing infant could contract AIDS from breast-feeding. Casual skin contact with infected breast milk would not lead to AIDS.

19. Can I continue to work if I have AIDS?

Initially, yes. Since AIDS is a progressive disease and may cause varying symptoms, it is important to discuss this with your doctor on a regular basis.

20. Can I touch someone with AIDS?

Yes. AIDS is not spread by touching, hugging, or shaking hands.

21. Can I get AIDS from a pool?

No. AIDS is not spread by swimming or using hot tubs.

22. If I test positive for AIDS, what can I do to help myself?

Maintain a healthy lifestyle, which includes good nutritional habits, and plenty of rest and exercise. Avoid stress, drugs, alcohol, and exposure to individuals with infections and sexually transmitted diseases. Contact your local AIDS support group to share information and reduce feelings of isolation, loneliness, and possible depression. See your physician every three months; and tell your dentist and all physicians of positive test results. If you continue to feel depressed or suicidal, seek help immediately.

23. Is my diagnosis of AIDS protected by rules of antidiscrimination?

The president's commission on AIDS called for nondiscrimination against AIDS patients, but no new federal laws have been passed to that effect. Some states, California among them, have passed their own antidiscrimination laws. Some states have also extended antidiscrimination provisions for the handicapped to HIV-infected persons.

24. What should I tell my teenagger about AIDS?

Encourage your teenager to say no to illegal drugs and to sex, and educate her or him thoroughly about AIDS.

25. How can I help my friend or family member who has AIDS?

Continue to be supportive. Let him or her express her anger, sadness, and anxiety. Encourage him or her to grieve, knowing that this is a healthy process. An AIDS support group or a religious or community resource group can also be helpful. Simply be there as a friend.

Gonorrhea

Gonorrhea, the best known and most widely reported venereal infection, affects two million people annually. Gonorrhea is caused by a bacterial organism, called *Neisseria gonorrhoeae*, which thrives in a warm, moist environment, such as the mucous membranes. In women, this organism is usually found in the cervix or urethra. Rectal infections can also occur (without rectal intercourse), and gonorrhea can infect the throat of men or women after oral sexual activity with an infected person.

Symptoms

Twenty percent of women with gonorrhea have nonspecific symptoms of vaginal discharge or irritation or slight discomfort urinating. These symptoms usually occur within two to seven days after exposure. Eighty percent of women with gonorrhea, however, have no symptoms at all. In contrast, the majority of men with gonorrhea will have painful urination or a discharge from the penis. Women exposed to gonorrhea often become aware of their infection only when notified by their respective partners. Symptomless infections in both men and women (known as the *carrier state*) make this disease difficult to control. In less than three percent of individuals, gonorrhea may spread to the blood, causing fever, rash, and arthritis. The most serious complication of gonorrhea, pelvic inflammatory disease (see later in this chapter), occurs in approximately 17% of women with this infection and is a major cause of sterility in women.

Table 40 — THE COST OF SEXUALLY TRANSMITTED DISEASE

Sexually Transmitted Disease	Estimated Number of Cases 1987	Estimated Treatment Costs 1986
AIDS (1981 through 2/88)	17,000 (52,000)	$1.7 billion ($4.1 billion)
Chlamydia	4 million	
Trichomoniasis	3 million	
Gonorrhea	2 million	
Genital Herpes	500,000	$4 billion
Syphilis	100,000	
Other	2.4 million	

Sources:
American Social Health Association
Centers for Disease Control
Public Health Report

Diagnosis

The clinician cannot tell by examination whether or not you have gonorrhea, and there is no blood test for this infection. Sometimes a gram stain, a special slide test of cervical secretions, may suggest this diagnosis. A firm diagnosis, however, requires a laboratory technique known as a culture, in which a cotton-tipped swab is dipped into the cervix and then sent for evaluation to the pathology lab. The diagnosis is confirmed if, in twenty-four to seventy-two hours, bacterial growth of the specific gonorrhea organism is identified.

Effect in pregnancy

Gonorrhea acquired early in pregnancy slightly increases the risk of premature labor, stillbirth, and postpartum uterine infection. Also, the newborn may acquire serious eye infection if gonorrhea is present during delivery. To prevent this infection, newborns routinely receive an antibiotic eye ointment after delivery. In pregnancy, most gonorrhea infections remain in the cervix and rarely spread to the uterus or tubes. This is probably due to the cervical mucus plug which acts as a barrier to infection.

Table 41 EARLY SYMPTOMS OF SEXUALLY TRANSMITTED DISEASES

Disease	Symptoms in Men	Symptoms in Women
Gonorrhea	None in 10% to 15%; usually thick discharge from penis or painful urination	Often none; slight vaginal irritation, itching, or discharge; burning with urination
Chlamydia (nonspecific urethritis)	May be none; slight discharge from penis or mildly painful urination; eyes, when involved, become red and irritated	Usually none; may be slight vaginal irritation, itching, or discharge; burning with urination; eyes, when involved, become red and irritated
Trichomonas vaginitis	Usually none; sometimes burning with urination	May be none; usually foul-smelling vaginal discharge with itching; burning or painful urination
Condylomata acuminata (venereal warts)	Small wartlike growths around genital area	Small wartlike growths around genital area
Genital herpes	May be none; usually painful ulcers in and around genital area	May be none; usually painful ulcers in and around genital area; painful urination
Syphilis	Painless ulcer around genital area or mouth; may be unnoticed	Painless ulcer around genital area or mouth; may be unnoticed
Parasitic skin infections: lice ("crabs"), scabies	Intense itching and sometimes rash around the pubic area	Intense itching and sometimes rash around the pubic area

Treatment

Gonorrhea has traditionally been treated by penicillin or by tetracycline if the patient is allergic to penicillin. However, the recent emergence of both penicillin- and tetracycline-resistant strains of gonorrhea has led to the use of newer drugs. Currently, the recommended treatment for gonorrhea is ceftriaxone (Rocephin), which is given as a single injection. For patients who cannot take Rocephin, alternative single-dose drugs that can be given orally include cefixime (Suprax), ciprofloxacin (Cipro), or ofloxacin (Floxin). Both Cepro and Floxin are contraindicated in pregnancy, however. Since chlamydia infection (see below) is present in up to 45% of women with gonorrhea, a separate antibiotic, doxycycline, is also administered to protect against the possible coinfection with this organism. A seven-day oral course of doxycycline (or erythromycin if you happen to be pregnant) effectively protects against chlamydia. Treatment is the safest approach if you suspect exposure to gonorrhea regardless of whether a positive culture is confirmed, because in a small percentage of cases the gonorrhea culture is a "false negative"—that

is, for some reason the organism cannot be grown and cultured.

A gonorrhea attack confers no immunity to subsequent infection. "Ping-pong" gonorrhea—successful treatment, reinfection, and repetition of the cycle—is common. If you suspect your sexual partner may be a carrier (if symptoms or a positive culture persist after you have had treatment), encourage him to use a condom and to seek medical attention. Condoms, while not one hundred percent effective, do decrease the probability of infection. Whether or not your symptoms persist, you should obtain a repeat gonorrhea culture after treatment to make sure the infection is gone.

Syphilis ("bad blood," lues)

The incidence of syphilis in the United States increased dramatically in the 1980s and early 1990s, especially in urban areas. The rate of neonatal syphilis has recently reached its highest peak in fifty years. Three states—New York, California, and Florida—lead the United States in reported syphilis cases, which are especially concentrated among blacks, Hispanics, and the urban poor. Syphilis is spreading faster among women than among men regardless of ethnic background. This represents an ominous trend for pregnant women, as syphilis affects about 40% of babies born to mothers with this disease.

In adults, syphilis can lead to blindness, mental deficiency, or some other serious problem. Approximately 20,000 cases of syphilis are reported annually in women.

Symptoms

Symptoms of syphilis are classified into three stages. In the *primary* stage, the microorganism (*Treponema pallidum*) causing this disease causes formation of a hard, oval-shaped, painless sore known as a *chancre* (pronounced "shanker') from two to twelve weeks after exposure. If the chancre occurs in the vagina, a woman may not even notice this painless ulcer, which disappears on its own two to four weeks later. Although the majority of chancres affect the genital area, five percent occur on the lips, breasts, or mouth. If primary syphilis is untreated, *secondary* syphilis (the second stage) develops one to two months later, when the organism spreads into the bloodstream. At this time, a painless rash (often involving palms of the hands and soles of the feet), swollen lymph glands, and fever may occur. These symptoms, too, may go unnoticed and subside by themselves. During *latent* syphilis, the secondary symptoms have subsided and the only evidence of infection is a positive blood test. After one year of latent syphilis, the person is not likely to be infectious, an exception being the pregnant woman, who may infect her unborn child. The most serious stage, *tertiary syphilis* (the third stage), develops from one to twenty-five years after the secondary stage. In tertiary syphilis, serious, irreversible damage to the liver, bones, brain, heart, and other organs may occur.

Diagnosis

Syphilis, like gonorrhea, cannot be diagnosed by examination alone. The diagnosis requires laboratory tests involving either the use of a special microscopic technique (dark-field examination) or, more commonly, a blood test. Blood tests for syphilis include one called the VDRL (which stands for Venereal Disease Research Labs) and another called the RPR (rapid plasma reagin). These so-called *screening* tests may not become positive for up to six weeks after exposure to syphilis or for three weeks after the chancre appears; therefore, a blood test immediately after exposure to this disease may not be positive for syphilis and should be repeated several weeks later if the initial test comes back negative. The clinician orders a *specific* blood test for syphilis if you have a positive screening test to make sure the original test is not a "false positive"— that is, the test is positive as a result of conditions (viral infections, for example) not caused by syphilis. A scraping of the lesion (performed like a Pap smear) can immediately diagnose syphilis. However, this test requires a special dark-field microscope, which is not available in most doctors' offices.

Effect in pregnancy

Untreated syphilis in the pregnant woman may result in miscarriage, stillbirth, birth defects, or severe infection of the newborn. For this reason, clinicians routinely check the mother for syphilis at the beginning of pregnancy and sometimes in the last three months of pregnancy as well. Unlike gonorrhea and herpes, which rarely affect the newborn prior to delivery, syphilis may directly infect and damage the fetus during pregnancy, especially in the second half.

Treatment

Penicillin, the standard treatment for syphilis, is very effective in the primary and secondary stages of this disease. Penicillin treatment for syphilis requires an injection containing a special, long-acting form of this drug. It is important to realize this fact since oral forms of penicillin prescribed to treat gonorrhea may not be effective against syphilis, if you happen to have syphilis as well. Unlike oral penicillin, Rocephin is likely to be effective against incubating syphilis. However, it is not the most effective drug for treating this disease. A woman treated with oral penicillin for gonorrhea should be tested six weeks later for syphilis. Anyone with primary or secondary syphilis should not have sexual intercourse for one month after receiving treatment. Condoms, while usually protective against gonorrhea, do not offer adequate protection against syphilis.

Genital Herpes

An estimated 40 million Americans have genital herpes, and about 500,000 new cases occur each year. In addition to physical symptoms, this disease, like most sexually transmitted infections, often causes emotional strain, taking the form of depression related to a sense of loss of control or of anxiety due to fear of transmitting herpes to a partner. In a few individuals, the diagnoses of herpes may lead to more prominent and sometimes persistent psychological symptoms.

Herpes infections are due to viruses that may be of two types. The herpes simplex virus type I (HSV-I) generally causes cold sores or fever blisters on the lips and mouth. HSV-I is rarely acquired by sexual contact. Herpes simplex virus type II (HSV-II) generally occurs in the genital area. Although either virus strain can spread to other parts of the body, nearly 90% of genital herpes is due to HSV-II, which is usually acquired by sexual contact.

Genital herpes is highly contagious whenever the blisters (see below) are present, both at the time of an initial attack and at the time of a recurrence. In addition to infection by sexual transmission, the virus can spread from one area to another on the same person (autoinoculation). Fingers and eyes are especially vulnerable.

Symptoms

Many cases of genital herpes are acquired from partners who do not themselves know they have an HSV infection. This is because genital herpes produces few or no recognizable symptoms in most individuals with this infection. Typical symptoms, if they do occur, usually appear two to ten days following sexual contact with an infected person. At first, one or more fluid-filled blisters form in or around the genital area and burst in two or three days, becoming extremely painful ulcers (sores). In a woman painful urination is characteristic at this time. The sores heal by themselves in two or three weeks. If herpes involves only the cervix or upper vagina, symptoms may be minimal or nonexistent. However, during the first infection, generalized symptoms usually occur, including fever and swollen lymph glands in the groin. In the absence of symptoms, the herpes virus is believed to lie dormant along the course of the affected nerve.

Some people never have recurrences, some have a few, and others have recurrences on a regular basis. A recurrence of herpes is characteristically shorter and less severe than the first attack. Some women experience burning, itching, or tingling at the place of previous infection just before the herpes sores reappear. In rare instances recurrences may involve the cervix alone and may not be apparent to a woman or her partner, but she may nevertheless be infectious. Men, too, have been noted in a few case reports to be infectious in the absence of external sores, for a day or two just prior to or following a recurrence. A variety of factors may trigger genital herpes recurrences: colds, fever, menstrual periods, emotional stress, tightfitting clothing, and vaginal infections. Sexual contact is not necessary for a recurrence.

Diagnosis

The physician usually diagnoses genital herpes during a pelvic examination by the appearance of sores. This diagnosis is not always clear-cut, however, especially after the sores begin to heal. Three tests can confirm your clinician's diagnosis: 1) a Pap smear of open sores detects cell changes characteristic of herpes 60% of the time; 2) special herpes cultures—the most accurate means of diagnosis—also require material from early, non-healed sores; and 3) blood tests can measure herpes antibodies (see glossary) and confirm previous or present HSV-II infections. Once antibodies form—about two weeks after a first-time herpes infection—they remain permanently in the blood. However, blood testing may not be particularly helpful (*unless the result is negative*), since current methods frequently don't distinguish between HSV-I and HSV-II antibodies.

Effect in pregnancy

Serious newborn infection may occur if vaginal delivery is performed during or shortly after the active stage of the disease when blisters are present (see Chapter 20).

Treatment

Unlike some other sexually transmitted diseases, there is no cure for genital herpes. Present treatment of herpes aims to provide symptomatic relief and to prevent a bacterial infection from developing alongside the one caused by the herpes virus. Warm tub baths to which are added Betadine douche or solution (three tablespoonfuls) or Domeboro powder or tablets may provide relief. And you can sprinkle your underwear with cornstarch or talcum powder to keep the area dry. Your physician may prescribe a topical (applied locally) anesthetic or pain medication as well as antibiotics to prevent infection. It is important to avoid sexual activity for as long as sores persist and until they completely heal.

The drug acyclovir (Zovirax), taken orally, lessens the duration of pain, but it is not a cure. The pill is usually taken five times a day for seven to ten days to treat an initial episode and for five days to treat recurrences. Famvir and Valtrex have also been approved recently to treat recurrences. Suppressive therapy involves taking the drug for up to twelve months. Information regarding treatment with Zovirax for longer periods of time is still limited. Long-term effects and the possible development of viral resistance to the drug continue to concern researchers. Suppressive therapy should be considered only if you have frequent recurrences (more than six per year) and are using contraception, as the drug is contraindicated in pregnancy. The five-day, short-term treatment should be reserved for *severe* recurrences and started as soon as symptoms begin to develop —within two days of the appearance of ulcers. Zovirax cream has been found to be less effective than the oral form of the drug; its use is limited to initial episodes of herpes, in which the cream may have a slight effect in decreasing virus shedding.

Long-term effects of herpes

New studies indicate that people with herpes are at greater risk for acquiring AIDS. It is believed that the virus causing AIDS may enter the body more easily during sexual activity if open herpes sores are present in the genital area. For this reason, intercourse and oral sex should be avoided when genital sores are present.

In earlier studies a slightly increased risk of cervical cancer was reported in women who have had herpes infections. Current research suggests that herpes does not cause or lead to cervix cancer. Like most women, those with a history of genital herpes should have a Pap smear at least once a year.

Resources

For more information, call the National Herpes Hot Line at (919) 361-8488, or write to Herpes Resource Center, c/o American Social Health Association, P.O. Box 13827, Research Triangle Park, North Carolina 27709.

1 800 653 health

Nongonococcal Urethritis (Chlamydia Infection, Nonspecific Urethritis)

Nongonococcal urethritis (NGU) refers to several newly discovered types of sexually transmitted infections which are largely symptomless in the female and may cause mild burning on urination or a urethral discharge in the male, resembling gonorrhea—hence the term *nongonococcal urethritis*, which means inflammation of the urethra not due to gonorrhea. (In women, since the cervix rather than the urethra is the principal place affected, the term *urethritis* is somewhat misleading.)

Although several types of microbes cause NGU, the main one is *Chlamydia trachomatis*. For practical purposes, when the term *nongonococcal urethritis* is used, it usually means that a chlamydia infection is present. Chlamydia infection has now become one of the most common sexually transmitted diseases, affecting about 4 million men and women in the United States each year. The Centers for Disease Control estimates that infection with chlamydia occurs twice as often as with gonorrhea. Chlamydia often coexists with other sexually transmitted diseases, especially gonorrhea; these two "silent" forms of VD are often found together. A woman with gonorrhea, for example, has a 25% to 40% chance of also having a chlamydia infection in her cervix. When chlamydia spreads beyond the cervix, the infection can affect the Fallopian tubes and lead to pelvic inflammatory disease (see below). By causing tubal damage, chlamydia is a major cause of infertility and ectopic pregnancy. As with other sexually transmitted diseases, the factors that increase the risk of having chlamydia include being single, being under age twenty-five, having a new or more than one sexual partner, and a history (in you or your partner) of other types of VD, such as gonorrhea. The chance of acquiring chlamydia also increases if you exclusively use a nonbarrier method for birth control.

Symptoms

Chlamydia symptoms develop up to three or four weeks after exposure but are usually mild or nonexistent in women. Men often have mild burning with urination or a thin urethral discharge similar to a mild case of gonorrhea. Women may have mild vaginal irritation, burning, or discharge but more often a woman does not realize she is infected unless her partner mentions symptoms. Chlamydia may affect the eyes by direct contact with an infected area and produce redness, mild itching, or irritation (conjunctivitis). Eye infection does not require sexual contact.

Diagnosis

Chlamydia is a difficult infection to diagnose. The microbe cannot be detected by a pelvic exam and may be confused with other infections that produce vaginal discharge. A specific diagnosis for chlamydia requires a culture (obtained as for a gonorrhea culture); unlike other bacteria, however, the chlamydia organism is not easy to grow and it takes several days to achieve results. Recently, better screening methods have been available that use "immunoassay" and other newer technologies. These "nonculture" tests are performed much like a Pap smear and provide more rapid results, usually within twenty-four to forty-eight hours. Since 1993, the CDC has recommended increased use of such tests to screen asymptomatic women who may be at increased risk for chlamydia infections (e.g., adolescents and women with more than one sexual partner). If the nonculture test is positive for chlamydia, a confirming test (culture) may be done to be sure the initial test is not a false positive, but more often the physician just proceeds directly with antibiotic treatment.

Effect in pregnancy

The fetus carried by a woman with chlamydia is not likely to be affected before delivery. During childbirth, however, direct contact of the new-born with the chlamydia organism causes minor eye infections nearly 50% of the time, and pneumonia in a smaller percentage of cases. Women at increased risk for chlamydia (i.e., single women, teenagers) should have a culture test done during pregnancy. If the test is positive, the mother is treated with erythromycin to prevent chlamydia infection in the newborn.

Treatment

Doctors treat chlamydia with tetracycline or doxycycline for one to two weeks or with a newer drug, azithromycin, which can be given in a single dose. During pregnancy, since tetracycline is contraindicated, erythromycin is used. In women, early treatment is important to prevent spread of the disease to the ovaries and tubes. Treatment of chlamydia infection is often complicated by the fact that this infection may be misdiagnosed as or coexist with gonorrhea. In either case, penicillin, if prescribed, will not kill chlamydia organisms. For this reason, if your partner has a persistent discharge diagnosed as NGU, both of you need a course of treatment with tetracycline. You should be treated even if you have no symptoms, since over 50% of women exposed to men with chlamydia become infected. Even following appropriate tetracycline therapy, chlamydia may become a recurrent problem requiring further therapy.

Pelvic Inflammatory Disease

Inflammation or infection within the tubes (salpingitis) or ovaries (oophoritis) is known as *pelvic inflammatory disease* (PID). Such an infection occurs in at least 850,000 women annually and partially explains the increasing rates of infertility and tubal pregnancy, which have more than doubled in the last two decades. PID leads to sterility in approximately 60,000 young women every year. It is estimated that 75% of all pelvic inflammatory disease is initially sexually transmitted, involving a gonorrhea or chlamydia infection in most cases. At other times, PID follows infection associated with childbirth, abortion, or surgery involving the pelvic organs. Intrauterine contraceptive devices (IUDs) also have been associated with an increased chance of PID,

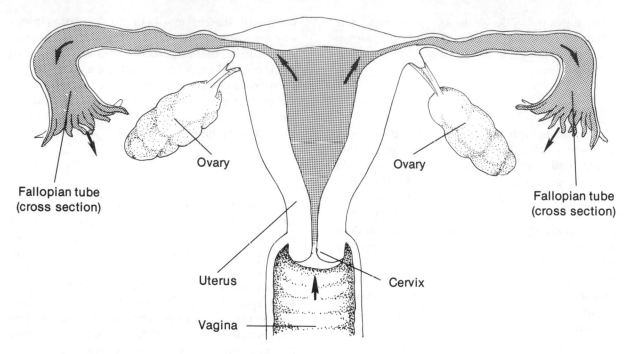

Ovary

Ovary

Fallopian tube
(cross section)

Fallopian tube
(cross section)

Uterus

Cervix

Vagina

Figure 32 *Pathways of pelvic infection. Gonorrhea and other types of VD can cause tubal infections (pelvic inflammatory disease).*

especially in a woman with a prior history of tubal infection.

PID usually starts with a cervical gonorrhea infection which then spreads into the uterine cavity and extends into the tubes (see Figure 32). Pus formation may remain in the tubes or extend to the ovaries. The result is adhesions and scar tissue within and around the tubes (see Figure 33). When infection is severe or inadequately treated, the chances for permanent tubal damage and sterility increase.

Not all infections respond to the initial antibiotic treatment; sometimes stronger drugs requiring hospitalization are needed. If the initial attack of PID is not controlled, chronic infection may develop with recurrent episodes of pain and infection not necessarily brought on by sexual activity. The development of chronic PID seriously threatens a woman's childbearing potential as the chance of infertility doubles with each new attack.

Symptoms

Pelvic inflammatory disease, even in its early stages, can make a woman acutely ill with symptoms of low abdominal (pelvic) pain, vaginal discharge, and fever. Pelvic pain is moderate to severe and frequently occurs within one week of

a menstrual period. Infection often follows the menstrual period, a time when the cervix dilates and facilitates passage of gonorrhea and other bacteria from the cervix into the uterine cavity.

Diagnosis

The clinician usually diagnoses PID by pelvic exam. Few specific diagnostic tests are available, aside from a culture of the cervix, which reveals gonorrhea up to 50% of the time. The physician can, however, confirm or rule out a diagnosis of PID by laparoscopy (see glossary).

Treatment

In its earlier stages, physicians successfully treat PID with oral antibiotics. In more advanced cases, the doctor may hospitalize you in order to give the antibiotics by IV (that is, intravenously), which allows higher blood levels of these drugs. Only if you have recurrent bouts of PID that are unresponsive to medical treatment, or a pelvic mass indicating abscess formation, will you require surgery. If the infection is localized, the surgeon may need to remove only the affected tube and ovary. Frequently, especially if both tubes are affected, removal of

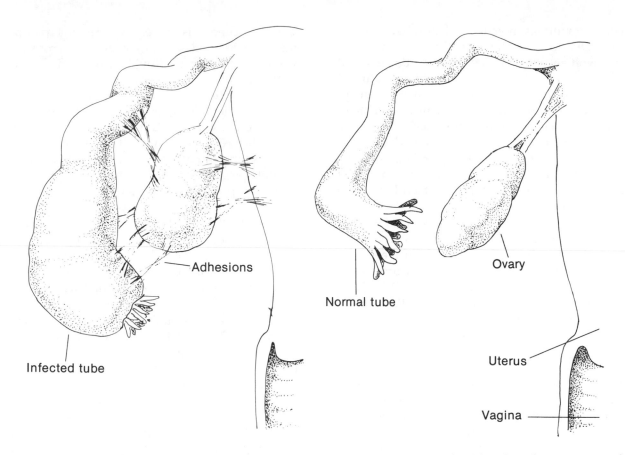

Figure 33 *The left tube shows signs of infection, swelling, and adhesions to the ovary. The right tube and ovary are normal.*

tubes, ovaries, and uterus is the only means of definitive treatment.

Effect in pregnancy

PID is a major cause of ectopic (tubal) pregnancies (see Chapter 83). Tubal scarring from previous infection makes a woman more susceptible to this complication of early pregnancy. Thus, ectopic pregnancy is at least twenty times more common in women with a history of tubal infections. However, during a normally progressing pregnancy, acute attacks of pelvic infection rarely occur, partly because of the mucus plug, which acts as a barrier to infection.

Human Papilloma Virus (HPV) Infection

Human Papilloma Virus (HPV) infection is a highly contagious sexually transmitted disease caused by any one of about seventy viruses belonging to the human papilloma group. HPV infection usually appears in one of two ways—either as venereal warts (small growths located on the vulva, rectum, vagina, or cervix) or as an abnormal Pap smear. HPV infection is believed to account for the majority of abnormal Pap smears and shows up in 1% to 2% of women having routine Pap-smear screening. This infection appears to be the fastest growing sexually transmitted disease in the United States today, with the number of office visits for genital warts having increased fourfold during the past fifteen years. During this time, doctor visits for genital warts have outnumbered visits for herpes by three to one.

In its most characteristic form, HPV infection appears as venereal warts or *Condylomata acuminata*. The incubation period for the warts, which may take up to three months, is much longer than for most other sexually acquired infections, and it can be much longer than three months from the time of sexual exposure until the warts appear. In many people the warts are "subclinical"; that is, they are too small to be seen except through magnification (see below). About 70% of the time, the male partner of a woman with this infection will also have the disease. Due to these statistics, the male partner of any woman with vaginal warts or documented HPV infection of the cervix should be evaluated by a physician. While a urologist may be an appropriate referral choice for males, dermatologists are sometimes more interested in and more used to dealing with HPV infections. Although HPV is considered almost entirely a sexually transmitted infection, some cases of nonsexual transmission (e.g., via hand contact) have been documented.

In addition to causing genital warts, HPV has now been linked to the more serious problem of precancerous changes and cancer of the cervix, vagina, and vulva. For this reason, women with genital warts as well as those with HPV-related abnormal Pap smears should have Pap smears performed at least annually.

Symptoms

The rampant spread of HPV infections can be attributed partly to the lack of symptoms that characterize most infections in both men and women. The warts are often microscopic, and in women with symptomless HPV infections of the cervix, Pap smears detect less than half of the actual cases. For this reason, it is believed that many if not most of the 10 million or more women in the United States with HPV infections are never diagnosed. When externally visible warts are present, they appear as painless, fleshy growths, often no longer than the tip of a pencil. When present in clusters, the warts have a cauliflower appearance. The warts may cause occasional mild irritation or itching around the vulva or rectum. Recurring warts are not unusual even in healthy, treated individuals. Chronic infection is also seen in immunosuppressed individuals, such as those on immunosuppression drugs or those who have AIDS.

Diagnosis

The Pap smear is often the way HPV infection is detected initially. When genital warts are present, the diagnosis of HPV infection is self-evident, although a confirming biopsy is sometimes done. When the only indication of HPV infection is an abnormal Pap smear "suspicious for HPV," a tissue sample or biopsy of the cervix is often performed using a colposcope.

This instrument is merely a large microscope that is positioned several inches away from the vaginal speculum to provide a magnified view of the cervix (see Chapter 37).

Traditionally, the cervical biopsy has been the basis for diagnosing both HPV infection and precancerous changes. Unfortunately, much confusion has resulted from the fact that the symptomless form of HPV, unassociated with obvious genital warts, may be difficult to diagnose, even with a biopsy. (Precancer, on the other hand, is much more clear-cut.) Many HPV experts believe that HPV, while still epidemic, has been overdiagnosed. This may have happened because the criteria for making a diagnosis of HPV through the microscope are nonspecific and somewhat open to interpretation. This problem is of special importance to couples who are mutually monogamous and have no history of genital warts. Fortunately, more specific tests for HPV are becoming available and can be expected to clear up many of these concerns.

Newer HPV tests identify the specific HPV virus type based on its DNA or genetic makeup. These tests are performed much like a Pap smear. "ViraPap," the first such test to have FDA approval, tests for the presence of any of the seven main viruses found in most HPV infections. The test does not distinguish between different types and is reported simply as "positive" or "negative." The ability to test for specific HPV types, which will soon become available through most labs and physician offices, is important because certain types (especially types 16, 18, 31, 33, and 35) are more likely to lead to cancer of the cervix or vagina, while others (types 6 and 11) usually do not. While not 100% accurate, and too expensive (roughly, $35 to $50) to be used for routine screening, tests like the ViraPap help in the diagnosis of HPV infection, especially if a woman has an abnormal Pap smear or cervical biopsy "suggestive of HPV."

Effect in pregnancy

In pregnancy, venereal warts tend to bleed, become infected, or grow in size. In rare cases, they may block the birth canal, making a cesarean delivery inevitable. There have been case reports of condylomata growths on the newborn's larynx, but otherwise no effect on the infant has been noted. Podophyllin treatments (described below) should not be taken during pregnancy because they may harm the newborn. However, laser surgery, if needed, can be used during pregnancy.

Treatment

The treatment of warts on the vulva with the chemical podophyllin has become less popular because the treatment is successful only about 20% of the time. In addition, the warts in the vagina cannot be treated due to the drug's toxicity. When podophyllin treatment is prescribed, sufferers should apply petroleum jelly to the skin around the edge of the area being treated because the drug is caustic to normal skin. To prevent burns, wash off the podophyllin in a warm bath four to six hours after application by the physician.

The simplest current methods to remove warts are electrical burning (electrocautery), chemical burning (with trichloroacetic acid, or TCA), or freezing (cryosurgery). These methods work best when only a few warts are present on the cervix, vagina, or vulva, and may require multiple treatments. Laser surgery (see Chapter 37) has been used successfully to remove venereal warts in patients who don't respond to the other methods. Laser surgery is also appropriate for first-time treatment when large numbers of warts are present. Recurrence rates, even with laser therapy, are at least 25%, and the procedure is costly. While such surgery removes the warts and associated precancerous changes, if present, it does not kill the virus. However, unlike herpes, which often recurs from time to time, venereal warts, once successfully treated, usually do not recur.

Newer treatments for venereal warts include the antitumor, antiviral drugs (Intron A) and 5-fluorouracil or 5FU (Efudex). Interferon is injected directly into the wart three times a week for several weeks. Various clinical trials involving interferon have found that in 36% to 62% of patients the warts were successfully eliminated, although there were a few recurrences after eighteen months. Side effects of interferon include a flulike syndrome that is usually mild.

A more practical treatment that appears promising is application of 5FU (Efudex) in a vaginal cream that is used in small quantities, either for several days or once weekly for several weeks. Like podophyllin, 5FU must be used sparingly to avoid tissue irritation and inflammation. Some physicians now use 5FU instead of the more expensive laser approach as a first-line treatment when multiple genital warts are present. Success rates with this cream are comparable or better than those with laser surgery. Recently, 5FU and laser surgery treatment have been combined, with the cream being given before and after laser surgery.

Table 42	WHAT TO DO AFTER POSSIBLE EXPOSURE TO A SEXUALLY TRANSMITTED DISEASE

Do's	Don'ts
1. Do seek early testing and treatment (even if only your partner has symptoms).	1. Don't wait for symptoms to occur before seeking treatment—*exposure* alone to venereal infection is an indication to be treated.
2. Do inform your partner(s) so he (they) can seek treatment.	2. Don't assume your clinician will routinely test for VD. You may have to ask specifically for a gonorrhea culture or a blood test for syphilis (repeat the blood test in six weeks).
3. Do take all the medication prescribed even if your symptoms subside before you have taken it all.	3. Don't resume intercourse or other intimate activity until you have been treated and your symptoms have gone.
4. Do find out when to return for a follow-up visit to have possible follow-up tests.	4. Don't blame yourself; sexually transmitted infection may produce little or no warning symptoms in either partner.

CHAPTER 25

Sexual Assault

The problem of sexual assault and adequate methods for helping the rape victim have received considerable attention over the last few years. Even so, most people do not discuss the subject of rape or rape prevention until they themselves or a person they know is involved. Most likely you will never experience rape, but it can happen to anyone. We discuss in this chapter some of the legal, medical, and emotional aspects connected with such a possibility, however small. Table 43 summarizes the steps you should take if you do become a victim of rape.

Sexual assault, more commonly called rape, is not, in general, considered a sex crime; it is considered a crime of violence. But we have nonetheless included this discussion on rape as part of this section on sexual issues because of the related problems—the possibility of venereal disease and pregnancy—and because for many women there exists a real concern that needs to be dealt with. "Date rape," which occurs when an unsuspecting woman is raped on a casual social occasion, is currently increasing and is reported more frequently than violent sexual assault.

Most communities have a twenty-four-hour crisis hot line, with people available who can advise you about obtaining medical care and about the police procedures involved in reporting rape. Write down, in a place where you can quickly find it, the telephone number of the nearest rape or other crisis center in case you ever need it.

Legal Aspects

If you are raped and you decide to press charges, you will need medical evidence to show that you were raped. You do not have to make the decision to press charges immediately, however. Have an examination by a physician trained to treat rape victims. This procedure is an involved one, not so much medically as legally, in order to adequately prepare medical findings for evidence at a later date. Legally, all evidence can be obtained only by a physician, as opposed to a nurse practitioner or another care provider. You don't have to have evidence of physical violence to be justified in reporting the assault. The presence of semen is not always needed, as some rapes are committed by men who cannot ejaculate.

Whether or not to bring charges against the attacker is your decision. The attack may be reported anonymously through your rape crisis center. Pressing charges in person is a lengthy process, and some women feel it is too traumatic emotionally. Women who do press charges against their attacker frequently do so on the basis that charging him with assault may prevent him from attacking again.

Unfortunately, rape is the only crime in our society in which the victim may be dealt with as if she were an accessory. Police officers or examining personnel may act as if you somehow "provoked" the rape. In general, people react uncomfortably toward rape victims, and this uneasiness may make your immediate medical examination more difficult. It is helpful to have a supportive person with you during this time.

Medical Care

If you have physical injuries, the physician will care for these injuries first. All injuries, no matter how slight, will be recorded. A pelvic examination is performed to search for evidence of recent trauma or intercourse and to test for gonorrhea, which may be detected in semen. Since evidence of sperm disappears from your cervix in approximately eight to ten hours, have your pelvic exam done as soon as possible. The vaginal secretions are tested for sperm cells as well as acid phosphatase, a substance produced by the male prostate gland.

The physician also checks for possible physical evidence, including hairs, bits of skin, dirt, blood, or grass stains on your clothing, under your fingernails, or on any other part of your body. (Because you may be feeling very vulnerable after a rape, this meticulous physical exam can be upsetting.) Your pelvic hair may be combed to further search for evidence of your attacker. Each piece of evidence will be labeled and sealed, in case you decide to press charges.

The risk of sexually transmitted disease (VD) is relatively high after rape, and you will be tested for gonorrhea, syphilis, hepatitis, and AIDS. Because these diseases cannot be completely ruled out immediately, you should return for repeat tests—in two weeks for a gonorrhea test, in six to eight weeks for a syphilis test, and in three to six months to repeat the other tests, assuming initial results were negative. A follow-up exam at the time of the syphilis test is also advisable to check for the presence of the other venereal diseases that may not show up until then.

The chance of pregnancy occurring as a result of rape is small. You will be given a pregnancy test to determine if you are already pregnant. If not, you may want to consider using the "morning-after" pill, which prevents conception when taken within seventy-two hours after intercourse (see Chapter 9). You should have a repeat pregnancy test at six to eight weeks, perhaps at the time of the follow-up exam mentioned above. Also, if you do not take the "morning-after" pill, you should avoid intercourse (or use some form of birth control) until you know this repeat pregnancy test is negative.

Emotional Reactions

Most attackers use a weapon to force their victims to submit to rape. When faced with the threat of possible death, most women feel they have no choice but to submit in order to stay alive. After it is over, you may feel both shock and relief for having survived this act of violence. In the case of "date rape," the elements of surprise, physical force, and mental intimidation make the rape possible. Afterward, you may feel disbelief and guilt that you were placed in such a vulnerable position.

Later you may find yourself feeling depressed, angry, and helpless. Some women, for weeks or months, deny it ever happened, but eventually the anger surfaces. You may feel ashamed, used, and bitter that this attack happened to you. Most women have the inner strength to work through the crisis of rape. It will help if you can acknowledge these feelings gradually and talk with a few close friends

---

Table 43   WHAT TO DO IF YOU ARE A RAPE VICTIM

1. Call someone close to you. This isn't a time to be alone.
2. Don't take a shower or bath, don't douche, and don't change clothes until after you have been examined by a physician, even though you may want to.
3. Call the nearest rape crisis center. They can help you through the next few hours *in a way no one else can*.
4. Go with your friend and perhaps someone from the rape crisis center to the nearest medical facility that handles rape victims. Bring extra clothing in case your clothing may be needed as evidence.
5. Don't feel you must decide now whether you will press charges. Take every legal precaution so that you can take legal action later if you decide to do so. You can report the rape immediately to the police and decide later if you want to press charges. Or you can have the rape crisis center report the rape, with or without using your name.
6. Return to a physician or medical facility for follow-up VD and pregnancy tests.

---

about what happened. Use a rape crisis center if available. Seek competent professional counseling if possible. The long-term psychological impact of rape should not be underestimated, especially when it involves a child or it is an initial sexual experience. A rape experience can be an underlying cause of sexual problems in later life.

Rape Prevention

Many communities have rape prevention classes or lectures sponsored by the community, a women's center, or a local service organization. If you do not have access to such a service or you do not wish to attend, here are some things you can do to minimize the risk of rape.

1. *In your car:* Keep your doors locked at all times, even if you are leaving your car for only a short time. If you have car trouble and must stay with your car (as on a limited access highway), raise your hood, get into your car, lock your doors, and wait for the police; it's usually safer not to accept help from a stranger. At night park in well-lighted areas. When you approach your parked car, walk confidently, have the key in your hand and look around and inside

your car before you get in. Don't pick up hitchhikers.

2. *At home:* Keep your doors locked (and, when possible, use a deadbolt) at all times even if you leave for just a moment. If possible, use a 180-degree peephole on your entry door; and avoid letting in anyone you don't know or aren't expecting (for example, service repairmen). Use initials rather than your first name on your mailbox and in the telephone directory. Leave your radio on while you are out, turned to a talk radio station.

3. *On the telephone:* Avoid giving out personal information or confirming your telephone number to someone you don't know. Never say on your answering machine that you are not home, or refer to the fact that you live alone. Leave a message such as: "We are not taking calls at this time; please leave your name and number and your call will be returned at our earliest convenience." Report any obscene telephone calls you receive to the telephone company and any personal threats you receive to the police. If you are receiving obscene calls, answer your calls with your radio turned on to a talk show so your caller will not know you are alone.

4. *Out-of-doors:* Avoid walking or jogging alone at night; if you do, follow well-lighted, well-traveled routes and vary both the time and the rate of your routine. Carry protective items such as Mace, where state laws permit, and a whistle. Avoid conversation with strangers even to give directions, especially if you are in a position where you could be cornered. Don't hitchhike. Don't accept rides from strangers. If you frequent recreational places alone or with other women, especially at night, be careful whom you leave the place with.

5. *Don't* put yourself in the position of being alone with someone you know only casually. When dating someone new, stick to public places until you know him well.

6. Don't give personal biographical information to someone you have just met. Always be aware that someone may take advantage of your compassion; don't assume that requests for money or physical help are legitimate.

7. Remember that your consent for a sharing of a social occasion is not a consent for sex.

How to Help a Friend Who Has Been Raped

When you know someone close to you has been raped, you will undoubtedly want to help her. The best kind of support you can give is the same as if she were the victim of any other kind of crisis. You can play an important role by providing the reassurance and support she needs. You can help by encouraging her to seek medical care and remaining with her, if she prefers, throughout the entire examination procedure. If you can, encourage her to talk about her feelings, but only after she is ready to do so. Sometimes a rape victim is afraid to talk about the attack for fear her family or friends will change their attitudes toward her. She may blame herself and think of what she could have done to prevent it. But this is not the time to reproach or reprimand her, which may reinforce her own self doubts. Perhaps the best help you can give her is to see that she gets competent medical care and to reassure her that it *is* possible to survive such a traumatic event.

Sexual Abuse in Children

Today, there is more awareness of family violence, including the problems of incest, physical assault, and sexual abuse in children. The majority of sexually abused children are girls (average age, five), and most often the abuse has been perpetrated by a relative or close family friend. It is important and necessary today to educate your children as preschoolers not only to be aware of strangers but to be protective of their "private" body areas. A good book for parents and young children to read together is *Private Zone,* by Frances S. Dayee. Children should know the difference between appropriate touching and "bad touching." Most importantly, children need to be encouraged to assertively "tell" when an adult touches their private area. If a child tells about such an incident, listen to and believe her; experts report that children do not lie about sexual assault. Reassure your child and seek help. Call your doctor or contact the National Child Abuse Referral Service, 1-800-422-4453.

Domestic Abuse

Marital violence is a serious problem in the United States, with one out of eight husbands physically aggressive at least once toward his wife. Nearly 2 million women are severely assaulted by male partners. Including acts by both partners, 8.7 million American couples (nearly one out of six) experience violence each year.

Violence often begins at the early stage of a relationship. Research has found that 30% of men are physically aggressive toward their partners in the year before marriage. Such behavior may involve only pushing or shoving, but it may continue into something worse if nothing is done to stop it. Up to 25% of all homicides in the United States are committed by a husband or wife. Marital violence has also been linked to psychological conditions such as depression, alcohol abuse, and post-traumatic stress disorder (see Chapter 47). Domestic violence is often associated with child abuse and may harm a child psychologically, even if it is not. Forced sexual activity is another form of physical abuse.

Verbal abuse usually precedes physical abuse. In a verbally abusive relationship, the abuser denies the abuse and it most often takes place in private. Witty sarcasm, manipulative coercion, angry outbursts, and unreasonable demands are common forms of verbal abuse. Recognizing and identifying verbal abuse has proven to be difficult for many people, especially those who grew up in an abusive household. Indeed, use of both physical and verbal abuse has been found to be linked from one generation of a family to the next. The periods of abuse are often followed by periods in which the abuser is kind and considerate toward his partner, leading the victim to become more emotionally involved and dependent on the abuser. The process is slow and insidious, with the victim becoming so entrenched in the relationship that it is difficult to "see one's way out." This leads to a confusing, isolated state for the woman, and she may somehow feel the abuse is all her fault.

The first helpful step for an abused woman is for her to share the situation with a friend, physician, or trusted family member. This relieves her isolation and provides some emotional support and perspective. Often a battered woman feels responsible—that there is something she can do to stop the violence. It is important to remember that the abuser is the person who is responsible for his violent behavior, not the victim. Violent behavior usually increases as the abusing partner realizes he has control of the situation.

Once a woman secures help, she can decide what is best for her own situation. Individual counseling is usually necessary for the abuser to change his behavior and for the woman to improve her self-esteem. Her physical safety is of the utmost concern. Most communities have resources available for abused women. If you feel you are involved in a relationship that threatens your well-being or that of your children, get help. No one deserves to be abused.

References for Section Five

Chapter 22—Female Sexuality

American College of Obstetricians and Gynecologists *Technical Bulletin* 211. Sexual dysfunction, Sep 1995.

Saultz, J. Common sexual complaints: how to elicit and evaluate them. *The Female Patient* 13(10):41–48, Oct 1988.

Kaplan, H. *The Illustrated Manual of Sex Therapy.* New York: Brunner/Mazel, 1987.

Master, W. *Human Sexual Response.* Boston: Little/Brown, 1966.

Brick, P. Toward a positive approach to adolescent sexuality, *SIECUS Report* 17(5):1–6, May/July 1989.

Smith, M. Health concerns of lesbian women. *The Female Patient* 14(7):43–50, July 1989.

Chapter 23—Sexuality and Pregnancy
Chapter 24—Sexually Transmitted Diseases

Reyes, M. Dealing with maternal and congenital syphilis. *Contemporary OB/GYN* 52–62, June 1995.

1993 Sexually transmitted diseases treatment guidelines. *Morbidity and Mortality Weekly Report, Recommendations and Reports* 42, no. RR-14. Sep 24, 1993.

Stratton P. Treatment options for HIV pregnancies. *Contemporary OB/GYN* 99–118, May 1994.

Cavanagh, D. AIDS in women: mentioning the unmentionable. *The Female Patient* 19:38, Nov 1994.

Heterosexual acquired AIDS—United States, 1993. *The Journal of the American Medical Association* (Reprint), vol. 271, no. 13, Apr 6, 1994.

Update: impact of the expanded AIDS surveillance case definition for adolescents and adults on case reporting—United States 1993. *The Journal of the American Medical Association* (Reprint), Apr 6, 1994.

Drugs for AIDS and Associated Infections. *The Medical Letter, on Drugs and Therapeutics* 37 (155.959): Oct 13, 1995.

U.S. Public Health Service recommendations for human immunodeficiency virus, counseling and voluntary testing for pregnant women *Morbidity and Mortality Weekly Report, Recommendations and Reports* 44, no. RR-7. July 7, 1995.

American College of Obstetricians and Gynecologists, Committee on obstetric practice, *Committee Opinion* 148. Zidovudine for the prevention of vertical Transmission of human immunodeficiency virus, Dec 1994.

American College of Obstetricians and Gynecologists *Technical Bulletin* 119. Gynecologic herpes simplex virus infections, Aug 1988.

American College of Obstetricians and Gynecologists *Technical Bulletin* 169. Human immunodeficiency virus infections, June 1992.

American College of Obstetricians and Gynecologists *Technical Bulletin* 190. Gonorrhea and chlamydial infections, Mar 1994.

Brown, H. Recognizing common sexually transmitted diseases in adolescents. *Contemporary OB/GYN* 33(3):47–64, Mar 1989.

Bump, R. Bacterial vaginosis in virginal and sexually active adolescent females: evidence against exclusive sexual transmission. *American Journal of Obstetrics and Gynecology* 158:935–939, 1988.

Faro, S. Trichomonas vaginitis: quick treatment plan for a persistent infection. *The Female Patient* 12:37–42, 1987.

Centers for Disease Control. *Morbidity and Mortality Weekly Report*, Update: universal precautions for prevention of transmission of human immunodeficiency virus, hepatitis B virus and other bloodborne pathogens in health care settings, 37(24):June 1988.

Richart, R. Human papilloma virus DNA: quicker ways to discern viral types. *Contemporary OB/GYN*: 112–133, Apr 1989.

Bistoletti, P. Genital papilloma virus infection after treatment for cervical intraepithelial neoplasia (CIN) III. *Cancer* 62(9):2056–2059, Nov 1988.

Schneider, A. Humana papilloma virus infection in women and their male partners. *Contemporary OB/GYN* 32(5):131–144, Nov 1988.

Dorsey, J. Condyloma acuminata: brief update on diagnosis and management. *Medical Aspects of Human Sexuality* 22:55–63, Mar 1988.

Experts urge OB/GYNs not to treat human papilloma virus in its subclinical stage. *ACOG Newsletter*: 5, Aug 1989.

Syphilis rate again soars to levels as high as during the 1950's. *ACOG Newsletter*: 9, Dec 1988.

Cohen, I. Chlamydia trachomatis in the perinatal period. *Contemporary OB/GYN* 33:22–34, June 1989.

Peng, T. Herpes simplex virus in the pregnant patient. *The Female Patient* 14(8):27–41, Aug 1989.

Pokorny, S. Pelvic inflammatory disease: an epidemic among American teenagers. *The Female Patient* 14(8):42–48, Aug 1989.

Chapter 25—Sexual Assault

American College of Obstetricians and Gynecologists *Technical Bulletin* 172. Sexual assault, Sep 1992.

Abel, G. Sexual abuse. *Psychiatric Clinics of North America* 18(1):139–53, Mar 1995.

Housekemp, B. Assessing and treating battered women: a clinical review of issues and approaches. *New Directions for Mental Health Services* 64:79–89, Winter 1994.

Gilbert, B. Treatment of adult victims of rape. *New Directions for Mental Health Services* 64:67–78, Winter 1994.

Beckmann, C. Treating sexual assault victims—a protocol for health professionals. *The Female Patient* 14(5):78–83, May 1989.

Boston Women's Health Book Collective: *The New Our Bodies, Ourselves.* New York: Touchstone, 1992.

Minden, P. The victim care service: a program for victims of sexual assault. *Archives of Psychiatric Nursing* 3(1):41–46, Feb 1989.

Hicks, D. The patient who's been raped. *Emergency Medicine* 20:106–110, Nov 1988.

Heinrich, L. Care of the female rape victim. *Nurse Practitioner: American Journal of Primary Health Care* 12(11):9–18, 1987.

A man who shoots up can be very giving.

He can give you and your baby AIDS.

Most babies with AIDS are born to mothers who shot drugs or who sleep with men who have.

Babies with AIDS are born to die.

If you're thinking of having a baby you and your partner need to get tested for AIDS. Only get pregnant when you're sure both of you aren't infected. Until then help protect yourself and your partner by using condoms.

And if your man shoots drugs, help him get into treatment now. It could save three lives, his, yours and your baby's.

STOP SHOOTING UP AIDS.
GET INTO DRUG TREATMENT.
CALL 1-800 662 HELP.

A Public Service of the National Institute on Drug Abuse, Department of Health and Human Services.

HEALTH CONCERNS DURING AND AFTER MENOPAUSE

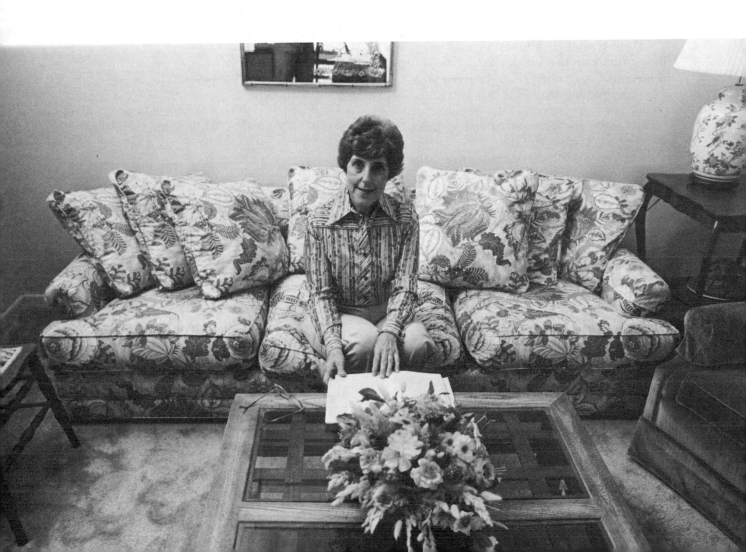

CHAPTER 26

Menopause

Menopause marks the time in a woman's life when menstrual periods cease. The hormone changes that occur at this time and the symptoms that may be produced as a result are discussed in this chapter. Elsewhere in this book we have touched upon other medical concerns of the middle-aged and older woman that are not related to the menopause.

Although the average age for menopause is fifty-one, menopause may occur anywhere between ages forty-one and fifty-five. For several years before menopause, hormone levels gradually decline, causing changes throughout your body. Menstrual periods, for example, become shorter, lighter, and less frequent (see Chapter 78). These changes in your cycle reflect a gradual decrease in estrogen production by the ovaries. Menopause is reached once your periods stop altogether for an entire year. It is helpful to keep a record of your periods to determine when you have reached menopause. After this time, you can no longer have children but you can continue to lead a perfectly normal life sexually and in every other way.

Menopause and Midlife

In a youth-oriented society, both older and middle-aged women sometimes suffer from the belief that a person's worth and talents are solely determined by age. As the number of midlife women grows, public awareness and respect for the intellectual contributions and capacities of older women should increase. Menopause is only a physical sign of having reached midlife, and the ways in which this physical and emotional event affects each woman vary greatly. Midlife is a time when many women find themselves free from the demands of young children and more able to creatively develop their own identity and interests. For many women, midlife is one of the most satisfying periods in life.

Today, about 40 million American women have reached menopause or are in their premenopausal years. With a life expectancy of seventy-eight years, many women now spend a third of their lives or more beyond the age of menopause. In order for you to stay well and enjoy these added years, it is more important than ever to maintain a healthy life-style. If you are a fitness late-bloomer, or just found out that your cholesterol level isn't where it should be, don't despair: it is never too late to start. Dr. Morris Notelovitz, Director of the Climacteric Clinic in Gainesville, Florida, has shown that regular aerobic exercise in his menopausal-aged patients improves cardiovascular fitness about 15%. Following a balanced diet that minimizes saturated fats and cholesterol can have a positive impact, too, since for every 1% decrease in your blood cholesterol, your risk for coronary artery disease goes down 2%. At this time in life a woman should be sure to have the frequent checkups along with the tests recommended by the American Cancer Society (see Table 3). Hormone replacement therapy is a question to be considered.

Symptoms of menopause

The ways in which women experience menopause vary greatly. While some women experi-

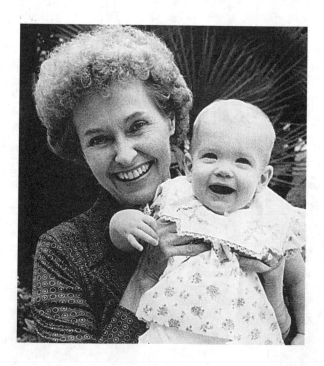

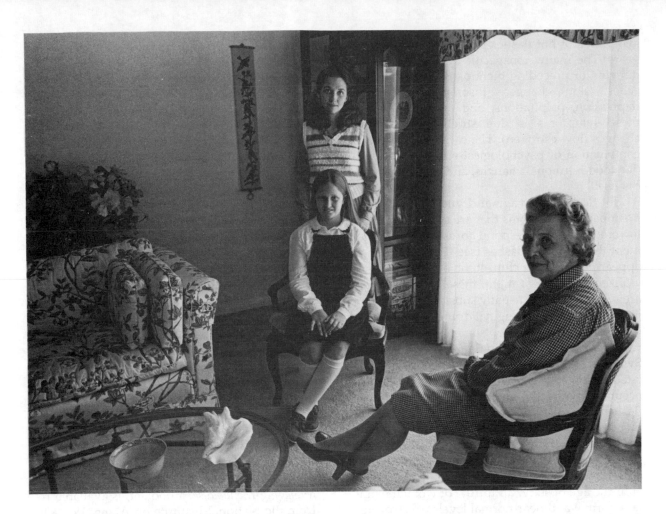

ence depression, others are hardly affected. On the other hand, loss of sleep and the fatigue associated with menopausal symptoms such as hot flashes is sufficient reason for a mild case of the blues in many people. How you react depends somewhat upon the way you have coped with change in the past and perhaps upon your mother's menopausal experience. It is reassuring to note that most women experience an increased sense of emotional well-being as the physical symptoms of menopause diminish. Sharing your feelings with friends can often greatly reduce your concerns about the normal symptoms accompanying menopause and aging.

Most women have very little difficulty with hot flashes and other menopausal symptoms. In fact, 25% of all women undergoing menopause have little in the way of symptoms aside from cessation of menses. Symptoms are more pronounced if menopause occurs abruptly (for example, as a result of surgery) as opposed to gradually over a period of one to two years. If hot flashes or other symptoms are present, they

often last only a few months while the body adjusts to lower estrogen levels. Declining estrogen levels cause physical changes—muscles lose some strength and tone, the bones become more brittle, and there is a loss of elasticity of tissue, including the tissue of the genitalia. Vaginal lubrication may decrease noticeably, and the vaginal tissue becomes thinner and more susceptible to irritation or infection. These gradual changes vary in severity, depending on the individual woman. Painful intercourse may be lessened by the use of water-soluble vaginal lubricants (such as K-Y lubricating jelly or Astroglide) and regular sexual activity. Nonhormonal vaginal moisturizers, such as Replens and Gyne-Moistrin, have become available and may provide longer-acting lubrication than traditional water-soluble lubricants. Painful and/or frequent urination is also a common experience in post-menopausal women. This condition is not caused by an infection but by changes in the urinary system as part of the aging process.

Only about 20% of menopausal women have

symptoms of hot flashes persisting over several years. The many nonspecific symptoms accompanying or preceding menopause include headaches, skin changes, insomnia, irritability, depression, palpitations, and fatigue. None of these symptoms is due strictly to hormone changes (low estrogen). The cause is probably a combination of psychological stress, poorly understood hormonal changes, and the aging process itself.

Hot flashes and vaginal dryness or irritation, menopausal symptoms that are a direct result of lowered estrogen, respond to estrogen replacement therapy. Hot flashes (see Chapter 70) may appear early in the climacteric along with generalized sweating at night; these two symptoms are self-limited and usually subside on their own in one or two years. Vaginal dryness can account for painful intercourse, sometimes associated with discharge or bleeding after sexual activity. Symptoms of vaginal dryness or irritation related to lowered estrogen levels usually do not occur until after the menopause and, unlike hot flashes, may persist and require periodic treatment (see Chapter 27).

Various hormone tests obtained during and after menopause show that not all women have a decline in estrogen below normal levels. Even after the age of sixty, up to 10% of women maintain normal and near-normal levels of estrogens. This maintenance of a normal estrogen level occurs in some women because the ovaries, adrenal glands, and fat cells in these women produce more estrogen than usual for reasons not understood. This individuality in body chemistry explains some of the variation in menopausal symptoms among different women.

Tests for the Menopause

Sometimes a woman experiencing hot flashes or lighter, less frequent periods wants to know whether or not she is approaching menopause. The most accurate way to answer this question is by a blood test to measure the brain hormones FSH and LH (see glossary). You should continue to use a method of birth control until you have this test, or until you stop having periods for at least a year. These hormones indirectly reflect the amount of estrogen produced by the ovaries.

This test confirms if you have reached menopause and no longer need to use contraception. Other blood tests to measure estrogen levels directly are less reliable since estrogen blood levels can vary widely each day. The *maturation index* is the simplest and least costly way to evaluate estrogen levels. The maturation index evaluates vaginal cells to determine your estrogen level. The cells are obtained like a Pap smear at the time of a pelvic exam. This test, too, is much less accurate than FSH in determining whether you have reached menopause.

Resource

Managing Menopause, a booklet, is available free from the National Institute on Aging. Write to:

National Institute on Aging Information Center
P.O. Box 8057
Gaithersburg, Maryland 20898-8057

CHAPTER 27

Hormone-Replacement Therapy

The practice of prescribing estrogen- and progesterone-containing drugs to replace the amounts of these hormones no longer being supplied by the ovaries during and after menopause is known as *hormone-replacement therapy* (HRT). In the past, physicians frequently prescribed estrogen not just to relieve menopausal symptoms such as hot flashes but also to achieve other results that long since have been discredited—for example, to "maintain youth." In the 1950s and early 1960s, estrogen was prescribed with near-blind enthusiasm; slogans like "feminine forever" characterized these practices. Beginning in the 1970s, however, it became clear that some women taking high estrogen dosages for many years would develop cancer of the uterus (endometrial cancer). During the 1970s and early 1980s, prescription of estrogen declined substantially as report after report linked long-term estrogen use to uterine cancer. Subsequently, numerous studies in the United States and worldwide have shown that the risk of uterine cancer could be all but eliminated by including several tablets of the hormone progesterone along with the estrogen. Progesterone's protective action results from the hormone's tendency to oppose the effect of estrogen on the uterine lining or endometrium. In fact, women on HRT that includes both estrogen and progesterone have been found to have a somewhat *lower* risk of uterine cancer than women not taking hormones. The potential uses of hormone therapy became extended in the 1980s. A number of studies have confirmed that modern combination HRT has long-term benefits such as prevention of osteoporosis and, to some degree, prevention of coronary artery disease. Such perceived benefits have once again led to widespread prescribing of these drugs since the mid-1980s. This is not to say that physicians have begun approaching the subject of hormone replacement with the same abandon as was common several decades ago. Today, most practitioners are keenly aware of side effects, certain risks, and the need to tailor therapy to suit each woman's individual needs.

Possible long-term effects such as stimulation of breast cancer in certain subgroups of postmenopausal women will have to be clarified in the years to come before HRT can be recommended unequivocally. Bearing all this in mind, hormone replacement appears to have more benefits than risks for many women in their menopausal years. It is reassuring to note that the overwhelming evidence indicates the use of estrogen after menopause for less then 10 years appears to have little, if any, effect on the risk of breast cancer. Still, the decision to take these hormones is an intensely personal one and needs to be thoroughly discussed with your doctor. During the 1990s, if prescription practices of OB-GYNs follow the recommendations that have been coming out of the leading medical journals, well over half of postmenopausal women will be taking some form of hormone therapy.

Possible Benefits of Estrogen

There are three FDA-accepted indications for the use of estrogen in menopausal women: treatment of hot flashes, treatment of symptoms of vaginal atrophy, and prevention of osteoporosis. In addition, an increasing number of practitioners believe the most important use of estrogen is in the prevention of heart disease. Recent research indicates estrogen may have other beneficial effects, including an improvement in memory and a lessening of insomnia, depression, and irritability in some women.

Hot flashes

Although hot flashes are not life-threatening, they may be debilitating to some women, producing secondary symptoms such as insomnia. The most effective treatment of hot flashes consists of estrogen, either in oral tablet form or in the new estrogen patch (see below). Although estrogens do relieve hot-flash symptoms, hot flashes usually subside on their own in most women in a matter of months.

Vaginal atrophy

Vaginal atrophy refers to thinning of the vulvar and vaginal tissue, which may become easily irritated and susceptible to vaginal infection (see Chapter 87 on atrophic vaginitis). As a result of these changes, painful intercourse or bleeding after intercourse may occur. Estrogen treatment can reverse the symptoms of vaginal atrophy. These symptoms are also at times associated with painful or frequent urination due to the thinning of the tissue in and around the urethra and bladder. These urinary symptoms are also due to a decreased supply of estrogen and may be relieved by taking estrogen if an infection or other cause is not present (see Chapter 88). Oral estrogen or oral estrogen plus estrogen cream provides the most effective treatment for vaginal atrophy. Estrogen creams are used along with the pill form if symptoms are severe. Estrogen creams are also used instead of oral estrogen if vaginal atrophy is the only reason you take es-

trogen and you want the least amount of the drug absorbed. Bear in mind, however, that even with the cream, some of the hormone will be absorbed. For this reason, if you have a contraindication to estrogen, the cream form may be contraindicated, too.

Osteoporosis

Osteoporosis, which results in progressive degeneration of the spine and other bones, occurs in approximately 50% of postmenopausal women, many of whom may then develop fractures of the backbone or hip as they age. Osteoporosis affects 25 million people, mostly women, and accounts for more than 1 million fractures per year. Osteoporosis also eventually produces nonradiating low back pain (see Chapters 51 and 83), curvature of the spine, and diminished height.

Osteoporosis has been one of the most widely studied diseases in recent years and has received great attention in the media. Proper nutrition, exercise, and adequate calcium intake are important in its prevention; estrogen has increas-

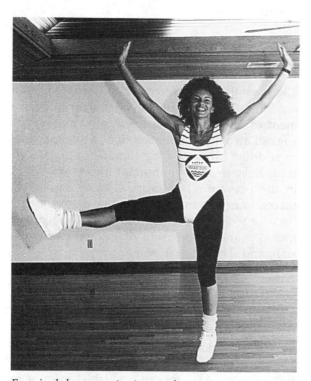
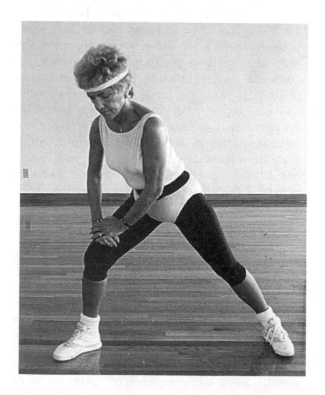

Exercise helps prevent osteoporosis.

ingly been seen as helpful in its prevention as well. A 1987 National Institutes of Health workshop clearly emphasized the importance of estrogen in stating that "calcium is not a substitute for estrogen replacement to retard bone loss in postmenopausal women."

To be effective, postmenopausal hormone replacement must begin soon after the woman ceases to have periods because a woman's bone mass, which peaks at age thirty-five, rapidly decreases in the years immediately following menopause. Bone loss is maximal in the first three years after menopause. At this time a woman loses approximately 2.5% of bone mass per year. Thereafter, the loss is 1% per year. Symptoms such as backache do not develop until fully 50% of bone loss has occurred; fractures begin after 70% of bone density is lost.

The chance of developing osteoporosis is associated with certain risk factors. While practitioners treat at-risk women with estrogen therapy, others also give estrogen to women without risk factors since they, too, may develop this disease. Women at greater risk for developing osteoporosis include thin white women as well as those with a family history of this disease, a sedentary life-style, or a diet low in calcium. Other risk factors include a history of early menopause, excessive alcohol or caffeine consumption, and a history of smoking, which may decrease estrogen levels.

One approach to identifying the woman at risk for osteoporosis-related fractures has been the use of bone-density tests. At present, no single screening test has proved cost-effective and accurate enough to be used routinely. Such screening may involve measurement of certain elements in the blood or urine, such as calcium or phosphate, to assess bone metabolism. Radiographic tests (called bone densitometry) seek to measure actual bone density. These tests usually involve passing a beam of light through a bone (such as the radius bone in the forearm) and then measuring the beam's intensity as it emerges. A computer converts the data and gives the bone calcium contents in grams per centimeter. This procedure is called "single" or "dual" photon absorptiometry. A faster, improved form of this technique called dual energy X-ray absorptiometry is slightly more accurate. All of these techniques produce minimal radiation exposure and are mainly used to follow the progress of women with osteoporosis or to screen menopausal women at risk for this disease (e.g., those who cannot or choose not to take estrogen).

Estrogen helps to prevent osteoporosis by maintaining calcium balance, both by aiding absorption of dietary calcium and by reducing bone loss of this mineral. In order to be effective in preventing this disease, a sufficient dose of estrogen is required. Premarin, the most widely prescribed product for estrogen replacement, comes in five dosages—.3 mg, .625 mg, .9 mg, 1.25 mg, and 2.5 mg. The .625-mg Premarin dosage is considered by most authorities to be the minimum daily dose for preventing osteoporosis. Other estrogens widely used to treat osteoporosis include the oral forms Estrace, Estratab, Menest, Ogen, and Ortho-Est. The "skin patch" forms of estrogen include Estraderm and Climara.

In addition to estrogen replacement, several other measures can be taken to prevent osteoporosis. Among the most important is the intake of a sufficient amount of calcium in the diet. Two or three glasses of vitamin D-enriched milk per day are recommended for women over forty. In addition to milk, active-culture yogurt can provide an excellent source of calcium. Several brands of low-fat yogurt contain approximately 400 mg of calcium per cup, as compared to 300 mg of calcium per cup of milk. Many women have an insufficient intake of dietary calcium because they avoid dairy products due to dieting or to milk intolerance. The average American daily dietary intake of calcium—500 mg—is well below dietary needs for calcium (about 1000 mg daily for women before menopause and 1500 mg after menopause.) Higher doses of calcium may contribute to kidney stones and should be avoided. The calcium requirement for postmenopausal women drops to about 1000 mg for women on estrogen replacement. Most women over forty need a calcium supplement. Calcium supplements such as Bio-Cal, Caltrate, and OsCal contain 500 to 600 mg of elemental calcium per tablet. Tums 500, which contains 500 mg of calcium per tablet, may be somewhat less expensive. Calcium should be taken with meals; a high-fiber diet may be helpful in avoiding any resulting constipation. Supplementation with vitamin D is generally not necessary in women under sixty-five years of age.

In addition to supplemental calcium, two other medications have been used to prevent osteoporosis: fluoride (a mineral) and calcitonin (a hormone). Fluoride's side effects, which include gastrointestinal bleeding and joint pain, have limited this drug's usefulness in the past. Calcitonin, which is less effective than estrogen in preventing osteoporosis, has been used mainly in the treatment of this disease. Concerning newer therapies for osteoporosis, a significant breakthrough occurred in 1995 with the approval of Fosamax, a new drug that acts specifically by inhibiting bone breakdown. In addition, a nasal spray (Miacalcin) recently has been approved for the treatment of osteoporosis. Both these drugs will be especially useful for postmenopausal women who cannot take estrogen.

Weight-bearing exercise such as weight lifting and walking can also help women to avoid osteoporosis. The mechanical forces in weight-bearing exercise seem to play an important role in bone formation. Such exercise should be regular and vigorous, and applied to both upper and lower body to prevent bone loss. Excessive exercise may itself cause damage, such as stress fractures, which sometimes occur in long-distance runners.

Resource

National Osteoporosis Foundation
1150 17th Street, N.W., Suite 500
Washington, D.C. 20036

This voluntary nonprofit health agency seeks to decrease osteoporosis through research, education, and patient advocacy.

Heart Disease and Hormone Replacement

Many clinicians now consider prevention of heart disease the most important reason for prescribing estrogen after menopause. Heart disease, which is responsible for ten times as many deaths in postmenopausal women as breast cancer, is the number-one cause of death in women over fifty. A major reason for the rise in heart disease after menopause is the loss of protection from the estrogen that keeps women relatively immune to heart disease in the first four decades of life. Recent large-scale studies such as the Nurses' Health Study from Boston, which involves 121,000 registered nurses, and the Lipid Research Clinic Study, a collaborative project of ten centers throughout the United States, have shown that postmenopausal women on hormone replacement have only one-third the risk of a heart attack compared to similar women not taking hormone-replacement therapy. Women who experience premature menopause (before age forty) as a result of surgical removal of the ovaries are at extremely high risk—with up to seven times the chance of heart disease if estrogen-replacement therapy is not begun after surgery. It is believed that estrogen's beneficial role in reducing the risk of heart disease comes about by the hormone's effect on lipoproteins—special "carrier" proteins that transport cholesterol and other fats to and from tissue. Estrogen increases blood levels of the so-called good cholesterol carrier—HDL—which transports cholesterol away from tissue. Estrogen decreases levels of the so-called bad carrier—LDL—which brings cholesterol to tissue, where it can form fatty deposits. It has been found that people with higher HDL levels and lower LDL levels are less likely to suffer from heart disease.

Considerations Before Taking Estrogen

1. Estrogen, progesterone, and breast cancer. At this time the exact relationship between estrogen (and progesterone) therapy and breast cancer remains unclear. At least twenty clinical research studies have indicated little or no increased risk of breast cancer among postmenopausal women using estrogen. Most authorities believe that any breast cancer risk associated with hormone therapy is relatively small and may be related to long-term use (i.e., greater than five years). For example, the recently published update of the Nurses' Health Study found that current estrogen users had a 32% increased risk of breast cancer, which increased to 46% if they had been using estrogen for five years or more. Similar statistics are reported for postmenopausal users of estrogen plus progesterone (*New England Journal of Medicine*, June 15, 1995). While the Nurses' Health Study is one of the largest to examine this question, other research linking hormones to breast

cancer remains inconsistent. Among the reasons for this are variations in study designs and case controls. For example, hormone dosages and schedules have changed over the years, and current methods and dosages are not necessarily comparable to previous ones. At this time, most OB/GYNs approach the subject of hormone replacement with the knowledge that there may be a small increase in risk of breast cancer, one that is often offset by a decrease in rates of heart disease and osteoporosis, especially among women at risk for these conditions.

2. Talk with your doctor if you have a previous history of blood clots associated with estrogen use (including estrogen in birth control pills). These include any that occurred in the leg (thrombophlebitis), in the lung (pulmonary embolus), in the brain (stroke or "cerebral vascular accident"—called a CVA), or in the heart (heart attack or coronary thrombosis). A history of blood clots unrelated to estrogen (or progesterone) is no longer considered a contraindication to the use of estrogen replacement, but rather an indication to use caution and to discuss your previous condition with your doctor before starting to take the drug. Confusion exists here because birth control pills—a more potent form of estrogen—have been linked to an increased risk of blood clots, which *are* a contraindication to taking birth control pills. But estrogen used to treat menopausal symptoms is not known at this time to cause blood clots or strokes, probably because the dosage and type of estrogen is less potent than that in birth control pills. In fact the opposite may occur. A report concerning this subject appeared in 1988 in the *British Medical Journal*, which reported that among 8,882 postmenopausal women, half as many estrogen users (twenty) died from stroke as compared to nonusers of estrogen (forty-three) who died from this disease.

3. Never take estrogen if you are or could be pregnant.

4. You should avoid estrogen if you have unexplained or abnormal vaginal bleeding.

5. Avoid estrogen if you have abnormal liver tests or liver disease such as chronic hepatitis.

6. Avoid estrogen (with rare exception) if you have had uterine or breast cancer.

How Progesterone Fits into Hormone-Replacement Therapy (HRT)

Initially, progesterone was added to estrogen-replacement therapy to prevent estrogen-induced overstimulation of the lining of the uterus (endometrium), an effect that could subsequently lead to uterine cancer. For some women who cannot take estrogen, progesterone alone has been successful in preventing hot flashes. When progesterone is combined with estrogen, the combination may have an enhancing effect in reducing the occurrence of hot flashes. Historically, progesterone has not been associated with serious side effects and, unlike estrogen, it has not been linked to blood clots in most scientific studies. (Nevertheless, the FDA, in product labeling, has required the listing of blood clots as a contraindication to the use of progesterone. Some clinicians feel this is inappropriate.) Other contraindications to progesterone use include known or suspected breast cancer, liver disease, and undiagnosed vaginal bleeding.

One potentially negative effect of progesterone is the hormone's tendency to alter blood lipids in a way that may increase the risk of heart disease. Depending on the specific progesterone drug and its dosage, this hormone may slightly lower the amount of "good" cholesterol, HDL, in the system. This tendency is an unwanted effect since the lower your HDL, the higher your overall risk of heart problems. It is not known whether this action is significant enough to reverse estrogen's heart-protective effect, which results from an opposite effect on lipid levels in the blood. For this reason, most physicians recommend prescribing estrogen replacement therapy *alone* in women who have had a hysterectomy, since the most important use of progesterone is in prevention of uterine cancer. This way, a woman who has had a hysterectomy will have the full benefit of the estrogen in protecting against heart disease. For women who have not had this surgery, progesterone should be prescribed as part of HRT. Any adverse lipid effects may be minimized by using the lowest possible dosage of this hormone and by using a proges-

Table 44 COMMON BRANDS OF ORAL ESTROGEN-CONTAINING DRUGS

Plain Estrogen	Estrogen Products Containing Testosterone	Estrogen Products Containing a Tranquilizer
Estrace	Estratest	PMB
Estratab	Premarin with Methyltestosterone	
Menest		
Ogen		
Ortho-Est		
Premarin		
Premphase*		
Prempro*		

* Also contains progesterone

terone such as medroxyprogesterone acetate (MPA). Typical forms of MPA prescribed today include Provera, Cycrin, and Amen. By using minimal dosages of progesterones in hormone-replacement therapy, (e.g., 2.5 mg of Provera instead of 10 mg), protection of the uterus can be achieved without significant unfavorable effects on your cholesterol level.

How Hormone-Replacement Therapy Is Prescribed

Estrogen and progesterone are usually prescribed separately and are not combined into one pill as in most birth control pills. (Exceptions include PREMPHASE and PREMPRO, products in which both hormones are combined within individual tablets.) Progesterone is nearly always given in oral tablet form. Estrogens in current use may be given orally, by means of a skin "patch," in a vaginal cream, or (rarely) by injection. (Injectable hormone shots are not used much today because they are inconvenient, costly, and impractical.) Estrogen creams (see Table 114) may be used instead of pills for some women who only have symptoms of vaginal itching (atrophic vaginitis) due to estrogen deficiency (see Chapter 89). Forms of estrogen that contain tranquilizers should be used with caution and awareness of potential sedative side effects.

Estrogen may not relieve menopausal symptoms in every woman. Some of these women are helped by estrogen preparations (e.g., Estratest) that contain small amounts of the male sex hormone testosterone—a hormone normally made in small amounts by the ovary. This combined estrogen-testosterone therapy has been used to increase sex drive and mood, but side effects, such as hair growth, may occur if too high a dose of the male hormone is used. This is not generally a problem, however, as a woman's natural testosterone levels usually decrease by as much as 50% during menopause.

There are numerous HRT prescription regimens. For example, estrogen may be prescribed for the first twenty-five days of the month, adding progesterone to the last twelve days during which estrogen is taken. During the pill-free interval after the twenty-fifth day, a woman often has a period. Due to the inconvenience and unpopularity of having periods, some physicians now encourage continuous therapy in which estrogen is prescribed daily and progesterone is added on the first twelve or last twelve days of the month or is given continuously (every day) using a lower dosage. The oral estrogens being prescribed today are listed in Table 44. The potency of these products—and thus the risks involved—is much lower than that of birth control pills. The proper length of time that a woman should remain on HRT therapy is still very much an individual matter and should be discussed with your physician. Recent data from the Framingham study in Boston suggests that a woman needs to take estrogen for at least seven years to prevent osteoporosis. Many physicians now recommend hormone therapy for at least this long, and others recommend this therapy "for life" to prevent osteoporosis and heart disease.

Table 45   QUESTIONS COMMONLY ASKED ABOUT ESTROGENS

Question	Yes	No	Comment
Are the estrogens commonly prescribed for hot flashes as strong as estrogens in birth control pills?		X	They are much less potent. Newer low-dose birth control pills can be prescribed (for contraception) until menopause in many healthy, nonsmoking women.
Are estrogens used in treating the menopause associated, like birth control pills, with blood clots, heart attacks, or stroke?		X	Estrogens used in treating menopausal symptoms are not known to cause blood clots. However, until this area is fully studied, the possibility of a very small risk of blood clots cannot be ruled out even in women without known risk factors.
Are heart attacks prevented by taking estrogen after the menopause?	X		Several large studies show the risk of coronary heart disease among postmenopausal women using estrogen to be about one-third the risk of nonusers.
If hormones (HRT) are stopped in a woman who has gone through menopause, will hot flashes subside eventually?	X		Usually in less than six months.
Are thyroid tests affected by estrogens?	X		Some thyroid tests are affected, but the amount of thyroid in the bloodstream is unchanged.
Are blood fatty substances (cholesterol) lowered in women taking estrogens?	X		This fact is important especially in women with risk factors for heart disease.
Should estrogen be stopped one month prior to elective surgery such as hysterectomy?	X		Stopping estrogen may decrease risk of blood clots associated with surgery.
Is the most common side effect of estrogen weight gain?		X	Nausea is more common.

Another vehicle for prescribing estrogen, the estrogen patch (Estraderm, Vivelle, Climara), may be preferable to oral estrogens for some women who have side effects such as nausea or bloating. Estraderm may prevent such side effects because it allows direct absorption of estrogen into the bloodstream, unlike pills, which are absorbed through the digestive tract. Also, in bypassing the liver, the patch system may reduce the chances of gallbladder problems. The Estraderm and Vivelle patches are applied to the skin and removed every three days, while the Climara patch is applied and removed once a week. An oral form of progesterone must be taken as well to avoid overstimulation of the uterine lining.

Tests Associated with Hormone-Replacement Therapy

Four types of tests may be appropriate in women receiving HRT. The *endometrial biopsy* (see page 282) may be performed any time abnormal bleeding occurs, and every year or so in women having regular withdrawal bleeding at the expected time. *Cholesterol screening* is important for all women over the age of twenty-five and especially upon initiation of HRT to serve as a baseline for comparison to subsequent cholesterol levels. *Bone-density screening* has not received widespread acceptance. However, in some women at high risk for osteoporosis, it may be an appropriate screening test. It may also be used for those already under treatment for osteoporosis to assess the progress of therapy. *Mammograms* should be performed regularly in accordance with the American Cancer Society guidelines (see Table 3) until the long-term effects of estrogen on the breasts are fully studied.

Precautions About the Use of Estrogen and Progesterone

Some conditions, while not absolute reasons to avoid estrogens, are likely to be made worse by taking this drug. Estrogen may stimulate the growth of *uterine fibroids* and produce symptoms of heavy menstrual bleeding or cramping. When these things happen and estrogen is then stopped, symptoms, including fibroid growth, usually subside without the need for surgery. *Jaundice* is also more likely to develop especially when estrogen is taken by a woman with a history of liver disease. *Gallbladder problems*, too, are more frequent. One study indicates a twofold increased risk of surgically confirmed gallbladder disease in women on estrogen. Estrogens and progesterones, by increasing fluid retention, may worsen or increase recurrences of certain conditions, such as *migraine headaches* or *epilepsy*, the control of which is depends upon preventing excessive fluid accumulation in certain parts of the body.

Side Effects of HRT

The most common side effects of estrogen are nausea, breast tenderness, and fluid retention. Infrequent effects which you should report to your doctor include vomiting, headaches, depression, pigmentation of facial skin, loss of hair, hair growth, skin rash, breast secretions, and intolerance to contact lenses. Also, be sure to notify your clinician of any abnormal or unscheduled vaginal spotting or bleeding. Progesterone usually causes fewer side effects. The most common ones are breast tenderness, abdominal bloating, acne, and depression.

Some women normally experience a period each month two or three days following the last estrogen pill (or the last progesterone pill in the case of combined estrogen and progesterone treatment). It is abnormal, however, to have spotting or bleeding during the days when the pills are taken; this condition is sometimes called breakthrough bleeding (see glossary) and may require a change in estrogen dosage. Any such abnormal bleeding should be evaluated by your physician. Abnormal bleeding in a woman over forty is best investigated either by endometrial biopsy (an office procedure; see glossary) or by dilatation and curettage (D & C; see glossary).

CHAPTER 28

Gynecologic Problems Related to Menopause

Around the time of menopause many women first notice certain symptoms that are associated with hormone changes that may affect the pelvic organs. These symptoms, known collectively as *pelvic relaxation*, may include frequent urination, vaginal or lower abdominal pressure, low back pain, or a feeling that "something is falling out." Pelvic relaxation refers to a gradual weakening of the vaginal muscles that support the uterus, bladder, and rectum. Weakening of these muscles may give rise to vaginal protrusions or hernias (see below), a "dropped" uterus (prolapsed uterus), or difficulty with bladder control (urinary stress incontinence; see glossary). Sometimes these problems begin before menopause, especially in women who have had difficult childbirth. Repeated childbirth, genetic factors, obesity, and conditions such as a chronic cough that continually strain pelvic muscles also cause a susceptibility to pelvic relaxation problems. Unless symptoms are severe, most women do not need surgical treatment. Surgery for any of the conditions is an elective procedure, the timing of which depends on the severity of the symptoms.

Vaginal Hernias (Cystoceles and Rectoceles)

Vaginal hernias (see also Chapter 88) appear as a bulge in the vaginal wall; your physician can diagnose them on pelvic examination. These painless protrusions represent a weakness in the muscles separating the vagina from the bladder (this one is called a *cystocele*) or the rectum (a *rectocele*). When these organs push against and bulge into the vaginal wall, completely emptying your bladder (in the case of a cystocele) or having a bowel movement (with a rectocele) sometimes becomes difficult. Symptoms of vaginal pressure and frequent urination (see Chapter 85) are common with cystoceles. Rectoceles cause symptoms less often but account for chronic constipation when a bowel movement becomes trapped in the rectocele and hardens.

About half of all postmenopausal women have at least mild degrees of these vaginal hernias, but fewer than 10% require surgery. You may need surgery for a cystocele if it causes chronic discomfort, frequent urination which interferes with daily activities, or incontinence (a condition where you are unable to hold in your urine). A rectocele may require surgical repair if you have frequent difficulty having a bowel movement. Rectoceles, even small ones, are sometimes associated with vaginal muscle damage, which gives rise to a sensation of vaginal looseness during intercourse, a problem that may also be surgically repaired.

Uterine Prolapse ("Dropped" Uterus)

Most women who have given birth have some degree of uterine prolapse, which is most often symptomless. Your partner may be the first to notice a more advanced prolapse if he feels "blockage" during penetration in intercourse. Moderate or severe prolapse may cause pressure or heaviness in the lower back or lower abdomen. Complete prolapse in which the uterus extends outside the vagina when the woman bears down is rare.

The clinician diagnoses uterine prolapse if the cervix visibly moves downward in the vaginal canal when he or she asks you to strain down during the speculum part of the pelvic examination. A dropped uterus in itself is not an indication for surgery especially if you have few or no symptoms and no related condition such as a vaginal hernia. However, this condition is one of the most common reasons given for hysterectomy. Vaginal hysterectomy (see Chapter 45) may be indicated, however, when prolapse causes severe backache or pelvic discomfort. To confirm this diagnosis, the clinician may attempt to reproduce your symptoms during the pelvic examination by pulling down on the uterus with a special clamp which attaches to the cervix. Another way to help establish that backache or other symptoms are due to prolapse and not to some other cause is to use a *pessary* (see below). If symptoms are then reduced, surgery is likely to relieve the discomfort.

A hysterectomy for mild prolapse is performed when other related surgery (such as for a vaginal hernia) is needed. In this case, hysterectomy improves the results of the associated surgery and prevents the need for a second operation in case prolapse symptoms become worse later. Hysterectomy also may be done if a woman desiring sterilization has symptoms of prolapse.

An alternative to surgery as a treatment for uterine prolapse is the use of a pessary, a rubber device which the clinician places into the vagina to support the uterus. Though not a permanent cure for the problem, a pessary prevents prolapse symptoms in women who do not want definitive surgery. The clinician removes and cleans the pessary every month or every two months to prevent vaginal infections, one of the complications of this device.

Urinary Stress Incontinence

A 1989 report of the Gerontological Society of America found that one in three perimenopausal (near menopausal-age) women aged forty-three to fifty experiences involuntary loss of urine at least once a month. In this survey of 541 randomly selected healthy women, more than one-half of the women having incontinence had the form of urinary loss known as *urinary stress incontinence* (USI). USI is the involuntary loss of urine during sudden activity that increases pressure inside the abdomen, such as coughing, laughing, or sneezing. From time to time, every woman normally experiences this problem, one which may have been previously underreported; USI also may occur more frequently during pregnancy. Frequent USI results from muscle weakness around the urethra and bladder. The term *urethrocele* refers to a displaced urethra, which often accompanies USI. This condition may be associated with urethrocele, cystocele, or uterine prolapse.

The physician diagnoses USI on the basis of a history of sudden loss of urine upon coughing, sneezing, laughing, or some other sudden strain. It is important for the clinician to differentiate this problem from other conditions affecting the urinary tract, such as infections, which are detectable by urinalysis or urine culture (see Chapters 85 and 86). USI may also be confused with a second type of incontinence—*urge incontinence*, in which the loss of urine is associated with a sudden urge to urinate rather than with some type of physical stress. Urge incontinence is usually due to other causes, such as bladder infection or anxiety, and does not respond to surgery. If there is any doubt about the diagnosis, a urologist may be consulted or the gynecologist may perform additional tests such as cystoscopy, an office or outpatient procedure used to examine the inside of the bladder for signs of inflammation or infection.

You may prevent the progression of this condition by doing an exercise (called Kegel's exercise) that will eventually strengthen your vaginal muscles. To do this exercise: Slowly contract (pull in) the muscle you use to control urination (as though you were going to stop the urine flow); hold it for three seconds and then gradually relax the muscle. Do this tightening-relaxing sequence as often as possible. The more often you do it, the better will be the result. Over a period of several months, you can build up your vaginal muscle tone and strength. Like any exercise, this program requires persistence and patience to get results. In the long run, this exercise will control mild degrees of urinary stress incontinence. (A possible added benefit is greater sexual satisfaction brought about by increased vaginal sensation and snugness during intercourse.)

Apart from these exercises there are a number of nonsurgical interventions and treatments that may help control stress incontinence. Any woman with this condition should avoid excessive fluid intake as well as caffeine-containing beverages. Respond right away to the urge to void so the bladder does not become distended. Biofeedback and other behavioral techniques have been helpful in some patients. Various types of vaginal pessaries that are used to treat uterine prolapse may also help to alleviate symptoms of stress urinary incontinence. In addition, prosthetic devices are now available to

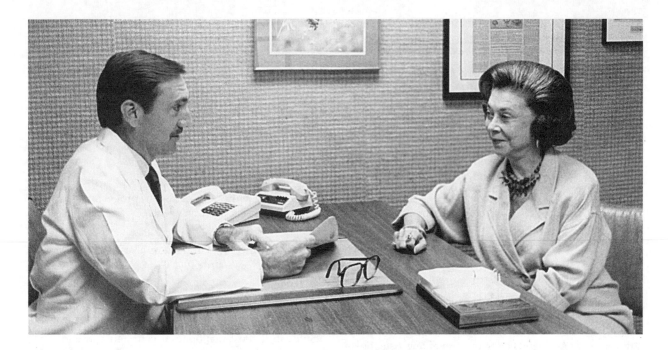

help support and restore bladder positioning without surgery. One such device is the INTROL Bladder Neck Support Prosthesis. Simply introducing a diaphragm or tampon may help some women with mild stress incontinence that occurs only with exercise.

When urinary stress incontinence becomes so severe that you need to wear a pad, or the problem becomes socially inconvenient or embarrassing, surgical treatment usually becomes necessary. This treatment involves a special operation performed through either the abdomen or the vagina to reposition the bladder and urethra. Both the abdominal and the vaginal operations have the same goal: to reposition the displaced urethra so that it functions normally. With either operation, there may be a recurrence of symptoms within five years 30% to 40% of the time. If there is a recurrence of symptoms, the need for additional surgery may then be evaluated.

Resource

For information on urinary incontinence write:

National Association for Continence
P.O. Box 8310
Spartanburg, South Carolina 29305-8310

References for Section Six

Chapter 26—Menopause
Chapter 27—Hormone-Replacement Therapy
Chapter 28—Gynecologic Problems Related to Menopause

American College of Obstetricians and Gynecologists *Technical Bulletin* 210. Health maintenance for perimenopausal women, Aug 1995.

American College of Obstetricians and Gynecologists *Technical Bulletin* 213. Urinary incontinence, Oct 1995.

American College of Obstetricians and Gynecologists *Technical Bulletin* 166. Hormone replacement therapy, Apr 1992.

American College of Obstetricians and Gynecologists *Technical Bulletin* 167. Osteoporosis, May 1992.

Reid, I. Effects of calcium supplementation on bone loss in postmenopausal women. *The New England Journal of Medicine* 328(7):460–464, Feb 18, 1993.

Effects of estrogen or estrogen/progestin regimens on heart disease risk factors in postmenopausal women. *The Journal of the American Medical Association* 273(3):199–240, Jan 18, 1995.

Petitti, D. Hormone replacement therapy. *The Female Patient* 19:93–104, Sep 1994.

Anderson, E. Characteristics of menopausal women seeking assistance. *American Journal of Obstetrics and Gynecology* 156:428–433, 1987.

Patterson, M. Menopause: salient issues for counselors. *Journal of Counseling and Development* 67:185–188, Nov 1988.

Castelli, W. Cardiac risks in women: what is the role of the OB/GYN. *The Female Patient* 14:54–66, 1989.

Ferguson, K. Estrogen replacement therapy: a survey of women's knowledge and attitudes. *Archives of Internal Medicine* 149:133–136, 1989.

Kannel, W. Metabolic risk factors for coronary heart disease in women: perspective from the Framingham study. *American Heart Journal* 114:413–419, 1987.

Indications for combining estrogen replacement therapy with testosterone therapy. *International Correspondent Society of Obstetricians and Gynecologists* 29(9): Sep 1988.

Grisanti, J. Some new views on preventing osteoporosis. *Contemporary OB/GYN* 33(5):60–78, May 1989.

Shephard, B. Hot flashes: not for women only. *Encyclopaedia Britannica Health Annual*, 1990.

Piziak, V. Osteoporosis: what can be done? *The Female Patient* 14:57–68, Feb 1989.

Brenner, P. The menopausal syndrome. *Obstetrics and Gynecology* 72 (supplement 5):6s–11s, 1988.

Hunt, K. Long-term surveillance of mortality and cancer incidence in women receiving hormone replacement therapy. *British Journal of Obstetrics and Gynecology* 94:620–635, 1987.

Prough, S. Continuous estrogen/progestin therapy in menopause. *American Journal of Obstetrics and Gynecology* 157: 1449–1453, 1987.

Judd, H. Efficacy of transdermal estradiol. *American Journal of Obstetrics and Gynecology* 156:1326–1331, 1987.

Speroff, L. Options in estrogen replacement therapy. *Contemporary OB/GYN* 31(3):190–210, Mar 1988.

Sullivan, J. Post-menopausal estrogen use and coronary atherosclerosis. *Annals of Internal Medicine* 108:358–363, 1988.

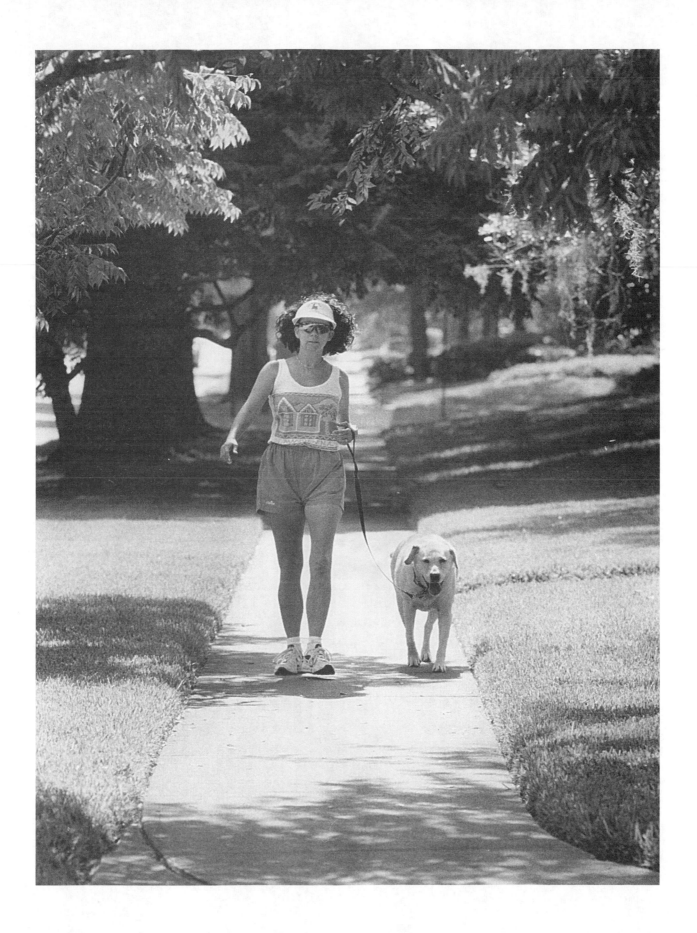

THE WOMAN CONSUMER AND DRUGS

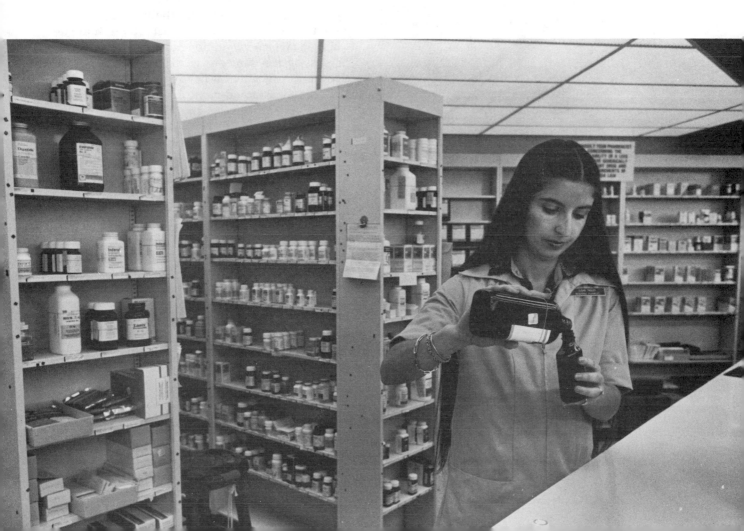

CHAPTER 29

Understanding the Drugs You Take

In 1995, U.S. doctors wrote more than 1.6 billion prescriptions; the majority were for women. Historically, women have been the major users of both prescription and nonprescription (also called over-the-counter) drugs. As the principal consumers of both prescription and nonprescription drugs, women have a personal responsibility to know the effects of the drugs they take and a financial stake in knowing some rules about medicine shopping. This section of the book will help you understand both of these areas.

Generic Versus Brand-Name Drugs

Every drug has a *generic*, or chemical, name. A *brand* or *trade* name is a name given to a drug product by the manufacturer who first developed the drug. The brand name is designed to be short and easy to remember. For example, the brand name of a common tranquilizer, Librium, is far easier to spell and to recall than its generic name, chlordiazepoxide. These brand-name drugs are allowed to be manufactured and sold only by the manufacturer that developed the drug, since that company usually acquires patent rights for seventeen years. During this period of time, the company that introduced the product has exclusive manufacturing rights and other manufacturers are prevented from marketing a drug with the same chemical structure. After the patent period has ended, the product can be manufactured by other drug companies and sold under its generic name or under the new manufacturer's own trade name.

Generic drugs cost less than brand-name drugs because they can be manufactured by a number of competing drug companies; this competition lowers prices. As a result of cheaper costs, generic drug prescriptions have been on the increase and accounted for about 50% of prescription-drug sales in 1995 compared to 14% in 1985, a near fourfold increase. Although more generic drugs are being prescribed, not all brand-name drugs are available by generic name because the patent rights have not yet expired.

Along with increased generic prescribing by doctors, generic substitution by pharmacists has become more frequent and is mandated by law in many states. In such states, the patient automatically gets the generic equivalent drug, which is usually cheaper, unless a brand name is specified. In other states, patients or their physicians must request that a generic drug be prescribed. HMOs and government programs like Medicaid may also require the use of generic drugs.

Two potential problems may arise when a generic drug is prescribed. One concern is that various allergic reactions, such as hives and wheezing, may result from the inert ingredients such as coloring agents, preservatives, and stabilizers, which vary among different generic versions of the same drug. The second area of concern is whether or not generic drugs work as effectively as brand-name drugs. While most generics appear to do so, exceptions may arise due to the relatively wide latitude the FDA has given drug manufacturers concerning *bioavailability*.

Bioavailability—the amount of the drug that reaches the bloodstream—is the usual criteria for deciding if the generic form and a brand-name preparation are essentially equivalent. The FDA accepts variations in bioavailability of up to 30% in either direction between the generic and a brand-name drug. This means that a total of 60% variation in bioavailability could arise between the brand-name and the generic version or between one generic version and another. Critics of generics argue that this broad standard leaves little room for individual patient variation and that generics that have the same bioavailability may still not have clinical equivalence in individual patients.

The American Pharmaceutical Association has stated that differences in quality of drug products from different sources may show significant variation in effectiveness, safety, or both. The effectiveness of varying generics may be of special importance to patients on long-term medication (such as those for heart disease or high blood pressure) who may be obtaining different generic versions with each refill. The problem is further compounded if the drug has a *narrow therapeutic range*, meaning that small variations in blood concentrations (within FDA standards) could result in a lack of effectiveness or in side effects. Two groups of medications prescribed for women that fall into this category are birth control pills and certain estrogens, such as Premarin, which are used in treating menopausal symptoms. For this reason, some physicians avoid generics when prescribing these hormones.

Nonprescription Versus Prescription Drugs

Over-the-counter (OTC) drugs differ from prescription drugs because they require no prescription for you to obtain them and they are generally cheaper and less powerful. No doubt, you take nonprescription drugs for relief of minor problems such as headache, diarrhea, and indigestion. Studies have shown that most consumers get their information on over-the-counter drugs from advertising rather than from labels on the drug itself. Currently drug advertisements are not regulated by the FDA; however, drug labels must provide all the directions needed by the average person. It is important that you carefully read the label as well as any accompanying information in the package.

Chronic use of OTC drugs for long periods, especially when they do not relieve your symptoms, can mask underlying illness, possibly delaying diagnosis and treatment. For this reason, you should avoid chronic self-medication. Use the two-week rule-of-thumb: If you have been taking, say, aspirin every day for two weeks for headaches and you still have headaches, make an appointment with your doctor. If you have questions about side effects or adverse (unfavorable) reactions of any OTC drugs you are taking, ask your pharmacist these questions.

Before You Take Prescription Drugs

1. If you regularly use antacids, laxatives, pain relievers, or diet aids, mention this use to your physician before he or she prescribes a drug for you. Many OTC drugs don't "mix" with prescription medicines.
2. Tell the clinician about any allergic reactions (such as itching, rash, vomiting, or difficult breathing) you have had to drugs in the past. Allergic reactions to certain drugs like penicillin tend to get worse each time you take the drug. You may want to take a special skin test to safely determine if you are allergic to penicillin (or any of its forms, such as ampicillin).
3. Inform your clinician of any past health problems as this may influence his or her choice of drugs for you. For example, certain drugs are dangerous for a person with chronic liver or kidney disease, since these organs are involved in eliminating the drug from your body. Some drugs affect chronic conditions in a harmful way. Birth control pills, for instance, may make migraine headaches, epilepsy, or heart disease worse because of increased fluid retention.
4. If there is any possibility of pregnancy, avoid drugs altogether unless specified by your doctor. (See Chapter 31, *Drugs and the Pregnant Woman.*) Seemingly harmless drugs, even aspirin, may be harmful to the fetus.
5. If you are breast-feeding, avoid using drugs if possible because almost all drugs can pass into the breast milk. Subtle drug effects on the newborn's growth, development, or behavior are difficult to measure and in most cases are unknown.

When You Are Given a Prescription Drug

Here are some questions you should ask your clinician when he or she has prescribed a drug for you.

1. What is the purpose of the drug? Has a diagnosis been made? If not, find out if drug treatment is really necessary or if the symptoms are likely to subside on their own. For example, birth control pills are often prescribed for adolescents to "regulate" their cycle although some menstrual irregularity is perfectly normal among teen-age women.

2. Are less costly OTC drugs available? For instance, for nonpregnant women, prescriptions for multiple vitamins and iron are practically never necessary and almost always more costly than OTC equivalents.
3. What are possible side effects to watch for? What should be done if they occur?
4. How often should the drug be taken? When a prescription reads "four times a day," does that mean this amount is the necessary dosage to get a curative effect, as with antibiotics, or does that indicate the maximum dosage per day for a drug to be taken only "when needed" as with pain medication?
5. For how many days should the drug be taken? Until this entire prescription is used up or less? Should I have the prescription refilled?
6. Could this drug interact harmfully with other prescription or OTC drugs I am taking? What are the symptoms to watch for? Find out if food or alcoholic beverages will affect the way the drug should be taken. For example, is it better to take this drug on an empty stomach, before meals, after meals? How many hours before or after I take the medication can I drink alcohol?
7. Can the generic equivalent be prescribed if one is available?

When Taking a Prescription Drug

1. Keep a record of the drug, dosage, and the time of day you take each dose. This record will accomplish at least two things: 1) it will remind you of when you took your last dose; and 2) if you are taking more than one drug and they shouldn't be taken at the same time, you can remember to separate the times you take them. Put the record where it will remind you to take the drug.

2. Ask your pharmacist for a copy of the manufacturer's package insert that accompanies prescription drugs. These inserts provide detailed information about the drug although not in layman language since they are intended primarily for the pharmacist or physicians. Other pamphlets written for patients may be available with certain prescription drugs.
3. Know how to store the drug. Some drugs have to be refrigerated and others have to be kept in a tight, dry container. Keep them safely out of the reach of small children—perhaps in a locked medicine cabinet or, when necessary to be refrigerated, in a part of the refrigerator that a child cannot reach.
4. Take the full course of the drug prescription if that is what your doctor's instructions are. Sometimes symptoms improve before the drug therapy has been completed and it is tempting to stop taking the drug. A relapse of symptoms can occur, as with certain vaginal infections.
5. Be familiar with harmful side effects. If they occur, stop the drug and inform your doctor.
6. If you are taking a drug chronically, get periodic checkups. Women taking prescription medication chronically for high blood pressure, thyroid conditions, contraception, or any chronic health problem should have a checkup at least annually.
7. If surgery is scheduled, review your prescription drugs with your physician. Oral contraceptives, for example, should be stopped one or two months prior to elective surgery, since blood clots after an operation are more common in users of birth control pills.
8. Discard drugs that you have not used. It can be dangerous to take old, outdated drugs.

CHAPTER 30

Avoiding Drug Abuse

Substance abuse represents an urgent health problem for many American women. Consider these three facts:

- Almost half of all women aged 15 to 45 have used drugs at least once in their life.
- More than 3.7 million women have taken prescription drugs nonmedically during the past year.
- More than 28,000 (70%) of the AIDS cases among women are drug-related.

The spectrum of substance abuse includes legal drugs, both prescription and nonprescription, illegal "street" drugs, and substances not always thought of as drugs, such as nicotine and alcohol. Drug abuse causes health problems for the woman, and if she happens to be pregnant, for her unborn child as well. While an exact definition of drug abuse is hard to come by, most experts agree that drug abuse occurs whenever an individual takes a drug routinely in order to function—to "get through the day."

Although limited research has been done in the area of women and drugs, the available literature indicates significant differences between male and female drug abusers. Characteristics of the female drug abuser frequently include problems with sexual identity, difficulty expressing anger directly (resulting in passive, indirect, or acting-out behavior), intense feelings of personal inadequacy, and fear of close relationships. There are certain critical times in a woman's life when drug abuse is more likely to occur: early in a marriage, with the birth of the first child, with an unwanted pregnancy, and during divorce, widowhood, menopause, or major surgery. Just being aware that you might be more susceptible to drug abuse during these times of crisis will hopefully help you avoid using drugs as a crutch. In such highly stressful times, it is important to seek out extra support from family or friends. In addition, you might want to consult a competent therapist.

Common Forms of Drug Abuse

According to national surveys, women are *less* likely than men to become involved with three of the most commonly abused substances: alcohol, marijuana, and cocaine. However, women are *more* likely than men to become involved with drugs in a fourth category: prescription psychoactive drugs. These are drugs that affect the mind, such as tranquilizers, sedatives, and diet pills. The most recent information on the ways in which men and women compare in the major categories of substance abuse in American society are listed below. Substance abuse involving nicotine and caffeine is discussed elsewhere (see Index). Drug abuse during pregnancy is covered separately in Chapter 31.

Prescription Psychoactive Drugs

Historically, women have been far more likely than men to have their physician prescribe mood-altering drugs. Men, however, are more likely to take these drugs for nonmedical purposes, without a doctor's prescription, or in greater amounts than prescribed.

The termination of chronic use of many psychoactive drugs, even "minor" tranquilizers like Valium or Tranxene, can result in withdrawal symptoms such as delirium, trembling, psychotic behavior, and exaggeration of reflexes. With repeated use of mood-altering substances, including most prescription tranquilizers, diet pills, and pain pills, *tolerance* may develop, resulting in diminished effect of the drug unless dosage is increased.

Why are women more prone than men to abuse prescription psychoactive drugs? This situation may be related to the fact that women are more likely than men to acknowledge psychological distress and to seek medical aid for it. Physicians' prescribing practices may also contribute to illegal abuse, depending upon how problems of male and female patients are perceived. Physicians who accept the sexual stereotype of women as "weak and helpless" may be more likely to prescribe tranquilizers for women

Table 46   SYMPTOMS OF DRUG ABUSE

	Symptoms of Excessive Use or Overdose	Symptoms of Withdrawal
Narcotics	extreme drowsiness or confusion loss of appetite slow, shallow breathing cold, clammy skin seizures coma	nausea, vomiting, stomach cramps excessive nervousness sweating hand tremor watery nose and eyes yawning
Barbiturates, sleeping pills, tranquilizers, and alcohol	slurred speech, staggering gait disorientation extreme drowsiness, falling asleep at work slow, shallow breathing cold, clammy skin coma	excessive nervousness insomnia hand tremor confusion seizures
Stimulants (diet pills, "crack," cocaine)	agitation or extreme nervousness excitation or irritability hallucinations, dilated pupils seizures	depression, apathy confusion irritability

with symptoms of anxiety and depression as opposed to recommending behavioral self-help strategies. Some drug companies may indirectly encourage such prescribing through advertisements that depict drugs as a solution to normal life stresses or that show women in stereotyped sex roles in which they suffer from nervousness and depression. Whatever the cause, the problem of misuse of prescription drugs is real.

Marijuana

Marijuana, the most widely used illicit drug in the United States, has been tried at least once by one-third of Americans over the age of eleven. More than 5.6 million women have used marijuana in their life. In the 1985 household survey by the National Institute on Drug Abuse (NIDA), usage rates were higher among males, 38% of whom reported using marijuana at least once in their lifetime, compared to 27% of females. Also, reported usage rates were higher for white women than for black or Hispanic women. Marijuana is also the most commonly used drug in the workplace; some companies now test prospective employees for this and other drugs before hiring. Motivation for using drugs such as marijuana may relate to unpleasant moods such as anxiety or depression, which

are more commonly reported among women. However, the drug may also induce these symptoms. The average potency of marijuana has increased in recent years, increasing the likelihood of withdrawal effects. Chronic marijuana use may cause or make worse a range of lung conditions ranging from bronchitis to emphysema. Perhaps the most dangerous effect of marijuana is that its use may lead to other more dangerous drugs, especially cocaine and narcotics.

Cocaine

More than 600,000 women have used cocaine. Cocaine is the most common form of stimulant abused in the United States today and is more likely than any other known drug to produce chemical dependency. Many users have a prior history of alcohol or marijuana abuse, addictions that have been called the "twin gateways to cocaine addiction." The desperate craving for this expensive drug has led some women to turn to prostitution to support their "coke" or "crack" habits. Prostitution, in turn, is often linked to various sexually transmitted diseases, such as hepatitis and AIDS, especially where IV drug use is concerned.

Cocaine use became widespread in the late 1970s and 1980s; as many as 12% of U.S. residents over the age of twelve have tried cocaine. The incidence is higher among certain age groups, such as those eighteen to thirty-four years of age, among whom one in four has tried cocaine at least once. Among individuals eighteen to twenty-five years old, 29% of males have tried cocaine compared with 22% of females, while among twenty-six- to thirty-four-year-olds, the usage rates were 30% for males and 18% for females. For those over thirty-five years old, only 7% of males versus 2% of females have tried the drug according to the 1985 national household survey. As for marijuana, these usage percentages were highest for white females as compared to either black or Hispanic females.

Cocaine overdose is a major cause of death among chronic cocaine users. Symptoms include sweating, nervousness, paranoia, hallucinations, and depression that may lead to suicide. Physical complications of overdose include heart attack and stroke. The intense craving of the cocaine addict makes the disease highly resistant to treatment. Stopping use of the drug is the most essential component of any form of therapy. Long-term follow-up is necessary, and successful treatment involves commitment to a life-style in which all mood-altering drugs are avoided. Counseling, both individual and group, as well as continuing attendance of support groups such as Narcotics Anonymous and Cocaine Anonymous, have been successful in helping some cocaine addicts.

Alcohol

Women experience the ill effects of alcohol earlier than men and at lower consumption levels.

Table 47   WARNING SIGNALS OF DRUG ABUSE

If you answer yes to any of the questions below, you may have a problem with drugs, alcohol, or both.

1. Are you defensive if a friend or relative mentions your drug or alcohol use?

2. Are you sometimes embarrassed or frightened by your behavior under the influence of drugs or alcohol?

3. Have you ever gone to see a new doctor because your regular physician would not prescribe the drug you wanted?

4. When you are under pressure or feel anxious, do you automatically take a tranquilizer or a drink or both?

5. Do you take drugs more often than recommended by your doctor or for purposes other than those recommended by your doctor?

6. Do you mix drugs and alcohol?

7. Do you regularly drink or take drugs to help you sleep?

8. Do you have to take a pill to get going in the morning?

This is because women have less water in their bodies than men so the alcohol is less diluted and has a greater impact. In addition, and perhaps due, in part, to estrogen, women do not metabolize alcohol as efficiently as men do, which may make women more vulnerable to the consequences of drinking. Drink for drink, women have a 30% higher blood alcohol level compared to men.

Several differences in the pattern of alcohol abuse among men and women have been noted by various research studies. Compared to men, for example, women start drinking and begin

---

Table 48   DRUGS WITH HIGHEST POTENTIAL FOR ABUSE*

Drug Family	Generic Name	Common Brand Names Containing This Drug	Medical Use
amphetamine (stimulant)	amphetamine	Dexedrine, Biphetamine, Desoxyn	lose weight**
analgesic (narcotic)	oxycodone	Percodan, Percocet, Tylox	pain relief
analgesic (narcotic)	meperidine	Demerol	pain relief
barbiturate (sedative)	pentobarbital	Nembutal	promote sleep

* Controlled Substances Act
** Not approved for this use in some states.

Table 49 DRUGS WITH INTERMEDIATE POTENTIAL FOR ABUSE*

Drug Family	Generic Name	Common Brand Names Containing This Drug	Medical Use
amphetamine-like (stimulant)	phentermine	Fastin, Ionamin	lose weight
amphetamine-like (stimulant)	fenfluramine	Pondimin	lose weight
amphetamine-like (stimulant)	phendimetrazine	Prelu-2	lose weight
analgesic (narcotic)	codeine	Empirin with Codeine (#3 & #4) Fiorinal with Codeine Phenaphen with Codeine (#3 & #4) Tylenol with Codeine (#2, #3, & #4)	pain relief, cough suppression
analgesic (narcotic)	hydrocodone	Triaminic Expectorant DH Tussionex	cough suppression
analgesic (narcotic)	opium	Paregoric	pain relief relief of intestinal spasm and diarrhea
analgesic (narcotic)	propoxyphene	Darvon Darvon Compound Darvocet-N Wygesic	pain relief
analgesic (nonnarcotic)	pentazocine	Talwin Compound Talacen	pain relief
barbiturate (sedative)	butabarbital	Butisol Phenobarbital	relief of anxiety
barbiturate (sedative)	butalbital	Fioricet	relieve tension headache
barbiturate (sedative)	butalbital	Fiorinal	relieve tension headache
sleeping pill	chloral hydrate	Chloral Hydrate	promote sleep
sleeping pill	ethchlorvynol	Placidyl	promote sleep
sleeping pill	flurazepam	Dalmane	promote sleep
sleeping pill	triazolam	Halcion	promote sleep
sleeping pill	methyprylon	Noludar	promote sleep
sleeping pill	temazepam	Restoril	promote sleep
tranquilizer	meprobamate	Equagesic	pain relief
tranquilizer	meprobamate	Equanil, Miltown	relief of anxiety
tranquilizer	chlordiazepoxide	Librium, Limbitrol	relief of anxiety
tranquilizer	lorazepam	Ativan	relief of anxiety
tranqulizer	oxazepam	Serax	relief of anxiety
tranquilizer	chlorazepate	Tranxene	relief of anxiety
tranquilizer	diazepam	Valium	relief of anxiety
tranquilizer	alprazolam	Xanax	relief of anxiety

* Controlled Substances Act

their pattern of alcohol abuse at a later age. However, they seek medical care at about the same age, suggesting either that women seek care earlier or that the course of alcohol problems is more rapid in women. Compared to men, alcoholic women are more likely to be divorced or to be living with an alcoholic partner. In addition, women alcoholics are more likely to have a history of suicide or of prescription substance abuse. In comparison to men, women alcoholics are also more likely to report symptoms of psychological distress, such as anxiety or depression, and are more likely to be victims of domestic violence, especially spousal abuse.

Women comprise one third of the 15 million alcoholics in the U.S. Late stage complications of alcoholism in women, such as liver damage (cirrhosis), anemia and malnutrition, develop more rapidly in women compared to men. Likewise the percentage of alcoholics who die from causes such as suicide, accidents and circulatory disorders is higher among women than men. Women

---

Table 50   DRUGS WITH LOWEST POTENTIAL FOR ABUSE*

For Diarrhea	*Contain small amounts of paregoric:*
	Parepectolin, Donnagel PG
For Cough	*Contain small amounts of codeine:*
	Actifed with Codeine
	Ambenyl Cough Syrup
	Capital with Codeine Suspension
	Dimetane DC
	Novahistine DH and Expectorant
	Phenergan VC with Codeine
	Robitussin A-C and DAC
	Triaminic Expectorant with Codeine
	Tylenol with Codeine Elixir

---

* Controlled Substances Act

alcoholics also experience heavier, more painful periods as well as higher rates of stroke, osteoporosis and infertility than do nondrinkers.

The variety of treatment programs for alcoholism mirror those for treatment of other serious drug problems and include individual and group therapy, and medical treatment of psychiatric problems, including anxiety and depression. The most important goal of treatment, as in any form of drug abuse, is to prevent relapse. Treatment programs often include lifelong membership in Alcoholics Anonymous. This organization offers one of the best and most successful resources for helping the alcoholic who has acknowledged that he or she has a problem and is ready to work on it.

The Controlled Substances Act

Legal drugs subject to abuse are regulated by the Controlled Substances Act. This Federal law specifies several different categories of prescription and nonprescription drugs according to how likely the drugs are to cause addiction and harmful effects as a result of excessive use. We have arranged these so-called controlled drugs by highest, intermediate, and lowest drug abuse potential in Tables 48, 49, and 50, respectively.

Table 48 includes the strongest of all prescription pain killers (analgesics), sleeping pills, and diet pills. Table 49 encompasses less potent and lower dose pain pills and cough suppressants. Also, milder barbiturates and sleeping pills, tranquilizers like Valium, and the least toxic diet pills are included in this group. Table 50 includes mainly drugs for cough and a few drugs for diarrhea. Many of the products in Table 50 may be purchased over-the-counter in most states simply by signing the pharmacist's register, specifying the type and amount of medication purchased. The ready availability of drugs in this group may make them subject to more frequent abuse compared to some of the more potent drugs in the other tables.

Resources

Local drug abuse or women's health centers: see your telephone directory.

For information about alcohol, drugs, or drug abuse write:

National Clearinghouse for Alcohol and Drug Information
P.O. Box 2345
Rockville, Maryland 20847

The Clearinghouse also maintains an updated directory of women's drug abuse treatment programs throughout the United States.

Resource groups for alcohol abuse:

If you are having a problem with alcohol abuse, no matter what your age is, you can contact:

Alcoholics Anonymous
Grand Central Station
P.O. Box 459
New York, New York 10163

For local meetings see your local telephone directory under Alcoholics Anonymous.

If a member of your family (any age) or a friend is having a problem with alcohol abuse, write:

Al-Anon Family Group Headquarters, Inc.
P.O. Box 862
Midtown Station
New York, N.Y. 10018-0862

For local Al-Anon meetings see your local telephone directory under Al-Anon Family Group. If you are a teenager (or younger) and a family member or friend is having a problem with alcohol abuse, *you* can get help with how to deal with the problem. Look under Alateen, or Al-Anon-Alateen, in your telephone directory.

For all of these alcohol programs (Alcoholics Anonymous, Al-Anon, and Alateen) you do not have to give your last name; you can attend meetings and can remain, as the name implies, anonymous.

CHAPTER 31

Drugs and the Pregnant Woman

The subject of drug use during pregnancy is beset with conflicting reports and controversy. The shocking realization of the effect of drugs on the fetus occurred in the 1960s following the thalidomide tragedy. Thalidomide was prescribed widely in Europe as a sedative for four years before it was found to cause profound limb deformities in the fetus when the drug was taken in early pregnancy. Although the drug had not been approved by the FDA for use in the U.S., the thalidomide story led to stricter drug regulation within the U.S. by the FDA. Today there is increasing concern about possible biochemical and long-term behavioral effects on the fetus of drugs taken during pregnancy as well as on physical malformations of the fetus.

Women are presented with new press reports every day about drugs potentially harmful to the unborn. At the same time a constant barrage of advertisements in the media encourage women to consume drugs for a variety of symptoms, many of which are common in pregnancy. The ready availability and lack of labels warning against use in pregnancy on most over-the-counter drugs may help account for the widespread use of these remedies by pregnant women.

You should ask your physician about *any* drug you are routinely taking when you become pregnant. The use of most drugs during pregnancy is associated with some risk to the fetus; this risk must be weighed against the expected benefits of the drug. There are several points to be considered when you make this choice:

1. Approximately 2% to 5% of all pregnancies result in birth defects. It is believed that most of these defects are due to a variety of interacting causes of which drugs are only one factor. In fact, it is estimated that drugs (excluding alcohol) cause only 1% to 3% of these birth defects.
2. Extremely few drugs are known to cause malformations. These include thalidomide (no longer marketed), sex hormones, and certain drugs used to treat cancer.
3. Some drugs are considered safe in pregnancy either because they are not absorbed or because long-term use has not been associated with harmful effects on the newborn (see Table 51).
4. The placenta is not a barrier. Most drugs travel across the placenta and reach the fetus. For this reason, it is difficult to completely exclude the possibility of harmful fetal effects for most drugs. Some effects may take years to show up, as in the case of DES (see Chapter 38), a drug now believed to cause vaginal cancer in young women who were exposed before birth, when their mothers were pregnant with

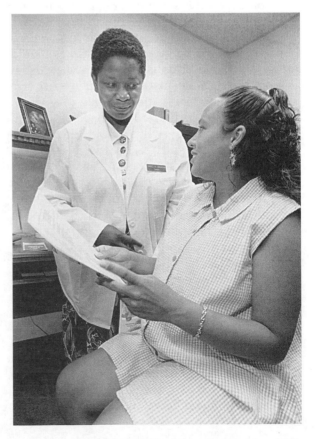

Table 51 DRUGS PRESENTLY CONSIDERED SAFE TO USE DURING PREGNANCY

Symptom	Drug
Pain (e.g., headache)	Acetaminophen (e.g., Tylenol, Datril)
Diarrhea	Kaopectate
Constipation	Certain laxatives (see Chapter 60 on constipation)
Heartburn	Antacids (but avoid antacids containing aspirin)
Itching; insomnia	Diphenhydramine (Benadryl)
Hay fever; sinus congestion	Chlorpheniramine (Chlor-Trimeton)

them and were given this drug to prevent miscarriage.

5. The effect of a drug on the fetus depends partly on the stage of pregnancy. In early pregnancy, especially during the first two months after conception, the fetal organs are forming and unnecessary drugs should be avoided. This is the stage when drug-induced malformations usually occur (see Table 52). In middle and late pregnancy, drugs may be harmful to the fetus's chemical functioning, which could result in adverse effects such as internal bleeding or growth retardation (see Table 53). Just prior to labor, drugs may affect the baby's capacity to adjust to life outside the uterus. Breathing difficulty may be encountered at birth in newborns exposed in late pregnancy to tranquilizers, sedatives, or excessive alcohol.

6. Certain medical conditions may necessitate the taking of drugs in pregnancy. Often the advantages of taking these medicines outweigh the fetal risks involved (see Table 54).

7. Drug use during breast-feeding may be associated with certain risks to the newborn although the quantity of most drugs in breast milk is very low (see Tables 55 and 56).

Table 52 DRUGS THAT MAY CAUSE FETAL ABNORMALITIES IN EARLY PREGNANCY

Not all drugs listed here are definitely known to cause birth defects in humans. However, the available evidence, including animal research, indicates the advisability of avoiding these drugs in pregnancy, particularly in the first three months.

Drug	Comments
Accutane	An acne drug known to cause birth defects
Alcohol	Associated with various birth defects (see text and Table 57)
Anticancer drugs	For example, Aminopterin and methotrexate; associated with various birth defects
Caffeine	Known to cause birth defects in animals but not, so far, in humans; FDA recommends avoiding caffeine-containing products or using them sparingly in pregnancy
Hormones	Androgens (male sex hormones) and certain progesterones may cause masculinization of female infants. An increased risk of certain birth defects has been reported with sex hormones (estrogen and progesterone) including the "pill"
Lithium	Associated with heart defects
Retinoic acid (Vitamin A)	High doses associated with miscarriage and certain birth defects (see Chapter 48)
Tranquilizers	For example, Librium, Tranxene, Valium; slight increased risk of birth defects has been reported
Warfarin	For example, Coumadin (an anticoagulant); known to cause various birth defects

Remember, it is important to consider carefully before you take any drug while you are pregnant. Because new research studies are constantly uncovering new information, it is a good idea to consult with your clinician on any new findings that would make advisable or inadvis-

Table 53 DRUGS THAT MAY CAUSE ADVERSE FETAL EFFECTS IN LATE PREGNANCY

Drug	Comments
Alcohol	Mental retardation, growth problems (see text and Table 57)
Antithyroid drugs (and drugs containing potassium iodide, an ingredient in some cough syrups and a few asthma remedies)	May cause fetal goiter or abnormal thyroid condition
Aspirin	Aspirin-containing drugs may cause fetal bleeding
Chloramphenicol	This antibiotic may cause "Gray Syndrome," a toxic, sometimes fatal, reaction in the newborn
Tetracycline	For example, Achromycin, Minocin, Sumycin, Vibramycin; may cause stained teeth and abnormal fetal growth
Warfarin	For example, Coumadin; may cause fetal bleeding
Water pills	Certain types, such as Diuril, Dyazide, Hydrodiuril, and others may cause fetal bleeding or jaundice

Table 54 DRUG USE DURING PREGNANCY FOR CERTAIN MEDICAL CONDITIONS

Condition	Comment
Asthma	Continue most medications; avoid drugs containing iodides as iodides may be harmful to the fetus; avoid steroids such as Prednisone and Aristocort unless advised by physician; safety of Cromolyn not established.
High blood pressure	Continue most medications under physician supervision. Avoid captopril and enalapril, which may cause serious injury to the fetus throughout pregnancy.
Diabetes	Avoid all oral medication—possibly harmful to fetus; use insulin only—dosage of insulin will increase during pregnancy.
Seizures	Dilantin and other drugs used in treating seizures have been associated with an increased risk of fetal malformation. However, the benefits of most of these drugs to prevent seizures outweigh the risks. A neurologist's consultation may be advisable.
Hypothyroidism (low thyroid)	Frequent thyroid blood tests are necessary to determine correct dosage.

able the use of any drug you plan to take while you are pregnant. This responsibility is yours; you owe it to yourself and your unborn.

Substance Abuse During Pregnancy

Substance abuse during pregnancy, like drug abuse in nonpregnant individuals, may take many forms: heavy smoking or drinking, abuse of prescription and nonprescription drugs, or the use of illicit street drugs, recreationally, compulsively, or as an addictive habit. Many individuals who use drugs intermittently or recreationally may stop or lessen drug use during pregnancy out of guilt or concern for the fetus. Unfortunately, such steps may come too late since pregnancy is often diagnosed well into the early months, when fetal organ development has already begun to occur. The use of "hard" drugs, including "crack," cocaine, heroin, and other narcotics, while occurring throughout American society, has become increasingly prevalent within the inner cities. This represents an additional problem for the urban poor, including poor women who happen to be pregnant. In 1993 the National Institute on Drug Abuse conducted the first large survey of drug use by pregnant women in the United States. The survey, which went to 52 hospitals, found an estimated 6% of pregnant women use illicit drugs such as marijuana and cocaine during their pregnancy.

Most drugs, including narcotics, barbiturates, cocaine, and alcohol, cross the placenta to the fetus. Except for alcohol, which is associated with a well-known syndrome of birth defects (see below), most illicit drugs cannot be linked to birth defects. This is partly because unlike alcohol, illicit drugs cannot be studied easily and

Table 55 DRUGS TO AVOID IF YOU BREAST-FEED

If you are breast-feeding and you take—	your baby may develop—
aspirin (high doses)	bleeding problems
atropine (antispasmodic drug)	constipation or more serious reactions
barbiturates (high doses)	drowsiness (baby will nurse less easily)
ergotamine (antimigraine drug)	nausea, vomiting, or diarrhea
Flagyl (for vaginitis)	low blood count
laxatives (stimulant type except milk of magnesia and Dulcolax)	diarrhea
Lithium	high blood levels of the drug
sleeping pills	drowsiness (baby will nurse less easily)
sulfa (antibiotic)	jaundice
tetracycline (antibiotic)	tooth discoloration (rare)
thiazides (water pills)	jaundice or bleeding (rare)
tranquilizers (for example, Valium, Tranxene, Miltown, Equanil)	drowsiness (baby will nurse less easily)

Table 56 DRUGS PRESENTLY CONSIDERED SAFE TO TAKE IF YOU BREAST-FEED*

Drug	Comment
Alcohol	
Antacids	Maalox, Mylanta, Rolaids, Tums, and others
Antibiotics (some)	ampicillin (for example, Principen, Omnipen, Polycillin), cephalosporins (for example, Keflex), erythromycin
Iron	
Laxatives (mild)	Dulcolax, milk of magnesia, Metamucil
Pain relievers	both nonnarcotic and narcotic in recommended doses
Stool softeners	Colace, Dialose, Kasof, Surfak
Vitamins	

* Newborn allergic reactions may occur but are uncommon. Newborns with problems such as prematurity may accumulate drugs and more readily develop side effects.

partly because individuals involved in drug abuse often consume a combination of substances. What is clear, however, is that regular drug use, especially involving narcotics, cocaine, or alcohol, is usually associated with severe nutritional deficiencies in the mother that often lead to anemia and growth problems in the fetus. Some of the maternal and fetal concerns surrounding use of the more common street drugs include the following:

Marijuana/Hashish

Birth defects have been shown to result in animals but not in humans. Smoking marijuana exposes the fetus to numerous chemicals. A 1989 report from *The New England Journal of Medicine* found that the use of marijuana in pregnancy significantly impaired fetal growth. In the mother, lung damage may be similar to that caused by smoking cigarettes.

Narcotics

Heroin addiction during pregnancy represents one of the highest risks to the fetus. Narcotic abuse is associated with growth retardation, preterm labor, and a potentially fatal withdrawal syndrome after birth. Since sudden narcotic withdrawal in pregnancy also can be fatal to the fetus, heroin-addicted mothers are often maintained on methadone during their pregnancies. Narcotic abuse, like other forms of drug abuse, is associated with decreased prenatal care; about 50% of drug addicts receive no prenatal care. The incidence of sudden infant death syndrome (SIDS) during the first year of life is increased ten times, from .4% to 4%, for infants whose mothers abuse narcotics. Maternal complications of narcotics abuse during pregnancy, as in nonpregnant individuals, may include hepatitis and AIDS (acquired immune deficiency syndrome), especially if IV drug use is involved.

Cocaine

This central-nervous-system stimulant causes the uterus to contract, which may be why preterm labor and abruptio placenta (see Chapter

Table 57   POSSIBLE EFFECTS ON THE NEWBORN FROM ALCOHOL ABUSE DURING PREGNANCY*

1. Low birth weight.

2. Abnormally small head.

3. Facial or joint deformity.

4. Heart defect.

5. Poor coordination.

6. Hyperactivity.

7. Learning disability.

8. Poor growth before and after birth.

9. Mental retardation.

* See text under Drinking Alcohol During Pregnancy.

55) occur much more often in cocaine users. Cocaine use is associated with increased rates of miscarriage, stillbirth, and birth defects, although a specific syndrome of birth defects has not been identified. A recent report on seventy women who used cocaine during pregnancy found that their drug use was associated with increased rates of prematurity and fetal growth retardation. Maternal complications of cocaine use are similar to those of nonpregnant women and include seizures, irregular heart rhythms, high blood pressure, and heart attacks. The risk of sudden infant death syndrome (SIDS) among cocaine-using mothers-to-be is exceedingly high —up to thirty times that found in women with drug-free pregnancies. A recent study showed that children up to two years of age had more difficulty and greater frustration in dealing with structured tasks than those in a control group whose mothers had not used cocaine.

Hallucinogens

LSD and PCP (angel dust) have been shown to cause birth defects in animals but not in humans. These hallucination-inducing drugs may cause psychotic episodes during pregnancy.

Amphetamines

Amphetamines, the main ingredient in most "diet pills," have been reported to cause birth

defects involving the heart in at least one study involving humans. Other reports have not confirmed this finding. These drugs may cause high blood pressure or irregular heart rhythm.

Tranquilizers

Barbiturates such as Seconal and Nembutal have not been linked with birth defects directly, but their use during late pregnancy may result in respiratory depression in the newborn. Newer benzodiazepine tranquilizers, which include Valium, Tranxene, Xanax, and others, have been linked to isolated reports of birth defects, but these findings have not been confirmed in other studies. If heavy use is involved during late pregnancy, the newborn may experience a withdrawal syndrome that includes irritability, loss of muscle tone, and impaired temperature regulation.

Drinking Alcohol During Pregnancy

An estimated 19% of pregnant women consume alcohol during their pregnancy, according to the 1993 National Institute on Drug Abuse National Pregnancy and Health Survey. Maternal alcohol use accounts for up to 5% of all birth defects and ranks with Down syndrome as a major cause of mental retardation. Chronic, heavy alcohol use during pregnancy may lead to a distinct pattern of physical and mental abnormalities in the fetus known as *fetal alcohol syndrome* (see Table 57). The complete syndrome probably occurs with a frequency of 1 to 3 cases per 1,000 live births, while other individual alcohol-related problems including miscarriage, stillbirth, low birth weight, and cerebral palsy, occur considerably more frequently.

Both animal and human research studies have singled out alcohol apart from smoking, poor nutrition, or other risk factors as the major influence in the development of the fetal alcohol syndrome. Alcohol readily crosses the placenta. The fetus receives as much alcohol as the mother; but since the fetus burns up alcohol half as fast as the mother does, the alcohol remains in the fetal system longer. Although we don't know how much alcohol is required to endanger the developing fetus, it is now believed that a woman who drinks more than six hard drinks per day, particularly in early pregnancy, clearly risks harm to the fetus. At this level of alcohol consumption, the risk of a serious problem in the fetus has been reported at between 30% and 50%. The effect on a fetus in mothers who consume three to six drinks per day is less than in mothers who consume more than six drinks per day. The effect on a fetus in mothers who drink less than three drinks per day is unclear, but a 1987 National Institutes of Health study failed to find an increased risk of birth defects among offspring of women who consumed one to two drinks per day or less. Nevertheless, since the level below which no risk is present is not known for sure, it is advisable that women who are pregnant or considering pregnancy abide by the Surgeon General's recommendation to avoid all alcoholic beverages.

For more information on alcohol and pregnancy, write to:

National Clearinghouse for Alcohol and Drug Information
P.O. Box 2345
Rockville, Maryland 20847

Smoking During Pregnancy

Numerous studies have detailed the hazards of smoking during pregnancy. A report from the National Center for Health Statistics, which reviewed records for 360,000 births, found that fetal and infant mortality rates increased by 56% in first-time mothers who smoked more than one pack per day during their pregnancies. It is estimated that among U.S. women of childbearing age, more than one in four smoke, and many of these women continue to do so during pregnancy. Reports from the Surgeon General's office over the past several years have repeatedly warned that cigarettes may slow fetal growth, double the chance of a baby with low birth weight, and increase the risk of having a stillborn child (see Table 58). These findings confirm data collected from the U.S. Collaborative Perinatal Project, which examined more than 50,000 pregnancies at twelve hospitals. Some of the most valuable information came from 227 women who were studied during two pregnancies but who smoked during only one of them. These women had smaller babies in the smoking pregnancy, a finding which tends to prove wrong the claims that constitutional differences

---

Table 58   POSSIBLE EFFECTS ON THE NEWBORN FROM SMOKING DURING PREGNANCY

1. Low birth weight of newborn.
2. Premature labor.
3. Miscarriage.
4. Stillbirth.
5. Birth defects.
6. Premature rupture of membranes.
7. Bleeding in late pregnancy.
8. Sudden infant death syndrome.
9. Infant respiratory illness, including pneumonia.

---

between women who smoke and those who don't smoke affect the baby rather than the smoking itself.

One of the reasons assumed for the slower growth of the fetus in smoking mothers is the effect of carbon monoxide, one of the substances in cigarette smoke. This gas inhaled by the mother forces oxygen out of her blood and, after crossing the placenta, does the same thing to the fetus's blood. In a heavy smoker, the fetal oxygen supply may be reduced by as much as 50%. Another ingredient in cigarette smoke, nicotine, has been shown to pass freely across the placenta where it constricts blood vessels and thereby diminishes the supply of nourishment to the fetus.

Although smoking is associated with the many adverse conditions listed in Table 58, these conditions affect nonsmokers as well. For this reason, the magnitude of the smoking risk in a given woman is difficult to judge. Conditions such as miscarriage and premature labor are known to be associated with a variety of factors of which smoking is only one. Since the number of cigarettes smoked directly affects the degree of impairment of the fetus, cutting back would be beneficial to the woman who feels she cannot quit completely.

For further reading:

DATA: Drug, Alcohol, Tobacco Abuse During Pregnancy. Contact:

March of Dimes Birth Defects Foundation
1275 Mamaroneck Avenue
White Plains, N.Y. 10605
(914) 428-7100

References for Section Seven

Chapter 29—Understanding the Drugs You Take

Physicians' Desk Reference, 49th ed. Rutherford N.J.: Medical Economics, 1995.

Physicians' Desk Reference for Nonprescription Drugs, 16th ed. Rutherford, N.J.: Medical Economics, 1995.

Wartak, J. Generic drugs: what's in a name? *Encyclopaedia Britannica Health Annual*: 459–460, 1988.

Lasagna, L. Therapeutic substitution: how will it affect medical practice? *Drug Therapy* 19(3):10–14, Mar 1989.

Chapter 30—Avoiding Drug Abuse

American College of Obstetricians and Gynecologists, *Technical Bulletin* 194. Substance abuse, July 1994.

Women and drugs: a new era for research. Research monograph series #65. National Institute on Drug Abuse, 1986.

Women and alcohol use: a review of research literature. National Institute on Alcohol Abuse and Alcoholism, 1988.

Blume, S. Women and alcohol—a review. *Journal of the American Medical Association* 256(11):1467–1470, Sep 19, 1986.

Parker, D. Alcohol use and depression symptoms among employed men and women. *American Journal of Public Health* 77(6):704–707, June 1987.

Litte, V. Cocaine abuse during pregnancy: maternal and fetal implications. *Obstetrics and Gynecology* 73(2): 157–160, Feb 1989.

Cocaine in pregnancy. *Genesis* 11(1):13, Jan/Feb 1989.

Verloove, S. Addicted mothers and pre-term babies: a disasterous outcome. *Lancet* 1:421–422, 1988.

Cherukuri, R. A cohort study of alkaloidal cocaine ("crack") in pregnancy. *Obstetrics and Gynecology* 72:147–151, 1988.

MacGregor, S. Substance abuse in pregnancy—a practical management plan. *The Female Patient* 14(1):49–63, Jan 1989.

Zuckerman, B. Effects of maternal marijuana and cocaine on fetal growth. *New England Journal of Medicine* 320:762–768, Mar 1989.

Program strategies for preventing fetal alcohol syndrome and alcohol-related birth defects. National Institute on Alcohol Abuse and Alcoholism, U.S. Dept. of Health and Human Services, 1987.

Chapter 31—Drugs and the Pregnant Woman

American College of Obstetricians and Gynecologists, *Technical Bulletin* 195. Substance abuse in pregnancy, July 1994.

American College of Obstetricians and Gynecologists, Committee on obstetrics: maternal and fetal medicine, *Committee Opinion* 114. Cocaine in pregnancy, Sep 1992.

Shephard, B. Say no to drugs (in pregnancy). *Encyclopedia Britannica Health Annual*: 419–423, 1994.

Gilstrap, L. Drugs and medications in pregnancy. *Williams Obstetrics*, Supplement 13, July/Aug 1987.

Mattison, D. Effects of drugs and chemicals on the fetus, Part I. *Contemporary OB/GYN* 33(3):163–176, Mar 1989.

Mattison D. Effects of drugs and chemicals on the fetus, Part II. *Contemporary OB/GYN* 33(4):97–110, Apr 1989.

Mattison, D. Effects of drugs and chemicals on the fetus, Part III. *Contemporary OB/GYN* 33(5):131–147, May 1989.

Berger, A. Effects of caffeine consumption on pregnancy outcome. *Journal of Reproductive Medicine* 33(12):945–954, Dec 1988.

DISEASES OF THE FEMALE REPRODUCTIVE SYSTEM

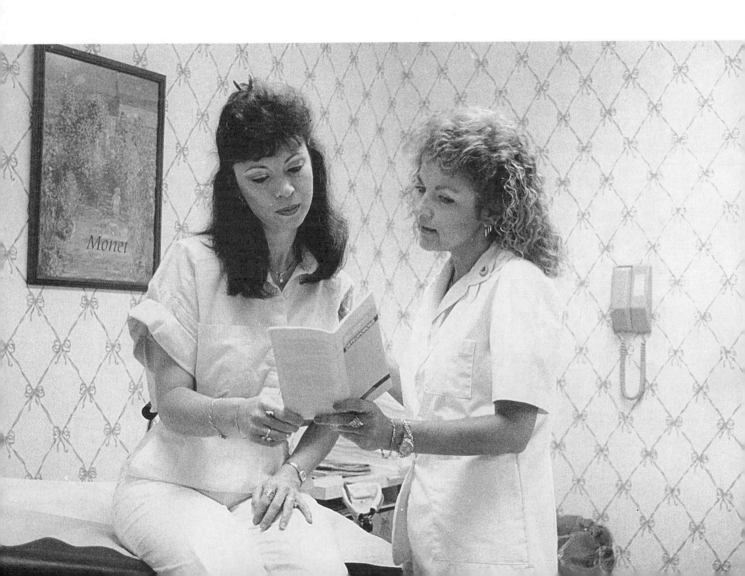

CHAPTER 32

Premenstrual Syndrome (PMS)

Premenstrual Syndrome (PMS) is a major concern for many women. Estimates of the frequency of PMS vary from 10% to 80% of menstruating women. Its causes are still not clearly understood, and no single treatment has been found effective. Among the various hypotheses to explain the disorder, one of the most discussed in medical literature is the *progesterone deficiency theory*. However, controlled studies have eliminated the possibility that PMS results from deficiency of a single hormone, such as progesterone, estradiol, follicle stimulating hormone, luteinizing hormone, testosterone, or prolactin. The syndrome was first given a name in 1931, although women have been aware of the symptoms for centuries. Basically, PMS consists of symptoms that begin after ovulation, peak prior to menstruation, and stop abruptly after menses begin.

The diagnosis of PMS has political implications. Some women feel that PMS is a way of reducing the status of women, by linking the normal ovarian cycle to a phenomenon that ostensibly reduces a woman's ability to cope. Psychologists and psychiatrists use the term Premenstrual Dysphoric Disorder (PDD) to describe severe PMS. Its main symptoms are described as extreme moodiness and depression that interfere with normal functioning. The moods must occur

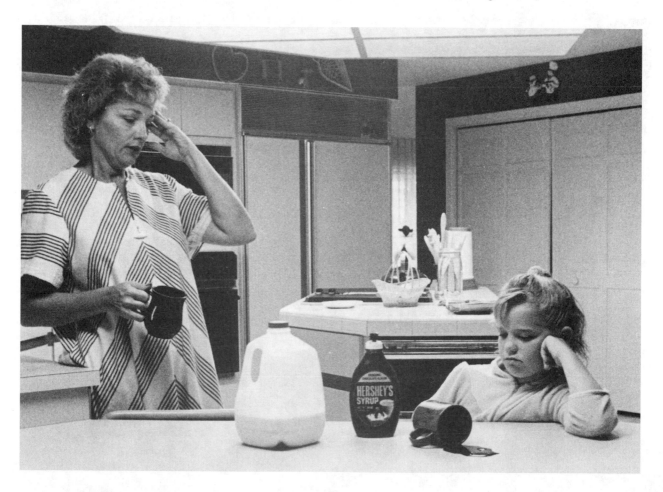

Table 59 — SAMPLE CHART FOR PMS DETERMINATION

Name _____ Beginning Date _____ Weight _____

Month	(Jan)			(Feb)			(March)		
Day	M	WT	SX	M	WT	SX	M	WT	SX
1									
2									
3									
4									
5									
6									
7									
8									
9									
10									
11									
12									
13									
14									
15									
16									
17									
18									
19									
20									
21									
22									
23									
24									
25									
26									
27									
28									
29									
30									
31									

M = menstruation—mark if menstruating

WT = daily weight—take at same time each day

SX—symptoms. Chart these at the same time each day, using abbreviations if necessary (i.e., H = headache, T = tension, C = crying).

You may also want to keep a basal temperature chart at the same time and mark down the day you ovulate.

in relation to the menstrual cycle and not be the result of any underlying mental disorder.

The National Institute of Mental Health describes PMS as a condition in which an otherwise healthy woman experiences physical and/or emotional symptoms severe enough to impair her functioning at work or in a social situation. Some 200 different symptoms have been reported; the most common are abdominal bloating, breast tenderness, acne, appetite changes and cravings, swelling of the extremities, headache, and gastrointestinal upset. Psychological symptoms include fatigue, irritability, moodiness, depression, oversensitivity, crying spells, social withdrawal, forgetfulness, and difficulty concentrating. A marked increase in anger has been shown to be one of the most significant symptoms of PMS. PMS occurs rarely in adolescence, more commonly in the twenties, and most commonly in the thirties and forties. Some women report experiencing it from the onset of puberty, but the majority develop it in later years following a significant interruption of the hormonal cycle, such as after stopping birth control pills or following a pregnancy. It has been estimated that one in ten menstruating women suffers enough from PMS to require medical treatment.

To help in diagnosing PMS, a woman should keep a daily record of symptoms for at least two and preferably three months to see if the timing of the symptoms is related to the menstrual cycle (see Table 59). Treatment then depends upon which symptoms are identified as well as their severity. Initial treatment may include stress management, increased exercise (less strenuous exercise such as walking may help reduce symptoms), increased rest, and changes in diet. Nutritional modifications include limiting intake of alcohol, caffeine (including coffee, tea, and caffeine-containing soft drinks), salt (to reduce swelling), and sugar. Eating smaller, more frequent, meals to minimize fluctuations in blood-sugar levels, as well as increasing complex carbohydrates, may also be helpful. Some women with PMS benefit from diets that limit dairy products, reduce saturated fats (to less than 20% of total calories), or increase complex carbohydrate intake (to 60% or more of daily calories). Such dietary changes usually require that you consume more green leafy vegetables, whole grains and cereals, and fish and poultry.

Various medications, from pain-relievers to "water pills" (diuretics), alleviate specific PMS symptoms but have not been found effective in relieving the entire disorder or in preventing it. Among over-the-counter products, Vitamin B_6 (pyridoxine) has been reported (inconsistently) as helpful, but the high dosages typically used may lead to diarrhea or other side effects. Other nonprescription drugs to treat PMS often contain multiple ingredients that used to be popular in cold remedies. This "shotgun" approach to

PMS is found in products like Premsyn PMS, which contains acetaminophen (the pain killer found in Tylenol), an antihistamine (for its sedative effects), and a weak diuretic (the same level found in a cup of tea). In general, consumers should be wary of multi-ingredient products, although they may help some PMS sufferers. Evening Primrose Oil (linoleic acid, gamma linoleic acid, and vitamin E) given at 1.5 grams twice daily may help those with significant breast pain or tenderness. The use of 1,000 milligrams of magnesium per day during the premenstrual phase has improved some symptoms.

Progesterone, taken orally or vaginally, has been used widely in the treatment of PMS, especially in England, with mixed success; reports in the United States have not confirmed the benefits of such therapy. In addition to diuretics for bloating and edema, prostaglandin inhibitors (see Chapter 79) and antidepressants, such as Prozac, Zoloft, and Paxil, may be helpful in relieving pain and mood disorders respectively. The use of tranquilizers such as Xanax should be limited to short-term use, as many of these drugs may be habit forming. Recently, some success in relieving PMS symptoms has been found in the use of GnRH agonists such as Lupron (see Chapter 36). Both danazol and bromocriptine (see Index) have been used to treat PMS-related breast tenderness and bloating, though side effects such as nausea and dizziness are common. Oral contraception for suppression of ovulation has helped some women. Whatever your choice of treatment, it is useful to keep daily diaries before and during treatments.

Whatever the course of treatment, it is important that you feel confident in your physician's ability to deal with PMS. Not every physician can. The doctor-patient relationship is especially important in helping women with this syndrome. A strong relationship can help you with the feelings of helplessness and loss of control that are so unpleasant with PMS. Sometimes counseling is helpful in developing a more effective coping style. Local PMS support groups are also very useful. For more information contact:

PMS Access
P.O. Box 9326
Madison, Wisconsin 53715

CHAPTER 33

Toxic Shock Syndrome

The use of tampons has been associated with a rare and sometimes fatal disease called *toxic shock syndrome* (TSS). This mysterious illness first received wide public attention in early 1980 when the Centers for Disease Control reported several studies linking the use of Rely brand tampons with an increased risk of developing TSS. Although Rely was ultimately withdrawn from the market, other cases of TSS have occurred with tampons produced by all the other major manufacturers. However, the risk with these brands has been lower than with Rely. Since 1982 the Food and Drug Administration (FDA) began requiring tampon manufacturers to place warning labels about the association between TSS and tampons on their products. Since March 1990, the FDA has required standardized absorbency labeling. This labeling makes it easier for consumers to compare brands and select low-absorbency products, which may be safer.

Toxic shock syndrome is a name given to a disease characterized by a collection of symptoms experienced most often by women during their menstrual period. Although the exact cause of TSS is unknown, a bacterium called *Staphylococcus aureus* has been identified in many women experiencing this disease. It has been theorized that tampon use may favor the growth of this bacterium in the vagina because the natural flow of blood is blocked by the tampon. Once absorbed into the bloodstream from the vagina, the staph bacteria or their toxins (poi-

sonous substances) may then cause the symptoms of toxic shock: rash, high fever, vomiting, and diarrhea followed by a sudden drop in blood pressure. Penicillin drugs are usually effective in treating TSS, but in some cases the bacteria are resistant to the antibiotic.

According to the Centers for Disease Control, 85% of TSS cases involve women. The proportion of total cases associated with menstruation, however, has declined from 85% in 1981 to about 55% in 1989. Also, the overall incidence of TSS has gone down from 6 to 7 cases per 100,000 people in 1981 to less than 1 case per 100,000 people in 1989. Cases of TSS have been reported in diaphragm users.

The American College of Obstetricians and Gynecologists has offered these guidelines for women using tampons:

1. Change tampons often—at least as frequently as every six to eight hours.
2. Use medium or regular tampons instead of super-absorbent ones (often designated as "Super" or "Super Plus").
3. Alternate tampon use with sanitary napkins (or mini- or maxi-pads) during a given menstrual period.
4. If symptoms of high fever, vomiting, diarrhea, or sunburnlike rash occur, discontinue tampon use and immediately consult your physician.

Based on the theory that certain tampons may scratch the mucosal lining (surface) of the vagina and thus lead to the staphylococcal infection, Dr. S. A. Kaufman from Lenox Hill Hospital, New York City, has added the following guidelines:

1. On days when secretions in the vagina are scanty, use a water-soluble lubricating jelly on the tampon applicator to avoid nicking the vaginal mucosa.
2. Use tampons with no applicators or with cardboard applicators, because plastic applicators may be more likely to cause mucosal scratches.

CHAPTER 34

Breast Diseases

Benign Breast Conditions

Fibrocystic disease, sometimes called cystic mastitis (see also Chapters 58 and 59), is the most common breast disorder and the most frequent cause of a breast lump in a woman under the age of twenty-five. Characteristic symptoms include lumpy, tender breasts, particularly during the week before menses. Occurring predominantly in women between thirty and fifty, fibrocystic disease usually involves both breasts. Only a small subgroup of these women—those with *atypical cell changes* (atypical hyperplasia)—are at increased risk, and this can only be diagnosed by breast biopsy. Since this finding is fairly uncommon, women with fibrocystic breast disease do not require a biopsy unless the woman or her doctor feels a distinct lump (see Chapter 58) or her mammogram is abnormal.

A variety of hormones—including birth control pills, progesterone, androgens, and danazol—have been used to treat fibrocystic breast disease. Danazol has been among the more successful, improving symptoms in nearly 80% of women after two to eight months of treatment; breast tenderness is relieved in more than 50% of women, and another 25% show some improvement. Any persistent thickening or lumpiness after danazol or other medical therapy may need to be biopsied. Disadvantages to danazol treatment include cost and possible unwanted side effects, including absent menstrual periods, acne, and slight weight gain. Some form of birth control other than the pill should be used during danazol therapy, since the drug is contraindicated in pregnancy. Some studies indicate that vitamin E in dosages of 400 to 600 international units per day, as well as a diet low in foods containing caffeine, may relieve the symptoms of this condition (see Chapter 59).

The most common breast tumor in women younger than twenty-five is the benign (noncancerous) fibroadenoma. Most predominant in women fifteen to thirty, this tumor produces a firm, movable, nontender lump. Fibroadenomas are removed both to confirm the diagnosis and to prevent damage to breast tissue from localized tumor growth.

Breast Cancer

In the 1980s, the frequency of breast cancer, the most common cancer in women, increased by about 1% each year. This increase in rate may be due to more frequent use of both breast self-examination and mammography than to an increased frequency in the disease itself. In 1995, breast cancer accounted for 18% of cancer deaths among women, second only to lung cancer (see Table 71 for information on frequency statistics and other factors associated with breast cancer).

Approximately one woman in eight will develop breast cancer in the course of a lifetime. The disease, however, is rare before the age of thirty-five; 85% of the tumors occur in women over forty.

The five-year survival for this disease depends a great deal on the stage of the cancer when it is first detected. The five-year survival with disease localized to the breast may be as high as 93%. Table 61 gives more information on five-year survival rates.

Most clinicians believe that the best hope for attacking this disease is through early diagnosis, which can be achieved through more aggressive efforts to screen and identify women at risk for breast cancer (see Table 60).

Screening for breast cancer

Since early breast cancers rarely cause pain or other symptoms, the importance of screening techniques cannot be overemphasized. A monthly breast self-examination, periodic examination by your clinician, and selective use of mammography (X-ray) are your best preventive health measures.

The American Cancer Society recommends that women over twenty-five examine their breasts monthly after menses. For women past menopause the examination should be done on a regularly scheduled monthly basis. In fact, over 90% of breast cancers are detected by women themselves. Table 62 indicates abnormal breast changes you should report to your doctor. Symptoms of breast disease include breast discharge and breast lumps (see Chapters 57 and 58).

Breast X-rays (mammography)

It is now believed that most breast cancers are present for six to eight years before they become larger than a pea and can be felt. Mammography, an X-ray technique that provides a picture of the breasts, is the best screening method currently available for detecting nonpalpable tumors (ones that can't be felt).

Currently, the National Cancer Institute and the American Cancer Society Breast Cancer Demonstration Projects have detected increasing numbers of nonpalpable small breast cancers, using mammography. Mammograms accurately identify breast cancer 85% of the time. Compared to tumors found by physical examination

alone, those detected through mammography are more likely to be in an earlier stage and not yet spread beyond the breast.

The mammogram procedure involves compressing the breast between two flat discs. Most women have only slight discomfort during breast compression, while a few describe it as moderately painful. Two X-rays are taken of each breast: one from above the breast, known as a *craniocaudal* view, and one from the side, called a *lateral* view. Women who menstruate may want to schedule their breast X-rays the week after menses, when cyclic breast tenderness or swelling is least likely. Mammograms are now widely available outside of hospitals (which usually charge the most)—in doctors' offices, in free-standing X-ray facilities, and even in traveling X-ray mobiles. The better facilities use "dedicated" equipment—i.e., mammography equipment designed specifically and exclusively for breast X-rays; these facilities are often approved by a new accreditation program for breast X-ray facilities. The program, established in 1988 by the American College of Radiology (A.C.R.), sets minimum standards that assure some degree of consistency and quality in technique. It is worth knowing if the breast X-ray facility you use is A.C.R. approved.

There is a general consensus that women over fifty should receive annual mammograms to screen for breast cancer. The benefits of routine mammography for women in their forties is also becoming apparent. The A.M.A., the American Cancer Society, and the American College of Radiology now recommend mammograms every one to two years for all women beginning at age forty. Large-scale studies have clearly shown about a 30% decrease in breast-cancer mortality among women over fifty who receive annual mammograms. Screening women in their forties will save some lives, but the numbers will be smaller in this younger age group.

Several years ago the safety of mammography was questioned because of the possibility that radiation exposure during the mammography could itself cause breast cancer. This risk has essentially now been eliminated as a result of improved X-ray imaging, which delivers a minimal dose of radiation (less than 1 rad) to the breast.

The cost of annual breast X-rays (an item often not covered by insurance) makes price shopping worthwhile. There may be emotional costs as well—for example, when the mammogram

---

Table 60   RISK FACTORS ASSOCIATED WITH BREAST CANCER

Highest Risk Factors:

1. Personal history of breast cancer.
2. Family history of breast cancer in a close relative (mother or sister).
3. History of breast biopsy showing "proliferative" or "atypical" cell changes.
4. History of mammogram suspicious for breast cancer.

Other Risk Factors:

1. First pregnancy after age thirty (or never had children).
2. Family history of breast cancer in a distant relative (maternal aunt or grandmother).
3. History of menstrual periods before age twelve.
4. History of fibrocystic breast disease.
5. Obesity or a high-fat diet.
6. History of an abnormal thermogram.
7. Previous endometrial cancer.
8. Menopause after age fifty.

Possible Risk Factors—Not Proven:

1. Estrogen hormones
2. Being a DES mother (see Chapter 38).
3. Plastic surgery to enlarge breasts using implants*.

---

* Risk not associated with implants but with possible decreased ability to detect breast lumps through physical examination after such surgery.

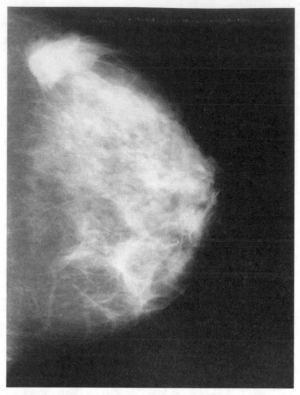

A mammogram can detect breast cancer early, when it is more likely to be fully curable.

reveals an "abnormal" finding, such as calcium deposits, that must be watched and that necessitate repeating the X-rays in six months. This period of waiting is necessary to see if the questionable area represents an early malignancy. In women under fifty, especially, mammogram interpretation may be more difficult and result in more "borderline" readings, as breast ductal patterns are more complex and variable than in older women. Fortunately, most difficult-to-interpret mammograms turn out to be negative on breast biopsy, although the risk increases with age—the chance of a positive biopsy is one in sixteen among women thirty-five to thirty-nine years of age, increasing to one in three in women age seventy to seventy-four.

Sonography and Thermography

Sonography is a technique that produces an image of the breast by using sound waves rather than radiation. This procedure is used to more clearly define suspicious areas on the mammogram rather than as a screening test. Sonog-

raphy's main value is in distinguishing fluid-filled cysts, which are usually benign, from solid growths, which sometimes represent cancer. Thus, a questionable area that turns out to be a cyst can often be seen, while a solid mass may need a biopsy.

Thermography takes advantage of the fact that some breast cancers cause an increase in the breast skin temperature. Thermography provides a photographic image of the heat patterns on the breast surface. A heat-detecting device maps and records hot spots or areas of increased blood distribution. While it avoids the risks of X-rays, thermography has very limited usefulness because it does not distinguish well between cancer and other breast diseases. The result is a high percentage of "false positive" thermograms. Consequently, mammography is the main screening technique for breast diagnosis today.

Myths About Breast Cancer

Everything we know about breast cancer suggests that controlling this disease depends upon one factor: early diagnosis (see Table 61). Yet it is estimated that only four out of ten women regularly practice breast self-examination and that many women over forty have never had a mammogram. While women give many reasons for not taking these preventive steps, the cause is often lack of information. We suggest that every mother tell her teenage daughter about breast self-examination and stress that it should be done routinely in adulthood. Many myths still surround the subject of breast cancer, including the following:

Myth: Breast cancer develops only after age fifty.
Fact: 30% of all breast cancers occur in women under fifty.
Myth: Most breast cancers are found by breast X-rays.
Fact: Most breast cancers are detected by the woman herself through breast self-examination.
Myth: A lack of family history of breast cancer means little or no risk for this disease.
Fact: 80% of breast-cancer patients have no family history of breast cancer.

Table 61   THE FIVE STAGES OF BREAST CANCER

Stage	5-year survival rate
In situ Can be diagnosed by mammograms but can't be felt	95%
Stage I Remains localized to breast and smaller than 2 cm; has not spread to lymph nodes under arm	85%
Stage II Growths are 2 to 5 cm and have not spread to lymph nodes	66%
Stage III Growths are over 5 cm or have grown into chest wall, skin, or distant lymph nodes	41%
Stage IV Growths have spread to other parts of the body	10%

Myth: Breast cancer can't be present unless a lump in the breast can be felt.

Fact: Early, more curable, tumors are often first detected by mammogram. The average size of a lump found by periodic mammogram is ⅛ inch, while that found on average by women practicing regular self-examination is ¼ inch.

Diagnosis and treatment of breast cancer

Although a doctor may suspect a diagnosis of breast cancer after examination or mammography, it is ultimately diagnosed by a breast biopsy, in which a small sample of breast tissue is removed and examined with a microscope. The primary treatment of breast cancer is surgery—either by a breast-removal operation (mastectomy) or by local removal of the tumor (lumpectomy). This surgery may be performed immediately following a positive biopsy, thereby avoiding the need for a second anesthetic and second operation later. More often today, however, patients choose a two-step approach, in which the biopsy and subsequent sur-

gery are performed as separate procedures at separate times. This method enables the woman to have a better opportunity to examine her treatment options thoroughly and perhaps to obtain a second opinion.

In the past ten years, there has been considerable debate as to the best surgical method of treating breast cancer. Most surgeons now agree, however, that there are relatively few indications for the classical procedure known as *radical mastectomy*, in which the entire affected breast, the chest muscles underneath, and the lymph nodes under the arm are removed. A less extensive procedure, the *modified radical mastectomy* (also called *total mastectomy*), without removal of the chest wall muscles, has been the standard operation for most breast cancers.

Other types of mastectomy include *simple mastectomy* (complete removal of the breast but not the lymph nodes under the arm or the chest wall muscles), and *segmental mastectomy* (or *lumpectomy*) in which only a portion of the breast is removed, including the cancer and a surrounding margin of breast tissue.

Lumpectomy accompanied by removal of the underarm lymph nodes and usually with subsequent radiation therapy has become the dominant alternative to modified radical mastectomy. In this instance, radiation therapy is used after surgery to eliminate any remaining cancer cells. Most surgeons limit lumpectomy to women with small, well-defined tumors—less than 1 to 2 inches in diameter. This breast-conserving surgery is now under continued study in a number of cancer centers to determine whether lumpectomy can achieve long-term results comparable to total mastectomy. So far, results appear very promising.

The role of *adjuvant therapy*, which includes both anti-cancer drugs (chemotherapy) and hormone therapy, has changed in recent years. In fact, the entire subject of breast-cancer treatment is in a state of flux as of this writing, as the findings of various clinical trials both in the United States and worldwide are being reported. These trials include studies with the drug tamoxifen (Nolvadex), a form of chemotherapy traditionally used for advanced disease. Currently, a number of studies are underway at the National Cancer Institute, seeking to determine whether the use of tamoxifen will benefit some premenopausal women with very early cancers, as well as women who are at high risk for devel-

Table 62	BREAST CHANGES TO REPORT TO YOUR DOCTOR

The following are possible signs of breast cancer:

Change	Comment
Breast lump or lumps	especially if painless and involving only one breast and if lumps do not become smaller following menses
Breast discharge	especially if bloody or involving only one breast
Skin changes	flaking, crusting, or "weeping" eruptions around the nipple; dimpling or retraction of skin over a portion of one breast

Table 63	PERIODIC MAMMOGRAMS

When are periodic* mammograms (breast X-rays) recommended for women without symptoms of breast disease?

Under 40 years	Not generally recommended unless highest risk factors are present (see Table 60)
40 to 50 years	Every 1 to 2 years
Over 50 years	Every year

* Recommended by the American College of Obstetricians and Gynocologists

oping breast cancer, but have not yet been diagnosed as having the disease. Whether or not more aggressive use of adjuvant therapy in women with breast cancer will prolong survival will take 10 or 15 more years of study in the United States to determine. However, European chemotherapy trials with longer follow-up already support this approach. In the future, the use of early chemotherapy and hormone therapy may be an important factor in reducing the death rate from this disease.

Because technical knowledge affecting treatment of breast cancer changes so rapidly, any woman with this disease should consider referral to a major cancer center, which will have the latest, specialized methods to diagnose and treat the disease.

Rehabilitation after breast surgery

During rehabilitation, physical therapy may be necessary. Often plastic surgery can be performed to reconstruct the breast. Following less radical forms of surgery, breast reconstructive surgery may be relatively easy. At other times, the plastic surgery may involve taking skin and other tissue from another part of the body, such as the thigh, and grafting it onto the breast (see Chapter 46).

After the initial crisis of a mastectomy has passed, there is a continuing need for emotional support. Support groups, such as the American Cancer Society's Reach to Recovery Program composed of women who have experienced mastectomy, help women cope with the emotional problems associated both with the loss of a breast and with being afflicted with a serious disease. It is encouraging to note that a recent study assessing psychological and social adjustment to mastectomy found that 70% of the women studied felt they had made a satisfactory emotional adjustment one year after their surgery.

Resources

For more information about all forms of cancer, including breast cancer, contact the following groups:

1. Cancer Information Service, telephone 800-422–6237. This is a national, toll-free telephone network of the National Cancer Institute which provides information about cancer and cancer-related resources to the general public.

2. Office of Cancer Communications. This organization provides information on all aspects of cancer research, operates the Cancer Information Service, and distributes free publications on cancer to the general public. Write to:

    Office of Cancer Communications
    National Cancer Institute
    Building 31, Room 10A-16
    9000 Rockville Pike
    Bethesda, Maryland 20892

3. Your local chapter of the American Cancer Society. The A.C.S. can provide helpful educational material as well as information on local and regional resources including the "Reach to Recovery" Program. Or write to:

   American Cancer Society, Inc.
   1599 Clifton Road, N.E.
   Atlanta, Georgia 30329

4. Mammatech Corporation. This organization runs MammaCare, a unique learning system that allows women to detect early breast abnormalities through the use of special breast models and physician instruction on breast self-examination. Cost: $60 to $90 for a training session at a local MammaCare Center or through a physician participating in the MammaCare program. Or write to:

   MammaTech Corporation
   930 N.W. 8th Avenue
   Gainesville, Florida 32601
   800-MAM–CARE

5. Y-ME, telephone 800-221–2141 (9 A.M. to 5 P.M., Central Time, weekdays). This line is staffed by counselors who have had breast cancer.

6. American Society of Plastic and Reconstructive Surgeons, telephone 800-635–0635. This organization can provide information on plastic surgery and suggestions for selecting an appropriate surgeon for breast reconstruction.

7. *NABCO News.* This quarterly newsletter of The National Alliance of Breast Cancer Organizations provides information on the latest research and treatment. Membership ($40) includes a resource list, newsletter, and special mailings. Write to:

   NABCO
   9 East 37th Street, 10th Floor
   New York, New York 10016
   (212) 719–0154

8. Books:
   Choices: Realistic Alternatives in Cancer Treatment. Marion Morra and Eve Potts, 1994, Avon Books, New York ($15).
   Breast Cancer—The Complete Guide. Y. Hirshaut and P. I. Pressman, 1993, Bantam, New York ($12.95).
   What to Do If You Get Breast Cancer. L. Komarnicky and A. Rosenberg, 1995, Little, Brown and Co., Boston ($10.95).

CHAPTER 35

Uterine Fibroids

Uterine fibroids, the number-one cause of an abnormally enlarged uterus, are found in 20% to 25% of women of reproductive age. These growths are also the most common reason for hysterectomy. Fibroid tumors, composed of muscular and fibrous tissue, originate in the wall of the uterus (see Figure 34). The size, shape, location, and symptoms of uterine fibroids are tremendously variable, sometimes making it difficult or impossible to differentiate them from an enlarged ovary. Fibroids, single or multiple, usually grow slowly, if at all. They may increase in size under the influence of estrogen produced during pregnancy. When estrogen production stops following menopause, fibroids tend to decrease in size.

Fibroids are nearly always benign growths, with only one out of two hundred containing uterine cancer. It is not known whether such cancers represent a malignant transformation of the fibroid itself or merely arise as coincidental, spontaneous growths within the uterus. Although usually symptomless, large fibroids may cause chronic backache, pelvic pain, and heavy or prolonged periods. Some research suggests that fibroids located within the uterine cavity may also contribute to impaired fertility, repeated miscarriage, or premature labor.

Diagnosis

Uterine fibroids are usually detected during a routine pelvic exam because they result in an enlarged, irregular uterus. Sonography may help to localize and identify fibroids when the diagnosis is in doubt. This may occur if the fibroid's position or size prevents a thorough pelvic examination of the ovaries or if the woman is overweight. Another test, hysterosalpingography, may provide helpful information about fibroids located within the uterine cavity. Fibroids are sometimes detected inadvertently at the time of a D & C (see glossary). The fibroids produce an irregular surface along the uterine cavity that the doctor can feel during this procedure.

Treatment

Fibroids that are not causing any symptoms can be managed "expectantly" for the most part. This usually means having a pelvic examination at least every six months to check for fibroid growth. Treatment is indicated for women with fibroids that cause symptoms of pain, bleeding, or pressure or who have infertility or recurrent miscarriage attributable to these growths.

The treatment of fibroids has four basic approaches. Each approach has its advantages and disadvantages and must be individualized according to the patient's age, her symptoms, and her childbearing goals.

1. *Medication.* Nonsteroidal anti-inflammatory drugs, which are often used to treat arthritis (see Chapter 73), may help with symptoms of heavy menstrual flow or menstrual pain. Low-dose birth control pills also may reduce these syptoms, although there have also been reports of pill-induced fibroid growths.

   A relatively recent medical approach for treating fibroids involves the use of the drug leuprolide (Lupron), which in clinical trials has been found capable of shrinking fibroids and reducing their symptoms prior to surgery. Leuprolide is a synthetic form of gonadotropin-releasing hormone (GnRH), a hormone that plays a major role in regulating a woman's menstrual cycle. Leuprolide causes a decrease in estrogen production by the ovaries and leads to a temporary menopausal-like state. This medication, however, does not permanently reduce the fibroid size; indeed, fibroids usually regrow to their pretreatment size two to three months after stopping therapy. Your physician may consider using this drug under three types of situations: prior to surgery to cut down on blood loss; to stop bleeding or allow anemia to be corrected prior to surgery; and in older women, to control fibroid growth until natural menopause occurs. Side effects of leuprolide include hot flashes and temporary negative calcium balance, which can be treated with calcium supplements—so-called add-back therapy. The drug is given as a monthly intramuscular injection.

2. *Myomectomy.* This "conservative surgery" involves removing the fibroid and repairing the "defect" in the uterus. After myomectomy you will continue to have menstrual periods and the operation preserves a woman's fertility. Today in the United States over 20,000 myomectomies are performed annually. The operation is more likely to be successful when there is a single, isolated fibroid that does not involve a large amount of the uterine wall. Following myomectomy and repair of the uterus, many women who subsequently become pregnant will require cesarean births. The usual surgical approach employs a regular abdominal incision (laparotomy). A somewhat more controversial approach to myomectomy utilizes laparoscopy (see Chapter 41). Fibroids may be removed piece by piece through the laparoscope, although the process is time-consuming and may be as costly as the traditional operation.

3. *Hysteroscopy* (see Chapter 41). This technique enables removal of fibroids located within the uterine cavity. While there are relatively limited occasions for using this specialized form of myomectomy, it may offer the best option when symptom-producing fibroids are mostly "inside" the uterus rather than mainly within or outside the uterine wall.

4. *Hysterectomy.* While this is the most radical approach, it is often ultimately the most effective one for some women with symptomatic fibroids unresponsive to medical therapy. Like all medical decisions, this one deserves your full understanding and participation. One out of every five hysterectomies are performed for uterine fibroids, and while most are beneficial and "indicated," certainly some are not. A second opinion is one of your best assurances against unnecessary surgery. See Chapter 45 for more information on hysterectomy.

Table 64   POSSIBLE REASONS FOR FIBROID SURGERY

1. Persistently heavy periods, often with anemia, despite medical therapy.
2. Persistent pain, backache, or severe menstrual cramps despite medical therapy.
3. Increase in fibroid growth especially in a woman not taking the pill or other estrogen-containing drug.
4. When the diagnosis is in doubt making it impossible to distinguish between a uterine and an ovarian tumor.

Figure 34
Different types of fibroid tumor.

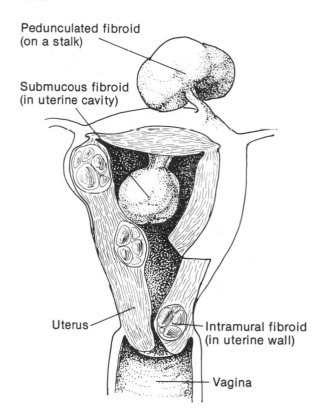

Pedunculated fibroid (on a stalk)

Submucous fibroid (in uterine cavity)

Uterus

Intramural fibroid (in uterine wall)

Vagina

CHAPTER 36

Endometriosis

Sometimes the tissue that lines the uterine cavity (this lining is called the *endometrium*) implants at other places, such as the ovaries, the tubes, or outside the uterus. When this condition occurs, the disorder is called *endometriosis*. A chronic, characteristically progressive condition, endometriosis occurs only during the reproductive years and is most prevalent among women in their thirties and forties. Endometriosis affects as many as 10% of women of reproductive age and is now being actively studied through the recently formed Office of Research on Women's Health and the National Institute of Health.

Exactly how endometrial tissue gets to these places is unknown, but it is believed that during menstruation portions of the endometrium are displaced from the uterine cavity into the Fallopian tubes and from there into the abdominal cavity. These endometrial deposits adhere to the surfaces of other organs, such as the ovaries and intestines, and sometimes form large cysts.

Because endometrial tissue responds to hormonal influences during the menstrual cycle, women who have this disorder often feel pain just prior to or during menstruation. The character and severity of endometriosis pain, however, varies considerably, depending on where the endometrial tissue is deposited. Although some women have no pain at all, others chronically experience pelvic pain or painful intercourse. Aside from pain, the other important health problem associated with endometriosis is infertility, which is found in about 30% of women with this condition. Endometriosis may contribute to infertility by interfering with ovulation or by causing tubal blockage.

Endometriosis is more likely if you have a close relative who has the disease. Pregnancy tends to prevent or lessen the symptoms of endometriosis, while delayed childbearing may predispose to this disease.

Diagnosis

Endometriosis is probably underdiagnosed because in its early stages there may be few or no symptoms. A doctor often presumes a woman has endometriosis if, during a pelvic examination, he or she feels nodular, tender areas behind or beneath the cervix. No laboratory tests are available to confirm the diagnosis, however. Only by seeing the pelvic organs during surgery can a doctor be certain that endometrial deposits exist. (Even when a woman with endometriosis experiences severe chronic pelvic pain, there may be no abnormal physical findings.)

The usual procedure for confirming the diagnosis of endometriosis is laparoscopy. During this surgery, the doctor views the pelvic organs with a small, telescopelike instrument. Often the physician can then remove small endometrial implants as well as larger areas of endometriosis through *operative* laparoscopy (see below).

Treatment

Standard initial treatment for endometriosis consists of hormones to prevent ovulation. These drugs cause a remission of the disease for several months or even years. Often, however, symptoms resume after treatment stops. Hormone therapy is often used in two situations: when the disease is considered "mild" as judged by laparoscopy; or to complement surgical therapy, in which case hormones may precede or follow surgery. The main hormones used are progesterone, combinations of estrogens and progesterone (as found in most oral contraceptives), danazol (a testosterone derivative), and, most recently, a new group of drugs called GnRH agonists.

The woman who has not started or completed her family should not delay treatment for endometriosis if the disease is moderate or severe since it may progress, with symptoms of increasing pain and greater likelihood of impaired fertility. However, it has been recognized that women with minimal disease—usually with just a few spots of endometriosis covering the ovaries and other surfaces but no adhesions or cysts—have about the same rate of fertility one year after the initial diagnosis of endometriosis whether they are treated or not. For this reason, expectant therapy—no drugs or surgery—is the standard approach of many physicians for the first twelve to eighteen months after diagnosis of *mild* endometriosis, unless the woman is in her later childbearing years or has significant pain.

Birth control pills probably represent one of the oldest forms of hormonal therapy. These pills are sometimes given continuously, instead of for three weeks at a time with an interval break in between, as when the pill is taken for contraception. Another hormonal drug, danazol, is sometimes used for moderate to severe endometriosis. Although danazol is costly, the drug appears to offer one of the most effective hormonal treatments for women with severe pain or infertility due to endometriosis. Danazol's side effects, however, may include weight gain, acne, and on rare occasions, increased hair growth. Like other hormonal therapies, danazol must be taken for three to six months to be effective, and pregnancy is contraindicated during this time. Approximately 70% to 90% of the women taking danazol obtain relief from pain symptoms, and 50% to 70% of women taking the drug overcome infertility and can become pregnant following danazol therapy.

One of the most promising types of medical therapy for endometriosis includes a group of drugs called GnRH agonists (see also Chapter 35). These drugs are synthetic replicas of one of the major hormones involved in regulating menstruation—gonadotropin-releasing hormone. In a normal menstrual cycle, this hormone, which is produced in the hypothalamus at the base of the brain, stimulates the ovary to release estrogen. When given in therapeutic doses, however, GnRH has an opposite effect and inhibits estrogen release for as long as the drug is given. This produces a so-called hypoestrogenic state resembling menopause, including hot flashes and the absence of periods. Such side effects may persist as long as the drug is given but subside upon its withdrawal. GnRH may be given by monthly injection (Lupron or Zoladex) or by twice-daily nasal spray (Synarel) for three to six months. Several reports suggest that pelvic pain after GnRH treatment is significantly reduced, about the same as for danazol, but with fewer side effects such as weight gain and acne.

When hormonal drugs fail to relieve symptoms of pain or endometriosis has progressed to the point of forming large cysts, a woman may require surgical evaluation. Surgery, as opposed to hormonal therapy, may be the first step in treatment if endometriosis is severe or the woman is in her late childbearing years and desires to take every possible step toward conceiving as soon as possible. There are at least three different ways to approach this surgery. Your gynecologist should discuss the alternatives with you so you can select the option that best suits your needs.

The most popular approach currently involves laparoscopy to confirm the diagnosis, establish the extent of the disease, and remove as much endometriosis as possible. Today, more and more gynecologists are treating endometriosis as well as diagnosing it through the laparoscope. Through *operative* laparoscopy (see page 290) deposits of endometriosis as well as more extensive disease involving cysts and adhesions can be removed using either electrocautery (burning) or a laser. The laser uses a high-intensity light beam for precise destruction of abnormal tissue—in this case, areas of endometriosis. Fertility rates after surgery approach 70% if only mild disease is present. If the endometriosis cannot be treated with laparoscopy, further surgery may be put off until you have the opportunity to discuss the surgeon's findings and possible alternatives with your doctor.

The second surgical approach involves limited or *conservative* surgery. Operating through a regular abdominal incision, the surgeon removes endometrial cysts, adhesions, or other evidence of endometriosis that cannot be removed during laparoscopy either because of the size and extent of the disease or because the surgeon is untrained in operative laparoscopy. The laser may be used here as well and sometimes in combination with microsurgery (see Chapter 13). Only time will tell whether the laser technique is more effective than traditional electrocautery in the treatment of this disease. It should be kept in mind, however, that as good as the fertility rate with conservative surgery is, women with *mild* endometriosis have up to a 60% fertility rate without therapy in the first year after diagnosis.

The most radical surgery, as well as the only definitive cure for endometriosis, involves a complete hysterectomy; that is, removal of the uterus, both Fallopian tubes, and the ovaries. Removal of the ovaries, especially, is needed to prevent further hormonal stimulation and is the key to controlling this disease. Because such surgery eliminates childbearing potential, it may be best suited for the woman who has already completed her family, since endometriosis can recur after limited surgery. However, if infertility rather than pain is the primary problem, consideration should be given to conservative surgery without removing the uterus. This option would allow pregnancy through in-vitro fertilization (see Chapter 13) using an egg from a donor.

Resource

Endometriosis Association
8585 North 76th Place
Milwaukee, Wisconsin 53223
800–992–ENDO

CHAPTER 37

Cervical Abnormalities and the Pap Smear

What You Should Know About Your Pap Smear

Cervical abnormalities can be detected early, thanks to Pap smear screening. The Pap smear is a painless procedure for obtaining cells from the cervix, which are then sent to a laboratory for microscopic analysis. The technique, however, is just a screening device, and only a cervical biopsy can establish a firm diagnosis if the Pap smear is abnormal. The Pap smear is an effective screening tool because precancerous changes usually occur over a number of years before cervical cancer develops. Pap smears also can detect about 50% of endometrial (uterine) cancers and a much lesser percentage of other tumors in the female reproductive tract. Approximately 45 out of every 1,000 women screened have abnormal Pap smears, but many of these are due to infections, not to cancer or precancerous changes. Such precancerous changes are called *dysplasia*.

Dysplasia is classified as *mild*, *moderate*, or *severe*. Severe dysplasia is the most likely of the three to become cancerous, while milder forms sometimes go away on their own. Over a period of many years, about one-third of the women with moderate or severe dysplasia will develop cervical cancer if the condition is not treated. Severe dysplasia characteristically progresses first to surface cancer, or *carcinoma-in-situ*, involving only the outer layer of the cervix. Both dysplasia and carcinoma-in-situ, readily detected by Pap smears, can be cured nearly 100% of the time with appropriate therapy.

Using traditional terminology, dysplasia and carcinoma-in-situ are sometimes referred to collectively as cervical intraepithelial neoplasia (CIN). In the "CIN" classification the different grades of dysplasia are given a number based on severity—for example, mild dysplasia would be equivalent to "CIN₁" and carcinoma-in-situ would be equivalent to "CIN₃."

Pap smears previously have been classified by number, name, and descriptive term indicating the most likely cause for an abnormality when there is one (see Table 65). This system has been replaced by a newer, simpler one called the "Bethesda System" (see below). However, we will describe the older "traditional" Pap smear classification here as well.

In the traditional system, most women would have a normal, or Class I, so-called negative, smear. All other classes denote an abnormal condition, which is not necessarily a cancerous or precancerous one. The second most common Pap smear result, a Class II smear, was often referred to as "atypical" or "inflammatory" to reflect underlying cervical or vaginal infection. A Class III or "suspicious" smear would indicate about a 50% chance of cervical cancer, while Class IV and V smears represented surface cancer (carcinoma-in-situ) and invading cancer, respectively.

The "Bethesda System" of classifying Pap smears was developed under the auspices of the National Cancer Institute at a workshop in Bethesda, Maryland, in 1988. The format of reporting Paps consists of three elements:

1. A statement of whether the specimen is *adequate for diagnosis*. (Previously "inadequate" Paps, where insufficient cellular material was obtained, were referred to as Class "O." Such Paps are simply repeated because of technical problems in obtaining the sample.)
2. A *general categorization* of the diagnosis as "normal" or "other." "Other" could refer to simple infections (bacterial, viral, etc.), inflammations, or cell abnormalities.
3. A *descriptive diagnosis* explaining what was found under "other." All degrees of dysplasia (and CIN) fit under one of two categories:
—Low-grade squamous intraepithelial le-

Table 65   PAP SMEAR CLASSIFICATIONS—OLDER TERMINOLOGY

Number	Name	Descriptive Term*	Is Cervical Biopsy and/or Colposcopy Indicated?
I	normal	"negative," sometimes "mild inflammation"	no
II	atypical	usually "inflammation," occasionally "dysplasia"	yes, if repeat Pap smear is still abnormal after treatment of infection
III	suspicious	usually "dysplasia," sometimes "carcinoma-in-situ" (surface cancer), rarely "invasive carcinoma" (cancer)	yes
IV	positive	usually "carcinoma-in-situ" (surface cancer), sometimes "invasive carcinoma" (cancer)	yes
V	positive	usually "invasive carcinoma" (cancer)	yes

* New terminology refers to dysplasia or carcinoma-in-situ as *cervical intraepithelial neoplasia* (CIN).

sions (includes mild dysplasia as well as CIN 1).
—High-grade squamous intraepithelial lesions (includes moderate dysplasia, CIN 2, severe dysplasia, carcinoma in situ, and CIN 3).

Cancer, spread beyond the epithelium, continues to be described according to type—either squamous cell carcinoma or adenocarcinoma. The Bethesda System has introduced greater consistency and uniformity in Pap smear reporting, a change which, hopefully, will improve patient care in this area.

In 1987, the American Cancer Society revised and clarified its guidelines concerning the frequency of Pap-smear screening. The guidelines state that all women who are or have been sexually active, or have reached the age of eighteen, should have an annual Pap test and pelvic examination. After a woman has had three or more consecutive negative smears, the frequency of further Paps may be a joint decision made between you and your doctor. However, regular Pap-smear testing—at least annually—is recommended for all women who are at high risk for any of the conditions that could lead to cervical cancer (see Table 66). It is important that women with risk factors for cervical cancer—especially the fastest growing risk factor for cervix cancer, HPV infection (see Chapter 24)—should continue to have Pap smears every year—in some cases, more often. It is estimated that 50% to 80% of American women are in one of the high-risk

categories for this disease. In addition, the American Cancer Society continues to recommend annual breast and pelvic exams for all women over the age of forty.

Cervigrams (high-magnification photographs of the cervix) may be used to complement the Pap smear as a screening test. While not widely used at this time, partly due to cost, the cervigram may serve as an intermediate step between the Pap smear and an eventual biopsy when the Pap smear is initially abnormal. Cervigrams use a microscope with a camera to photograph the cervix. Due to the presence of many false positive cervigrams and the slightly greater cost of cervigrams in comparison to Pap smears, this technique is not presently widely accepted.

Evaluation of Abnormal Pap Smears

Depending on the type of abnormal Pap smear, the physician may elect to obtain more information by performing a cervical biopsy (see Figure 35) or just repeat the Pap smear after a short interval, say three to six months. Some debate exists as to when to biopsy and when to perform another Pap smear when the initial Pap smear is just slightly abnormal. This question comes up most often with smears known under the Bethesda System as "atypical squamous cells of uncertain significance" (ASCUS). Most physicians will manage such Paps by treating any existing cervix infection and by repeating the Pap smear since dysplasia is usually not present in ASCUS smears. A cervical biopsy is obtained if the repeat Pap again comes back ASCUS. Biopsies are also done for most initial smears that come back "squamous intraepithelial lesion," especially if it is a "high-grade" one. The biopsy is usually preceded by *colposcopy*, a painless office procedure using a colposcope, a special type of microscope that allows the doctor to examine the cervix and vagina more closely. This method enables the physician to take the most accurate cervical biopsy possible by selecting tissue from the most abnormal area. When combined with cervical biopsy, colposcopy usually eliminates the need for more extensive and costly surgical procedures, such as the "LEEP" procedure and the cone biopsy (see below). However, cone biopsy may still be necessary if the findings up to this point cannot explain the abnormal Pap smear.

A more aggressive medical approach to abnormal Paps is only one reason why a woman is more likely to end up having a cervix biopsy when she sees her gynecologist for checkups. Another major factor is the epidemic of sexually transmitted infections, especially human papilloma virus (HPV) infections, which have been linked to precancerous and cancerous changes in the cervix. While an HPV infection cannot be diagnosed with certainty by Pap smear, it causes specific microscopic changes in the cells that may make a clinician suspect this diagnosis. In such cases, the Pap smear under the Bethesda System will be reported as "changes associated with HPV." This notation will be added to the report of either a "low grade" or "high grade" squamous epithelial lesion (SIL), whichever is appropriate, if features of dysplasia or "CIN" are present. If no features of dysplasia or "CIN" are present, the HPV notation may be listed separately or (more likely) will be included under the "low-grade SIL" designation. Such changes in the reporting of HPV are an improvement, as they appropriately focus attention upon whether *precancerous* changes (dysplasia or "CIN") are present—not just whether HPV may be present, the significance of which is less certain. The treatment of HPV changes alone is also unclear as presently no treatment to eliminate the HPV virus from the genital tract is available. Instead, the treatment goal is to remove HPV-related precancerous changes (i.e., dysplasia).

A separate screening test for HPV infection has been developed. It works like a Pap smear and may ultimately change the way physicians manage the 50 million women who get Pap smears every year. The HPV test, called "ViraPap" (see Chapter 24), is more sensitive than the Pap test for detecting HPV infections, which have been linked to cancer of the cervix. As many as one-third of women with HPV infections may have precancerous changes of the cervix.

In addition to the HPV virus, other sexually transmitted infections such as chlamydia and herpes (see Chapter 24) may also be suggested by certain microscopic findings on a Pap smear. However, the diagnosis is by no means conclusive without a confirming culture or other specific test.

Recently, media attention has focused on high rates of false-positive and negative Pap smears. You may want to ask your physician about the pathology lab he or she uses. The College of American Pathologists recommends that you ask if the lab is licensed, accredited, and inspected, and if it is close enough to your doctor's office to allow easy communication with the pathologist. (It's better to avoid out-of-town, high volume "Pap smear mills," where quality control may be substandard.) Also, ask whether an unsatisfactory specimen—for example, one with too few cells—prompts a request for another sample. In such instances, you should have a repeat Pap, which will most likely be done without an additional charge.

Evaluation of the Cervical Biopsy

Ultimate treatment of an abnormal Pap smear depends upon what the cervical biopsy reveals—inflammation, precancerous changes (dysplasia), or, rarely, cancer. Inflammation of the cervix (cervicitis) may be associated with a vaginal infection or discharge that requires only local treatment with vaginal creams or suppositories. Therapy for dysplasia depends upon its severity and usually consists of cryosurgery, cone biopsy, or the "LEEP" procedure (see below).

Cryosurgery

Cryosurgery, or so-called cold cautery, destroys tissue by freezing. In recent years, cryosurgery

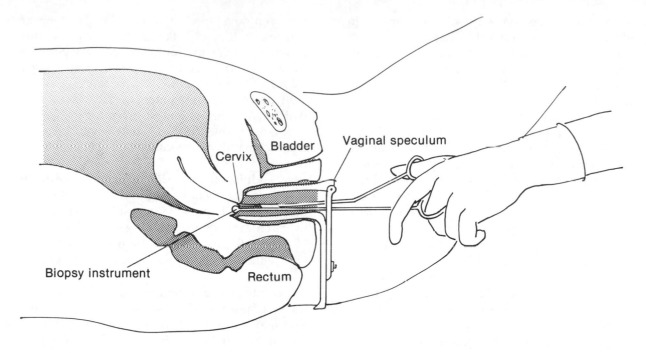

Cervix Bladder Vaginal speculum

Biopsy instrument Rectum

Figure 35 *Biopsy of the cervix. The doctor uses an instrument to biopsy, or remove, a small piece of tissue from the cervix.*

has become popular in treating cervical infections, benign cervical growths, such as polyps, and some forms of dysplasia. Cryosurgery is most often used to treat mild or (sometimes) moderate dysplasia. A few clinicians, who rely heavily on their expertise as colposcopists, also treat severe dysplasia or even surface cervical cancers with cryosurgery. This latter approach is controversial because its long-term effectiveness has not been studied. Most gynecologists believe severe dysplasia and surface cervical cancer call for a more aggressive form of therapy such as

---

Table 66 RISK FACTORS ASSOCIATED WITH CANCER OF THE CERVIX

1. First intercourse, marriage, or pregnancy at an early age.

2. Multiple sex partners, or a partner who has had multiple sex partners.

3. History of human papilloma virus (HPV) infection (including vaginal warts).

4. Large family size (many pregnancies).

5. Daughters of women who took DES during pregnancy (see Chapter 38).

"cold knife" cone biopsy, laser surgery, or the "LEEP" (see page 273).

Cryosurgery has the advantage of producing little or no discomfort. It also poses little risk of complications, such as bleeding, further infection, or (rarely) infertility from scarring. Following cryosurgery, a watery vaginal discharge may occur for about two weeks. Most clinicians recommend avoiding intercourse, douching, and the use of tampons during this time.

Cone biopsy (conization)

A cone biopsy is an extended form of cervical biopsy, which derives its name from the cone-shaped wedge of tissue that is removed from the lower cervix (see Figure 46, in Chapter 45). Although a cone biopsy removes the same tissue as would be destroyed by cryosurgery, the biopsy usually removes a *deeper* section of tissue.

A cone biopsy is both diagnostic and therapeutic, as it provides tissue for an accurate diagnosis as well as remove the abnormal tissue. There is much less need for performing cone biopsies today than in prior years because of the widespread use of colposcopy and biopsy, which can nearly always identify the abnormal tissue adequately. But if further tissue samples are needed, often the physician can obtain them using the newer "LEEP" (see below) rather than resorting to the more expensive cone biopsy operation. However, a cone biopsy may still be necessary if the lesion cannot be seen very well with colposcopy, or if there is suspicion of an invasive cancer. Cone biopsy is more expensive than office colposcopic or "LEEP" biopsies since it is performed in a hospital or outpatient facility, usually under general anesthesia.

Laser surgery

Laser surgery was widely used in the 1980s in the treatment of dysplasia and carcinoma-in-situ. The laser uses a high-intensity light beam for precise destruction of abnormal tissue. The procedure is really a specialized form of cone biopsy and is usually performed on an outpatient basis. In experienced hands the laser appears to be as effective in treating dysplasia and carcinoma-in-situ as the other methods but because of the significant cost, its use to treat CIN disease has fallen off considerably.

The "LEEP" Procedure

More recently, another approach to abnormal cervix biopsies—the "LEEP" procedure—has become very popular. LEEP, which stands for Loop Excision Electrosurgical Procedure, amounts to taking a "super biopsy" from the cervix by a technique using a special form of high frequency current. The procedure also goes by "LLETZ," which stands for Large Loop Excision of the Transformation Zone. The physician uses a hand-held wire loop that, when activated by an electrosurgical generator, cuts across the cervix with the same precision as a laser beam. The tissue sample derived by LEEP or LLETZ is larger and more uniform than the tiny cervical biopsies obtained with colposcopy. The "LEEP" procedure may be indicated when the cervix biopsy shows moderate or severe dysplasia (CIN II or III). This method is superior to cryosurgery because in addition to providing treatment a generous diagnostic tissue sample is obtained. The "LEEP" can be accomplished safely in the doctor's office using local anesthesia. The cost of the procedure is a fraction of that using either laser surgery or hospital cone biopsy.

The tissue diagnosis from the "LEEP" procedure or cone biopsy indicates whether further treatment is necessary. If the tissue diagnosis shows mild or moderate dysplasia, then no further treatment is indicated but careful follow-up is essential. If severe dysplasia or carcinoma-in-situ is found, however, hysterectomy may be considered in a woman who has completed her childbearing. If she does plan to conceive, the "LEEP" or cone biopsy may be considered a cure, at least for the time being, although a recurrence occasionally happens years later. Finally, if invasive cancer of the cervix is found, prompt treatment, either by surgery or radiation therapy, is the recommended approach (see below).

The most common complication of the cone biopsy and the "LEEP" procedure is postoperative bleeding, which occurs about 10% of the time and may develop as late as two weeks after surgery. Much less often, these procedures may lead to narrowing or blockage of the cervical canal and this, with removal of glands lining the cervix, may result in impaired fertility. An extensive or deep cone or LEEP may weaken the cervix's ability to remain closed during pregnancy and, on rare occasions, may cause a woman to be more susceptible to miscarriage or premature labor. Another problem with cone biopsy is that it makes follow-up of the patient more difficult in that disease can be hidden both from the Pap smear and the colposcope.

A woman with a history of dysplasia or carcinoma-in-situ should, following treatment, have Pap smears and colposcopic assessment more regularly than women without cervical disease. One rule of thumb in following treatment for biopsy-proven CIN or dysplasia is to repeat the Pap smear at least every six months for three to five years, and yearly thereafter. Following a cone biopsy, laser surgery, or cryosurgery, a woman should not have her next Pap smear for three or four months, since these procedures may cause temporary cell changes that could produce falsely abnormal Pap smears.

Cancer of the Cervix

Cervical cancer is one of the most common pelvic cancers in women. The incidence of invasive cervical cancer, where the tumor extends into deeper tissue layers or spreads to other organs, has decreased about one half in the past twenty years. However, the incidence of carcinoma-in-situ, which involves only the outer portion (surface layer) of the cervix, has risen steadily. Overall survival from cervical cancer has steadily improved over the past ten years, more so than for any other malignancy in women. The statistics have been attributed in part to early detection of precancerous changes through Pap smear screening. (See Table 71 for information on frequency statistics and other factors associated with cervical cancer.)

Invasive cancer rarely occurs in women who have regular checkups. But when it does, it may cause a blood discharge between periods or spotting after intercourse. By the time carcinoma-in-situ has become invasive, there is likely to be an abnormal growth on the cervix. Cervical biopsy is then performed to establish the diagnosis. Carcinoma-in-situ alone usually does not produce symptoms or abnormal physical findings.

Cervical cancer of the usual "squamous" type is sometimes referred to as a venereal disease because risk factors consistently relate to sexual intercourse and the cancer rarely occurs in the absence of regular intercourse. The disease hardly ever occurs, for example, in nuns, other celibate women, or lesbians. Risk factors for cervical cancer include multiple sex partners, first intercourse at an early age, early marriage, large family size, and possibly long-term use of birth control pills (more than five years). Although the sexually transmitted agent in cervical cancer has yet to be identified, the HPV virus has been suspected of playing a major role since women with these infections have an increased risk of developing this malignancy. The rising rate of HPV infections in recent years is becoming a major concern to thousands of young women who have a history of this viral disease. Even more alarming are estimates from DNA studies which suggest that 30% to 40% of sexually active women in the United States harbor the HPV virus and most have no symptoms. Among nearly 50 million U.S. women with this infection only about 5% to 10% are ever diagnosed as having HPV. For this reason alone, women with one or more risk factors (see Table 66) should have Pap smears at least annually. Fortunately, with regular checkups, invasive cancer—even in high-risk women—should be completely preventable.

Treatment

Treatment of cervical cancer depends on the tumor's stage when diagnosed. Carcinoma-in-situ may be treated with cone biopsy in a woman who has not completed her family. However, definitive treatment of carcinoma-in-situ requires hysterectomy because surface cancer can recur in 5% to 10% of the women treated with cone biopsy alone. Even after hysterectomy, 2% have a recurrence in the vagina, so these patients require follow-up for the rest of their lives.

Invasive cancer may be treated by a more extended hysterectomy, called *radical hysterectomy*, in which the upper portion of the vagina and the pelvic lymph nodes are also removed, or by radiation therapy. Most women with cervical cancer can be cured, including up to 95% of those with early invasive cancers and nearly 100% of those with carcinoma-in-situ.

CHAPTER 38

The DES Story

Between 1938 and 1971, in an attempt to prevent miscarriages, millions of expectant mothers took synthetic estrogen drugs called DES, which stands for diethylstilbestrol. (DES and DES-related drugs are listed in Table 67.) Twenty years later, seven young women developed vaginal cancer called *clear cell carcinoma*, a malignancy hardly ever reported before. An investigation of the women and their families showed a definite relationship between treatment of pregnant women with DES-type drugs and the development in their daughters of a variety of uterine and vaginal abnormalities, including vaginal cancer. Fortunately, the incidence of this cancer has turned out to be much lower than originally feared, the estimated frequency being about 1 in 1,000 exposed daughters.

Benign Changes in DES Daughters

Up to 80% of DES daughters have benign changes involving the cervix or vagina as a result of exposure to this drug. These abnormalities include slight, symptomless anatomical changes involving the upper vagina and cervix. These would go unnoticed if pelvic examinations were not done. An examination may reveal that the cervix is surrounded by a fold of vaginal tissue, sometimes known as a *vaginal collar*. In addition, the glands normally found only in the cervix appear in small numbers in the vagina as well. This condition, called *adenosis*, occasionally leads to a slight increase in vaginal discharge. It has been theorized that vaginal cancer may develop in areas of adenosis since 90% of the women who have vaginal cancer have adenosis as well.

Several investigators report a possible link between DES exposure in utero (that is, a

Table 67   DES-TYPE DRUGS*

Amperone	Diethylstilbestrol Dipropionate	Menocrin	Oestromon	Stilpalmitate
Benzestrol		Meprane	Orestol	Stilphostrol
Chlorotrianisene	Diethylstilbenediol	Mestilbol	Pabestrol D	Stilronate
Comestrol	Digestil	Methallenestril	Palestrol	Stilrone
Cyren A	Domestrol	Metystil	Restrol	Stils
Cyren B	Estan	Microest	Stil-Rol	Synestrin
Delvinal	Estilben	Mikarol	Stilbal	Synestrol
DES	Estrobene	Mikarol forti	Stilbestrol	Synthoestrin
DesPlex	Estrobene DP	Milestrol	Stilbestronate	
Di-Erone	Estrosyn	Monomestrol	Stilbetin	Tace
Diestryl	Fonatol	Neo-Oestranol I	Stilbinol	Teserene
Dibestil	Gynben	Neo-Oestranol II	Stilboestroform	Tylandril
Diethylstilbestrol Dipalmitate	Gyneben	Nulabort	Stilboestrol	Tylosterone
	Hexestrol	Oestrogenine	Stilboestrol DP	Vallestril
Diethylstilbestrol Diphosphate	Hexoestrol	Oestromenin	Stilestrate	Willestrol
	Hi-Bestrol			

* From *DES Exposure in Utero*, (former) Department of Health, Education, and Welfare, Publication No. (NIH) 76-1119.

woman's exposure to the drug when she was a fetus in her mother's uterus) and certain malformations of the daughter's uterus that may make the daughter susceptible to complications during pregnancy, especially premature labor.

Des Daughters and Cancer

As early as 1978 and subsequently in 1985, task forces on DES (formed by the Department of Health and Human Services [HHS]) verified the link between DES exposure in utero and increased risk of vaginal cancer. In fact, approximately 600 DES daughters have been found to have cancer of the vagina. The disease may be symptomless in its early stages, or a woman, as young as a teenager, may experience abnormal bleeding.

Considerable controversy surrounds the question of whether cancer of the *cervix* or precancerous cervical changes (dysplasia) are related to DES exposure. A definite relationship is yet to be established, and the increased risk of *cervical* cancer, if present, is believed to be extremely small.

Overall, the chances of a DES daughter developing vaginal or cervical cancer are slight. But, because the long-term effects of DES exposure are unknown, some physicians recommend that DES daughters minimize their exposure to estrogen, whether in the form of birth control pills, postmenopausal estrogens, or postcoital (after intercourse) contraceptives. Estrogens are not absolutely forbidden, but they should be taken only after careful discussion of alternatives with your clinician.

Evaluation of DES Daughters

If a woman was possibly exposed to DES-type drugs before birth, an attempt should be made to verify the information from medical records. The physician who cared for the mother during her pregnancy should have them. A DES daughter should, starting at the age of fourteen (or earlier if there is abnormal vaginal bleeding or discharge), have a pelvic exam at least once a year (see Table 68). Her checkup should include a regular Pap smear, as well as a Pap smear of the upper vagina since this is where vaginal can-

---

Table 68 RECOMMENDATIONS FOR DES DAUGHTERS

1. Have an annual pelvic examination, including Pap smear and iodine staining of the vagina, starting at age 14.

2. If your Pap smear is abnormal, make sure that a colposcopic examination is performed. You'll also need more frequent examinations—every six months.

3. Report abnormal or irregular vaginal bleeding to your clinician.

4. If you become pregnant, be especially alert for signs of premature labor. Ask your clinician to perform frequent pelvic examinations during your pregnancy to check for early dilation of the cervix.

---

cer would arise. She should also have an iodine staining of her vagina and cervix to identify abnormal areas and possible adenosis. If adenosis is suspected, a biopsy (removal and examination of tissue) is necessary to confirm this diagnosis. Such biopsies cause very little discomfort. To help identify suspicious cervical or vaginal areas, many gynecologists will also perform colposcopy (see Chapter 37, under Evaluation of Abnormal Pap Smears). This procedure is not essential, however, because most, if not all, DES-related abnormalities are easily seen or felt on pelvic exam or by iodine staining. If the clinician does find benign cervical or vaginal abnormalities, including adenosis, no specific therapy is indicated. The woman should, however, have frequent checkups, usually about every six months, depending on the severity of the findings. These checkups should include both the Pap smear and iodine staining. Abnormal Pap smears should, of course, be evaluated and treated as discussed in Chapter 37.

DES Mothers

Controversy exists surrounding the relationship between DES exposure during pregnancy and the development of breast cancer in mothers who were originally treated with this drug. Since the original 1978 DES report, a subsequent DES task force in 1985 noted four new studies that suggested that women who used this drug during pregnancy may have an increased risk of breast cancer. However, the task force did not find enough evidence to conclude that a cause-and-effect relationship between DES and subsequent breast cancer exists. Most professionals recommend that DES mothers take the same precautions concerning breast disease as women who did not take this drug in pregnancy—i.e., have regular annual breast and pelvic examinations, perform self-examinations of their breasts every month, and have periodic mammograms as recommended by the American Cancer Society (see Table 63).

DES Sons

Recent studies have shown an increase in genital and possibly urinary tract abnormalities in males exposed to DES. The abnormalities include lowered sperm counts, undersized pe-nises, small or undescended testes, and testicular cysts. Young men and boys who were exposed to DES in utero should have their primary care physician or a urologist examine them to determine if they have any of the problems associated with DES exposure.

Resources

For further information about DES write to:

Office of Cancer Communications
National Cancer Institute
Building 31, Room 10A-16
Bethesda, Maryland 20892

DES Action USA
1615 Broadway, #510
Oakland, California 94612

Des Action is a consumer group that represents DES-exposed people and publishes a quarterly newsletter and brochures related to DES.

CHAPTER 39

Ovarian Cysts and Tumors

An enlarged ovary may result from a variety of different kinds of tumors. A tumor is a swelling or an abnormal tissue growth, and the great majority are benign. Some tumors are solid, while others, known as *cysts*, consist of a thin-walled sac filled with fluid (see Figure 36). In children or in women over forty, *neoplasms* (new growths) usually cause the tumors. In women of child-

bearing age, however, an enlarged ovary usually results from ovarian cysts which are nonneoplastic—not representative of new growth. Rather, these ovarian cysts are the byproducts of hormone changes that occur during the normal functioning of the ovaries.

Each time the ovary produces an egg, a small cystlike structure (the *follicle*) forms. Typically, the follicle ruptures at ovulation when the ovary releases the egg. Occasionally, the follicle fails to rupture and instead continues to grow, forming a *follicle cyst*. Follicle cysts rarely require treatment. Most regress (return to normal) or occasionally may rupture later on. Sometimes multiple tiny follicle cysts are found in both ovaries. This fairly common condition, known as *polycystic ovary* syndrome (see Chapter 78), occurs because of a hormone imbalance associated with infrequent or absent menstruation. After ovulation, the follicle normally becomes a small hormone-producing structure, known as the *corpus luteum*. Occasionally, the corpus luteum continues to grow, forming a *corpus luteum cyst*.

Ovarian cysts and neoplasms may produce pelvic pain if they rupture, twist, bleed, or become infected. Most of these tumors, however, are symptomless and are first detected during a pelvic examination.

Evaluation of an Enlarged Ovary

Evaluation of an enlarged ovary depends on a woman's symptoms, age, and the characteristics of the tumor at the time of examination. Most ovarian cysts found in women of childbearing age tend to be small (usually less than two inches in diameter) and, in the absence of pelvic pain, can be reevaluated after the next menstrual period. Some clinicians recommend hormones (often birth control pills) to suppress cyst growth for one or two months. If the cyst does not regress during this time, surgery is indicated.

Women with tumors that are larger than three inches in diameter are usually operated on without delay. In a woman past menopause, any ovarian enlargement is abnormal and considered an indication for surgical diagnosis. Only by means of biopsy (tissue removal) can a clinician determine the exact cause of an enlarged ovary. Sometimes a doctor cannot clearly differentiate an ovarian enlargement from a uterine

Figure 36
Noncancerous cyst involving the left ovary.

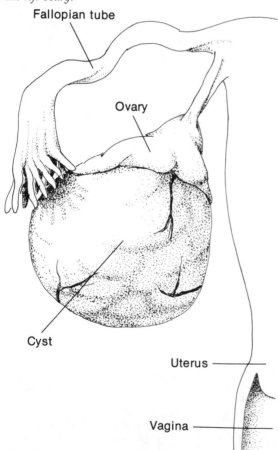

Fallopian tube

Ovary

Cyst

Uterus

Vagina

enlargement during the pelvic examination. This distinction is important because uterine growths are less likely to be malignant. Sonography (see glossary) has now replaced the abdominal X-ray as the best means to distinguish the two. If an ovarian tumor can be ruled out, surgery may be unnecessary.

Many ovarian tumors require exploratory surgery (laparotomy) performed through an abdominal incision. The physician may also attempt to establish a diagnosis through laparoscopy, a much less involved procedure, which may be performed on an outpatient basis (see glossary). Laparoscopy is commonly done to assess cystic growths in women under forty or in situations where the clinician cannot determine from the pelvic examination or sonography whether the enlargement originates from the ovary or from the uterus. Sometimes the laparoscopy procedure uncovers unsuspected disease, such as pelvic infection or endometriosis. These conditions may account for symptoms of pelvic pain previously attributed to an ovarian cyst.

An ovarian tumor which appears suspicious at the time of surgery is biopsied to find out if the tissue is cancerous. The surgeon may remove a small area of tumor at the time of laparoscopy. If a regular incision has been made, the biopsy usually consists of removal of the entire tumor. Either way, the tissue is sent to the hospital pathologist for an immediate preliminary evaluation, known as a *frozen section*. If the tissue is cancerous, further surgery can be done without delay.

Nonmalignant tumors may require no further treatment, depending somewhat on the woman's age and childbearing plans. During the childbearing years, most benign ovarian cysts can be removed without damaging the affected ovary (see Figure 37), and no further surgery need be done. However, if you are over forty or if you have completed your family, your doctor may recommend more aggressive treatment, depending upon the tumor's microscopic appearance. The problem is that certain types of ovarian growths cannot be classified as strictly benign or malignant. These types are sometimes described as having "intermediate," or borderline, potential for becoming cancerous later and are sometimes managed by removal of one or both ovaries (oophorectomy; see glossary) as well as the tumor itself. For this reason desire

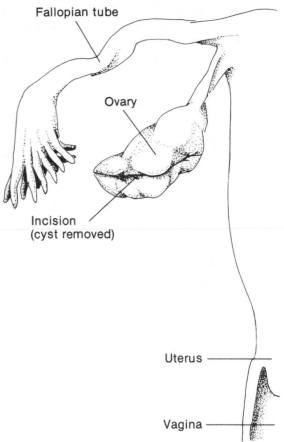

Figure 37
Many benign ovarian cysts can be surgically removed without removing the entire ovary. Normal hormone production continues in the remaining part of the ovary.

for future childbearing is a particularly important issue that a woman should discuss thoroughly with her surgeon *before* the operation. In a young woman, removal of just the affected ovary is often done for treatment of these borderline tumors if future childbearing is desired.

Ovarian Cancer

Although less common than cancers of the uterus or cervix, ovarian cancer is the leading killer among gynecologic malignancies, accounting for over 14,000 deaths in 1995. Approximately one woman in seventy may develop ovarian cancer, although rarely before the age of thirty. The overall five-year survival rate of about 35% has improved only slightly in the past thirty-five years. (See Table 71 for information on frequency statistics and other factors associated with ovarian cancer.)

Although at present specific screening tests are unavailable for early detection, periodic pelvic examinations provide some assurance that ovarian cancer will not go undetected. Research on screening tests such as sonography and the CA-125 blood test continue, but these tests are currently not used routinely in women without symptoms. Ovarian cancer characteristically spreads silently and rapidly to other organs within the abdominal cavity and is discovered in a late stage approximately two-thirds of the time. Unlike breast and uterine cancer, ovarian malignancy is associated with a very few known risk factors. Women who have never given birth or have a family history of gynecologic cancer or who consume a high-fat diet may be at slightly increased risk. A family history of ovarian cancer is especially significant in a woman's mother or sister. Recent studies from 1992 and 1994 have suggested a possible link between ovarian cancer and the use of fertility drugs like clomiphene. This association is far from proven at this time, however.

Early symptoms of ovarian cancer may include pelvic pressure, abdominal swelling, gas pains, indigestion, and vague abdominal discomfort. Rarely are any of these symptoms, however, attributed to an ovarian tumor since they are usually due to other, benign causes.

The treatment for ovarian cancer is surgery. Occasionally young women who have early tumors involving just one ovary and who have not completed their families may be treated by removal of just the tube and ovary on the affected side. Definitive treatment, however, requires removal of the uterus as well as both tubes and ovaries. Because it is a particularly aggressive cancer, physicians often have previously recommended removing the ovaries during elective pelvic surgery being done for some other reason in women over the age of forty-five. This position is now being reconsidered (see Chapter 45).

Few ovarian cancers, even the most advanced, are inoperable. Even if the tumor spreads beyond the abdominal cavity, survival is related directly to the amount of cancerous tissue removed, even if all of it cannot be reached. Following surgery, chemotherapy has been increasingly used to lessen the symptoms and improve the prognosis for women with this disease.

CHAPTER 40

Uterine Cancer

Because uterine cancer most commonly begins inside the womb in the tissue lining the uterine cavity (endometrium), the tumor initially cannot be seen or felt during a pelvic examination. While the Pap smear can detect cervical cancer at least 90% of the time, it is unlikely to uncover uterine cancer in more than 50% of the women tested.

Characteristically, uterine (endometrial) cancer afflicts a woman at or past menopause. It is rare before age forty, but about 25% of these cancers do occur in premenopausal women, causing abnormal bleeding between periods or heavy, prolonged menses.

The incidence of endometrial cancer, the fourth most frequent cancer in women, has increased in the past two decades, with 33,000 cases estimated for 1995—nearly double the in-

---

Table 69   RISK FACTORS ASSOCIATED WITH UTERINE (ENDOMETRIAL) CANCER

1. Family history of uterine cancer.

2. Obesity.

3. High blood pressure.

4. Diabetes.

5. Polycystic ovaries.

6. Infrequent periods (less than four per year) or infertility due to lack of ovulation.

7. Menstrual periods continuing after age fifty.

8. Infertility or never pregnant.

9. Prolonged treatment with estrogen alone (not with progesterone).*

10. Use of tamoxifen (anticancer drug used in chemotherapy for breast cancer).

---

* Not including oral contraceptives.

Table 70   RECOMMENDATIONS TO MINIMIZE UTERINE CANCER RISK IN WOMEN WHO TAKE ESTROGEN

If you take estrogen:

1. Ask your clinician to perform a periodic (for example, annual) endometrial biopsy or aspiration (see glossary) to evaluate the uterine lining.

2. Use the lowest possible dose which relieves symptoms (for example, Premarin 0.3- or 0.625-mg pills instead of 1.25 or 2.5 mg).

3. Ask your clinician about prescribing progesterone (for example, Provera) for several days each month.

4. Consult your clinician if abnormal vaginal bleeding occurs (any vaginal bleeding after the menopause is abnormal).

---

cidence twenty years earlier. The extent to which rising uterine cancer rates in the 1980s reflect an aging population, more aggressive cancer screening, or the enthusiasm for high-dose estrogen-only hormone replacement therapy prior to the 1970s is not clear. However, this disease appears to have leveled off in frequency during the 1990s and accounts for less than 3% of all cancer deaths among women. Fortunately, most of these tumors are detected at an early, curable, stage. (See Table 71 for information on frequency statistics and other factors associated with uterine cancer.)

There are various factors that increase a woman's chances of developing uterine cancer (see Table 69). But while one or more of these conditions apply for many women, only a very few women are likely to develop this malignancy. Still, some authorities now recommend that women of menopausal age who have one or more risk factors should be screened annually by means of one of the procedures for sampling endometrial tissue (see Diagnosis, page 282).

Estrogen and Uterine Cancer

The association between long-term estrogen use (without the additional hormone progesterone) and the development of endometrial cancer was established in the 1970s. Since 1975, a number of studies have revealed a strong association between estrogen treatment for menopausal symptoms and endometrial cancer. The link was clarified in 1979 by a National Institutes of Health (NIH) task force, which found that women who took estrogen alone increased their risk for uterine cancer severalfold. The type of uterine cancer associated with estrogen therapy is usually the slower-growing type, which is easier to detect and cure. During the 1980s, subsequent studies found that the risk of developing uterine cancer in postmenopausal women taking estrogen is essentially prevented by taking a second hormone, progesterone, during several days of each cycle. This practice has become an integral part of hormone-replacement therapy (see Chapter 27). Table 70 gives a number of recommendations to minimize the risk of uterine cancer in postmenopausal women receiving hormonal therapy.

Diagnosis

Uterine cancer may be diagnosed by endometrial biospy or endometrial aspiration (see glossary), two office procedures which evaluate the tissues and cells lining the uterine cavity. It may also be detected by dilatation and curettage (D & C), a surgical procedure performed in a hospital or an ambulatory care facility.

With an endometrial biopsy, the clinician removes samples of endometrial tissue with a curette. Endometrial aspiration is usually a less painful procedure during which the physician washes out the uterine cavity with a syringe that is connected to a small tube that contains a sterile solution. The fluid is then drawn back into the syringe for later laboratory evaluation of uterine cells.

In a woman over forty who is bleeding abnormally but exhibits no other physical symptoms, such as uterine enlargement, an endometrial biopsy or aspiration is usually performed first. These procedures are very reliable in detecting endometrial cancer. A D & C and hysteroscopy (see Chapter 41) may be done in the postmenopausal woman when the office biopsy does not produce a diagnosis or if abnormal bleeding persists.

Sometimes the pathology report from a uter-

Table 71 FREQUENCY STATISTICS AND OTHER FACTORS ASSOCIATED WITH CANCER OF THE REPRODUCTIVE ORGANS*

	Location			
	Ovary	Uterus	Cervix	Breast
Estimated number of new cases in 1996 (U.S.)	26,700	34,000	15,700**	186,000
Estimated number of deaths in 1996 (U.S.)	14,800	6,000	4,900	45,000
Percent of all cancer deaths in women	6%	2%	2%	17%
Average age	62 (rare before age 40)	57 (rare before age 40)	46 (very uncommon before age 40)	54 (very uncommon before age 40)
Is tumor growth stimulated by estrogen drugs?	no	sometimes***	no	sometimes***
Do periodic examinations allow early detection?	sometimes	definitely	definitely	often
Frequently tumor is detected by:	routine pelvic examinations	endometrial biopsy for abnormal bleeding	Pap smear	self-examination

* See also Figure 38.

** Not including surface cancer (carcinoma-in-situ).

*** However, no data has established that estrogen-containing drugs cause breast or uterine cancer.

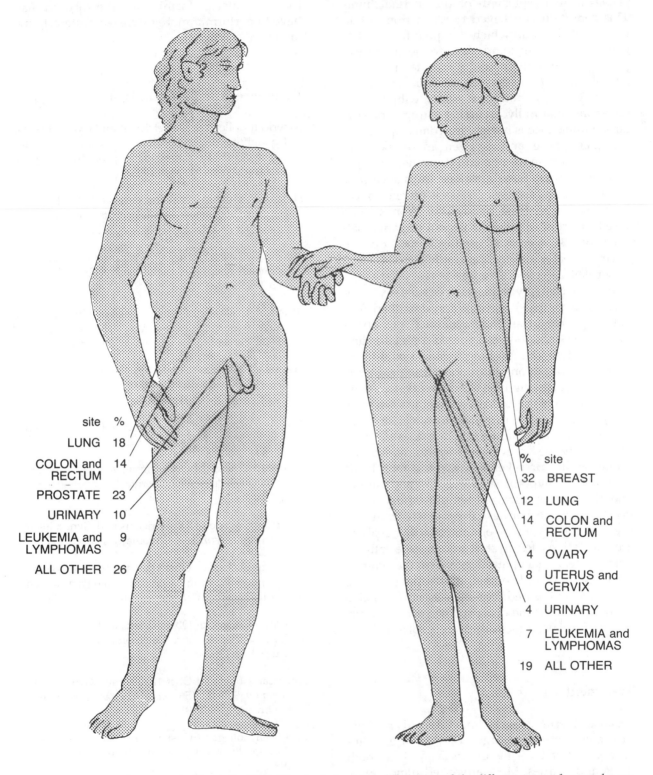

site	%
LUNG	18
COLON and RECTUM	14
PROSTATE	23
URINARY	10
LEUKEMIA and LYMPHOMAS	9
ALL OTHER	26

%	site
32	BREAST
12	LUNG
14	COLON and RECTUM
4	OVARY
8	UTERUS and CERVIX
4	URINARY
7	LEUKEMIA and LYMPHOMAS
19	ALL OTHER

Figure 38   *Estimated cancer incidence for 1996. The chart shows the distribution of the different types of cancer by sex. For example, breast cancer accounts for 31% of all cancers in women. Percentages are based on projections from the National Cancer Institute's Surveillance, Epidemiology, and End Results Program. Carcinoma-in-situ, or surface cancer, of the cervix is not included in the statistics.*

ine biopsy or D & C will reveal *endometrial hyperplasia*, an overgrowth of the uterine lining. This condition is believed to result from a hormone imbalance in which the quantity of estrogen is excessive in comparison to the quantity of progesterone. Endometrial hyperplasia may occur by itself, or it may result from prolonged use of estrogen hormone alone, without progesterone. Naturally occurring estrogen-progesterone imbalance is normal in women approaching menopause and is even more likely in infertile or obese women and in women with polycystic ovaries. Such hormone imbalance may account for the increased risk of uterine cancer in women with these conditions. Women who take birth control pills—which all contain a balance of estrogen *and* progesterone—do *not* have a greater risk of developing endometrial hyperplasia.

Endometrial hyperplasia occasionally progresses to uterine cancer. When described in a pathology report as "adenomatous" or "atypical," it is definitely considered premalignant. The condition can often be reversed by administering progesterone hormones. The progesterone counteracts the effect of excessive estrogen stimulation on the uterus. In women who are being treated with estrogen to alleviate postmenopausal hot flashes, endometrial hyperplasia can be prevented by administering progesterone for several days each month. (If endometrial hyperplasia develops and subsequently persists, estrogen should be discontinued.) Most authorities believe recurrent or precancerous types of endometrial hyperplasia are indications for hysterectomy, especially in women near menopausal age. For the woman who has not completed her family, progesterone therapy may be tried; but such therapy remains controversial for the older woman with a recurrent or precancerous form of hyperplasia.

Treatment

Because uterine cancer may spread rapidly, treatment for early stages of this disease involves removal of the uterus as well as both tubes and ovaries. More advanced tumors may be treated with radiation or chemotherapy, in addition to surgery. A gynecology cancer specialist (gynecologic oncologist) is usually consulted if uterine cancer spreads beyond the cavity of the uterus. In this case, the surgeon may have to perform a more extensive hysterectomy, known as a *radical hysterectomy*.

References for Section Eight

American College of Obstetricians and Gynecologists, Committee on gynecologic practice, *Committee Opinion* 152. Recommendations on frequency of Pap test screening, Mar 1995.

Hillard, P. Human Papillomavirus and the abnormal Papanicolaou smear in adolescents. *The Female Patient* 19:48–60, Dec 1994.

Nuovo, G. Lowering risks of recurrent cervical intraepithelial neoplasia. *Contemporary OB/GYN*: 9–19, Feb 1995.

American College of Obstetricians and Gynecologists Current Journal Review, Vol. 7 No. 6. *Oncology*: 35–36. Screening for early ovarian cancer, 1994.

Teneriello, M. Early detection of ovarian cancer. *CA-A Cancer Journal for Clinicians, Ovarian Cancer* 45(2): 71–85, Mar/Apr 1995.

Cancer statistics 1995. *CA-A Cancer Journal for Clinicians*, 46(1):8–12, Jan/Feb 1996.

American College of Obstetricians and Gynecologists *Technical Bulletin* 192. Uterine leiomyomata, May 1994.

American College of Obstetricians and Gynecologists *Technical Bulletin* 184. Endometriosis, Sep 1993.

American College of Obstetricians and Gynecologists *Technical Bulletin* 183. Cervical cytology: evaluation and management of abnormalities, Aug 1993.

American College of Obstetricians and Gynecologists *Technical Bulletin* 162. Carcinoma of the endometrium, Dec 1991.

American College of Obstetricians and Gynecologists *Technical Bulletin* 156. Nonmalignant conditions of the breast, June 1991.

American College of Obstetricians and Gynecologists *Technical Bulletin* 158. Carcinoma of the breast, Aug 1991.

American College of Obstetricians and Gynecologists *Technical Bulletin* 155. Classification and staging of gynecologic malignancies, May 1991.

American College of Obstetricians and Gynecologists *Technical Bulletin* 141. Cancer of the ovary, May 1990.

American College of Obstetricians and Gynecologists *Technical Bulletin* 138. Diagnosis and management of invasive cervical carcinomas, Dec 1989.

American College of Obstetricians and Gynecologists, Committee on gynecologic practice, *Committee Opinion* 131. Diethylstilbestrol, Dec 1993.

American College of Obstetricians and Gynecologists, Committee on gynecologic practice, *Committee Opinion* 127. Office mammography, Aug 1993.

American College of Obstetricians and Gynecologists, Committee on gynecologic practice, *Committee Opinion* 117. Genetic risk and screening techniques for epithelial ovarian cancer, Dec 1992.

American College of Obstetricians and Gynecologists, Committee on gynecologic practice, *Committee Opinion* 100. Second-look surgery for ovarian carcinoma, Nov 1991.

Goldfarb, H. Removing uterine fibroids laparoscopically. *Contemporary OB/GYN* 50–72, Feb 1994.

Berkley, S. The relationship of tampon characteristics to menstrual toxic shock syndrome. *Journal of the American Medical Association* 258:917–920, 1987.

FDA proposes standardized absorbency labeling for tampons. *ACOG Newsletter* 2: Dec 1988.

Bope, E. Screening for breast cancer. *The Female Patient* 14(3):75–86, Mar 1989.

Frankle, G. Screening mammography: why wait? *The Female Patient* 12:55–60, Dec 1987.

Greenspan, E. Toward the chemoprevention of breast cancer. *The Female Patient* 14(4):110–113, Apr 1989.

Willis, J. Why women don't get mammograms (and why they should). *FDA Consumer*, May 1987.

Dershaw, D. Mammography after prosthesis placement for augmentation or reconstructive mammoplasty. *Radiology* 170:69–74, 1989.

Townsend, C. Management of breast cancer—surgery and adjuvant therapy. *CIBA Clinical Symposia* 39(4): 1987.

Gidwani, G. Endometriosis in the adolescent. *Contemporary OB/GYN* 33(4):75–89, Apr 1989.

Henzi, M. Administration of nasal nafarelin as compared with oral danazol for endometriosis: a multicenter double-blind comparative clinical trial. *New England Journal of Medicine* 318:485–489, 1988.

Seibel, M. Does minimal endometriosis always require treatment? *Contemporary OB/GYN* 34(1):27–40, July 1989.

Friedman, A. Clinical experience in the treatment of fibroids with leuprolide and other GnRH agonists. *Obstetrical and Gynecological Survey* 44(5):311–313, May 1989.

Hill, G. Clinical experience in the treatment of endometriosis with GnRH agonists. *Obstetrical and Gynecological Survey* 44(5):305–307, May 1989.

Friedman, A. Leuprolide acetate: applications in gynecology. *Current Problems in Obstetrics, Gynecology and Infertility* XI (6):209–244, Nov/Dec 1988.

Nelson, J. Cervical intraepithelial neoplasia, and early invasive cervical carcinoma. *CA-A Cancer Journal for Clinicians* 39(3):157–178, May/June 1989.

Kwikkel, H. Treating CIN—laser vaporization or cryotherapy? *Contemporary OB/GYN* 33(3):29–46, Mar 1989.

Morrison, B. The significance of atypical cervical smears. *The Journal of Reproductive Medicine* 33(10):809–812, Oct 1988.

Lee, D. Accuracy of pap smears—art or science? *Journal of Reproductive Medicine* 33(10):795–798, Oct 1988.

Holloway, R. The carbon dioxide laser: a guide to its use in lower genital tract disorders. *The Female Patient* 13:74–81, July 1988.

Piver, M. Preventing deaths from cervical cancer: the Pap smear controversy. *The Female Patient* 13(10):19–37, Oct 1988.

Winguard, D. Longterm effects of exposure to diethylstilbestrol. *Clinical Medicine* 551–554, Nov 1988.

Linn, S. Adverse outcomes of pregnancy in women exposed to diethylstilbestrol in utero. *Journal of Reproductive Medicine* 33(1):3–7, Jan 1988.

Senekjian, E. Reproductive function in DES-exposed women. *Female Patient* 13(4):12–15, Apr 1988.

Cloitre, M. The psychological impact of prenatal DES exposure in women: a comparison of shortterm and longterm effects. *Journal of Psychosomatic Obstetrics and Gynecology* 8:149–168, 1988.

Dalton, K. *Once a Month.* Claremont, CA: Hunter House, Inc., 1987.

Rubinow, D. Changes in plasma hormones across the menstrual cycle in patients with menstrually-related mood disorder and in control subjects. *American Journal of Obstetrics and Gynecology* 158:5–11, 1988.

Maxson, W. The use of progesterone in the treatment of PMS. *Clinical Obstetrics and Gynecology* 3:465–477, 1987.

Sarno, A. Premenstrual syndrome: beneficial effects of periodic low-dose danazol. *Obstetrics and Gynecology* 70:33–36, 1987.

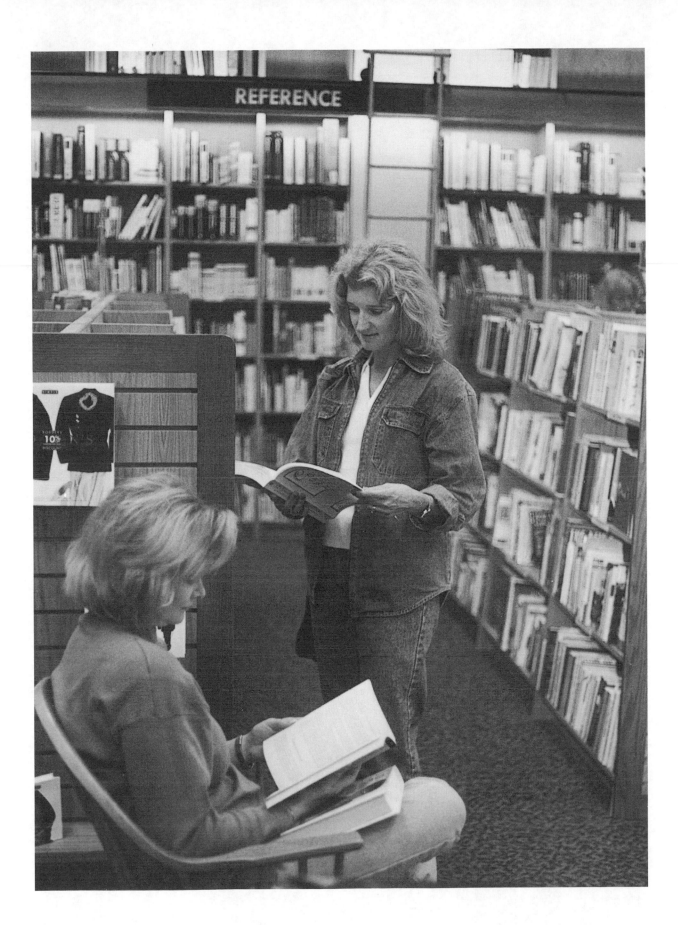

GYNECOLOGIC SURGERY

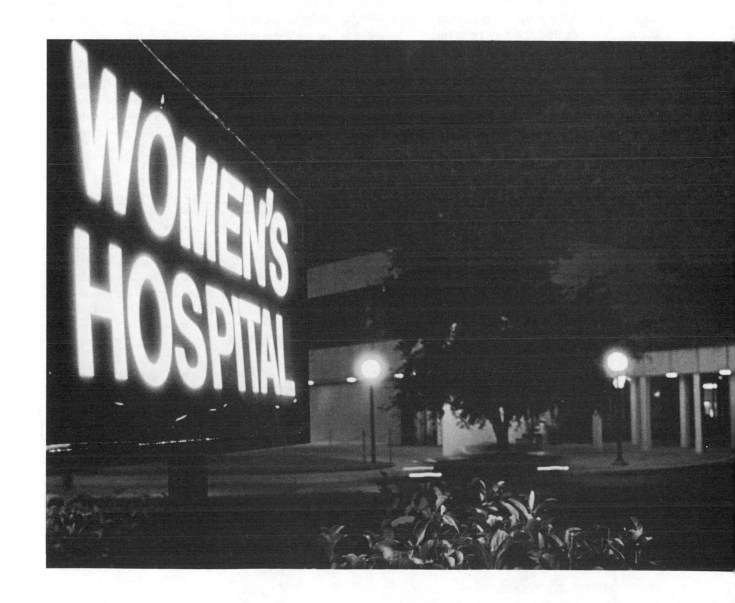

CHAPTER 41

Deciding About Surgery

Surgery involving the female pelvic organs is now safer than ever before. Better anesthesia, newer antibiotics, and increased numbers of board-certified obstetrician-gynecologists have improved the technical side of gynecologic surgery. And by obtaining second opinions and becoming better informed before surgery, women have learned to avoid unnecessary operations. This chapter will help you decide whether or not you need surgery—including the newer forms like laser surgery—and what to expect if you do.

New Surgical Technologies

Since the mid-1980s and well into the 1990s, three related techniques—laser surgery, operative laparoscopy, and hysteroscopy—have dominated new technology in gynecologic surgery. Each technique in its own way either complements or replaces the need for major gynecologic surgery. These techniques have the potential for cost savings by allowing for shorter, sometimes outpatient, hospital stays.

The word *laser* is an acronym for *light amplification by stimulated emission of radiation* and refers to a type of light that forms a concentrated beam and directs heat to one tiny spot. Advantages of laser compared to traditional surgical techniques include more precise dissection of tissue, less tissue damage (compared to electrocautery), and the ability to remove abnormal tissue (e.g., endometriosis) in "hard-to-reach" areas. Laser surgery includes three subtypes covered in different parts of this book (see index). The simplest form of laser surgery involves treating conditions of the lower reproductive tract—i.e., the vulva, vagina, and cervix. Here, the laser is used to burn off or "vaporize" condylomata (genital warts) or to remove precancerous tissue from around the cervix (see Chapter 37). More recently, laser therapy has been used in another way—in association with abdominal surgery, either with the abdomen opened surgically or, more often, via laparoscopy, in which the abdomen is essentially closed and the laser beam is directed through a laparoscope (see Chapter 43). Laser laparoscopy, as this second laser technique is called, requires only a tiny abdominal incision, which reduces recovery time. But the technique requires extensive experience with lasers and most problems can be treated equally well with traditional electrocautery. The third technique employs the laser to treat conditions inside the uterus using a special instrument called a hysteroscope (see below).

Laser surgery, which dominated new gynecologic technology during the 1980s, lost some of its luster in the 1990s. The use of lasers is now being reevaluated. Ongoing clinical studies are showing that often simpler, less costly techniques such as electrocautery can have the same effectiveness as lasers in treating conditions such as endometriosis, infertility, and pelvic pain. And in the treatment of abnormal Pap smears, a new procedure, also using electrocautery, has begun to replace laser surgery already (see the "LEEP" procedure, Chapter 37).

Operative laparoscopy, sometimes called pelviscopy—though this term really includes laser laparoscopy as well—represents another technical advance in female surgery. Pelviscopy is essentially an extension of laparoscopy—a technique that in the United States has traditionally been used either to *diagnose* problems, to treat relatively minor problems (e.g., to cut adhesions), or to perform tubal sterilization. As developed in Germany, pelviscopy carries the technique of laparoscopy further by using multiple small incisions (up to three or four, including the umbilical incision used in traditional laparoscopy) to enable the surgeon to perform major procedures such as the removal of an ectopic pregnancy or an ovarian cyst. An "incisionless" hysterectomy can be accomplished by combining laparoscopy techniques with vaginal hysterectomy in patients who need this surgery (see Chapter 45). This type of hysterectomy, called laparoscopic-assisted vaginal hysterectomy, avoids the long abdominal incision previously used routinely in patients having hysterectomies for ovarian disease, endometriosis, pelvic inflammatory disease, or pelvic

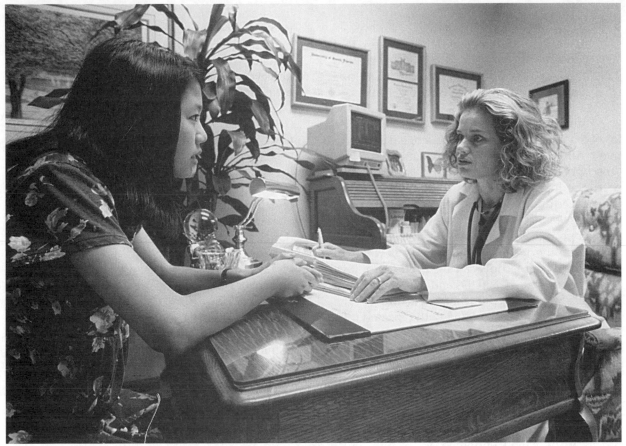

Obtaining a second opinion—an option to consider before you have surgery.

adhesions. Some of the common uses of laparoscopy include the following:

1. Endometriosis (see also Chapter 36). Endometriosis deposits may be removed by laser or by using electrosurgery. Large endometrial cysts may be drained and excised. Treatment of extensive endometriosis requires great skill and experience on the part of the operator; for some gynecologists this condition may be best handled by traditional surgery through a regular abdominal incision.
2. Tubal surgery for infertility. Adhesions surrounding the tubes and ovaries can often be removed and the blocked ends of Fallopian tubes opened using these techniques. However, removal of obstructions within the middle of the tube or surgery to reverse tubal ligation requires a larger incision and is better accomplished with microsurgery. Fallopian tube catheterization, on the other hand, may open tubes that are blocked where they *leave* the uterus. In this new procedure, called trans-cervical tuboplasty, a small tube containing a fine wire (or inflatable balloon) is passed into the uterine cavity and directed toward the obstructed tube, where a new opening is created.
3. Adhesions (fibrous bands that cause structures to stick together, sometimes creating pain). Many adhesions can be removed with laser therapy or pelviscopy (using an electrical current). Care must be used to avoid nicking such vital structures as the bowel and ureter (the tube connecting kidney and bladder).
4. Ectopic pregnancy. Laser or pelviscopy may be used to remove many ectopic pregnancies. This has been one of the more successful and widely practiced forms of operative laparoscopy.
5. Removal of benign-appearing growths. Both ovarian cysts and uterine fibroids (see Chapters 39 and 35) have been removed using these techniques. In Germany, ovarian cysts are commonly removed through

laparoscopy. In the United States this practice is increasing, tempered by concern that rupture of the cyst may cause painful chemical irritation or, if malignant, the spread of cancerous cells to other areas.

A third type of new technology, *hysteroscopy*, involves inserting a thin, telescopelike instrument called a hysteroscope (resembling a laparoscope) through the vagina and into the uterus. A local anesthetic is all that is needed for this procedure, which frequently accompanies a D & C (see Chapter 42). Hysteroscopy is used to treat abnormal bleeding or to remove growths within the uterus, such as polyps or fibroids. In addition, hysteroscopy can be used to remove foreign bodies such as IUDs and to check for and correct abnormalities in the structure of the uterus that may be associated with repeated miscarriage or infertility. Instruments—even laser fibers—may be inserted through a hysteroscope as with a laparoscope. The endometrial lining of the uterus may be destroyed with a hysteroscope in the patient who experiences excessive bleeding and is no longer interested in pregnancy and yet wishes to retain her uterus. This procedure is called endometrial ablation. Hysteroscopy, although adding to the cost of a D & C, often accompanies the procedure in the search for causes of abnormal bleeding. In the future, hysteroscopy may be used as a means of sterilization (see Chapter 43).

The benefits, risks, and costs of the new technology used in female surgery are presently being studied. To date, these approaches have not always been proven to be more effective than traditional surgery. For example, endometriosis may be treated equally well by traditional surgery as by laparoscopic laser, and the risks of the latter may be greater in inexperienced hands. As a rule, the skill of the operator rather than the instrument or technique is more important in determining the success and safety of a particular type of surgery. The convenience and potential for rapid recovery is the major benefit of pelviscopy and laser laparoscopy. A disadvantage of these surgeries is that they are very time-consuming, a factor that may increase anesthesia-related risks as well as cost. Visualization using these techniques as well as hysteroscopy can be a definite problem, even with the best optical systems available. In addi-

tion, the newer gynecological procedures tend to carry hefty price tags, sometimes as much as traditional surgery. This may be counterbalanced, however, by a much shorter (often outpatient) hospital stay.

Getting a Second Opinion

Seeking a second opinion may be one way to make sure you get the best possible care. A second opinion is especially desirable if your diagnosis is uncertain, if the need for surgery is not clear to you, or if the problem is a chronic one for which surgery was not previously advised. If you want a second opinion, ask your doctor or your local medical association to refer you to a board-certified obstetrician-gynecologist. You need not worry about offending your physician if you ask for a referral for a second opinion. Today physicians have come to expect such requests as a standard precaution against unnecessary surgery.

Informed Consent

Before you decide to have surgery and sign a legal-consent form, you need to know the answers to the five questions listed below. These make up the elements of what is called *informed consent*, a legal term meaning that you are informed of all the relevant facts surrounding your surgery and, on that basis, you consent to have the operation.

1. Why is surgery necessary?
2. What alternative treatment is available?
3. What exactly is to be done?
4. How can I expect to benefit from this surgery?
5. What complications may occur?

Even though you sign an operative consent, you can always change your mind, right up until the moment before surgery.

People differ as to how much they want to know about risks and complications, depending on how they cope with stress and whether they like to consider all aspects of a problem or put details out of their minds. However, it's a good idea to discuss specific worries about surgery with your doctor. You should have a clear understanding of the proposed operation and be able to summarize in your own words what exactly is to be done. Be sure you know the operation's likelihood of accomplishing what it is intended to do. For example, a hysterectomy may not always cure symptoms of pain, but the same operation relieves symptoms of abnormal uterine bleeding one hundred percent of the time. You may also want to ask your surgeon what kind of recovery period you can expect. And, finally, you should discuss with your surgeon what you would want if *unexpected findings* occurred. In deciding how to approach this issue, consider these questions:

1. Do you want to become pregnant in the future?
2. How important to you is maintaining childbearing potential relative to the discomfort caused by your symptoms?
3. If surgery to relieve these symptoms is unexpectedly required, for example, a hysterectomy, would you still want the surgery?
4. If it also required removal of your ovaries, would you still want it?

Answering these questions will help you make a sound and rational decision about surgery.

When You Enter the Hospital

Bring only essentials with you to the hospital. If you will be staying overnight, these items include your toothbrush, slippers, robe, nightgown, less than five dollars including change for phone calls and snacks, your medical insurance cards, and perhaps a book or magazine. Leave valuables, such as jewelry (including rings) and credit cards, at home.

After you arrive on the floor, a nurse (and perhaps a resident physician if your hospital is affiliated with a medical school) will visit you and take medical histories. The nursing history is taken and used by the nurses to develop a plan which aims at personalizing your hospital stay.

This is a good time for you to get to know the nursing staff, especially the head nurse on your floor, since they will take care of you after surgery. The licensed practical nurses (LPNs) and nurse's aides will provide most of the bed-side nursing, including periodic checking of your blood pressure, pulse, temperature, and so on. Registered nurses (RNs) are responsible for the care given on their floor and are always available should a problem arise. RNs can answer many questions about your surgery and often teach preparatory classes beforehand. If you have a problem after surgery—anytime, day or night—it is the RN's job to contact your physician and explain the problem. If you have requests, such as a particular diet or room change, tell any of the nurses. If the problem persists or you have difficulty making your needs known, ask to speak with the head nurse on your floor. Keep in mind that many hospitals are somewhat understaffed because of nationwide nursing shortages—this factor might be responsible for a problem going unrecognized. Most nurses will help you once they know you have a problem.

A day or so prior to surgery your physician will order some tests necessary to get you ready for surgery. A complete blood count (see glossary), urinalysis (see glossary), and pregnancy test are routine. Other blood tests, a chest X-ray, and a cardiogram are often ordered for women over age thirty-five.

The evening before or morning of your surgery, the anesthesiologist stops by and usually asks the same questions you answered before. This repetition, though perhaps annoying, usually works to your advantage, especially if it uncovers previously overlooked details such as a drug allergy. Be sure to mention *medications* you are currently taking, *drug allergies, past serious illnesses*, and any *present* or *chronic conditions* you have, especially any involving your heart or lungs. These areas may influence the type of anesthetic drug used. You can usually choose the type of anesthesia you want unless you have a particular medical problem. Discuss with the anesthesiologist your feelings about being awake or asleep during the operation. Keep in mind that the anesthesiologist you see the night before surgery may not be the same one who gives you your anesthesia since, in most hospitals, they work rotating shifts. Your own doctor will probably come by sometime before surgery, but if you have any last-minute questions, mention to the nurses that you want to see your doctor to ensure that he or she does stop by.

The night before major surgery you may need to take an enema to prevent difficulty having a bowel movement immediately after your operation. If you are going to have general anesthesia, you won't be permitted to eat or drink anything after midnight the night before surgery because your stomach has to be empty.

The Morning of Surgery

The morning of surgery, someone will shave (prep) the skin surrounding the surgical area if you are to have abdominal surgery. Only the pubic hair is shaved for vaginal operations. Many physicians no longer routinely order a prep, so discuss the prep beforehand with your surgeon.

You will be asked to remove all makeup and nail polish so that your skin color can be more closely observed in surgery. Remove contact lenses and any dentures as well. You will probably not be permitted to wear any rings during the surgery. A tube may be inserted into your bladder prior to surgery either in your hospital room or in the operating room after you are asleep. This tube, a catheter, prevents your bladder from filling up during surgery and thereby allows better visualization of your pelvic organs. About an hour before surgery the nurse gives you a sedative injection to make you drowsy and relaxed. Also you may notice your mouth becoming dry from the atropine which is usually given with the sedative. Atropine drugs dry up secretions in the lungs and keep the air passages free of mucus during administration of general anesthesia.

Just before surgery, you will be wheeled by stretcher to a holding area outside the operating room. At this time, a physician or nurse will start an intravenous infusion (IV). This involves inserting a small needle into a vein in your hand. The needle is connected by plastic tubing to a bottle containing the fluids you need during and after surgery. If blood is needed during the surgery, it is administered through the IV.

The Operating Room

Once in the operating room, which is significantly cooler than outside, you will notice that everybody wears surgical gowns, caps, masks, and gloves to prevent contamination of the sterile operating field. If you are having a general anesthetic, the anesthesiologist or nurse anes-

thetist usually administers sodium pentothal through your IV tubing to put you to sleep. After you fall asleep, an anesthetic gas which you breathe is administered either by mask or through a tube inserted into your windpipe. This so-called endotracheal tube, used for longer operations requiring deeper anesthesia or for surgical procedures like laparoscopy, prevents any stomach contents from reaching the lungs during surgery. If an endotracheal tube is used, don't be surprised if you have a sore throat for a day or two after surgery.

The Recovery Room

Depending on the length and type of operation, you spend about one or two hours in the recovery room, where visitors are not allowed. However, you can and should arrange for a close friend or relative to meet your surgeon after your surgery. Find out from your surgeon where this person should wait and when he or she can expect to hear from your doctor. After talking with your surgeon following the operation, this person can wait for you in your hospital room.

In the recovery room, specially trained nurses will monitor your physical condition closely and encourage you to "turn, cough, and deep breathe" frequently to expand your lungs, as well as to bend and move your legs to improve circulation. After major gynecologic surgery, you are likely to have two tubes attached: your IV and a urinary catheter tube. The catheter, which may produce a sensation that you have to urinate, continuously drains your urine into a portable bag that hangs on the side of your bed. After a general anesthetic, you are likely to be groggy and may not remember the recovery room at all. As anesthesia wears off, the nurse gives you pain medication to keep you comfortable. You may request this medication, ordered automatically by your surgeon, if you need it. After you are stable and you begin to awake from anesthesia, you will be transferred to your room, or sent home if you have had surgery as an outpatient.

Recovering in the Hospital

In the immediate postoperative period after major surgery (for example, vaginal hysterectomy

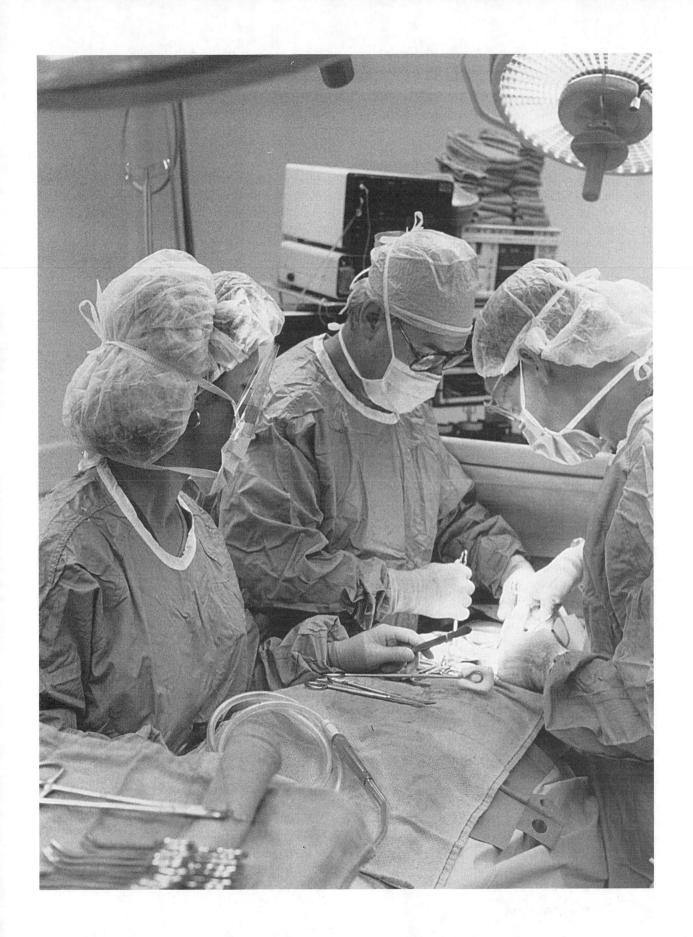

or any operation requiring a regular abdominal incision), your surgeon will come around to check on your general condition and perhaps examine your lungs and abdomen. Your doctor will write orders in your chart concerning four areas: activity, diet, tubes, and medication.

It is a good idea for you to become familiar with what these orders are. Hospital nursing staffs are busy, and you should be aware of what's planned for you: what and when medication is to be given, what you are allowed and not allowed to eat and drink, what your activity limitations and your doctor's recommendations are. Don't be afraid or embarrassed to ask questions. You have a right to know, for example, what the medication is that you are taking, what it is for, and what side effects you may expect. If you think you will be physically unable to handle this responsibility, arrange beforehand to have a relative or close friend ask questions and monitor your recovery procedures.

Activity

If you have had a general anesthetic, you will be encouraged to cough and take deep breaths to help expand your lungs. You can expect to be out of bed and walking (with your IV and catheter if they are still in use) the day after surgery. Early walking and moving about helps your lungs expand after a general anesthetic and promotes good circulation. Walking also helps you pass intestinal gas, a discomfort accompanying most abdominal operations on the second or third postoperative day. The first time you walk, someone will assist you. As soon as you are walking comfortably and feeling stronger and your IV and catheter have been removed (about the third or fourth postoperative day), you can shower and wash your hair. If you have an abdominal dressing, it will need changing after your shower.

Diet

Your diet normally progresses from clear or full liquids during the first twenty-four hours after surgery to a regular diet by the second or third postoperative day. Your diet can be progressed as fast as you are ready, but you should not force yourself if you are not hungry or if you feel nauseated. Gas pains often occur on about the second day, an expected sign that your in-

testines are starting to function normally. If gas pains are not relieved by walking, a mild laxative or enema may be ordered.

Tubes

The catheter (tube) draining the bladder, if used, is usually removed the next morning. However, if bladder surgery was performed, the catheter remains for several days. Your IV is removed when you can tolerate a clear liquid diet and if you don't need the IV for drugs, such as antibiotics. When vaginal or abdominal drains are used, these soft rubber tubes designed to prevent infection are moved outward a little each day from their position just inside the incision and completely removed within a few days of your operation.

Medication

Pain shots are replaced by milder pain pills as soon as you are ready, usually on the second or third day after surgery. Pain medication is a common source of nausea; if nausea occurs, ask for a change of medication as well as something for the nausea. You may want to ask for a sleeping pill as well when you switch from pain shots to pain pills. If you experience something you think may be a side effect, tell one of the nurses. You might be having a bad reaction to some medication.

When You Go Home

We have outlined the basics of what to expect before and after surgery. Your situation may be different depending on your surgery and your doctor's routine. If you have questions about your diet, activity, or medications, don't hesitate to ask. Find out what limitations your doctor thinks you should have, as, for example, in the areas of climbing stairs, driving, and resuming your normal physical activities. If your physician is not immediately available, ask a nurse.

Recovery from major gynecologic surgery often requires a hospital stay of two to five days after the operation. It takes most people this long to gain enough strength to begin to manage at home. However, cost pressures are forcing earlier discharges than ever before. Before you leave the hospital, certain medical requirements

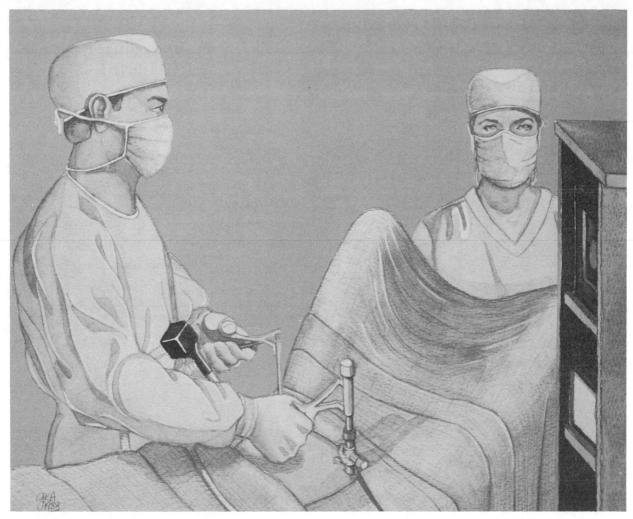

The technique of pelviscopy, using video camera and monitor.

must usually be met: you must not have signs of infection, such as fever, within the twenty-four hours before you are discharged; you must have resumed normal bowel and bladder function and your normal diet; if you have an abdominal incision, it must appear clean and uninfected; and your blood count must be reasonably normal.

Upon discharge, you are normally given instructions as to what you can and cannot do; at this time you may get a prescription for pain or antibiotic drugs. If you have had an abdominal operation, you may have clips or stitches, which are usually removed from five to eight days after surgery. In vaginal operations, the stitches are absorbed and do not need removal. Before you go home, schedule your follow-up visit, ask about the purpose and side effects of any new medications, and ask if you should watch out for any particular symptoms that might necessitate a call to your physician.

Short-Stay Procedures

Outpatient surgery saves you time and money and minimizes the upset of your home life and employment. Many gynecologic operations that previously required overnight stays can now be performed safely and effectively in an outpatient surgical setting.

In short-stay surgery, you can still have general anesthesia and go home the same day, usually within six hours of your arrival at the hospital. You will need someone to take you home after outpatient surgery, and you should avoid driving for twenty-four hours from the time you leave the hospital if a general anesthetic is used. The same general procedures are followed before outpatient surgery as for major surgery; the difference is that the postoperative recovery is at home. Table 72 lists operations that can be performed on an outpatient basis.

Table 72 OPERATIONS THAT CAN BE PERFORMED ON AN OUTPATIENT BASIS

1. Dilatation and curettage (D & C).

2. Therapeutic abortion.

3. Laparoscopy.

4. Tubal sterilization by laparoscopy, mini-laparotomy, or vaginal tubal ligation.

5. Cone biopsy.

6. Breast biopsy.*

7. Breast plastic surgery.*

8. Vaginal hysterectomy/laparoscopic-assisted vaginal hysterectomy (some cases).

---

* Usually performed by general surgeons.

CHAPTER 42

Dilatation and Curettage (D & C)

Gynecologists perform dilatation and curettage (D & C) more often than any other surgical procedure because it diagnoses and treats many pelvic problems. *Dilatation* is the gradual widening of the cervix, accomplished by placing progressively wider metal rods into the cervical opening (see Figure 39). *Curettage* refers to the insertion of a special, spoon-shaped instrument, called a *curette*, through the dilated cervix to curette, or scrape out, the tissue that lines the uterine cavity (see Figure 40). Another instrument shown in Figure 40, called a *tenaculum*, is used to grasp and steady the cervix during this procedure. Minimal anesthesia (usually a light general anesthetic, though a local or spinal may be used) is required for a D & C, which takes about fifteen minutes to perform and gives most women little or no postoperative discomfort. Shaving of pubic hair is no longer routinely done by most surgeons—check with your doctor.

When Is a D & C Indicated?

Dilatation and curettage (D & C), which used to be the only accepted method for diagnosing abnormal uterine bleeding, is performed less frequently today because of the availability of simpler, less costly office procedures. (A D & C is usually done in a hospital or outpatient surgical facility.) Office procedures like endometrial biopsy and endometrial aspiration (see glossary) are now the initial choice for evaluating abnormal bleeding in many women. A somewhat more involved office test, hysteroscopy, is often performed to diagnose and treat abnormal uterine bleeding that has not responded to traditional medical therapy (see Chapters 13 and 77).

Hysteroscopy allows the surgeon to visualize and biopsy the inner surface of the uterus and detect abnormalities a blind D & C may miss. Hysteroscopy may also be performed at the time of a D & C and, if so, should be listed as a separate procedure on your consent form. Hysteroscopy has become a useful way to diagnose and sometimes remove polyps or fibroids located inside the uterus. These more complex "operative" hysteroscopies are usually performed under general anesthesia in a hospital or outpatient facility, whereas the less involved office hysteroscopy requires only a local anesthetic.

If the physician obtains insufficient tissue from either the endometrial or the hysteroscopy biopsy, or if abnormal bleeding persists, then a D & C is usually performed. In women over forty who have abnormal heavy or frequent periods, the importance in having an endometrial tissue sample of some kind lies in excluding the possibility of a malignant tumor.

As a therapeutic measure, gynecologists perform a D & C most commonly after a miscarriage to prevent (or stop) hemorrhage or subsequent infection. Sometimes a D & C is needed after an abortion complicated by bleeding caused by retained tissue not removed during the abortion procedure.

Recovering from D & C

Recovery after a D & C is nearly immediate. You may experience slight vaginal bleeding and mild pelvic cramping for a few hours but rarely for more than a day. You can usually resume normal activity within a day or two. Most clinicians permit intercourse, douching, and the use of tampons within a week or two. Your first period after the operation may be earlier or later than expected. You should have a checkup a few days after the operation to discuss the surgical findings with your clinician.

Complications

D & C is associated with fewer complications than any other gynecologic surgical procedure.

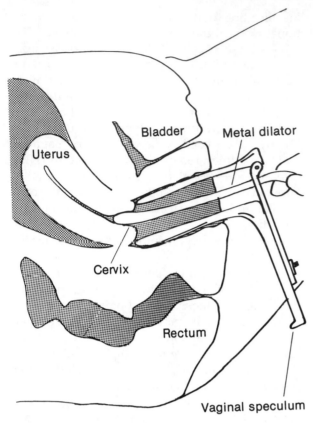

Figure 39
A metal dilator is used to widen, or dilate, the cervix during a D & C.

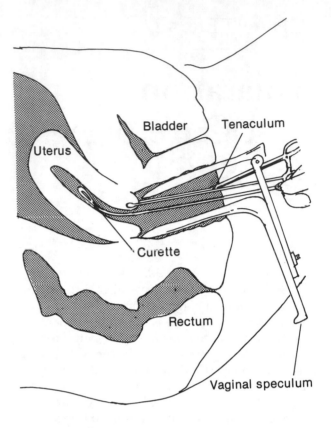

Figure 40
A curette is used to remove tissue from inside the uterine cavity during a D & C.

The main serious complication of a D & C is pelvic infection, which is more likely to occur if the procedure is performed while you *presently* have an infection of your reproductive system. (A sexually transmitted infection or any other infection of the uterus, tubes, or ovaries should be fully treated *before* you have a D & C.) After a D & C, immediately report to your clinician any symptoms of pelvic infection, such as pelvic pain, fever, or a bad-smelling vaginal discharge. Serious complications, such as bleeding from uterine injuries, are rare.

CHAPTER 43

Sterilization Options

Since 1970 more than 25 million U.S. women have opted for sterilization; that is, they have chosen by means of a surgical procedure to utilize a permanent method of birth control. In 1970, women accounted for only 20% of sterilizations. By 1989, this percentage had increased to over 50%, making surgical sterilization the number one method of birth control for married women over the age of twenty-nine.

When your family size is complete or you have medical reasons to avoid pregnancy, voluntary sterilization appears to be the safest, least expensive, and most effective method of female contraception.

Deciding About Sterilization

The decision to become sterilized by means of a surgical procedure is a voluntary decision that you should be absolutely certain about making. Although you can change your mind at any time prior to surgery, it is the kind of choice that should leave no doubts in your mind as to whether to have it done. A decision about sterilization should be made only after careful consideration and only after you have had the opportunity to fully discuss your questions and concerns with your clinician, preferably more than once.

The reason you must be sure about your decision is because the operation is considered irreversible. Only a small percentage of women who ask to have the condition reversed (that is, to have their tubes "untied") can successfully become pregnant. If there is any possibility that you may want to become pregnant in the future, perhaps because of remarriage, then choose a reversible contraceptive method instead. If you are past childbearing age, say in your mid-forties, you, too, may want to use another method of birth control, since fertility declines rapidly at this age, requiring contraception for only a few more years at most.

You and your partner or spouse may want to consider the option of male sterilization, called *vasectomy*. Keep in mind that vasectomy is slightly less risky, less costly, and only slightly less effective than female sterilization procedures, and just as irreversible. If, after considering all other forms of birth control, you decide on female sterilization, there are several operations from which to choose.

Operations for Female Sterilization

Female sterilization prevents pregnancy by blocking or dividing the Fallopian tubes and thereby preventing union of the sperm and the ovum, or egg—that is, preventing the egg from being fertilized by the sperm. This blocking or dividing of the tubes is achieved surgically by what is known as *tubal ligation*—which means "tying" the tubes. There are various methods for accomplishing this "tying," which we will discuss below. Hysterectomy, a much riskier procedure than tubal operations, is not usually performed for purposes of sterilization unless other pelvic conditions also require this surgery.

Excluding hysterectomy, there are basically five different methods of female sterilization, discussed below.

1. *Laparoscopic tubal ligation* (so-called *Band-Aid* or *bellybutton surgery*), an outpatient procedure, is the most popular method of female sterilization in the United States because it has the shortest recovery period of any method and it leaves only a tiny scar just inside the navel (see Figure 41). (This procedure will be referred to as *laparoscopy* throughout this chapter.)

   After giving the patient a general anesthetic, the surgeon makes a small (one half inch) incision just inside the navel. Then the surgeon inserts a needle through the abdominal incision and slowly injects carbon dioxide gas, which repositions the intestines so that your uterus and tubes can be seen clearly. The surgeon then removes the needle and introduces the *laparoscope*, a telescopelike instrument with a light

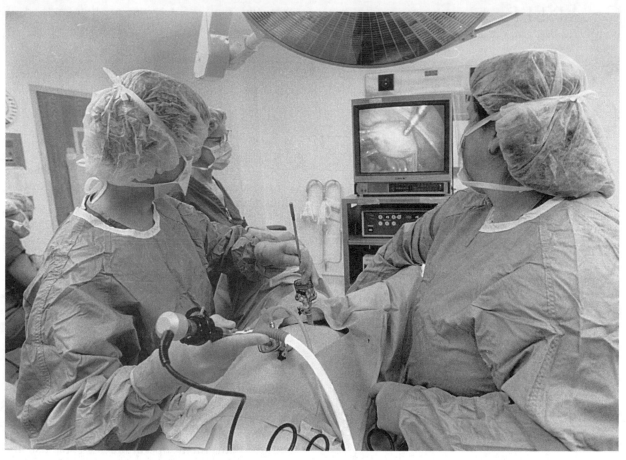

During laparoscopy, the surgical team views the operation on a video monitor. The surgeon (left) manipulates the uterus with an instrument in her left hand while holding the laparoscope and camera in her right.

source, through the navel incision. Next, the surgeon inserts a second instrument through an opening within the laparoscope (see Figure 42). Or this second instrument may be inserted through another tiny incision just above the pubic hairline. This "sealer" instrument blocks the tubes by electrical or nonelectrical means. In the most common method, electrocoagulation, an electric current seals (burns) the tubes by "clumping" them together (see Figure 43). In nonelectric techniques, a metal clip or silicone rubber band constricts the tube by binding the tube around the outside of it. This method has the advantage of avoiding accidental burns to other internal organs and has greater potential for reversibility (that is, restoring fertility) than electrocoagulation. However, clips and bands seem to produce slightly more postoperative pain. After completing the

procedure, the surgeon releases the carbon dioxide gas and places a Band-Aid over the tiny incision after closing it with a single suture.

Immediate postoperative side effects may include slight abdominal discomfort and distention (a bloated feeling) or shoulder pain, which usually subsides within forty-eight hours but may last for up to a week. The shoulder pain results from the pressure of any leftover gas. You may also experience slight vaginal bleeding for a few hours from the manipulation of the uterus necessary to visualize the tubes during laparoscopy. Occasionally redness and swelling occur around the incision several days later. You can clear up this condition rapidly by cleaning the area with peroxide and applying warm, moist gauze compresses four or so times a day. Most women who undergo laparoscopic sterilization resume their usual activities after a day or two.

In fewer than one percent of these operations, the surgeon finds unexpected pelvic adhesions during laparoscopy. If these adhesions dangerously obscure the surgeon's view of your tubes, he or she must make a regular abdominal incision to complete the operation safely.

Rare major complications of laparoscopy usually relate to anesthesia, internal bleeding, or damage to internal organs. Electrocoagulation, the most common laparoscopic method of tubal occlusion (blocking), has been associated with a very slight risk of accidental intestinal burns. If your surgeon does electrocoagulation, ask him or her to use *bipolar* coagulation forceps. The newer bipolar system uses less electric current than the unipolar type and decreases the risk of burns. Only one laparoscopy in three hundred requires major surgery to treat complications related to bleeding, burn injury, or damage to internal organs. If you have had previous abdominal surgery, especially with a vertical scar below the navel, there is an increased risk of intestinal damage during laparoscopy. The possibility of intestinal damage results from the fact that after previous abdominal surgery the intestines are more likely to adhere to the abdominal wall and not fall back out of the way at the time of laparoscopy. Many laparoscopy complications can be prevented by avoiding the procedure when these relative contraindications exist: pronounced obesity (increases technical difficulty of laparoscopy), serious heart disease, or chronic respiratory illness (the carbon dioxide gas may cause a tendency to irregular heartbeats or to breathing difficulties).

2. *Mini-laparotomy* differs from laparoscopy in that the surgeon uses no visualizing instrument. Although some women have local anesthesia for a mini-laparotomy, most surgeons recommend general anesthesia since many patients otherwise experience some discomfort. The physician begins the "mini-lap" with a small, one- to two-inch incision at or just above the pubic hairline (see Figure 41). With the help of an assistant who uses an instrument inserted

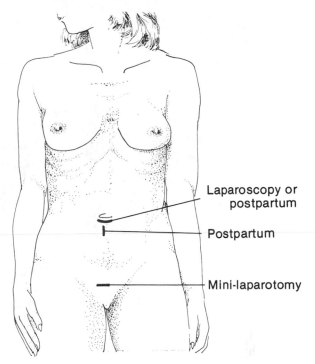

Figure 41
Types of tubal sterilization incisions. The incision for the laparoscopic tubal ligation (laparoscopy) is made just inside the navel. Postpartum tubal ligations can be performed through a small incision just inside the navel or through a slightly longer vertical incision below the navel. The incision for the mini-laparotomy is made at or just above the pubic hairline. Not shown are incisions for abdominal tubal ligation (see Figure 45) and for vaginal tubal ligation.

through the vagina and positions the uterus and its tubes near this incision (see Figure 44), the surgeon simply lifts the tubes through this incision and blocks them by the desired method. Usually the tubes are tied (ligated) using a suture, although bands and clips sometimes are used.

Increasing in popularity in the United States, the mini-laparotomy is considered by some authorities the safest procedure for female sterilization. This operation is ideally suited for women who cannot undergo laparoscopy because of previous

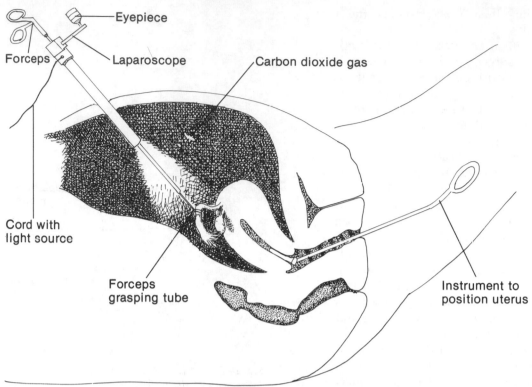

Eyepiece

Forceps

Laparoscope

Carbon dioxide gas

Cord with
light source

Forceps
grasping tube

Instrument to
position uterus

Figure 42   *Laparoscopy method of tubal sterilization. Laparoscopy alone, without use of the sealer instrument, is commonly used as a diagnostic procedure in the evaluation of pelvic pain, pelvic tumors, or infertility.*

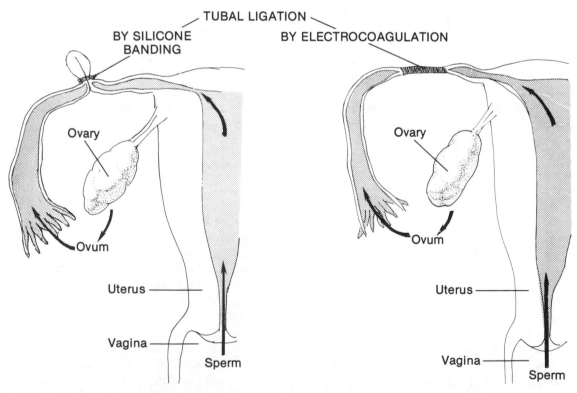

TUBAL LIGATION

BY SILICONE
BANDING

BY ELECTROCOAGULATION

Ovary

Ovum

Uterus

Vagina

Sperm

Ovary

Ovum

Uterus

Vagina

Sperm

Figure 43   *Depending on the technique used, the tubes may be blocked in a number of ways. Shown above are the two commonest methods used during laparoscopy tubal ligation: banding and electrocoagulation.*

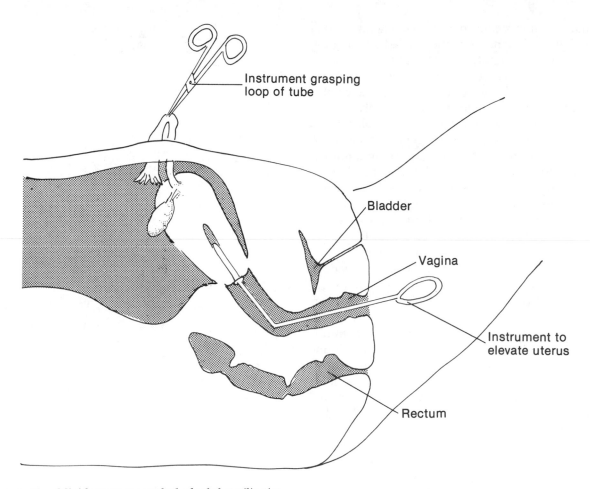

Instrument grasping
loop of tube

Bladder

Vagina

Instrument to
elevate uterus

Rectum

Figure 44   *Mini-laparotomy method of tubal sterilization.*

abdominal surgery or serious heart or respiratory illness. The small incision utilized
in mini-laparotomy allows rapid recovery
within two to three days. Although the procedure may be performed on an outpatient
basis, most patients stay overnight because
of greater discomfort with this procedure compared to laparoscopy. The major drawback of
mini-laparotomy is the technical difficulty of
operating through a tiny incision. For this
reason, if you weigh over 20% of ideal body
weight (see Table 116) or have a history of tubal
disease such as endometriosis or tubal infections, you should consider another method of
sterilization.

3. *Vaginal tubal ligation (colpotomy)* may be best
suited for women who have contraindications to
laparoscopy, such as previous abdominal surgery, or who are not ideally suited for mini-laparotomy because they are overweight. However,
many gynecologists have not been trained in this
technique, which is technically more difficult

than other sterilization procedures. For colpotomy, the surgeon makes a one- to two-inch incision in the vagina below the cervix. The
surgeon then draws the tubes through this incision and ligates them with suture material. As
with laparoscopy, the surgeon will resort to an
abdominal incision if, as a result of scarring or
adhesions, he or she cannot adequately visualize
the tubes.

Compared to abdominal incision methods in
which the skin is scrubbed with an antiseptic solution and made nearly sterile, the vagina's high
bacterial count makes the patient more susceptible to infection. As a result of such infections
about 2% to 3% of women experience painful
intercourse up to several months following vaginal tubal ligation. Advantages of vaginal tubal
ligation include the fact that the procedure can
be performed under local or spinal anesthesia,
instead of general anesthesia, and the absence of
a visible scar. Recovery from vaginal tubal ligation, while less rapid than for laparoscopy,

usually requires only one or two nights in the hospital, and sometimes the procedure may be performed on an outpatient basis.

4. *Abdominal tubal ligation* (using *laparotomy*—an incision in the abdomen) usually requires an abdominal incision made either vertically below the navel or horizontally just at the pubic hairline (see Figure 45). The surgeon may recommend laparotomy if you require abdominal surgery for other reasons or have had recent or chronic tubal infections or endometriosis. These conditions often cause adhesions or scarring, making it technically difficult or impossible for you to undergo sterilization by one of the other methods. For most women, laparotomy represents the least desirable method of sterilization because of its greater risks, longer hospital stay (three to five days), and prolonged recovery period.

5. *Postpartum tubal ligation*, essentially a mini-laparotomy that follows childbirth, is the second most commonly requested sterilization procedure. In this method, the surgeon makes a one- or two-inch incision inside or just below the navel (see Figure 41), draws part of each tube through the incision, and ligates the tubes using suture. Laparoscopy is seldom used immediately following childbirth because of the increased risk of damage to the uterus, which lies directly underneath the bellybutton at this time.

Postpartum tubal ligation usually does not prolong your hospital stay. The operation may be performed any time during the first three days postpartum, but it is most often done immediately after you deliver—in which case the same anesthetic (for example, epidural) may be used. This operation is associated with the same general risks as mini-laparotomy.

Although postpartum tubal ligation is convenient and avoids an additional hospitalization later, many women prefer to wait six weeks or more before making their final decision. It is unwise to base a decision to be sterilized on assumptions about the newborn's condition at birth. Problems in an apparently healthy baby may not show up until a day or two later. If you and your husband are considering sterilization, it makes sense to consider your options during pregnancy rather than at the time of labor and delivery or during the stressful postpartum period. You don't want to have to make this choice just before an emergency cesarean section, in the middle of a stressful labor, or when you are ad-

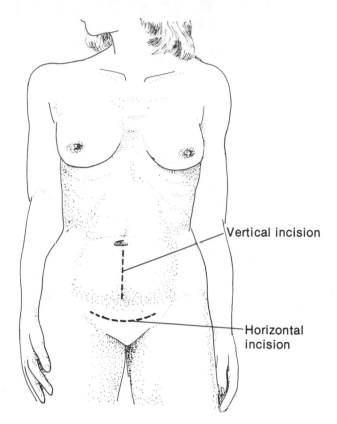

Figure 45 *Most gynecologic operations performed through the abdomen use either a vertical (midline) or a low horizontal (Pfannenstiel) incision.*

justing to the demands of a tiny newborn. Such conditions may make sound, objective decision making difficult.

Safety of Female Sterilization

Although no surgical procedure is without risk, tubal sterilizations are among the safest operations performed. The risk of death from this one-time operation is extremely low and no more than the *yearly* risk involved from the use of the pill or an IUD. Major complications, such as infections, bleeding, and damage to the internal organs as well as complications from anesthesia, occur in fewer than one percent of all surgeries. Although the various sterilization operations have slightly different benefits and risks, the skill and experience of your surgeon has much more to do with a safe, successful result than the type of operation you select. As with other surgeries, the safety of tubal sterilization depends somewhat upon your own health. If you tend to be overweight, smoke, or have serious medical problems such as heart disease, your chances of surgical complications increase. Also, if you have had previous tubal infections, any surgical procedure which manipulates the tubes can cause the infection to flare up.

Effectiveness of Female Sterilization

Because of inconclusive research, it is impossible to state precisely the exact effectiveness of each sterilization procedure. Although the chance of fertility is remote, pregnancy has occurred after tubal sterilization operations, at a rate of two to three per one thousand operations. Many of these pregnancies occur not as a result of surgical failure but because the woman was pregnant at the time of surgery. As a precaution, most hospitals perform pregnancy tests prior to any surgery. To be sure you are not pregnant—and to avoid the possibility of a "false negative" pregnancy test—it is advisable to have your sterilization operation within the first two weeks following the start of a normal period.

After Female Sterilization

Since the ovaries are not involved in tubal sterilization, hormone production is not interrupted. You will therefore continue to menstruate and ovulate (the egg, after release, becomes absorbed inside the abdomen). Most authorities agree that abnormal bleeding following tubal ligation usually means that the woman had a prior tendency to have this problem and that it is thus not a direct effect of the operation itself. Sometimes, however, tubal surgery may lessen the blood supply to the nearby ovaries and may then account for subsequent hormone imbalance and the accompanying symptoms of irregular or heavy periods. Tubal ligation has no direct effect, bad or good, on aging or sexual functioning. The predominant psychological effect in a woman who comfortably made the decision is great relief from fear of unwanted pregnancy, a feeling which often facilitates sexual enjoyment and emotional well-being. However, a woman who rushed into the decision for sterilization may regret it and later experience some depression.

Choosing the Right Operation

Which operation you choose depends upon individual circumstances—your physical condition, the type of anesthesia you want, and whether or not you plan to have the surgery immediately after childbirth. Among female sterilization procedures, the laparoscopy method and the mini-laparotomy method offer the greatest safety (assuming they are not inadvisable for you) and, when done on an outpatient basis, cost the least. If you plan to have your tubes tied after childbirth, you will avoid a second hospitalization later; but don't make this decision dependent on the baby's health at delivery.

Finally, if you have a history of pelvic disease such as tubal infections or endometriosis, remember that you have a greater chance of medical complications with laparoscopy, mini-laparotomy, or vaginal tubal ligation. When you have planned to have any one of these three procedures performed, discuss in advance with your surgeon what you want done if unexpected findings occur. For example, if the surgeon finds adhesions, it may be necessary for the surgeon to terminate the procedure or to perform a regular incision in order to tie your tubes. In rare circumstances, the clinician may find a so-called frozen pelvis, where dense scarring or tubal damage makes tubal sterilization impossible, even through an abdominal incision. In the event that this occurs, you must make it clear in advance whether you want the original procedure stopped or you want to have more extensive surgery done, usually including a hysterectomy.

Table 73 summarizes the important factors concerning the various methods of tubal sterilization.

Concerning future methods of sterilization, the most promising new technology involves surgery using hysteroscopy (see Chapter 13). Presently, the FDA is reviewing the use of the silicon plug (currently marketed in Europe). The plug, along with some silicon, is inserted by means of the hysteroscope into the end of the tube where it opens into the uterus. Hysteroscopy sterilization can be performed in a doctor's office using only local anesthesia. Success rates, however, are still not as good as with traditional sterilization procedures, and some surgeries may need to be repeated. Complication rates

Table 73   COMPARISON OF TUBAL STERILIZATION METHODS

	Laparoscopic Tubal Ligation (Laparoscopy)	Postpartum Tubal Ligation	Mini-laparotomy
Incision	½ inch, inside the navel	1 to 2 inches; inside or just below navel	1 to 2 inches, at or just above pubic hairline (horizontal)
Hospital stay	outpatient	1–2 nights	usually overnight; may be outpatient
Recovery period	24–48 hours	one week	one week
Intercourse may be resumed	24 hours	4–6 weeks	2–3 days
Anesthetic	general; may be local or epidural	general, epidural, or spinal; rarely local	general, spinal, or occasionally local
Major advantages	rapid recovery	same anesthetic as for childbirth may be used; rapid recovery	avoids risks of laparoscopy; may use local anesthesia
Major disadvantages	rarely, serious complications may occur	newborn's subsequent condition cannot be predicted at birth, which may affect sterilization decision	somewhat longer recovery period compared to laparoscopy
Area shaved (if any)	around naval or not at all	around navel or below	only hair over pubic bone

also appear to be somewhat higher for hysteroscopy sterilization. Complications include severe pain in some instances and may include bleeding and infection. Other approaches to sterilization by hysteroscopy include the use of the laser in sealing the tubes (instead of using plugs) and the introduction of chemical agents through the hysteroscope to produce tubal scarring and blockage. These investigational methods are presently under review by the FDA.

Resources

Resources for information on sterilization include the following:

Association for Voluntary Sterilization, Inc.
79 Madison Avenue
New York, New York 10016
(212) 561-8000

This association provides information on sterilization and referrals to qualified specialists.

Planned Parenthood Federation of
    America, Inc.
810 Seventh Avenue
New York, New York 10019
(212) 541–7800

Write for literature on sterilization and the location of the office nearest you if it is not listed in your telephone directory.

Vaginal Tubal Ligation (Colpotomy)	Abdominal Tubal Ligation (Laparotomy)
1 to 2 inches, within the vagina	3 to 4 inches, horizontal or vertical abdominal incision
usually overnight; may be outpatient	2 to 3 nights
1–3 weeks	2–6 weeks
4–6 weeks	2–6 weeks
general or spinal; rarely local	general or spinal
avoids any abdominal incision; alternative if laparoscopy or mini-lap is contraindicated	best visualization of pelvic organs
increased risk of infection	longest recovery period; highest number of complications
pubic hair around vagina	abdominal area of incision

CHAPTER 44

Terminating Pregnancy

This chapter is for the pregnant woman who, after carefully examining her alternatives, chooses to have an abortion. Abortion, the voluntary termination of pregnancy, was legalized by the U.S. Supreme Court in 1973. Since that time, the number of women requesting this procedure has steadily increased while the mortality rate associated with abortion has decreased to less than one death per 30,000 abortions. A woman may choose to have this procedure performed for a variety of reasons involving personal, medical, and other factors. The National Institutes of Health reports that approximately 50% of pregnancy terminations are associated with some form of contraceptive failure. Some women elect abortion when prenatal tests indicate a birth defect but by far the largest number of these procedures occur in association with an "unintended pregnancy," especially among the young, the poor, and the unmarried. In 1991, for example, among the 1.5 million women having abortions that year, 80% were single and 21% were teens.

Emotional Effects of Abortion

Women vary in their emotional reactions to abortion. When abortion is indicated for medical reasons, or after the diagnosis of a birth defect, a woman's grief may understandably be profound. Regardless of the circumstances, however, most women feel varying degrees of ambivalence and emotional distress about the decision. Fortunately, severe depression happens to very few women after a pregnancy termination. Rather, after the initial conflicts, the majority soon return to their previous emotional balance. In fact, some women report a sense of great relief after abortion along with some of the same mixed feelings that went into making the decision. Other women, who experienced abortion as teenagers or as very young women, report that it is only as they became older that they fully realized the emotional effect of their decision. Whatever the reasons for this decision, it is never an easy one to make.

It is normal after an abortion to experience feelings of depression and loss, and women vary in the intensity with which these emotions are felt, depending upon numerous complex factors. It is natural, perhaps even necessary, to feel sad at this time as you adjust to no longer being pregnant. However, it's usually better not to keep such emotions entirely to yourself as this may lead to a sense of isolation and further distress. It may help to share your feelings with a close friend, relative, or counselor who will help you acknowledge and accept these emotions, thereby starting the process of returning to "normal life."

In some circumstances, the emotional aftermath of abortion is more severe. Experience shows that later abortions, especially the saline type, tend to cause more prolonged grieving and other problems such as insomnia or intestinal upsets. Abortion may also be more stressful in the absence of a supportive family or partner, or when the woman feels she was forced because of external circumstances to make the decision to terminate pregnancy. If you feel you may need some help handling the conflicts associated with your abortion, you should seek abortion counseling *before* and *after* termination of pregnancy. Such counseling is usually provided by women's centers and Planned Parenthood centers as part of the overall cost of the procedure. Counseling or referral to a qualified counselor should be available through your clinician if he or she is performing the operation.

Methods of Terminating Pregnancy

Abortion becomes increasingly hazardous with each additional week of pregnancy after the first three months, so it's best to obtain early medical attention. Be sure that the clinical setting you choose (see Chapter 2) has adequate *follow-up care* in case you develop complications later. Women with serious health problems such as diabetes, heart disease, or bleeding disorders should seriously consider having the abortion in a hospital setting, where emergency equipment is immediately available.

When this operation is performed in the first three months of pregnancy, the doctor uses some type of suction (called *suction abortion*) to remove the embryo from the uterine cavity. If the woman is between 13 and 16 weeks pregnant, the operation performed is called *dilatation and evacuation* (D & E), a procedure to dilate the cervix and remove the fetus and placenta. After 16 weeks, most clinicians accomplish abortion by instilling a substance such as saline (a salt solution) into the amniotic sac around the fetus to stimulate labor and delivery (called *instillation abortion*).

Suction abortion, performed in women who are up to 12 weeks pregnant (first trimester), may be performed in a clinic, an office, an ambulatory care facility, or a hospital (usually on an outpatient basis). There are two types: *menstrual extraction* and *vacuum curettage*.

Menstrual extraction is an abortion procedure performed as early as one week after conception but no later than two weeks after a missed period. A woman considering this procedure must obtain a blood pregnancy test to verify pregnancy because a urine test is likely to be negative this early in pregnancy. (A negative blood test means that you are not pregnant and do not need the procedure.) Menstrual extraction, unlike other suction abortion methods, requires little or no dilation of the cervix. You may not need anesthesia if you have been pregnant before. In women with first-time pregnancies, however, injection of a local anesthetic around the cervix (paracervical block) prevents cramping. The physician performs menstrual extraction by placing a soft, flexible tube through the cervix and into the uterine cavity. The free end of the tube is connected to a hand-held syringe which provides suction as the doctor pulls back on it. Since this method has a failure rate of 2.5%, it is important to have a follow-up exam in one to two weeks so the clinician can confirm that you are no longer pregnant. Because of this failure rate, some doctors recommend waiting until seven or eight weeks of pregnancy when a standard suction abortion may be carried out with a failure rate of less than 1%.

Vacuum curettage, the usual method of first trimester abortion (also known as *suction curettage*, or *suction D & C*), is normally performed between 7 and 12 weeks of pregnancy, counting from the first day of your last menstrual period. Either local anesthesia (paracervical block) or general anesthesia is used. If the abortion is done under local anesthesia, the doctor may give you a sedative, such as Valium, a few minutes before the procedure to lessen your anxiety. Almost all women who are awake experience some degree of discomfort from the procedure, depending on how well the block "takes."

First the doctor will swab the vagina with an antiseptic. Shaving the pubic hair is unnecessary and you may specifically request that this be avoided. He or she then places a metal clamp on the cervix to steady the uterus and dilates the cervix using small, blunt, metal rods of progressively increasing diameter (see Figure 39). The cervix can also be dilated by means of laminaria (a kind of small, tubular marine plant); the clinician places a laminaria rod into the cervix the day before surgery and removes it at the time of the operation. The use of laminaria, which have been used widely in Japan and Europe, promotes slow, relatively painless, cervical dilation that results from the unique moisture-absorbing property of these rods that causes them to swell in diameter. After dilation, and removal of the laminaria, the doctor positions a plastic tube through the dilated cervix and attaches its free end to an electric suction pump. The suctioning empties the uterine cavity in three to five minutes. Most surgeons then examine the uterus with a metal instrument called a curette to ensure that no tissue remains. If you desire, the physician will insert an IUD following this abortion procedure. Recent reports indicate that immediate postoperative IUD insertion is safe and effective.

Dilatation and evacuation (D & E) is the procedure of choice between 13 and 16 weeks of pregnancy (second trimester). An abortion after 12 weeks usually involves significantly greater medical risk, emotional distress, and cost compared to procedures performed in the first three months of pregnancy. The physician often orders a sonogram (see Chapter 16) to determine the exact stage of gestation if you are more than 12 weeks by pelvic examination, because the bimanual examination cannot reliably evaluate uterine size after the first three months of pregnancy. D & E is usually performed in the hospital on an outpatient basis. General anesthesia is recommended although some clinics perform this procedure using local anesthesia. Many clinicians insert one or more laminaria rods the day before surgery. Since the cervix must be dilated more than with early abortions, the use of laminaria helps to prevent forceful cervical dilation using instruments that may damage the cervix. Such damage has been linked to subsequent pregnancy complications including an increased risk of premature labor and late miscarriage. The D & E is performed much like the D & C (see Chapter 42) but with special instruments to remove the larger volume of tissue encountered at more advanced stages of pregnancy.

Instillation abortion methods, performed between 16 and 24 weeks of pregnancy, initially involve injection of one of three substances: a salt solution (saline), a drug (prostaglandin), or a chemical compound (urea) into the amniotic fluid sac. To accomplish this, the clinician numbs the skin with a local anesthetic and then inserts a needle through the lower abdomen and *instills* (puts in drop by drop) the substance. Labor pains start within a few hours, and delivery of the fetus occurs from eight to seventy-two hours later (usually within twenty-four hours), so that a one- to two-day hospital stay is not unusual. The physician may shorten the time from instillation to delivery of the fetus by using laminaria to facilitate cervical dilation or by using an intravenous drug called oxytocin to stimulate uterine contractions when saline or urea is used. Delivery of the placenta is delayed in 30% to 40% of instillation abortions. If the afterbirth does not follow the delivery of the fetus within one to two hours, severe bleeding may occur. Therefore, if the doctor cannot manually remove a delayed placenta, he or she may perform a D & C to complete the abortion procedure.

Of the three substances used in instillation abortions, each has its own drawbacks. The saline method may result in fluid retention, making this type of instillation potentially hazardous for women with serious heart or kidney disease. As compared to the saline method, prostaglandin instillation is associated with a higher incidence of nausea, vomiting, and diarrhea, which affects at least 50% of women. No woman with lung disease, such as asthma, should undergo prostaglandin installation, because this hormone may cause spasms of the breathing tubes (bronchi) in the lungs. The urea method has the longest instillation-to-abortion time and thus requires additional drugs (oxytocin or prostaglan-

din), which may pose other risks such as clotting abnormalities. Studies comparing the safety and effectiveness of the instillation methods of abortion are ongoing.

Comparison of D & E with instillation abortion

Instillation abortion poses more risk, greater costs, and more emotional trauma to the woman than does the D & E performed earlier in pregnancy. In the past, women beyond the 12-week cutoff date for standard suction abortions waited until 16 weeks or more when instillation methods became technically feasible to perform. Studies indicate that at 13 to 16 weeks an *immediate* D & E is safer than waiting until 16 weeks to have a saline abortion. D & E lasts only a few minutes and spares the woman several days of hospitalization and the emotional trauma of labor and delivery of the fetus. Also, fewer infections and bleeding complications are associated with D & E as compared to saline instillations. Despite the relative advantages of the D & E, not all physicians are trained to perform this procedure, an important consideration to keep in mind if you are more than 12 weeks along and require an abortion. Find a surgeon experienced in this procedure to lessen the risk of uterine damage, a possible hazard with D & E even in the most skilled hands. *After* 16 weeks of pregnancy, a D & E is no safer than other methods of abortion.

Other methods of second trimester abortion

Older methods of abortion after 12 weeks of pregnancy require major operations through an abdominal incision. These include hysterectomy (removal of the uterus) and hysterotomy, a surgical procedure in which the fetus is delivered through the incision in the uterus. Because of the greater frequency of medical complications, these operations are rarely used today for pregnancy termination.

Another approach utilizes intramuscular injections or vaginal suppositories containing the hormone prostaglandin, which stimulates uterine contractions. Prostaglandin injections cause a high rate of side effects, especially nausea, vomiting, and diarrhea. These reactions are less likely with the suppository form of the drug.

After Your Surgery

Following an abortion, you should expect the mild cramping and slight vaginal bleeding to subside almost completely within an hour. A nurse or another assistant will monitor your pulse, your blood pressure, and your general condition until you are ready to go home. If you are Rh negative, the physician or nurse will administer a small dose of RhoGAM at this time to prevent Rh complications in future pregnancies (see Chapter 20). The physician may prescribe pills to help your uterus contract, antibiotics to prevent infection, or analgesics to lessen pain. If you will be taking birth control pills, ask for the prescription at this time so that you can start taking them one week after your abortion.

Many clinics and physicians provide a checklist of *do's* and *don'ts* during the recovery period following abortion. Some information you will need to know until your follow-up visit in one or two weeks is provided in Table 74.

Your Follow-up Visit

At your follow-up visit, the clinician will examine your uterus, making sure there are no signs of infection or enlargement. At this time, in addition to any questions you may have concerning contraception or future pregnancy, be sure to ask about your pathology report, which is your assurance that pregnancy was successfully terminated. If the report fails to indicate *fetal tissue, products of conception,* or *chorionic villi* (the technical name for microscopic placental tissue), the likeliest explanation is that you still have a uterine pregnancy that was "missed" at the time of your procedure. In such instances, after conferring with the pathologist to make sure nothing was overlooked, the clinician would probably repeat the procedure or first obtain a sonogram to rule out tubal pregnancy (see Figure 51 and Chapter 83).

Complications of Abortions

In general, an abortion is one of the safest procedures in medicine. Most complications are minor. *Major* complications, such as bleeding requiring a transfusion, occur least often for early

Table 74 RECOMMENDATIONS AFTER A PREGNANCY TERMINATION

From the time of your abortion until your follow-up visit in one or two weeks:

1. Know the telephone number of the physician who will be available (or the clinic) if you have a problem.

2. Take your temperature four times a day for about the first three days. Report to your clinician a rise in your temperature to 100.4° or more that occurs at any time before your follow-up visit.

3. Report any of these warning signs to your clinician: heavy bleeding (more than three or four pads in twelve hours), prolonged bleeding (for three days or more), severe abdominal pain, chills, bad-smelling vaginal discharge.

4. Don't douche, use tampons, or have intercourse for two weeks.

5. Follow any specific instructions that may have been given you by your doctor or the clinic or hospital.

suction abortion (0.6%), to a moderate degree for D & E (1%), and most often for instillation methods (2% to 3%).

Table 75 indicates mortality risks for various methods of abortion. The risk of death from early abortion is less than one-tenth the risk of childbirth, while the risk of instillation abortion methods is significantly greater.

Immediate complications

Early complications occurring within the first twenty-four hours of abortion include bleeding, uterine damage, and anesthesia-related problems. Incomplete emptying of the uterus causes bleeding and ultimately requires a D & C in less than 1% of all suction abortions and 10% of second-trimester procedures. Laceration (tearing) of the cervix from the clamp used to steady the uterus is easily treated by a single suture. Uterine perforation (passage of one of the instruments through the uterine wall), a potentially serious injury, occurs two to three times per one thousand abortions, with most patients requiring no more than careful overnight observation in the hospital. Anesthesia complications, though uncommon, can occur, and general anesthesia is just as safe as local anesthesia.

Table 75 MORTALITY RISKS FOR VARIOUS METHODS OF PREGNANCY TERMINATION

Method	No. of Deaths Per 100,000 Cases, 1979–1985
Suction abortions up to 12 weeks	0.5
Dilatation and evacuation (13–15 weeks)	1.8
Instillation methods (saline or prostaglandin—after 15 weeks)	5.8

Delayed complications

The most frequent delayed complications are bleeding and uterine infections. Therefore, you should contact your doctor for these signs of uterine infection: pelvic pain, heavy bleeding, fever (100.4° or more), chills, or foul-smelling vaginal discharge. These symptoms, which may begin several days to two weeks after the abortion procedure, usually respond well to oral antibiotics. If you are not feeling better twenty-four to forty-eight hours after treatment or if bleeding is heavy for several days (strongly suggesting that some tissue still remains inside the uterus), the clinician will perform a D & C. In rare instances, infection following abortion may spread to your tubes and require hospitalization for intravenous antibiotic treatment to prevent serious tubal damage, which could lead to chronic pain or sterility.

Long-term Effects

Future fertility is rarely impaired after pregnancy termination. Most authorities presently agree that a single abortion performed in the first 12 weeks of pregnancy does not threaten future childbearing potential. There is some evidence, however, that *repeat* abortions pose some risk to future child-bearing. A recent World Health Organization study reports that women who underwent two or more abortions had a two- to three-times-greater chance of miscarriage, premature delivery, or low birth weight infant. Considering its possible effects on reproductive potential, abortion as a means of contraception is very undesirable.

RU-486

RU-486, also known as the "abortion pill," has attracted worldwide interest as well as controversy, since it represents a medical alternative to the surgical methods of abortion. RU-486 is a derivative of a synthetic form of the hormone progesterone. The drug was first developed in France in 1982 and marketed there as well as in China since 1988. The drug blocks the action of progesterone, the hormone necessary for allowing the fertilized egg to implant itself into the uterus. In the absence of progesterone, the endometrium breaks down and sloughs as in the normal menstrual period. RU-486 is 95% effective when taken within forty-nine days of a woman's last menstrual period and followed in one to two days by a shot or suppository of a second drug, prostaglandin. Because the dose of prostaglandin is low (much lower than that used in an instillation abortion), side effects such as nausea and vomiting are generally not a problem. The induced period may be heavy and lasts about eleven days. Complication rates with RU-486 appear to be lower than those of abortions performed either by suction D & C or by D & E. RU-486 probably will not be available in the United States for some time due to the political controversy surrounding abortion and the FDA's long and costly drug-approval process.

Resources

For information about abortion services in your area contact your physician or your local county health department, women's center, or Planned Parenthood office. For information about an abortion provider near you, write or call:

National Abortion Federation
1436 U Street, N.W., Suite 103
Washington, D.C. 20009
800–772–9100

CHAPTER 45

Hysterectomy and Its Alternatives

In the past, 50% to 60% of all women in the United States had a hysterectomy at some point in their lifetime. Today 40% of U.S. women age fifty-five and older have had a hysterectomy and nearly one woman in three will have had a hysterectomy by age sixty-five. Hysterectomy is still the second most frequently performed major operation in the United States, although the frequency of this surgery has dropped since the late 1970s. According to the National Center for Health Statistics, the U.S. hysterectomy rate reached an all-time high of 725,000 per year in 1975, but has steadily declined since, with 547,000 of these surgeries performed in 1991. Despite this decline, the United States still has the highest hysterectomy rate in the world at a cost of $6 billion annually. Insurance companies and employers alike are increasingly sensitive about such statistics. One study by Blue Cross/Blue Shield of Illinois in 1990 found one out of three hysterectomies were unnecessary according to criteria established by the insurance company. Consumer groups have drawn attention to other concerns about this surgery, such as reports of immediate complication rates of over 25%. Reported long-term complications include decreased sexual functioning, depression, and pelvic pain. While more data pertaining to hysterectomy and complication rates are needed, a growing consensus, including the authors of this book, believe a significant number of these surgeries must be questioned. On the other hand, quite a number of truly indicated operations involve "quality of life" issues that must be determined by each woman's individual circumstances. This chapter attempts to tell you when hysterectomy is necessary and when you should avoid it and instead select among the various medical and surgical alternatives to it. Being better informed will help you ask crucial questions, evaluate alternatives, and feel more secure in whatever decision you make.

In our culture, the uterus has been seen as a symbol of reproductive ability or as an expression of femininity. The only physiologic function of the uterus, however, is to house the growing fetus during pregnancy. In fact, this operation has major *medical* impact only on the woman of child-bearing age because she will no longer menstruate or be able to conceive. Contrary to popular belief the uterus does not produce hormones, enhance sexual responsiveness, control weight, or prevent hair growth. Consequently, none of these factors are affected by removal of the uterus. However, removing the ovaries (a separate procedure sometimes accompanying a hysterectomy) in premenopausal women may cause temporary hot flashes, which can be prevented by estrogen replacement therapy (see Chapter 27).

Depending on circumstances discussed later in this chapter, the surgeon removes the uterus either through the abdomen or through the vagina. Either method may involve additional surgery. Here are common terms that describe each type of hysterectomy and possible related surgery.

Total abdominal hysterectomy refers to removal of the uterus (and cervix) through an abdominal incision.

Vaginal hysterectomy refers to removal of the uterus (and cervix) through a small incision in the vagina.

Laparoscopic-assisted vaginal hysterectomy (LAVH) and *laparoscopic hysterectomy* refer to new procedures that use a dual approach combining laparoscopy (see Chapter 41) with a modified version of vaginal hysterectomy.

Either total abdominal hysterectomy or vaginal hysterectomy is sometimes also referred to as *simple, incomplete,* or *partial hysterectomy.* Either operation is in reality a total *hysterectomy* since both the uterus and cervix are removed (see Figure 46) in both of these operations.

Bilateral salpingo-oophorectomy refers to removal of both tubes and ovaries and may accompany abdominal hysterectomy. Although the name is technically incorrect, the combination of these two procedures (removal of tubes and ovaries plus removal of the uterus and cer-

vix) is often referred to as *total hysterectomy* (see Figure 46).

Unilateral salpingo-oophorectomy refers to removal of the tube and ovary on one side only.

Radical hysterectomy, an operation performed only for certain pelvic cancers, refers to extended hysterectomy, which includes removal of the uterus (along with the cervix) and upper vagina as well as the adjacent pelvic lymph nodes.

Regardless of the approach (abdominal or vaginal), the surgeon detaches the uterus from the Fallopian tubes and ovaries and from the upper vagina. The ovaries and Fallopian tubes remain basically in the same location as before hysterectomy since they retain their attachment to the pelvic side wall after this operation. The surgeon then closes the vaginal opening from which the uterus was detached, restoring the vagina to its original shape and position. The intestines then fill in the space where the uterus was.

Whether or not the surgeon removes your ovaries during hysterectomy depends largely upon your age, family history, and the condition of your ovaries. You should especially consider having your ovaries removed if you have a strong family history (involving two close relatives such as a mother and sister) of breast or ovarian cancer. If you do have your ovaries removed before age fifty, you will need to take the hormone estrogen, which protects against the development of osteoporosis and heart disease.

Many gynecologists routinely recommend removal of both ovaries if hysterectomy is performed after the age of forty-five. However, this approach is now being reconsidered. Current research shows that premenopausal women who have their ovaries removed and cannot tolerate or who do not take replacement estrogen face greater risks of heart disease than they would of dying from ovarian cancer. For this reason some women having a hysterectomy while in their forties are electing not to have the ovaries removed unless there are medical indications, such as endometriosis or chronic pelvic pain. In such instances it may be preferable to remove the ovaries if they are damaged at all because pelvic pain may be a subsequent problem. In fact, recurrent pelvic pain accounts for 80% of all subsequent operations to remove ovaries that were left in at the time of hysterectomy. It is important to discuss all of these considerations in advance with your surgeon.

Abdominal Hysterectomy

Abdominal hysterectomy, which is accomplished through a regular incision in the lower abdomen, allows the surgeon better visualization of the pelvic organs and greater operating space than a vaginal hysterectomy. Therefore, if you have a large pelvic tumor or a suspected malignancy, your doctor may use this approach. The main disadvantages of abdominal hysterectomy compared to the vaginal approach are greater immediate postoperative discomfort, the presence of a visible scar, and a slightly longer hospital stay. Usually the surgeon can make a horizontal (so-called bikini) incision, which extends across the top of the pubic hairline. This incision is less noticeable than a vertical one which goes from below the navel to the top of the pubic bone.

Vaginal Hysterectomy and Laparoscopic-Assisted Vaginal Hysterectomy

Compared to abdominal hysterectomy, vaginal hysterectomy is technically more difficult because of the limited space in which the surgeon has to operate. This approach is ideal when the uterus is not enlarged or when the uterus has "dropped" as a result of the weakening of surrounding muscles and ligaments (see Chapter 28). Often, vaginal surgery to repair a cystocele or rectocele (see glossary) can be done at the time of vaginal hysterectomy. A variation on vaginal hysterectomy, laparoscopic-assisted vaginal hysterectomy (LAVH), is a new alternative for patients who usually have ovarian disease but previously could be offered only an abdominal hysterectomy with its long incision. With LAVH, ovarian abnormalities like endometriosis or pelvic adhesions are first removed through tiny incisions using laparoscopy. Then, depending on the technique used, the upper attachments to the uterus are next released. Finally, the remaining surgery is done from below, through the vagina, just like a vaginal hysterectomy.

Indications for Hysterectomy

Urgent indications for hysterectomy may include pelvic cancers, severe pelvic infections, or un-

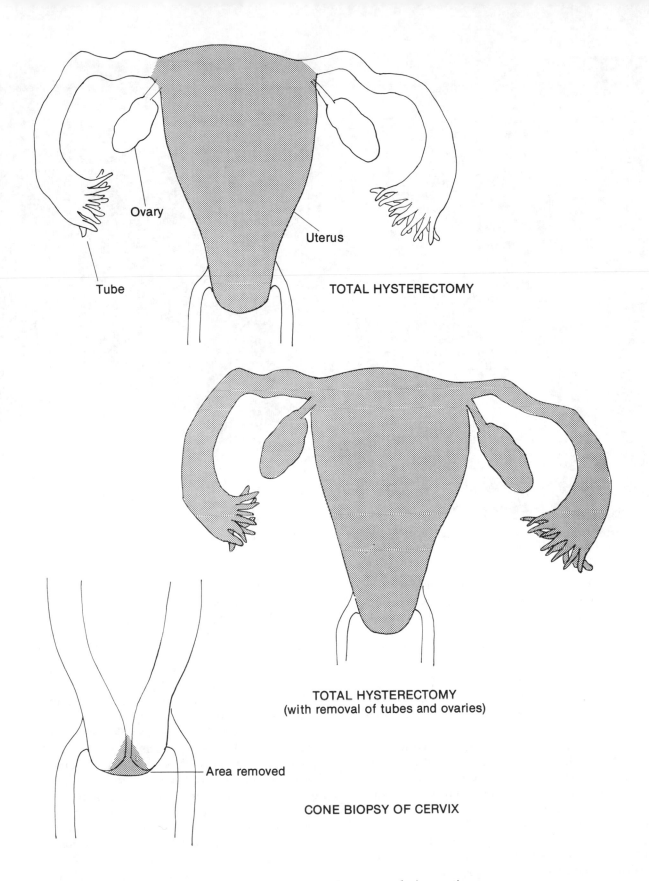

Ovary

Uterus

Tube

TOTAL HYSTERECTOMY

TOTAL HYSTERECTOMY
(with removal of tubes and ovaries)

Area removed

CONE BIOPSY OF CERVIX

Figure 46 *The shaded areas show what is removed in different gynecologic operations.*

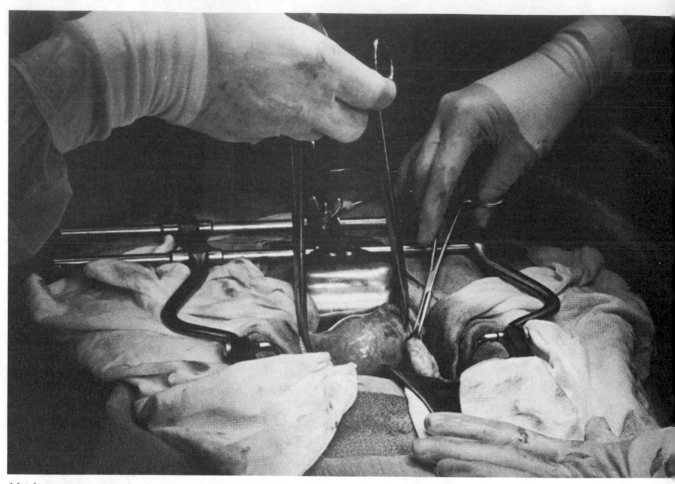

Metal retractors are used to keep an abdominal incision spread apart to provide the necessary exposure for surgery. The uterus can be seen in the center of the operating field.

controllable bleeding. In these instances, a hysterectomy may be lifesaving. Most often, however, the timing of hysterectomy depends upon the severity of your symptoms. Table 76 indicates conditions which may require hysterectomy and possible alternative therapy. Remember that pelvic pain and vaginal bleeding—the most common symptoms leading to hysterectomy—do not necessarily mean that something is wrong with your uterus or that you need this surgery. For instance, scar tissue from a condition like endometriosis may be removed through a relatively minor procedure, laparoscopy (see Chapter 13), which may relieve pain while preserving fertility. The term *female reconstructive surgery* has been applied to the many operations, like laparoscopy, which provide viable alternatives to hysterectomy, a far more radical procedure. For example, bleeding prob-

lems, which account for 40% of hysterectomies, may now be treated by a new outpatient technique called *endometrial ablation*. In this procedure, the lining of the uterus (endometrium) is cauterized or burned using a laser inserted through the cervix. The instrument through which the laser is inserted is called a *hysteroscope*. The scar tissue formed within the uterine lining from this procedure stops periods altogether in 50% of patients and reduces the bleeding in another 40%. At this time, relatively few gynecologists are familiar with endometrial ablation. The technique has not been as popular as other newer procedures, partly because hysterectomy is essentially 100% effective in treating abnormal uterine bleeding. Complications of endometrial ablation include perforation of the uterus as well as bleeding problems. For more information on the conditions requiring and alterna-

Table 76   CONDITIONS THAT MAY REQUIRE HYSTERECTOMY

Condition	When to Consider Hysterectomy	Alternative Therapy
Fibroids	• persistent, heavy menstrual bleeding, especially if severe anemia is present or if childbearing is not desired. • fibroid growth • fibroids greater than 12-weeks size	• myomectomy (surgical removal of fibroid tumor only) • hysteroscopy (if fibroid is inside uterine cavity) • stopping all estrogen medication, including the pill • iron for anemia due to blood loss • hormone therapy (Lupron—see Chapter 35).
Bleeding problems	• lack of response to alternative therapy, especially if severe anemia is present or if childbearing is not desired	• hormones (e.g., progesterone, the pill) • antibiotics for uterine infection • IUD removal • D & C or endometrial biopsy • endometrial ablation (hysteroscopy— see Chapter 41)
Uterine prolapse ("dropped uterus")	• persistent or severe pelvic pain, pressure, or backache after other causes have been ruled out • if surgery for urinary incontinence (e.g., bladder surgery) is planned and childbearing is not desired	• pessary (see glossary)
Carcinoma-in-situ (CIS) or severe dysplasia	• hysterectomy may be recommended for CIS if childbearing is not desired	• cone biopsy or "LEEP" surgery (see Chapter 37)
Cancer of uterus, ovary, or cervix	• hysterectomy is recommended unless radiation or chemotherapy is treatment of choice	• often none (radiation or chemotherapy in select cases)
Pelvic inflammatory disease (tube or ovary infections)	• if chronic pelvic pain or infection persists, especially if future childbearing is unwanted or is prevented by this disease	• antibiotics • conservative surgery (e.g., remove adhesions or one tube and ovary; tubal microsurgery if tube(s) are preserved and pregnancy is desired)
Endometriosis	• if chronic pelvic pain persists, especially if future childbearing is unwanted or is prevented by this disease	• hormones (e.g., progesterone, the pill, LH agonists—see Chapter 36) • conservative surgery to remove only endometriosis deposits and adhesions (see Chapter 36)
Desire for sterilization	• if any of the above conditions are present	• tubal sterilization or vasectomy

tives to hysterectomy, see Table 76 or refer to the index about the specific item in question.

When to Avoid Hysterectomy

Second opinion programs and greater consumer awareness about the risks of major surgery have reduced the number of unnecessary hysterectomies in recent years. One difficulty in deciding whether to have this operation is that the patient herself must supply some of the input as to the reasons for having it (for example, pain, bleeding) and must also consider the expected benefits to be derived. Truly informed consent (discussed in Chapter 41) is all-important: Will your pain be relieved? Will sexual enjoyment increase? Will you have more energy and more time free of disabling symptoms? The answers will most often be a qualified yes. In other words, there are a good many instances when

Table 77   CONDITIONS THAT DO NOT JUSTIFY HYSTERECTOMY

Avoid hysterectomy . . .	Because . . .	Unless . . .
to "prevent" cancer	the risks of surgery outweigh any so-called preventive benefits	you already have precancerous changes of the cervix (severe dysplasia) or uterus (atypical endometrial hyperplasia) (see Chapters 37 and 40)
for sterilization	the risks of hysterectomy surgery are much higher than for tubal sterilization or vasectomy	you also have one of the conditions named in Table 76 and hysterectomy is the treatment of choice
for bleeding problems if a D & C or endometrial biopsy is not done first	a uterine cancer requiring different treatment may be diagnosed	
for a "dropped" bladder or uterus if you have little or no discomfort or other symptoms	there is no indication for surgery	
for pelvic pain without a definite diagnosis	the pain may not be relieved by hysterectomy	diagnostic tests are first done, possibly including X-rays and laparoscopy (see Chapter 83)

the results of this surgery cannot be fully determined in advance.

There are, however, specific instances when you should avoid or delay having this operation. For example, to have a hysterectomy to prevent cancer of the cervix or uterus (in the absence of risk factors) makes no sense because the risks of having this major surgery outweigh the so-called cancer-protection benefits. Similarly, hysterectomy is not considered the first choice for sterilization in most healthy women. One of the tubal ligation operations (or vasectomy) is cheaper, easier, and safer unless other gynecologic conditions are present. At other times, hysterectomy may be premature if your problem has not had adequate diagnostic evaluation. Pelvic pain, for example, may be due to conditions involving the urinary tract, skeletal system, or digestive system; but you won't know unless appropriate tests and X-rays have ruled out these possibilities (see Chapter 83). Even then, a diagnostic laparoscopy may identify a problem that can be solved with surgery short of hysterectomy. To name another example: hysterectomy should be avoided in a postmenopausal woman with bleeding until after a D & C (see Chapter 42) is first done. The D & C might indicate the need for therapy different from hysterectomy or might itself be sufficient therapy. Finally, medical conditions such as obesity, high blood pressure, and diabetes increase the risk of any major surgery, including hysterectomy. For

this reason alone, some women should avoid exposure to such risks unless strong indications for hysterectomy warrant it (see Table 76). These and other examples of when to avoid hysterectomy are summarized in Table 77.

Deciding About Hysterectomy

Your decision regarding hysterectomy must take into account both the severity of the problem and your desire for future children. Although hysterectomy may improve your quality of life by relieving chronic symptoms such as pain or bleeding, where there is a choice some women are willing to tolerate these symptoms instead of having surgery. When deciding whether or not to have a hysterectomy, here are essential questions to ask your doctor:

1. Is alternative therapy available? If not, what will happen if I don't have a hysterectomy? If so, is alternative therapy likely to cure the problem or will relief be only temporary?
2. If alternative therapy includes conservative surgery short of hysterectomy, what are my chances of needing hysterectomy later?
3. What are the risks of alternative therapy and of hysterectomy?
4. If I want to become pregnant, is it possible or safe to get pregnant?

5. Is this condition likely to improve on its own or get worse?
6. Is hysterectomy *medically necessary* or is it *recommended* to relieve my symptoms?

Here are some questions to ask yourself and to discuss with your husband or partner before you decide on elective hysterectomy:

1. Do I want to become pregnant in the future?
2. What are my feelings about my no longer having a uterus?
3. How will my job and life style be affected by a major operation at this time?
4. What is my husband's or partner's attitude about this surgery?

Risks of Hysterectomy

Although hysterectomy is one of the safest operations, no major surgery is without some risk. Fever and infection, the most frequent of the complications of hysterectomy, occur more often with vaginal hysterectomies. Infection usually involves the bladder or upper vagina and almost always responds promptly to antibiotic therapy. Serious complications such as blood clots or severe bleeding occur less than one percent of the time. Damage to other organs such as the intestines or bladder also occurs infrequently and is usually repaired at surgery. Such injuries may prolong your stay in the hospital, however. Mortality from hysterectomy is related to your general condition and the reason for having surgery. Overall, approximately one death occurs for every two thousand hysterectomy operations. This frequency is considerably lower for women without chronic health problems such as heart disease or high blood pressure.

Recovering from Hysterectomy

In the past most women stayed in the hospital for four to six days following a hysterectomy. Now, with pressure from insurance companies and others paying health care bills to reduce hospital costs, postoperative stays are becoming shorter. Now, many patients go home by the third day after abdominal hysterectomy and by the first or second day after either vaginal hysterectomy or laparoscopic-assisted vaginal hys-

terectomy. The vaginal procedures involve less postoperative pain, quicker recovery, and the shortest possible hospital stay compared to the traditional abdominal operation.

Complete recovery from abdominal hysterectomy or other major abdominal surgery in which a regular five-inch ("laparotomy") incision is used usually takes up to six to eight weeks, with a gradual increase in activities as follows: during the first two weeks at home, get plenty of rest and do only the simplest tasks which require little or no lifting. You will probably feel tired, perhaps more so than you expected. It is generally safe to climb stairs, shower, and wash your hair. In the third and fourth weeks following surgery, you can gradually increase your activities, including light chores and driving; and if you work outside the home you may consider returning to your job part-time as long as heavy lifting is avoided. In the fifth and sixth postoperative weeks, you may gradually return to your preoperative activities, except for vigorous exercise. By the sixth week, and sometimes before, you may take tub baths and resume sexual activity.

The time required to recover from surgery varies from individual to individual. Because of this fact and the difficulty in forecasting how you will feel, schedule your postoperative checkup no later than four weeks after surgery. If you have any questions about your activity limitations, call your physician before this checkup. Most women can return to work by the sixth week after surgery and often earlier. You may, however, want initially to resume work half-time, especially if heavy lifting or strenuous activity is part of your job.

Long-term Effects of Hysterectomy

Many misconceptions and unnecessary fears surround the subject of hysterectomy and its possible effects—hormonal, sexual, and emotional. Following hysterectomy, a woman will not go through the menopause any sooner than nature intended unless both ovaries are removed, because hysterectomy alone causes no change in hormone levels. Surgical removal of both ovaries in women who have not reached menopause usually causes hot flashes, which can be prevented with estrogen replacement therapy (see Chapter 27). You will not need hormone replacement if one ovary is preserved, because one ovary functions well enough for two. Removal of the ovaries in women already past menopause will not cause hot flashes or other menopause symptoms.

Some women report fatigue, insomnia, and weight gain following a hysterectomy, but research has not supported a causal connection between these symptoms and this surgery. Decreased sexual desire, less intense orgasms, and slower arousal have also been reported. The loss of uterine contractions during orgasm may reduce sexual pleasure for some women. For most women, however, hysterectomy, with or without removal of the ovaries, has not been associated with these symptoms. For many, relief from fear of pregnancy results in heightened sexual enjoyment following hysterectomy. Vaginal dryness, which may occur following removal of the ovaries, can be relieved by estrogen pills or creams or by using a water-soluble lubricant like K-Y lubricating jelly. Occasionally, hysterectomy shortens vaginal length and results in slight discomfort during intercourse.

The emotional impact of hysterectomy, like that of other major operations, depends on the woman's preparation, the nature of the problem requiring surgery, and the support of friends and family. As with the surgical removal of any organ, it is normal to go through an adjustment period and to experience feelings of loss. The adjustment to hysterectomy, however, is often more difficult. It is encouraging to note that in a carefully designed study by Coppen and others, sixty women who underwent hysterectomy experienced an improvement of mood and a general sense of well-being following this surgery (see reference list at the end of this section). However, most older studies show that twice as many individuals are likely to experience serious depression following hysterectomy as compared to other forms of surgery. Such depression is more likely when the woman is younger than forty or if the condition requiring hysterectomy interfered with desired childbearing (for example, pelvic infection leading to sterility). Depression is also more common when the operation is performed for a serious disease (such as cancer) or if a woman feels she had little choice in making this decision (in an emergency, for instance). Don't hesitate to seek help from friends, other women who have undergone hysterectomy, your clinician, or a counselor if depression seems prolonged. Even the woman who is well prepared for hysterectomy and accepts the necessity for the surgery may experience some mental stress. However, women who have reacted to previous stress with positive efforts—recognition that feelings of loss are temporary, discussion of feelings with friends, realization of worthwhile results from surgery—may expect to respond similarly to hysterectomy.

CHAPTER 46

Cosmetic Surgery

As women age, they must come to terms with their changing appearance and with others' reactions to it. We live in a society in which the media emphasize youthful beauty and overwhelm us with advertisements for hair dyes, face-lifts, diets, and fashions that emphasize a youth-oriented ideal. Men are often depicted as aging more attractively than women. For many women, especially those whose self-esteem is closely allied with their physical beauty, looking older may be very difficult. Women may experience a concern about looking older starting in their late thirties, even though they may like the experience of being older (feeling more confident and independent and valuing their inner qualities more). Body changes resulting from health problems may be a concern. These issues may lead women to consider plastic surgery.

A growing number of cosmetic procedures are being performed today. Annually, more than half a million people in the United States have some type of plastic surgery. Unfortunately, this is a medical area subject to an increasing amount of sophisticated Madison Avenue–consumer-oriented advertising. As in ads for weight loss, such marketing often finds its way into print ads in local newspapers and magazines. So be cautious. Some points to keep in mind if you are considering cosmetic surgery are listed at the end of this chapter.

Plastic and reconstructive surgery is a surgi-

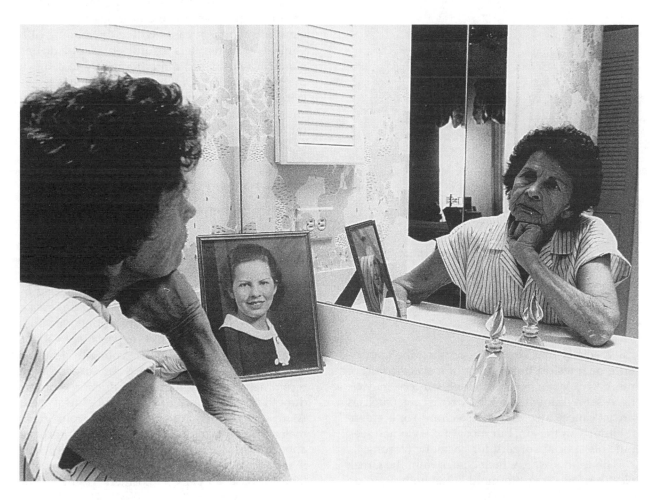

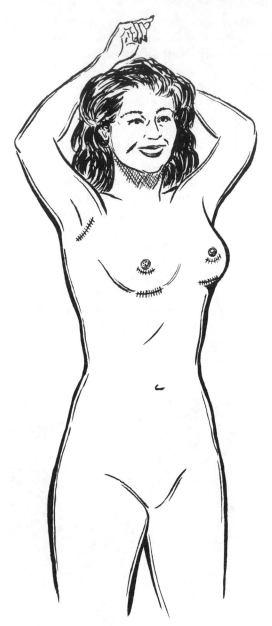

Figure 47
The three possible surgical approaches to breast augmentation (breast enlargement): peri-areolar (incision under nipple), axillary (incision in armpit), inframammary (incision under breast).

cal specialty that aims at improving the appearance or physical functioning of a specific part of the body. Major reconstructive surgery may be necessary following injury or disease (such as breast cancer treated by mastectomy) or accidental injury on the job, but most often, women seek out this special surgery for cosmetic reasons.

The term *plastic*, which comes from the Greek *plastikos*, meaning "to mold," has nothing to do with the type of synthetic materials used in plastic surgery today. Plastic surgeons use the same techniques basic to other surgical specialties but place much more emphasis on the healing process to keep scar tissue to a minimum. A plastic surgeon must know just how much tissue stretching or suture-line tension is enough to create the desired result. And while some scar tissue will always be left behind, a good plastic surgeon will know where and how to place an incision so that the skin heals in the least noticeable way. Incisions are placed in natural laugh lines, pre-existing wrinkle lines (such as in front of the ear), or in lines of expression, shadow areas, or hair-bearing areas such as the scalp, where scars may be easily concealed. More involved plastic procedures, such as breast reconstruction, may require some rearrangement of tissue, which may be removed from one area of the body and grafted onto another. In such grafting involving soft tissue, all of the tissue must come from the patient's own body. This prevents rejection as well as the need for the potent immunity-suppressing medications used in organ transplants. In cases where the amount of a patient's own tissue is insufficient, synthetic implants are now used quite frequently to achieve the desired result. One example is the use of silicone implants for chin and cheek enlargements and a combination of silicone and saline breast implants for breast enlargement.

Some of the more commonly performed cosmetic surgeries are discussed below.

Breast Augmentation (Breast Enlargement)

This is one of the more popular procedures among women having cosmetic surgery. Breast augmentation may be considered to enlarge small breasts or breasts that have diminished in size after childbearing, or to correct a difference in breast size. If you are considering this surgery, be sure to discuss expectations about breast contour and size with your physician. If breast sagging is a problem, your surgeon may recommend an additional "reduction" procedure to reshape and reduce breast tissue as well. As in any cosmetic operation, keep your goals realistic. Breast augmentation usually improves appearance and can renew self-confidence, but it won't change your personal or professional life. Likewise, a "perfect" cosmetic result cannot be relied upon—the final outcome can be somewhat variable, depending upon your anatomy and your surgeon's ability and technique.

There are three possible incisions used in breast augmentation. Regardless of which type a woman chooses, the procedure involves first developing a pocket either directly under the breast or under the chest-wall muscle. Then, an implant or prosthesis is placed into the pocket.

The peri-areolar approach

This approach uses a semicircular incision made under the nipple, usually just within the darker pigmented area of the nipple line. The advantage of this technique is the inconspicuous scar in most cases. Disadvantages include the necessity of damaging some of the milk ducts, which may affect breast-feeding; and possible loss of some sensation as a result of interruption of sensory nerves to the nipples. Also, if the scar becomes thicker in this area, it may be more obvious.

The axillary approach

This approach is a popular technique which, when successful, results in the least noticeable incision of all, as it is located in the armpit. However, scars in the armpit can be troublesome and sometimes visible. The surgeon's view is more limited in this procedure. If another procedure becomes necessary due to a complication, this approach may require an inframammary incision (see below), leaving the patient with two scars.

The inframammary approach

This approach is the one most frequently used today and offers avoidance of injury to the sensory nerves. The biggest disadvantage of the inframammary approach is that the scar is relatively visible under the breast crease. In most patients, however, the scar becomes less conspicuous with time and is not very troublesome.

The risks of breast augmentation are relatively few. The most important risk, perhaps, is that hardening or "capsulization" may occur, causing the tissue around the implant to become scarred and hardened. Loss of nipple sensitivity also may occur, but some sensation usually returns. This breast surgery may make cancer detection slightly more difficult, and until radiolucent breast implants are developed, patients having mammograms should have an additional "pinch" view taken in which the breast tissue is pulled forward while the implant is displaced against the chest wall. The principal ingredient in many breast implants—silicone—became the focus of considerable media attention in 1995, when three drug companies agreed to pay $4 billion to women who had problems with silicone implants. Some women and clinicians have claimed these devices can cause medical problems, including autoimmune disorders such as rheumatoid arthritis and lupus erythematosus. However, most research, including two studies reported in 1995 at the annual meeting of the American College of Rheumatology, cast considerable doubt on this theory. The great majority of women with silicone implants have had no problems. Women who have these implants and have concerns or who are considering breast implants in the future should discuss the subject with their plastic surgeon.

Mastopexy (Breast-Lift)

In situations where excessive sagging of the breasts is present, the breast implant is usually not a good choice. In such women, where the level of the nipple sags below the breast crease, the operation of choice is a *mastopexy* or breast-lift. This procedure is designed to preserve all the underlying breast tissue and results in a fuller, more compact breast situated back on the chest wall, with the nipple elevated into a normal position. Mastopexy is more involved than breast enlargement and leaves a more prominent scar, although the scars generally fade within a year or two.

Reduction Mammoplasty (Breast Reduction)

Reduction mammoplasty is generally the operation of choice in women who have massively enlarged breasts and require removal of ten ounces or more of breast tissue on each side. This operation is generally performed for discomfort, such as shoulder and back pain caused by excessively heavy breasts, but in some cases

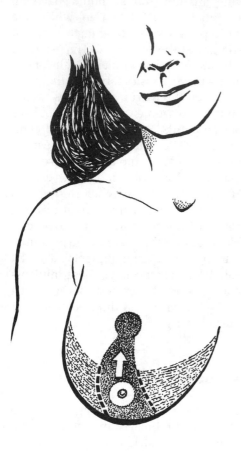

Figure 48
Reduction mammoplasty (breast reduction). Excess breast tissue in shaded area is removed and nipple is repositioned.

it may be considered for cosmetic purposes. Reduction mammoplasty is usually performed in a hospital under general anesthesia and is technically more involved than breast enlargement. However, the risks of infection and the need for a second operation for scar revision are fairly low, especially if postoperative instructions are followed closely. Reduction mammoplasty scars are much more conspicuous than those from breast enlargement, but the improvement in symptoms and appearance is generally worth it. The ability to breast-feed after reduction mammoplasty is unpredictable, a factor that must be borne in mind by women who have not completed their families. Unlike most cosmetic surgeries, reduction mammoplasty may be covered in part by insurance if the surgery is done for symptomatic relief as opposed to cosmetic reasons.

Other than the operations listed above, most surgeries for cosmetic improvement of the breast may have little value and can be downright hazardous. For example, free injection of fat and silicon is not only ineffective, but may also result in catastrophic complications and irreversible deformities. The recovery time for most breast surgery is several weeks. As a rule, rapid and stressful arm activities should be avoided in the first two weeks after surgery. Strenuous activities such as aerobic dance, tennis, and jogging should not be attempted for at least six to eight weeks.

Breast Reconstruction

Twenty years ago, a request for surgical breast reconstruction after mastectomy was considered unusual. Many women were instead fitted with an external breast prosthesis. Today, breast reconstruction has become a major part of the overall care of patients having a mastectomy or other breast surgery for cancer. Breast reconstruction is a rewarding experience for most women who need it. However, realistic expectations of what is involved are important, as two to three operations over the course of several months may be required to obtain the best results.

Breast reconstruction can be performed at the time of the mastectomy or at a later date. Most women choose to have it done following their initial surgery in order to allow time to consider the various procedures available. These procedures depend considerably upon a woman's anatomy and the extent of her initial surgery. Also, she may wish to select a plastic surgeon to do the reconstructive procedure, as the general surgeon who performs the initial surgery is often not trained in many of the cosmetic techniques used in breast reconstruction. Finally, a woman who waits before having this surgery allows for time to complete any radiation therapy or chemotherapy that may interfere with the more extensive wound healing often involved in cosmetic procedures.

The simplest procedures involve inserting silicon implants underneath the chest-wall muscle as is done in breast-enlargement operations. This procedure can be performed after lumpectomy, simple mastectomy, or even following modified mastectomy.

A more involved procedure for patients who need more soft tissue for reconstruction of the breast involves the use of a *tissue expander*. This device is a specialized envelope containing a silicon implant with an attached valve that extends to the outside of the body. Over several weeks, a sterile salt solution is gradually added to the tissue expander. This causes the overlying skin to stretch, and under this tension, new cell growth occurs and new skin tissue is created. Then, in a subsequent operation, the surgeon inserts a larger silicon implant than was possible formerly.

The most complex operations for breast reconstruction, which are used when maximal soft tissue is required, involve the use of tissue "flaps"—portions of skin, fatty tissue, and underlying muscle from nearby areas, including the upper back, abdomen, or buttocks. When transferred to the chest area, these large flaps of tissue usually appear very natural and heal well. However, complications, such as infections, wound breakdown, and scarring around the implant, sometimes occur.

An additional step in the process of breast reconstruction—such as a breast-lift or reduction of the opposite breast—is often needed to make the breasts symmetric. Finally, nipples can be reconstructed as a separate procedure from grafts of skin taken from the inner thigh or by sharing nipple tissue from the opposite breast. When all the stages of reconstruction are complete, the results are generally quite satisfactory, and most women report an enhanced body image.

Eyelid Surgery (Blepharoplasty)

Blepharoplasty, one of the simpler and more common plastic procedures, involves removal of excessive skin and fat tissue from the upper and lower eyelids. Sagging upper eyelids and lower-lid fullness are markedly improved by this procedure, which usually leaves imperceptible hairline scars. Uncommon complications may include difficulty closing the eyes or dry eyes. Blepharoplasty generally takes less than two hours. Skin bruising around the eyelids, which lasts up to fourteen days, may be dealt with by applying cosmetics. Blepharoplasty can usually be performed under local anesthesia on an outpatient basis.

Abdominoplasty

The abdominoplasty or "tummy tuck" is a procedure used to remove excess wrinkled skin and fatty tissue from the mid and lower abdomen. The result is usually a flattened lower abdomen from which excess skin has been removed. In addition, the abdominal muscles are strengthened.

This procedure best suits patients who have lost as much weight as possible. It is not a substitute for weight loss. Unlike many other cosmetic procedures, abdominoplasty sometimes requires two to three days in the hospital. The

Figure 49
The incision used for an abdominoplasty ("tummy tuck"). Following removal of excess skin from the lower abdomen, the navel is reconstructed.

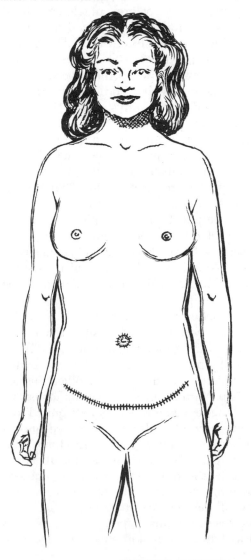

rather long incision for this surgery extends from hip to hip horizontally across the lower abdomen, just above the pubic hairline. During the procedure, the navel is essentially relocated as a result of excising the excess abdominal skin. This surgery, which requires a general anesthetic, is an extensive one, and dissection extends all the way to the rib margins, creating considerable postoperative discomfort in some patients. Another concern is that the navel may occasionally be slightly misplaced. Serious complications such as infection and blood clots are uncommon.

Liposuction (Suction-Assisted Lipectomy)

Liposuction is one cosmetic procedure about which the wise consumer must be wary. Although liposuction has enjoyed wide popularity, disturbing reports of preventable complications and deaths continue to be noted in the media. According to a task force of the American Society of Plastic and Reconstructive Surgeons, risks are more common when the procedure is used in conjunction with "body sculpturing" procedures and if the physician is inadequately trained in the technique.

Liposuction is a procedure for removing diet- and exercise-resistant fat deposits. The procedure is not a substitute for weight reduction. It is designed to remove localized fat from hips, buttocks, thighs, the lower abdomen, and other areas. Complications such as infection or collections of blood are uncommon with experienced physicians. More serious complications may include blood clots and fat embolism, a situation in which fat blocks the flow of blood to the heart, brain, or lungs.

Liposuction begins with a ½-inch incision in the area where the fat deposit is located. Then, using a blunt, tubular instrument, the fat is removed by mechanical disruption and suctioned under high vacuum pressure. When this operation is performed in the lower abdomen, wearing a long-legged girdle may be required for two to three months afterwards to enhance skin shrinkage. However, suction lipectomy will not flatten your stomach if excessive skin is present, in which case abdominoplasty is also necessary. Following liposuction, there may be some rippling of the skin or an uneven effect, and in some cases, sagging. Liposuction is more likely to leave an uneven skin effect in older persons,

who generally have less skin elasticity. In such cases, the excessive skin may need to be removed by a second procedure. With liposuction, as with any cosmetic surgery you are considering, it's a good idea to ask your surgeon how much experience he has had with the operation and to obtain more than one opinion.

Face-Lift (Rhytidectomy)

The face-lift has become one of the most popular elective surgeries in the United States, especially among women. This surgery is intended to remove excess or sagging skin from the face and neck. Face-lifts are most commonly performed on women in their forties and early fifties, although it is not uncommon for either younger or older individuals to request this procedure. A face-lift can help make a woman look good for her age, but it won't change your basic looks or make you look as much as twenty years younger. Maintaining good health habits, such as eating properly and not smoking, improve the results of this operation, but the outcome also depends on the elasticity of your skin, a partly hereditary characteristic. For most women, the benefits of this surgery will last up to ten years, after which time your face will again begin to show effects of aging.

The face-lift procedure can have many variations, from the standard lift, which involves elevating flaps of skin in front of the ears and sides of the neck, to incorporation of the scalp

Figure 50
Face-lift incisions are located in less noticeable hairline areas as much as possible.

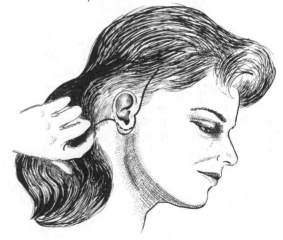

lift and lifts under the chin. Other additions to the face-lift include tightening of sagging muscle and connective tissue, and liposuction to remove excess fat along the sides of the face and neck. Most face-lifts are performed in conjunction with the blepharoplasty procedure (see above).

Serious complications, while uncommon, can include blood clots, facial nerve damage, and infection. The operation may be performed under local or general anesthesia, and recovery requires about six weeks before your "new face" can emerge without the bruising and swelling that normally accompanies this surgery. Scars from a face-lift are generally inconspicuous and fade with time or are located within hairline areas.

If you are considering plastic surgery, keep the following points in mind:

1. Keep your goals realistic, and discuss them with your physician. Be sure you know what risks the surgery involves.
2. Mention any medical problems to your physician. Certain problems, such as diabetes or bleeding disorders, may be of special importance for wound healing.
3. Discuss any medication you are taking with your doctor; medications containing aspirin and some anti-inflammatory drugs used for menstrual cramps may prolong bleeding and affect scar healing.
4. Know your insurance coverage. Most companies don't cover cosmetic surgery, so be prepared to write a check or pull out a credit card.
5. Most importantly, obtain more than one opinion before selecting a plastic surgeon. A useful resource is the American Society of Reconstructive and Plastic Surgery (800-635-0635).

References for Section Nine

Chapter 41—Deciding About Surgery

American College of Obstetricians and Gynecologists Technical Bulletin 146. Laser technology, Sep 1990.

American College of Obstetricians and Gynecologists, Committee on ethics, Committee Opinion 108. Ethical dimensions of informed consent, May 1992.

Park, R. Confronting troublesome GYN surgery trends. Contemporary OB/GYN 83–97, Sep 1994.

Feste, J. The laser in gynecologic procedures: advantages and pitfalls. The Female Patient 14:69–82, Jan 1989.

Richart, R. Using the carbon dioxide laser for genital surgery. Contemporary OB/GYN 34(1):106–141, July 1989.

Lomano, J. Laser hysteroscopy: new benefits, new risks. Contemporary OB/GYN 32(2):71–83, Aug 1988.

Nezhat, C. Video laparoscopy and video laseroscopy—alternatives to surgery? The Female Patient: 46–56, Sep 1988.

Carson, S. Operative hysteroscopy. Contemporary OB/GYN Special Issue 34:35–52, June 1989.

Johns, A. Consider the laparoscope for an ectopic gestation. Contemporary OB/GYN Special Issue 34:67–78, June 1989.

Vietz, P. The value of pelviscopic myomectomy. Contemporary OB/GYN Special Issue 34:105–110, June 1989.

Chapter 42—Dilatation and Curettage

American College of Obstetricians and Gynecologists Technical Bulletin 191. Hysteroscopy, Apr 1994.

Gimpelson, R. A comparative study between panoramic hysteroscopy with directed biopsies in dilatation and curettage: a review of 276 cases. American Journal of Obstetrics and Gynecology 158: 489–492, 1988.

Grimes, D. Diagnostic office curettage—heresy no longer. Contemporary OB/GYN 96–103, Jan 1986.

Chapter 43—Sterilization Options

American College of Obstetricians and Gynecologists, Committee on obstetrics: maternal and fetal medicine, Committee Opinion 105. Postpartum tubal sterilization, Mar 1992.

American College of Obstetricians and Gynecologists, Technical Bulletin 113. Sterilization, Feb 1988.

Rioux, J. Sterilization revisited. Contemporary OB/GYN 80–104, Aug 1987.

Pritchard, J. Williams Obstetrics, 17th ed. New York: Appleton-Century-Crofts, 1985.

Chapter 44—Terminating Pregnancy

Aguillaume, C. Current status and future projections on use of RU-486. Contemporary OB/GYN 23–40, June 1995.

American College of Obstetricians and Gynecologists *Technical Bulletin 109*. Methods of midtrimester abortion, Oct 1987.

Machol, L. Adoption services for your pregnant patient. *Contemporary OB/GYN* 33(3):114–126, Mar 1989.

Rosenfield, A. RU-486 and the politics of reproduction. *The Female Patient* 14(3):69–74, Mar 1989.

Nieman, L. The progesterone antagonist RU 486: a potential new contraceptive agent. *The New England Journal of Medicine* 316:187–191, 1987.

The antiprogesterones are coming—update on RU 486 (editorial). *The American Journal of Gynecologic Health* 3(1):7–8, Jan/Feb 1989.

Chapter 45—Hysterectomy and Its Alternatives

American College of Obstetricians and Gynecologists, Committee on gynecologic practice, *Committee Opinion* 146. Laparoscopically assisted vaginal hysterectomy, Nov 1994.

American College of Obstetricians and Gynecologists *Technical Bulletin* 214. Pelvic organ prolapse, Oct 1995.

Telinde's Operative Gynecology Updates, vol 1, no. 12. Indications for hysterectomy, 1993.

Pruitt, A. Advantages of laparoscopic-assisted vaginal hysterectomy. *Contemporary OB/GYN* 23–28, Feb 1995.

Renshaw, D. Sexuality and hysterectomy revisited. *The Female Patient* 13:45–46, Dec 1988.

Sanz, L. Myomectomy—an option for the fertile woman. *Contemporary OB/GYN* 32(1):129–140, July 1988.

DeCherney, A. Endometrial ablation for intractable uterine bleeding: hysteroscopic resection. *Obstetrics and Gynecology* 70:668–670, 1987.

Marchant, D. Hysterectomy: current trends. *The Female Patient* 13(5):71–92, May 1988.

Eisenberg, M. Endometrial laser ablation for menorrhagia: an effective alternative to hysterectomy. *The Female Patient* 13(5):38–49, May 1988.

Chapter 46—Cosmetic Surgery

Stephenson, J. Silicone implants and illness: Research doesn't support link. *OB/GYN News* 3–4, Dec 15, 1994.

Batoosingh, K. Implant settlement doesn't bring end to dispute. *OB/GYN News* 7–8, Nov 1, 1994.

Maxwell, G. Plastic and reconstructive breast surgery. *Clinics in Plastic Surgery* 15(4): Oct 1988.

Scheflan, M. Advances in breast reconstruction. *Clinics in Plastic Surgery* 11(2): Apr 1984.

Argenta, L. Tissue expansion. *Clinics in Plastic Surgery* 14(3): July 1987.

Marsh, J. Postmastectomy breast reconstruction. *The Female Patient* 13:41–47, Feb 1988.

Bostwick, J. Breast reconstruction following mastectomy. *CA-A Cancer Journal for Clinicians* 39(1):40–49, Jan/Feb 1989.

LaRossa, D. Surgical alteration of breast size. *Woman's Wellness* 1(5): Nov 1987.

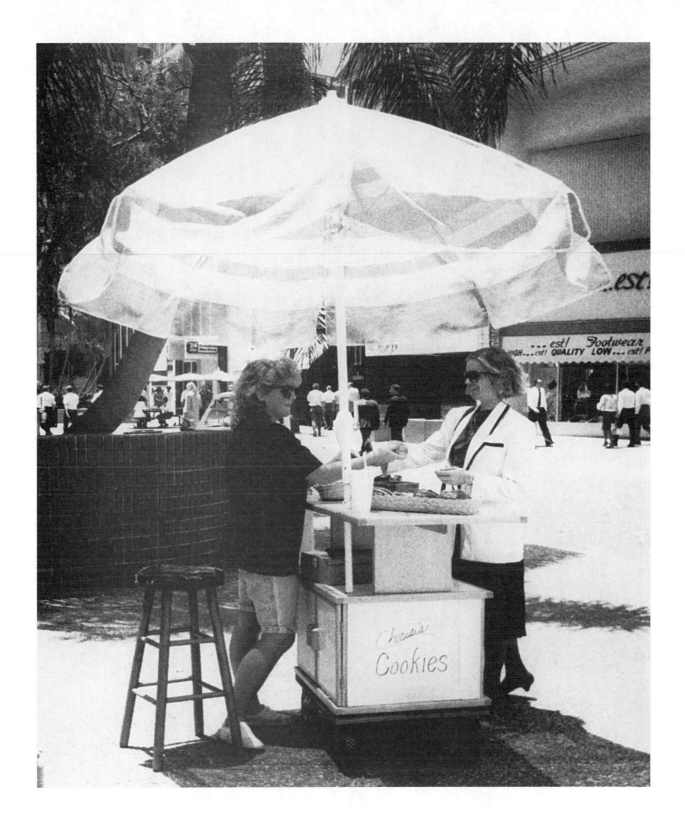

A HEALTHY
LIFESTYLE

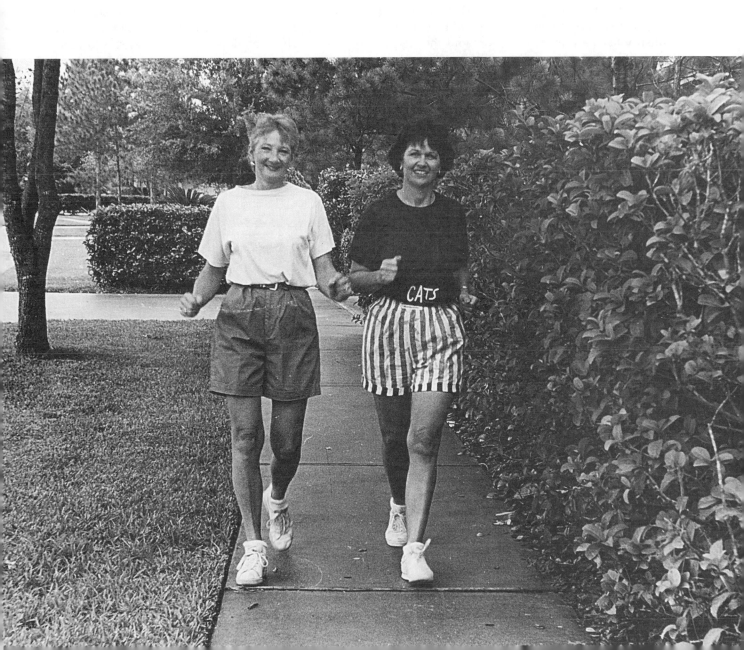

CHAPTER 47

Staying Healthy

Just what is good health? It can mean different things to different people, often depending upon their history of previous illness. People who have not lived with a chronic health problem might view good health as the absence of acute illness, such as colds and flu. Older persons might say that good health consists of having the energy and the physical capability to accomplish what they want to do without the restrictions imposed by serious illness, like heart disease. To a person with severe arthritis, being well might mean a few days without pain in the joints. In general, we can say that good health is a condition of physical and mental well-being, free from disease, pain, or defect, that enables us to live our lives with choices and with vitality.

Whatever our definition of good health, one thing is for sure: it's easy to take good health for granted as long as we have it. Sometimes it is only after we become ill or unexpectedly disabled that our health becomes more of a concern; we may then concentrate on getting "well" or getting "back to good health."

The question now comes up: How much of good health results from chance, determined purely by luck, and how much results from our own decisions, our own responsibility? Certainly a genetic predisposition to, say, heart disease, diabetes, or obesity is real. Disablement that results from an accident is an unfortunate happening. But to what extent can chronic illness and degenerative diseases associated with aging be prevented or delayed? Since the late 1970s, there has been increasing evidence that an individual's preventive health practices can promote health and prevent disease. Studies have shown that there *are* certain actions we can all take to promote a state of good health and consequently live longer, more productive lives with greater freedom from disease. Although the experts don't always agree, there is a good deal of consensus in three areas: there is value in getting adequate, regular exercise, in eating a nutritious diet regularly, and in avoiding smoking.

Recent research indicates the following factors also increase your life expectancy: seven to eight hours of sleep a night, regular meal taking, daily breakfast, maintenance of normal weight, and no more than moderate alcohol intake.

Another aspect of healthy living is the growing trend toward self care. This concept views good medical care as a partnership between patient and physician. Self care means the individual assumes an increasing role in health care decisions, such as whether to have certain diagnostic tests, medical treatments, or elective surgery, like hysterectomy. New drugstore products have encouraged the self-care trend. One company, Biotel, produces easy-to-use home screening tests for kidney disease, diabetes, and urinary tract infections. Other drugstore tests include ovulation detection kits, colon cancer screening tests, and home pregnancy tests. And some drugs, previously only available by prescription, are now available and FDA approved for over-the-counter purchase. These include ibuprofen (Advil and Nuprin) for menstrual cramps, and more recently Monistat 7 and Gyne-Lotrimin for vaginal yeast infections.

Self care is especially relevant to women today as social- and work-related pressures increasingly target women for stress-related illness, such as peptic ulcer and heart disease. Today more women are employed outside the home than ever before and often must assume multiple roles in society as workers, homemakers, wives, and mothers. The stress involved in assuming these various roles will no doubt take its toll, particularly in the area of heart disease. Women become more vulnerable to coronary (heart) disease after menopause as a result of decreasing amounts of estrogen. Before menopause, this hormone seems to provide some "natural immunity" to heart disease. As they catch up with men in rates of heart disease as well as other stress-related illnesses, American women, perhaps more than ever before, must use all of the resources at their disposal to preserve wellness.

Just what *should* you do to bring about and maintain good health? We discuss, either below or in separate chapters that follow, several topics relevant to the maintenance of good health. In all of these areas you can take much of the responsibility for your own continued wellness.

Good Nutrition

Eating a well-balanced diet on a regular basis and staying at your ideal weight are critical factors in maintaining your emotional and physical well-being. Chapter 48 tells you some of the things you need to know about good nutrition. Maintaining your ideal weight is very important; the obese person is much more likely to develop certain chronic conditions such as diabetes, high blood pressure, and heart disease. Chapter 89, Weight Gain and Weight Loss, discusses the subject in some detail and tells you how to determine your ideal weight based on your height and body frame.

Regular, Adequate Exercise

Benefits of a consistent exercise program, an essential part of health maintenance, usually include some loss of weight (especially in overweight individuals) and a lowered blood pressure, in persons with high blood pressure. Chapter 49 discusses the subject of physical exercise in some detail.

Have Regular Checkups

Table 3 lists the American Cancer Society's guidelines for periodic checkups. Having the recommended exams and tests can help physicians diagnose various forms of cancer at an earlier stage, when a cure is more likely. While most women are well informed about the need for regular Pap smears, many women are still not having mammograms as often as recommended by the Cancer Society.

Minimize Risk Factors for Heart Disease

Cardiovascular disease, especially heart disease and stroke, is the leading cause of death of women in the United States, claiming more lives than cancer, accidents, and diabetes combined. Every year approximately 250,000 women die from heart attacks and nearly 100,000 from strokes. Women are four times as likely to die of heart disease than of breast cancer. There is a misconception that heart disease is uncommon among women, when the fact is that the fre-

quency of heart disease is less for women compared to men *prior to menopause*. After that time, women have about the same chance of heart attacks and other forms of cardiovascular disease. Much depends upon risk factors—habits, traits, or conditions in an individual that are associated with an increased chance of developing a disease. High blood cholesterol is one of three main *controllable* risk factors for heart disease. The other two main controllable risk factors are high blood pressure and cigarette smoking. Any one of these factors increases a woman's chance of developing heart disease, and all three together may greatly increase the risk of heart disease, perhaps by ten times or more. Removal of the ovaries before menopause, obesity, and diabetes are other risk factors.

It is important to know whether your blood pressure is normal or not. Blood pressure is considered elevated if the first number, the systolic reading, is 140 or greater or if the second number, the diastolic reading, is 90 or greater. Like-

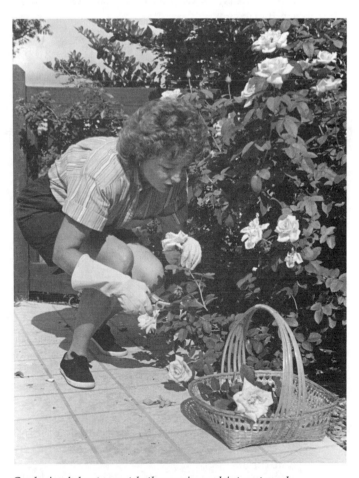

Gardening helps to meet both exercise and interest needs.

wise, every woman over the age of twenty should know the level of her blood cholesterol. The National Cholesterol Education Program, a national public-health initiative, has stressed the value of controlling cholesterol as a risk factor for heart disease. This program has established as a general guideline that an adult's cholesterol level should be less than 200 mg/dl and that higher levels warrant further testing and/or treatment. And yet about 50% of the women age fifty-five have cholesterol levels over 240 mg/dl, increasing their risk for heart disease. Both high blood pressure and high cholesterol can be treated with diet, and if that is unsuccessful, by drugs (see Chapters 69 and 48).

No Smoking

The best way to avoid smoking is never to start; but, unfortunately, studies show that smoking by women is on the rise. The numbers of teenage smokers, as well as older women smokers, are increasing.

Cigarettes contain nicotine, a drug that exerts a dependency action on the body, creating a habit that is hard to break. Just one cigarette upsets the flow of blood and air in your body by temporarily constricting blood vessels and paralyzing the little filaments (cilia) in the lung that normally move back and forth continuously to rid air passages of tiny dirt particles from the air we breathe. Clear-cut evidence from numerous studies indicates that smokers, both men and women, have a much greater risk of getting lung cancer, emphysema, bronchitis, and coronary heart disease.

When a pregnant woman smokes, she puts her baby's health at risk as well as her own. Smoking hurts the baby before, during, and after birth. Each puff introduces carbon monoxide into the fetus's blood, decreasing the oxygen-carrying capacity in the mother and her baby. Smoking during pregnancy increases the chances of complications such as vaginal bleeding, miscarriage, stillbirth, and prematurity. On the average, a smoker's baby weighs seven ounces less than a nonsmoker's baby and is a half inch shorter in length. Babies of smokers are at greater risk for cerebral palsy, various forms of brain damage, and sudden infant death syndrome.

The Surgeon General's report in 1986 on the adverse health effects of environmental tobacco smoke concluded that exposure to passive smoking was a contributing cause of lung cancer and heart disease. Studies have shown that infants and children exposed to passive smoke appear to be at increased risk for pulmonary problems, such as bronchitis, pneumonia, and asthma. Of course, children of smokers are more likely to become smokers, and teenage daughters tend to smoke if their mothers do—even if their fathers do not. Thus, it is not a good idea to smoke when your children are present.

Recently, there has been an increase in all forms of smokeless tobacco—"plug," "leaf," and snuff, especially "dipping snuff." This is a highly addictive habit and one that exposes a woman to levels of nicotine similar to those found in cigarettes. Oral cancer occurs more frequently among those who use snuff as compared to nontobacco users; an increase in cancer of the cheek and gum is also reported.

Quitting smoking is a difficult task but well worth it. It is estimated that a smoker who quits will live up to six years longer as a result. Quitting immediately instead of tapering off has proven to be the most effective method. Check with your local office of the American Cancer Society or American Lung Association for stop-smoking programs in your area. For more information, see Chapters 31 and 61.

Avoidance of Drug Abuse

Drug abuse involves misuse of any substance that can alter the chemical functioning of the body or mind and includes over-the-counter medications and, of course, alcohol. Section Seven (Chapters 29, 30, and 31) discusses the subject of women and the use of drugs.

Stress Management

Stress, it seems, is here to stay. For women, stress often results from having dual roles that compete. The working woman, more often than not, still comes home to clean house and take care of her kids. Finding a workable balance between these competing needs to allow more time for relaxation and rest is one of the main goals of stress management. Certain relaxation techniques, such as yoga, meditation, biofeedback, and hypnosis, used routinely, have been shown to be effective ways of coping with stress. It helps often to have some individual counseling as well if you are experiencing symptoms such as nervousness, anxiety, insomnia, or depression. But you need not have any of these symptoms to benefit from stress management, which has become popular among small businesses and corporations alike as a way of reducing stress in the workplace. However, the goal is not necessarily to become more efficient, but rather, more relaxed, more fulfilled, by resetting your priorities. This might mean less efficiency at work, less tidiness at home, and more "quality time" with family and friends as you learn to forget the "musts," "oughts," and "shoulds." Don't try to be a superwoman! In the end there are no "perfect" parents, single career women, dual career marriages, or grandparents!

If you find yourself caught up in a majority

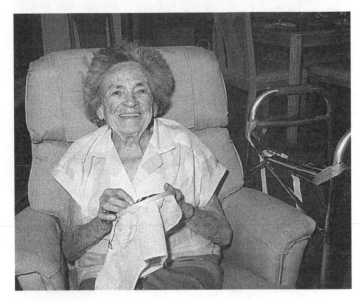

Stress management at ninety.

Table 78   WARNING SIGNALS OF TOO MUCH STRESS

You're doing too much if . . .

1. You find yourself impatient when standing in a slow line or following a slow, cautious driver.

2. You feel impatient and often interrupt people.

3. You find yourself feeling uncomfortable with the extra minutes you achieved by arriving someplace early.

4. You notice an increase in headaches or find yourself routinely starting off your day with aspirin or Tylenol.

5. You scream loudly at your kids when they accidentally spill their milk, feeling you can hardly tolerate this interruption.

6. You find yourself concentrating on winning every time, even when playing Candyland with your four-year-old.

7. You feel constantly hurried and try to do at least two things at once.

8. You feel uncomfortable about planning a vacation of only relaxing activities for a week, feeling you must "do" something.

9. Your intake of caffeine or cigarettes starts to climb markedly.

10. You find you can't relax at night because of worrying about all you have left to do.

11. You find you don't have time to keep up with your friends or attend your child's yearly open house at school.

---

of the behaviors, it's time to stop and reevaluate your priorities. Stress may be getting the best of you.

Stress and violence

One extreme consequence of stress is domestic violence, which has become pervasive in our society. Yet only recently has abuse of women become recognized as a national health problem. Elder abuse, parent abuse, sibling abuse, sexual assault, and partner abuse have been shown to occur at every level of American society. It has been estimated that at least 2 million women each year are battered by their intimate partners, and such physical abuse is the major cause of injury to American women (see Chapter 25).

Avoidance of Environmental Hazards

Environmental hazards are present everywhere. Because almost three of every five women seventeen and older are in the labor force today, hazards in the work world are an important consideration in women's health maintenance. Safety hazards, air as well as noise pollution, hazards from vibrations, frequent temperature changes, and the daily effect of working among smokers have all been shown to have potential health risks. We need to make ourselves aware of the possible specific hazards in our own environment, and we need to learn how to deal with them sensibly and safely.

Another environmental hazard that dermatologists have been warning us about for years is the sun. All forms of sun tanning and sun exposure are potentially hazardous to the skin. The sun's rays contain ultraviolet (UV) light, which has a radiation effect upon the skin. The American Cancer Society considers the sun the greatest single cause of cancer in the United States. Ultraviolet radiation consists of two types, A and B. The UV-A rays can penetrate the deeper dermis layer of the skin and cause changes in elastic tissues and blood vessels. The UV-B rays are the most harmful, may burn the skin, and are directly linked to skin cancer. Basal-cell carcinoma and squamous-cell carcinoma, the most common forms of skin cancer, are associated with frequent exposure to the sun over many years. These cancers are usually slow growing and easily curable. Melanoma, a fast-growing malignant skin cancer, has been associated with a single, blistering sunburn early in life. Researchers fear that the incidence of skin cancer will increase as the protective ozone layer is decreased by pollutants. Ultraviolet light also contributes to the formation of cataracts. The high-energy ultraviolet light from tanning booths can, if excessive, damage skin and can pass through the eyelids, causing irritation of the cornea, or even the retina.

Avoid direct exposure to sunlight, particularly between the hours of 10 A.M. and 3 P.M., when the sun's ultraviolet rays are strongest. Wear protective clothing or use a sunscreen lotion with a protective rating of 15 or more; the higher the number, the more protection. Applying a sunscreen thirty minutes prior to sunbathing helps to make certain it is absorbed. An opaque sunscreen is the most protective. If you must have a suntan, use a lotion containing PABA (para-aminobenzoic acid) to protect you from the sun. Choose the rating most beneficial to your skin; if you burn easily, choose a higher number. Wear sunglasses with a 100% UV-blocking coating. Contact lenses can be coated as well to screen out ultraviolet light. In general, avoid tanning parlors; if you do patronize them, wear protective goggles and be aware that tanning lamps can cause eye and skin damage as well as adverse reactions in people taking certain medications, such as antibiotics and anti-inflammatory drugs. Remember that the sun's rays are more intense the closer you are to the equator and that white sand, concrete surfaces, snow, and brightly painted surfaces reflect UV rays more efficiently.

Good Body Hygiene

Hygiene habits are established early in childhood; bad ones can be either eliminated or changed in adult life. Because women sometimes base their self-esteem on their appearance, they are often easy prey to the many pressures to buy numerous products—to keep "young looking," to be attractive, to have more energy, to be more "feminine," to look tan and "healthy," and so on and on.

The best rule for maintaining a healthy, clean body is to use common sense. Cleanliness with the use of a neutral soap and water and a moisturizer if you have dry skin are all that is usually necessary. (Studies haven't clearly shown one type of cosmetic to be more helpful than the rest—or everyone would be using it!) Take a long, hot bath if it relaxes you. Taking regular care of your nails, hair, and feet represents good hygiene and promotes a sense of well-being as well.

Regular douching is not an element of good hygiene and may at times be harmful. Concentrations of douche ingredients may not be listed on the package because some products are considered cosmetics instead of drugs. Among the ingredients in most douches are agents which act as local anesthetics (phenol, menthol), perfumes (eucalyptol), or substances which increase or decrease vaginal acidity. Many such ingredients may cause local allergic reactions or, by their local anesthetic effects, mask symptoms of infection, possibly delaying effective treatment. Single-ingredient douches containing either povidone-iodine or vinegar are sometimes used to supplement treatment of vaginal infections. However, most multi-ingredient douches and feminine hygiene products cannot be generally recommended since they have not been proven to be effective for either treatment or prevention of vaginal infections (see Chapter 87).

If you do douche, here are some precautions:

1. If you have symptoms of a vaginal infection which does not clear up after using Betadine douche for one week, get medical attention.
2. If you douche for hygiene purposes, do not douche more than twice a week.
3. If you are pregnant, avoid douching, especially in late pregnancy when your bag of waters could possibly be ruptured by use of the douche.
4. Do not use a douche as a contraceptive; it is a very ineffective method.
5. Do not douche within six hours of using a contraceptive cream or jelly since contraceptive effectiveness may be diminished.
6. Do not douche after intercourse if you are trying to get pregnant since some douche ingredients may destroy sperm.
7. Do not douche within twenty-four hours before a visit to your doctor for a routine pelvic exam, a Pap smear, an exam for a vaginal infection, etc.

Good Oral Hygiene

Oral hygiene, or regular care of your teeth and gums, is very important. We are mentioning it here because of the prevalence of periodontal disease. Periodontal disease affects three out of four adults. Surveys show that most people brush their teeth regularly but still get periodontal disease. The reason for this is that brushing alone does not necessarily get rid of plaque (the microorganisms that grow on the teeth). Plaque tends to accumulate at the gumline near the base of the teeth, areas that often are not well cleaned through typical toothbrushing. It usually is necessary to use an additional cleansing mechanism, such as dental floss, to remove the plaque. A proxabrush or gum brush is also helpful.

Periodontal disease usually shows itself initially as an inflammation of the gums (gingivitis); and, if it progresses, it destroys the alveolar bone and periodontal tissues supporting the teeth. With severe periodontal disease, loss of a tooth or teeth follows. Early signs of gingivitis include redness, swelling, and bleeding of the gums. Fortunately, this condition is reversible. It can be eliminated with proper home oral hygiene. It is best to discuss this condition with your dentist or dental hygienist *before* you have evidence of a problem.

Stress, hormonal changes, diet, pregnancy, menopause, and some medications can make a person's gums more susceptible to inflammation. Parents should start cleaning their child's teeth as soon as the baby teeth emerge; your child should be examined for cavities by age 2½. Early visits to a pediatric dentist will help you learn about caring for your child's teeth. Parents should floss and clean children's teeth daily until age eight to ten, when the child can do so himself. Good oral hygiene is based upon strong habits that are established during childhood. Gingivitis is common in children and adults who wear braces. Braces trap plaque; more than 75% of people who have braces have gingivitis.

Dentists recommend using a soft toothbrush with three or four rows of bristles that are rounded at the tips. Brushes should be replaced as soon as they begin to show wear. Mechanical toothbrushes such as Interplak are beneficial, as the groups of bristles move independently of each other for better cleaning. Use a toothpaste recommended by the American Dental Association (ADA). Their studies have shown that toothpastes with tartar-control formulas (for example, Crest with tartar control) are helpful. Since plaque requires twenty-four hours to build up in order to exert its harmful effects, at least one thorough plaque removal per day is needed. The ADA has found that Listerine and prescription Peridex (which causes darkened teeth stains that require teeth cleaning more often) are effective in significantly reducing the growth of plaque. See your dentist every six months for cleaning and evaluation, if possible.

Fluoridation

Community water fluoridation has been found to reduce the incidence of childhood dental cavities significantly. The Surgeon General recently reaffirmed that along with controlling the intake of sugars, the fluoridation of drinking water is the most important diet-related intervention in improving oral health. In areas where fluoridation is not available in the water, fluoride rinses or tablets can be used. There exists considerable scientific evidence that fluoridation is safe and effective in improving the health of the individual.

Adult Vaccinations

Infections for which vaccinations already exist kill 70,000 Americans per year. Historically, immunizations have been viewed as being for children only, but adults should get them, too. Your doctor should help you decide whether to become vaccinated; this usually depends upon your age, medical history, and the likelihood of a serious infection.

Researchers recommend a booster every ten years for those who have been vaccinated against tetanus or diphtheria. As many as 20% of Americans in their early twenties and thirties are susceptible to measles—either because they didn't get the virus as a child and have no natural immunity, or they received a weak measles vaccine. The possibility of contracting Rubella, or German measles, affects about 15% of women of childbearing age who do not have immunity to this virus. It is recommended that women considering pregnancy become immunized (if susceptible) by having the rubella vaccine (see Chapter 11) and the newly developed chicken pox vaccine as well.

Vaccines have been developed for flu, pneumonia, and hepatitis-B. The pneumococcal vaccine for the prevention of pneumonia caused by pneumococcal bacteria is a once-in-a-lifetime vaccine that is believed to prevent infection in two out of three persons who would otherwise become infected. Between 20,000 and 40,000 Americans die annually from this form of pneumonia. This vaccine is recommended for the elderly and chronically ill. The influenza (flu) vaccine is reformulated every year, may be taken annually, and is advised especially for women over sixty-five and for those suffering from chronic lung or heart disease. This vaccine is also advised for any adult who wants to lower the odds of getting the flu, which in a typical year kills 10,000 to 40,000 Americans. The vaccine prevents infection in 60% to 70% of recipients and lessens severity in most of the others. Hepatitis-B, a sometimes fatal liver infection, is declining in its spread in the United States because of the increased vaccination rate (see Chapter 20). The infection may be prevented by a vaccine that is administered in three doses over six months and is thought to provide lifetime immunity. This virus is transmitted by blood and blood products as well as by semen and saliva. Healthcare workers, IV drug abusers, homosexuals, and heterosexuals with multiple partners should be vaccinated. Ten percent of those infected become chronic carriers and carry the virus with them for the rest of their lives, sometimes unknowingly passing it on to others.

Resources

The following resources can be helpful in providing information about general health:

American Dental Association
Bureau of Health Education and Audiovisual
 Services
211 East Chicago Avenue
Chicago, Illinois 60611

American Public Health Association
1015 Fifteenth Street, N.W.
Washington, D.C. 20005

Council on Family Health
225 Park Avenue South, 17th Floor
New York, N.Y. 10003

National Mental Health Association
1021 Prince Street
Alexandria, Virginia 22314

CHAPTER 48

Nutrition

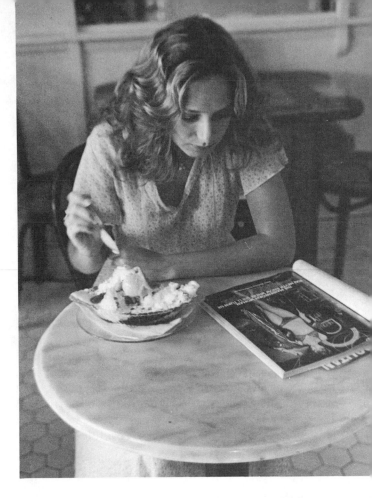

Nutrition plays a key role in maintaining health and in the prevention of many diseases. Dietary factors have been related to six of our leading causes of death: stroke, diabetes, heart disease, some cancers, hardening of the arteries, and cirrhosis of the liver. Today's American woman is concerned with a variety of issues relating to nutrition, from the proper use of vitamins to the health risks of food additives. She is bombarded daily with new books and magazine articles about various diets some of which promise easy answers to weight control or offer the prospect of controlling certain conditions, such as arthritis and heart disease. This chapter, because it discusses basic information we think most American women should know about nutrition, should help you to better evaluate what you read on the subject. For a discussion of nutrition and pregnancy see Chapter 16.

Nutrients

Nutrients are substances derived from food during the process of digestion. The major nutrients—proteins, carbohydrates, and fats—are needed by the body for growth, repair, maintenance, and energy. The amount of energy supplied by a nutrient is measured in calories, but the nutritive values of different foods cannot be measured by calories alone. Good nutrition requires a balance of the right nutrients, that is, getting the proper amount, or proportion, of each one. Nutrients can be classified as follows:

Proteins

Proteins are an essential part of every cell in your body. Proteins help to repair worn-out or diseased tissue and to build new tissue. Protein is used, for example, in the formulation of hormones, enzymes, red blood cells, and antibodies and in the formation of milk for breast-feeding. When digested, protein breaks down into smaller units called amino acids, some of which (the so-called essential ones) must be obtained from food. Proteins derived from animal foods, such as fish, meat, eggs, and dairy products, are "complete" proteins because they each contain all the amino acids, including the essential amino acids. Vegetable proteins are "incomplete" because each one lacks one or more essential amino acids. However, when vegetable proteins and proteins in whole grains are used in certain combinations of foods (such as dried beans and rice, or cereal and milk), they supply all the required amino acids.

Most nutrition experts believe that many Americans consume too much red meat in their diet and that more protein should be consumed from other, nonmeat sources. This is because red meat is a major source of undesirable saturated fat. You can cut down on this saturated fat by selecting leaner meats, by eating less red meat and more fish (as well as chicken without the fatty skin), and by eating smaller and fewer portions than usual. There are many good sources of nonmeat proteins such as lowfat dairy products, legumes, and whole-grain cereals.

Carbohydrates

Carbohydrates function primarily to provide energy, supplying about two-thirds of an individual's total energy needs. When insufficient carbohydrates are eaten, body fat and proteins are then broken down to meet the body's energy demands. Foods high in carbohydrates include grains, vegetables, fruits, and beans. Carbohydrates also include simple sugars found in sweets, candy, and pastries. Sugar is a "low-density" source of calories which are rapidly used up, thus promptly leading to a renewed desire for food. When used in moderate quantities, sugar isn't harmful as long as it doesn't replace other foods that have needed nutrients. Excess dietary sugar may lead to obesity, low blood sugar, and dental caries (tooth decay) and also has been linked to a possible increased risk of developing diabetes in later adult life.

Fats

The most concentrated source of food energy is found in fats, or lipids. They are necessary for the absorption and utilization of certain vitamins (A, E, D, and K). Fat deposits surround and protect body organs, such as the heart and liver, and help to maintain body temperature against outside environmental influences. Excess fat is stored in the body tissues and leads to weight gain.

High amounts of fat in the American diet have been linked to an increased risk for cancer and heart disease. The American Cancer Society announced results of a twelve-year study which found that excessive consumption of both saturated and unsaturated fats was linked to the development of breast and colon cancer. The American Heart Association (AHA) also suggests that Americans consume fewer dietary fats (no more than 30% of total calories). Two specific types of fat—saturated fats and cholesterol—are the most important to restrict because they tend to raise the level of cholesterol in the blood and a high cholesterol contributes to hardening of the arteries and heart disease.

Cholesterol

Cholesterol, a fatlike substance produced mainly in the liver, is involved in making essential body substances, such as cell walls and hormones. However, cholesterol is also a major contributor to the formation of waxy deposits in blood-vessel walls, a process called *atherosclerosis*. The deposits can create blockages in critical blood vessels; such a blockage in the coronary arteries can cause a heart attack. The link between blood-cholesterol level and heart disease has been noted by researchers for years. But only since 1984 has there been direct evidence that people could actually lower their blood-cholesterol counts by diet and, sometimes, drug therapy; this was the result of a landmark study (on men) by the National Heart, Lung, and Blood Institute. Since 1987, the federal government has recommended to the medical profession that all patients over the age of twenty have blood-cholesterol testing.

Cholesterol is measured in terms of milligrams per deciliter. A desirable cholesterol level is less than 200, borderline high is 200 to 239, and a count over 240—found in 25% of Americans—is considered high. Women with high cholesterol counts should have further screening consisting of measuring levels of special proteins in the blood called *lipoproteins*. Lipoproteins, which transport the cholesterol in the blood, consist of two basic types: high-density lipoprotein cholesterol (HDL) and low-density lipoprotein cholesterol (LDL). It is desirable to have a relatively high level of the "good" cholesterol, HDL, which is believed to take cholesterol away from the artery walls and transport it back to the liver for reprocessing. One way to help raise your HDL is through regular exercise. Women generally have higher levels of HDL than men, and this may explain in part why they have fewer heart attacks than do men. The "bad" cholesterol, LDL, contain the greatest amounts of cholesterol and may be responsible for depositing cholesterol in the artery walls.

Your blood-cholesterol level (including the lipoprotein cholesterols LDL and HDL) is directly and adversely affected by two factors: how much saturated fat and cholesterol are in your diet. Lowering blood cholesterol will reduce the risk of heart attack; a 1% reduction in total cholesterol roughly translates into a 2% drop in the risk of heart attacks, the number-one cause of death in the United States. Saturated fats are found in meats (especially red meats), in many whole dairy products, such as butter, cream, cheese, and whole milk, and in some foods of plant origin, such as palm and coconut oils. Cholesterol-rich foods include organ meats, liver, kidney, sweetbread (brain), and egg yolks, as well as certain shellfish, such as shrimp and lobster. Lesser amounts of cholesterol are found in animal meat, fish, poultry, and dairy products. It is important to remember that cholesterol is not the same as fat and that a food may contain substantial cholesterol but only a moderate amount of saturated fat (for example, shellfish). Foods of plant origin—vegetables, fruits, grains, seeds, and vegetable oils—have no cholesterol.

The National Cholesterol Education Program's Adult Treatment Report recommends a reduction in daily fat intake to less than 30% of calories rather than the present 40%. Less than 10% of total calories should come from *saturated* fat. The report recommended reducing dietary cholesterol to less than 300 mg per day—not much more than the amount found in a single egg. Practical guidelines to reduce the amount of saturated fat and cholesterol in your diet include the following:

- Avoid sausage and most processed lunch meats; instead, choose more fish, poultry (with skin removed), and lean cuts of meat. Eat moderate portions.
- Avoid cream, sour cream, ice cream, butter, and cheese, substituting lowfat dairy products such as skim or low-fat milk, low-fat or nonfat yogurt, low-fat cheese, etc.
- Bake, roast, or broil foods instead of frying.
- Add less fat and shortening to foods when cooking.
- Choose vegetable oils with the highest proportions of unsaturated fat. Avoid palm and coconut oil and hydrogenated shortening.
- Use margarine instead of butter.
- Read the nutrient section of food labels to choose items that are low in saturated fatty acids.
- Eat no more than three to four egg yolks per week.
- Consume more vegetables, fruits, grains, dried peas, rice, and pasta, which contain complex carbohydrates, little or no saturated fat, and no cholesterol.

Resource

For more information, write to:

Heart, Lung, and Blood Institute
   Information Center
P.O. Box 30105
Bethesda, Maryland 20824-0105

Fiber

Although, strictly speaking, fiber is not a nutrient, fiber plays a vital role in the digestive process by softening bile waste and speeding up the process of elimination of undigested food. Some research suggests (but has not been proven) that increased amounts of dietary fiber may help protect against the development of colon cancer. In older women especially, foods high in fiber, such as raw fruits and vegetables, may help prevent constipation and certain colon conditions such as diverticulitis (see glossary). In some individuals excessive fiber intake can be a problem, too, causing bloating, gas, and diarrhea.

Vitamins and Minerals

Vitamins are organic substances which have no caloric or energy value but which contribute to nutrition by allowing chemical reactions to occur normally throughout the body. These reactions, known collectively as metabolism, are responsible for numerous functions, such as converting fats and carbohydrates into energy and utilizing proteins to repair injured tissue. Vitamins act as essential catalysts in these processes.

Minerals are chemical substances, such as calcium, sodium, iron, and potassium, which participate in many chemical reactions essential in human nutrition. Minerals are similar to vitamins in that they don't directly provide energy; but, unlike vitamins, minerals do act as components of major body structures, including bones, teeth, blood, and soft tissue.

With a few exceptions, most healthy women don't need to take supplemental vitamins and minerals. The exceptions include women who are pregnant or breast-feeding (see Table 79), those on restricted or very low calorie diets (see Chapter 89), and women who consume moderate amounts of alcohol. Also, certain chronic illnesses and the use of certain medications may

HEALTHY SNACKS FOR A HEALTHY HEART

TRY THESE	INSTEAD OF THESE
FRESH FRUITS	FRUITS IN HEAVY SYRUP, PUDDINGS, CUSTARDS
WHOLE GRAIN MUFFINS AND CRACKERS	CAKES, COOKIES, PASTRIES
FROZEN YOGURT, SHERBET, ICE MILK	WHOLE MILK, ICE CREAM
POPCORN (UNBUTTERED, UNSALTED), PEANUTS AND WALNUTS IN THE SHELL, WHOLE GRAIN CEREALS	POTATO CHIPS, PRETZELS, CORN CHIPS
FRESH VEGETABLES	FRENCH FRIES, FRIED VEGETABLES
DRIED FRUITS INCLUDING APPLES, RAISINS, PRUNES	HARD CANDIES, CHOCOLATES, LOLLIPOPS

Reprinted with permission of Wyeth-Ayerst Labs.

make it advisable for a woman to take vitamin and mineral supplements. Although birth control pills slightly lower the blood level of certain vitamins, a supplement is usually unnecessary. Specific vitamin and mineral supplements may be needed as women get older. For example, menopausal women may need to take a calcium supplement to prevent osteoporosis (see Chapter 27), and elderly women may require a multiple vitamin and mineral supplement due to de-

creased absorption of certain nutrients like B_{12} and iron. In menstruating women, by far the most common dietary mineral deficiency is likely to be iron. Iron-deficiency anemia, associated with heavy menstrual periods, may necessitate the use of supplemental iron from time to time.

A few words should be said here about the absorption of iron by the body. Certain substances in some of the foods we eat, like the tan-

Table 79   U.S. RECOMMENDED DAILY ALLOWANCES OF VITAMINS (RDA)

Vitamin	For Adult Women	For Pregnant Women	For Breast-feeding Women
Vitamin A	800 mg*	800 mg	1,300 mg
Vitamin D	10 mg	10 mg	10 mg
Vitamin E	8 mg	10 mg	12 mg
Vitamin C	60 mg	70 mg	95 mg
Folic acid	0.18 mg	0.4 mg	0.28 mg
Thiamine	1.1 mg	1.5 mg	1.6 mg
Riboflavin	1.3 mg	1.6 mg	1.8 mg
Niacin	15 mg	17 mg	20 mg
Vitamin B$_6$	1.6 mg	2.2 mg	2.1 mg

* mg retinol equivalents

nic acid in tea, for example, inhibit the body's absorption of the kind of iron that is in plant foods. Certain other substances work in an opposite way and increase the amount of iron absorbed by the body from the foods we eat. These substances include high quality protein, like that provided by soybeans, and ascorbic acid (vitamin C), as found in orange juice. Not only do these substances increase the absorption of iron, they also reverse the inhibiting effects of substances like tannic acid. But in order for this reversal effect to take place, the foods must be eaten at the same meal. So if you drink tea, for example, with a meal, try to include some food high in vitamin C at the same meal.

The presumed beneficial effects of vitamins and minerals have been widely promoted by drug manufacturers. The consumer cannot easily evaluate the variety of claims being made for these products, and many of these claims are misleading. Vitamins do not, for example, provide energy or produce a sense of well-being. According to the FDA, vitamins are indicated only for the treatment or the prevention of deficiency states (see Table 81). Similarly, iron is indicated only when iron-deficiency anemia is present, but iron supplementation does not prevent listlessness or fatigue in individuals who are not anemic.

Vitamin preparations

There are numerous vitamin preparations available, some containing iron. If what you need is iron, you are just as well off and can save money by selecting an iron preparation with vitamin C (which helps the body to absorb the iron) rather than an iron and multiple vitamin combination. Vitamin products vary widely from expensive name brands which contain minerals rarely needed, such as manganese, to simple vitamin C. Over-the-counter products are almost always just as good as prescription vitamins. Neither are necessary in most healthy, nonpregnant women eating well-balanced diets.

Prescription vitamins, as distinguished from over-the-counter preparations, usually contain a larger dose of folic acid than is available in over-the-counter preparations. Multiple vitamins containing folic acid are now routinely prescribed for women planning to conceive. Folic acid, when taken during the months before pregnancy and in early gestation, has been found to help prevent spina bifida and other related abnormalities known as neural tube defects.

The whole practice of vitamin supplementation in pregnancy may be more of an expected tradition than a medical necessity in most healthy women. But because many vitamin preparations also contain the one mineral supplement that may be needed in pregnancy—iron—vitamins and iron tend to be prescribed and taken together in one pill, the so-called prenatal vitamins.

Table 82 answers some questions commonly asked about taking vitamins.

Megavitamins

Vitamins with a dose of more than ten times the Recommended Daily Allowance (RDA) (see below under Planning for Good Nutrition) are considered megavitamins. The megavitamin concept rests largely on the speculation that the vitamin needs of many people cannot be met from ordinary diets and on the belief that human nutrient needs vary over a range of greater than ten times the RDA. However, both human and animal studies have shown that maintenance of a satisfactory state of health seldom requires nutrient supplementation beyond the requirements of the RDA. Despite the many possible harmful effects of megavitamin dosages

Table 80   FAT AND CHOLESTEROL CONTENT OF DIFFERENT FOODS

Example of	Item	Saturated Fatty Acids (grams)	Total Fat (grams)	Cholesterol (milligrams)
Beef 100 grams (3½ ounces)	Top round, lean only, broiled	2.2	6.2	84
	Ground lean, broiled medium	7.3	18.5	87
	Beef prime rib, meat, lean and fat, broiled	14.9	35.2	86
Processed Meats 100 grams (3½ ounces)	Dutch loaf, pork and beef	6.4	17.8	47
	Sausage smoked, link, beef and pork	10.6	30.3	71
	Bologna, beef	11.7	28.4	56
	Frankfurter, beef	12.0	29.4	48
	Salami, dry or hard, pork, beef	12.2	34.4	79
Pork 100 grams (3½ ounces)	Ham steak, extra lean	1.4	4.2	45
	Pork, center loin, lean only, braised	4.7	13.7	111
	Pork, spareribs, lean and fat, braised	11.8	30.3	121
Poultry 100 grams (3½ ounces)	Chicken broilers or fryers, roasted:			
	• Light meat without skin	1.3	4.5	85
	• Light meat with skin	3.1	10.9	84
	• Dark meat without skin	2.7	9.7	93
	• Dark meat with skin	4.4	15.8	91
	• Chicken skin	11.4	40.7	83
Fin Fish 100 grams (3½ ounces)	Cod, Atlantic, dry heat cooked	0.1	0.7	58
	Perch, mixed species, dry heat cooked	0.2	1.2	115
	Snapper, mixed species, dry heat cooked	0.4	1.7	47
	Rockfish, Pacific, mixed species, dry heat cooked	0.5	2.0	44
	Tuna, bluefin, dry heat cooked	1.6	6.3	49
	Mackerel, Atlantic, dry heat cooked	4.2	17.8	75
Mollusks 100 grams (3½ ounces)	Clam, mixed species, moist heat cooked	0.2	2.0	67
	Mussel, blue, moist heat cooked	0.9	4.5	56
	Oyster, eastern, moist heat cooked	1.3	5.0	109
Crustaceans 100 grams (3½ ounces)	Crab, blue, moist heat cooked	0.2	1.8	100
	Lobster, northern, moist heat cooked	0.1	0.6	72
	Shrimp, mixed species, moist heat cooked	0.3	1.1	195
Liver and Organ Meats 100 grams (3½ ounces)	Chicken liver, cooked, simmered	1.8	5.5	631
	Beef liver, braised	1.9	4.9	389
	Pork brains, cooked	2.2	9.5	2,552
Eggs (1 yolk=17 grams) (1 white=33 grams) (1 whole=50 grams)	Egg yolk, chicken, raw	1.7	5.6	272
	Egg white, chicken, raw	0	trace	0
	Egg, whole, chicken, raw	1.7	5.6	272
Nuts and Seeds 100 grams (3½ ounces)	Chestnuts, European, roasted	0.4	2.2	0
	Almonds, dry roasted	4.9	51.6	0
	Sunflower seed kernels, dry roasted	5.2	49.8	0
	Pecans, dry roasted	5.2	64.6	0
	Walnuts, English, dried	5.6	61.9	0
	Pistachio nuts, dried	6.1	48.4	0
	Peanut kernels, dried	6.8	49.2	0
	Cashew nuts, dry roasted	9.2	46.4	0
	Brazil nuts, dried	16.2	66.2	0
Fruits 100 grams (3½ ounces)	Peaches, raw	0.010	0.09	0
	Oranges, raw	0.015	0.12	0
	Strawberries, raw	0.020	0.37	0
	Apples, with skin, raw	0.058	0.36	0

Example of	Item	Saturated Fatty Acids (grams)	Total Fat (grams)	Cholesterol (milligrams)
Vegetables 100 grams (3½ ounces)	Cooked, boiled, drained:	0.026	0.10	0
	• Potato, without skin	0.034	0.18	0
	• Carrots	0.042	0.26	0
	• Spinach	0.043	0.28	0
	• Broccoli	0.064	0.28	0
	• Beans, green and yellow	0.064	0.31	0
	• Squash, yellow, crookneck	0.197	1.28	0
	• Corn			
	• Avocado, raw, without skin or seed:			0
	Florida origin	1.74	8.86	0
	California origin	2.60	17.34	
Grains and Legumes 100 grams (3½ ounces)	Split peas, cooked, boiled	0.054	0.39	0
	Red kidney beans, cooked, boiled	0.07	0.5	0
	Oatmeal, cooked	0.19	1.0	0
Milk and Cream 1 cup (8 fluid ounces)	Skim milk	0.3	0.4	4
	Buttermilk (0.9% fat)	1.3	2.2	9
	Low fat milk (1% fat)	1.6	2.6	10
	Whole milk (3.7% fat)	5.6	8.9	35
	Light cream	28.8	46.3	159
	Heavy whipping cream	54.8	88.1	326
Yogurt and Sour Cream 1 cup (8 fluid ounces)	Plain yogurt, skim milk	0.3	0.4	4
	Plain yogurt, low fat (1.6%)	2.3	3.5	14
	Plain yogurt, whole milk	4.8	7.4	29
	Sour cream	30.0	48.2	102
Soft Cheeses 1 cup (8 fluid ounces)	Cottage cheese, low fat (1% fat)	1.5	2.3	10
	Cottage cheese, creamed	6.0	9.5	31
	Ricotta, part skim	12.1	19.5	76
	Ricotta, whole milk	18.8	29.5	116
	American processed spread	30.2	48.1	125
	Cream cheese	49.9	79.2	250
Hard cheeses (8 ounces)	Mozzarella, part skim	22.9	36.1	132
	Mozzarella, whole milk	29.7	49.0	177
	Provolone	38.8	60.4	157
	Swiss	40.4	62.4	209
	Blue	42.4	65.1	170
	Brick	42.7	67.4	213
	Muenster	43.4	68.1	218
	American processed	44.7	71.1	213
	Cheddar	47.9	75.1	238
Vegetable Oils and Shortening 1 cup (8 fluid ounces)	Canola oil	14.8	218.0	0
	Safflower oil	19.8	218.0	0
	Sunflower oil	22.5	218.0	0
	Corn oil	27.7	218.0	0
	Olive oil	29.2	216.0	0
	Soybean oil	31.4	218.0	0
	Margarine, regular soft tub*	32.2	182.6	0
	Margarine, stick or brick*	34.2	182.6	0
	Peanut oil	36.4	216.0	0
	Household vegetable shortening*	51.2	205.0	0
	Cottonseed oil	56.4	218.0	0
	Palm oil	107.4	218.0	0
	Coconut oil	188.5	218.0	0
	Palm kernel oil	177.4	218.0	0

*Made with hydrogenated soybean oil + hydrogenated cottonseed oil.

(Table continued on next page.)

Example of	Item	Saturated Fatty Acids (grams)	Total Fat (grams)	Cholesterol (milligrams)
Animal Fats	Chicken fat	61.2	205.0	174
1 cup	Lard	80.4	205.0	195
(8 fluid ounces)	Mutton fat	96.9	205.0	209
	Beef fat	102.1	205.0	223
	Butter	114.4	183.9	496

Table 81   SYMPTOMS OF VITAMIN DEFICIENCY

Vitamin	Early Symptoms of Deficiency	Food Containing Vitamin	Comment
A (Retinol)	night blindness, dry skin	liver, eggs, butter, whole milk, vegetables	deficiency rare
B_1 (Thiamine)	numbness, tingling, loss of sensation or shooting pains in the extremities, especially the legs	bran, whole grains, cereals, fruits, nuts, vegetables, fish	deficiency associated with excessive use of alcohol
B_2 (Riboflavin)	ulcer of mouth, cracking of lips, dimness of vision	liver, milk, eggs, vegetables	deficiency rare
B_3 (Niacin or Nicotinic acid)	weight loss, rough skin, mouth sores, burning of tongue, weakness, diarrhea	fish, meat, whole grains, cereals, vegetables	deficiency rare
B_6 (Pyridoxine)	depression, mouth soreness, dizziness, nausea	meat, vegetables, bran	deficiency rare but occasional depression is seen in women taking birth control pills
B_{12} (Cyanoco-balamine)	weakness, shortness of breath, numbness and tingling in fingers and toes	meat, fish, milk	deficiency rare; however, strict vegetarians should supplement their diets with this vitamin
C (Ascorbic acid)	gum bleeding, swelling, or infection; bleeding into the skin causing bruising	citrus fruits, fresh vegetables	deficiency very uncommon
D (Calciferol)	bowed legs, deformed spine	fish, egg yolks, vitamin D-fortified milk	deficiency rare; vitamin D is also formed in the skin from the sun's rays
E	none	vegetables, whole grains, cereals, fruits	no deficiency state known
Folic acid	weakness, numbness and tingling of fingers and toes, mouth ulcers, sore tongue	liver, vegetables, nuts, whole wheat	deficiency rare; supplementation needed in pregnancy and in women taking some anticonvulsant drugs
K	bleeding	vegetables	deficiency rare
Pantothenic acid	headache, fatigue, loss of coordination	liver, eggs, potatoes, vegetables	deficiency rare

Table 82   QUESTIONS COMMONLY ASKED ABOUT TAKING VITAMINS

Question	Yes	No	Comment
Are "natural" vitamins better than synthetic ones?		X	There is no evidence that they are.
Does vitamin E have any proven therapeutic value?		X	And vitamin E deficiency is virtually unknown. (See Chapter 59.)
Do I need to take vitamins while on the birth control pill?		X	Blood levels of folic acid and vitamin B_6 may be slightly but not significantly lowered.
Does vitamin A prevent or control acne?		X	The dosage required to prevent acne produces toxic side effects.
Is excessive alcohol intake associated with vitamin deficiency?	X		Especially thiamine.
Is B_{12} an appetite stimulant?		X	Injectable B_{12} has been used to improve mood and provide a sense of well-being—the effect is entirely placebo.
Does B_6 help to control nausea and vomiting in early pregnancy?	X		B_6 sometimes helps but no studies have been done to document its effectiveness.
Do vitamins provide energy?		X	They are organic compounds necessary for changing food into energy.
Do so-called average or normal eaters usually need supplemental vitamins?		X	Except perhaps during pregnancy.
Are cracked nails a common sign of vitamin deficiency?		X	Much more common causes are trauma to the nail base or a fungal infection of the nail.

(see Table 83), these dosages continue to be popular perhaps because of the placebo effect; that is, if both patient and doctor believe something will relieve a symptom, it often will. The National Nutrition Consortium, made up of a number of professional societies, has gone on record as recommending against large amounts of vitamins. Vitamin C megadose supplementation during pregnancy can lead to serious problems in the newborn. After having been exposed to large dosages of this vitamin before birth, the newborn may develop a relative deficiency state after birth, resulting in scurvy and possible life-threatening bleeding. Very high doses of vitamin A and vitamin D have been associated with birth defects in the newborn.

Iron preparations

You are much more likely to need and benefit from iron than from vitamins. Iron may be sold generically as ferrous sulfate, ferrous fumarate, or ferrous gluconate. These are the most eco-nomical forms of iron. The common side effects of iron are stomach irritation and constipation. Women who have a history of stomach ulcers should use iron preparations cautiously since such use sometimes brings on ulcerlike symptoms. Stomach irritation may occur as nausea, gas, or indigestion. Some iron products contain timed- or sustained-release forms of iron, which are less irritating to the stomach. The addition of vitamin C in the product may also decrease stomach irritation as well as increase iron absorption. For this reason, some iron preparations are sold in combination with this vitamin alone. Another way iron is prepared is in combination with a stool softener (sulfosuccinate). This combination may be helpful after surgery or childbirth when constipation is more likely to be a problem. All iron preparations may cause the formation of black-colored stool. See Table 84 for information on various types of iron preparations available and Table 85 for answers to questions commonly asked about taking iron.

Calcium Preparations

Dairy products (preferably low- or nonfat) and dark green, leafy vegetables are excellent sources of calcium, which may also be obtained as over-the-counter supplements. Calcium requirements for women vary during different stages of life. The recommended daily allowance for nonpregnant women is 1000 mg of calcium per day, increasing to 1200 mg during pregnancy. Many professionals recommend up to 1500 mg of calcium after menopause if you are not taking estrogen (1000 mg if you are). The risks of inadequate calcium in the diet leading to osteoporosis are discussed in Chapter 27, and calcium needs during pregnancy are discussed in Chapter 16. At this time, calcium supplements are not recommended for the prevention of high blood pressure, although some research indicates that inadequate calcium in the diet may be a contributing factor to this disease.

Planning for Good Nutrition

The five basic food groups

The Food and Nutrition Board of the National Research Council has noted that eating a variety of foods is the most important way to maintain good nutrition. Today dietitians often use the "food pyramid" as a visual aid to show how the five basic food groups should fit into our diet. These five food groups, which are shown in Table 87, contain the essential nutrients needed by the human body every day. The food pyramid is a nice way to show how the food groups should be balanced in terms of numbers of servings. A range of servings is noted in the table; the number you need depends upon your age, sex, activity level, and caloric intake. Many women will need more than the minimum number of servings from each of the five basic food groups. Pregnant women will also need an additional two servings from the milk and milk products group, and perhaps an extra serving or two from the bread and cereal group.

Optimum weight and energy balance

Your weight and energy balance are determined by three factors: the rate of your metabolism, the number of calories you eat, and the amount of

Table 83	POSSIBLE SIDE EFFECTS OF MEGAVITAMINS

Megavitamin*	Possible Side Effects
Vitamin C	diarrhea, kidney stones and kidney damage, increased susceptibility to gout, increased susceptibility to sickle-cell crisis in women with sickle-cell anemia
Nicotinic acid	flushing, itching rash, vomiting, jaundice, liver damage, peptic ulcer
Vitamin E	headache, nausea, dizziness, blurred vision
Folic acid	increased seizures in women with epilepsy
Vitamin A	headaches, diarrhea, blurred vision, nervous system damage, liver damage, bone damage
Vitamin D	headaches, weakness, nausea, blurred vision, nervous system or kidney damage
Vitamin K	decreases the effectiveness of blood thinners, such as Coumadin
Pyridoxine (vitamin B$_6$)	seizures

* 10 times Recommended Daily Allowance or more

exercise you get. The reasons for individual tendencies to gain weight are not always known. Individual variation with respect to metabolism is largely inherited so that some women never seem to have weight problems regardless of diet. Metabolism normally declines approximately 15% between the ages of twenty-five and seventy, representing a drop in calorie needs of about 1% every three years during this period. Metabolism is higher for males than for females at almost all ages. Obesity tends to start affecting women in their thirties whereas men are less likely to be affected before they reach their forties. During these times, a declining metabolic rate is likely to be paralleled by a decrease in activity. If the slow-down in metabolism and activity level in middle age is not accompanied by a decrease in calorie intake, weight gain occurs.

Obesity or excessive overweight is the number one nutrition problem in the United States today. New evidence suggests that *where* your fat is may be important too. Upper-body fat (on the abdomen, for example) seems to be riskier than lower-body fat (hips and thighs) as far as heart-disease risks are concerned. Excessive weight gain is not good for your health because it places an additional strain on your heart and may contribute to certain diseases such as high blood pressure, gallstones, and diabetes. The risk of uterine, breast, gallbladder, kidney, stomach, and colon cancer is also increased. Insurance statistics show that the lowest mortality rates among women are associated with a weight of 15% to 20% below ideal weight for height. Chapter 89 on weight gain and weight loss provides information about weight-loss dieting as well as on losing and keeping off extra pounds. Table 116 (in Chapter 89) shows suggested weights for heights.

Food labeling

New regulations by the U.S. Food and Drug Administration now require food labels that will help the consumer plan healthy diets. These new

---

Table 84   COMPARISON OF IRON-CONTAINING SUPPLEMENTS

Type of Iron	Common Brand Names	Comment
Simple iron, usually ferrous sulfate or ferrous fumarate	many brands	Many generics available and may be less costly. Liquid form generally costs more than capsule or tablet.
Timed-release iron products	Fero-Gradumet Fergon many other brands	Many generics available and may be less costly. Intended to prevent stomach irritation.
Iron plus a stool softener	Ferro-Sequels several other brands	Useful after surgery or childbirth.
Iron plus vitamin C	many brands	Vitamin C intended to promote absorption (slight effect) and decrease stomach irritation.
Iron plus multiple vitamins	many brands	Not needed in simple iron-deficiency anemia.

Table 85   QUESTIONS COMMONLY ASKED ABOUT TAKING IRON

Question	Yes	No	Comment
Do iron tablets usually require a prescription?		X	Almost never necessary.
Can iron overdose occur?	X		One of the more common fatal accidental poisonings in children.
Can iron interfere with absorption of tetracycline?	X		Avoid taking these products within two hours of each other.
Can I get enough iron during pregnancy by eating a well-balanced diet?		X	Iron is needed during pregnancy to double the amount of blood in your body and for the fetus. The amount of iron absorbed from food is limited.
Is iron deficiency the commonest cause of anemia in women, both pregnant and nonpregnant?	X		
Is one form of iron less likely to cause stomach irritation than another?		X	Stomach irritation is related to the total amount of iron rather than the specific type of iron taken.
Should iron be taken between meals to allow maximum absorption?	X		However, it may be taken just after meals if stomach irritation occurs.

Table 86 CALCIUM AND CALORIE CONTENT OF VARIOUS FOODS

	Calcium (milligrams)	Calories
Dairy sources		
Milk, whole (1 cup)	291	150
Milk, low-fat or 2% (1 cup)	297	120
Milk, skim or 1% (1 cup)	300	100
Cheese, American, pasteurized (1 oz)	174	105
Cheese, cheddar (1 oz)	204	115
Cheese, Monterey Jack (1 oz)	212	106
Cottage cheese, low-fat or 2% (1 cup)	155	205
Yogurt, plain, low-fat (1 cup)	415	145
Yogurt, plain, nonfat (1 cup)	452	125
Ice cream, 4% fat (1 cup)	176	185
Sherbet, 2% fat (1 cup)	103	270
Nondairy sources		
Almonds, whole (1 oz)	75	165
Broccoli, frozen, cooked (½ cup)	47	25
Kale, frozen, cooked (½ cup)	90	20
Salmon, pink, canned (3 oz)	167	120
Sardines, canned in oil (3 oz)	371	175
Snap beans, frozen, cooked (½ cup)	31	18

food labels represent the biggest change in nutritional information available to consumers in over twenty years. Food labels now carry a nutrition *information guide* on most packaged foods. The information includes serving sizes that more than ever before reflect the amounts people actually eat. The list of nutrients on the label covers those items most important to one's health, such as total fat, saturated fat, cholesterol, sodium, and total carbohydrate. For each item a percent of the daily value (DV) is noted. Daily value is a new dietary reference term that indicates the amount of major nutrients to consume on a daily basis.

Here's how it works. On each label the daily value for each nutrient is calculated for both a 2000-calorie diet and a 2500-calorie diet. Most women will probably want to use the 2000-calorie diet as their reference. In a 2000-calorie diet you should not exceed 65 grams of total fat, 20 grams of saturated fat, or 300 milligrams of cholesterol daily. These nutrient values are listed as maximums, but others, such as those for carbohydrates, are listed as minimums that should equal 300 grams or more per day in the 2000-calorie diet. Thus, this portion of the label tells you the total *maximum* or *minimum* amounts for each nutrient, which you can use as a reference

point to evaluate the *percentage* amount of each nutrient listed on the label of the product in question. These nutrition facts take a little getting used to, but as you get more familiar with the concept of daily value, you can use it to show how any given food fits into your overall daily diet.

Salt and other food additives

A food additive is any material other than the basic raw ingredients necessary for the production of a specific food. Additives are commonly used in most processed foods. Most additives are used for flavor, preservation of food, or color. Vitamin and mineral additives are used to enrich foods such as cereals, flour, and milk. Food additives are regulated by the FDA, which classifies them into two groups—newer additives and older ones which form the Generally Recognized As Safe list (GRAS). Sometimes older additives are reclassified by the FDA as possibly unsafe, as happened with saccharin. Ironically, saccharin was developed to avoid the presumed health risks of what is perhaps the most widely used additive—sugar. Although saccharin has not been found to cause cancer in humans, it has been linked to cancer in animals

Table 87   THE FOOD GUIDE PYRAMID—A GUIDE TO DAILY FOOD CHOICES

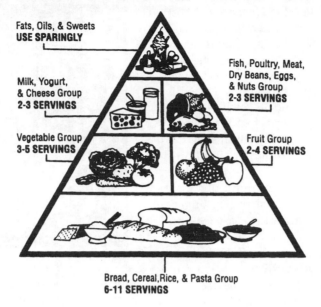

Fats, Oils, & Sweets
USE SPARINGLY

Milk, Yogurt,
& Cheese Group
2-3 SERVINGS

Fish, Poultry, Meat,
Dry Beans, Eggs,
& Nuts Group
2-3 SERVINGS

Vegetable Group
3-5 SERVINGS

Fruit Group
2-4 SERVINGS

Bread, Cereal, Rice, & Pasta Group
6-11 SERVINGS

> **The Food Guide Pyramid emphasizes foods from the five groups shown in the three lower sections of the pyramid.**
> **A good diet is low in fat, cholesterol, sodium, and sugars; and high in vegetables, fruits, beans, and whole grains. Eating well can make a real difference in your health and longevity.**

when very large doses were given. The risk of years of saccharin use in humans remains unclear.

Food additives may be a source of excess dietary salt. It is the sodium in salt that we need to be concerned with. Labeling on packages gives us the sodium content of the product, measured usually in mg (milligrams); 1000 mg is equal to 1 gram. Relatively large amounts of sodium are added as a preservative in most processed foods such as luncheon meats. More than sufficient sodium is obtained in the average American diet without adding salt at the table. The amount of sodium needed for healthy adults is 1 to 3 grams per day; the amount for you should depend on your physical activity and the amount of water you lose daily. Remember that the amount of sodium you consume will come from your total intake for the day, including those amounts "hidden" in foods (and some

antacids) and not just what comes out of your salt shaker. Ideally you should limit your sodium intake to 2 to 3 grams per day, but a more reasonable goal for most people would be to keep sodium intake to 6 grams or less. A salt-restricted diet has one gram of sodium or less daily. It has been estimated that the average American consumes much more salt than is needed for good nutrition. A heavy salt intake may be a health risk for some women, especially those with a personal or family history of heart disease or high blood pressure. Even in normal individuals, excess dietary salt is suspected of playing a contributing role in the development of these conditions. (See the reference list at the end of this section.)

Food snacks

Eating habits of Americans have changed enormously during the last twenty years. More meals are eaten on the run and often consist of so-called fast foods. Overall, the nutritional value of meals provided by fast-food chains is short on essential vitamins and minerals, and these meals give you far more fats, salts, and sugar than you would get if you selected from the five basic food groups in the right proportions. Even if you "have it your way," it is almost impossible to get sufficient fruits and vegetables at the hamburger, chicken, fish, and pizza fast-food chains. Snacking is one of the features of the American eating habits which plays a significant role—often detrimental—in the determination of the quality of our diet. Even less nutritious than fast-food meals are snacks consisting of sugar-laden "junk foods," such as candy, pastries, and soda pop.

As with your regular meals, it is best to choose low-fat alternatives with snacks. Current food manufacturing trends do emphasize low-fat and sugar-free foods. One word of caution—low-fat snacks are often high in sugar, while products advertised as sugar-free often contain more than their fair share of fat. Read labels on

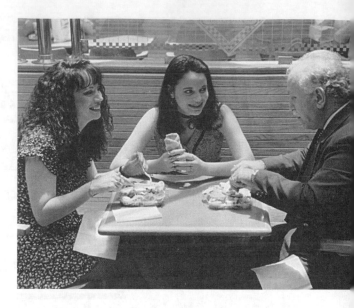

microwave food packages, too; some versions are more healthful than others. Here are some examples of snacks that we think are more on the healthy side:

Breads and cereals:	cheese wafers, graham crackers, sandwiches (use enriched or whole-grain bread)
Fruit and vegetables:	juices, dried fruits, fresh fruit and vegetables
Meat:	tacos, bean sandwiches, boiled eggs, meatballs, pizzas (with meat)
Milk (low fat):	cheese, ice cream, yogurt, milkshakes, pudding, milk-containing dips, cottage cheese

Food and Cancer

Much has been written recently about the subject of nutrition and cancer and anticancer diets. While there are clearly dietary risks for high blood pressure, heart disease, and obesity, the relationship between diet and cancer is not quite as well defined. However, the American Cancer Society notes seven dietary factors that may lead to a healthier life and, presumably, a lowered risk for cancer:

1. Eat more cabbage-family vegetables. This family of vegetables (known as *cruciferous*)

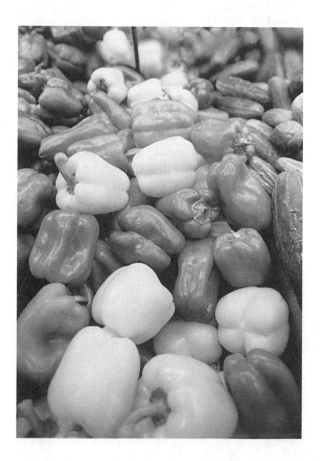

includes broccoli, Brussels sprouts, cabbage, and cauliflower. Studies indicate that regular consumption of these vegetables affords some protection against colon, stomach, and lung cancers.

2. Eat more high-fiber foods. Fiber is found in fruits and vegetables as well as in whole grains, which are present in whole-wheat bread and wheat and bran cereals. Fiber helps move food and waste products along the intestinal tract so that potentially cancer-causing toxins have less time to be exposed to the bowel. Some research indicates that people who eat a diet rich in high-fiber foods have a reduced risk of colon cancer.

3. Select foods rich in antioxidants like vitamins C and E and beta-carotene. Beta-carotene (the precursor to vitamin A) can be found in carrots, peaches, squash, and apricots, and may reduce your risk of cancer of the esophagus, larynx, and lungs.

4. Consume more vitamin C, which is found in citrus fruits and many fresh vegetables. A diet abundant in foods containing vitamin C may protect you against cancers of the esophagus and stomach.

5. Maintain a healthy weight. Obesity is linked to cancers of the breast, uterus, colon, and gallbladder.

6. Cut down on dietary fat. A high-fat diet has been linked to breast and colon cancer. Avoid fatty cuts of meat, cut down on red meat, eat more fish and skinned chicken, and select low-fat dairy products. Limit use of sweets and pastries.

7. Cut down on salt-cured, smoked, or nitrite-cured foods. Cancers of the esophagus and stomach are more common in countries where these foods are eaten in large quantities. Cut down on or practically eliminate such foods as bacon, ham, hot dogs, and salt-cured fish.

The last three factors (5, 6, and 7) also protect you against heart disease, which is associated with obesity, a high-fat diet, and excess dietary salt in the diet.

Nutrition in the Later Years

As women get older, they need the same essential nutrients but fewer calories, as a result of decreasing metabolism and lessened physical exercise. In recent years, certain specific nutritional needs of older women have become recognized. Dietary surveys have revealed that women, starting in their forties and fifties, often have deficiencies in calcium and ascorbic acid related to inadequate consumption of milk, fruit, and vegetables. Older women may benefit from increased amounts of dietary fiber. Fiber, which forms much of the undigested roughage in food, helps to prevent certain intestinal problems that increase with age, including diverticulitis and constipation.

Osteoporosis (see Chapters 27 and 51) is a debilitating illness affecting women in middle and older age and accounts for approximately five million fractures in women each year. Among the factors making a woman more susceptible to bone loss and, therefore, osteoporosis are the nutritional stresses of childbearing accompanied by

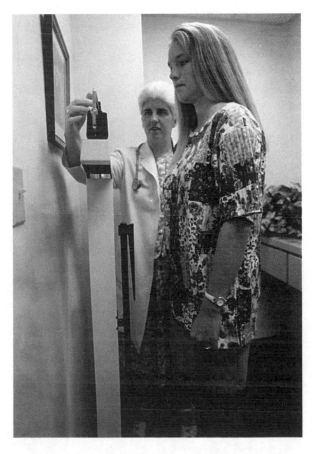

inadequate dietary calcium and sedentary lifestyles in later years. While the average nonpregnant woman needs at least 1000 milligrams of calcium daily before menopause and up to 1500 milligrams a day after menopause, it is estimated that most American women over the age of fifty consume barely half this amount in their diets. Older women are likely to decrease their consumption of calcium-rich dairy products when going on weight-loss diets or because of digestive intolerance to dairy products (such intolerance may cause diarrhea or cramping) that sometimes occurs with age. Another factor opposing adequate calcium utilization is the high content of phosphorus in the American diet. This mineral competes with calcium for absorption, with the result that the more phosphorous-rich foods you eat (such as meat, carbonated beverages, and processed foods), the less calcium is absorbed. To acquire the recommended daily 800 to 1000 mg of calcium from her diet, an adult woman should consume a quart (four 8-oz. glasses) of milk each day, or the amount of other dairy products that will yield an equivalent amount of calcium, or take a calcium supplement, such as calcium carbonate, or calcium citrate, available at most drugstores. Vitamin D helps increase calcium absorption. However, supplementation with this vitamin is probably unnecessary if you drink vitamin D–enriched milk.

It is difficult to define the exact requirements of the essential nutrients for one's later years. Following the adult requirements (U.S. RDA) is probably adequate. The greatest protection lies in consuming a wide variety of foods with as little processing as possible. Chronic conditions may require a special diet—for example, salt restriction with high blood pressure or heart disease. Be certain to find out from your clinician if any medications you are taking will affect your nutritional needs.

CHAPTER 49

Physical Fitness

Long ago in our society the physical demands of daily living were far greater than they are today. People then didn't have to be concerned with "creating" physical exercise to keep fit. Today, however, our jobs and daily lives, for most of us, place very few physical demands on us. As a result we must actively look for ways to keep in good physical condition.

Since the early 1960s, when President Kennedy recognized and promoted the need for increased physical fitness, Americans have shown a steadily increasing interest in maintaining good health through various forms of physical exercise. Women have become more and more involved in sports and fitness programs. With more women working than ever before and becoming, in some cases, the sole support of the family unit, women have come to realize that to get daily physical exercise, they have to plan for it.

How do you know what kind of physical shape you are in? You may notice the extra exertion required when an unexpected activity, such as running to catch a bus, leaves you feeling completely winded; or you may feel chronically tired and irritable after a day's work, with little energy left to enjoy your free time. *Hypokinesis* is the term used by physicians to indicate body deterioration or lack of proper physical fitness, which may be the cause of the symptoms just described.

When you decide that you do want to become more physically fit, where do you begin? Before you embark on any new physical exercise program, it is wise to have a physical examination and an EKG (electrocardiogram) to check for possible heart abnormalities. Most experts feel that if you are over the age of thirty-five, you should have a cardiovascular *stress test* (see glossary) before beginning a vigorous exercise program. If you have a family history of premature heart disease (that is, before age fifty) or are se-verely overweight, you should have a stress test, regardless of your age.

Physical Fitness and You

Physical fitness can be measured in different ways. It is often assessed by measuring heart rate after exercise. Fitness can also be measured in terms of muscular endurance or the strength of specific muscles required to perform a task such as lifting weights. Muscular flexibility is also a measure of fitness and refers to the range of motion of a particular joint. An example of this is how close you can come to touching your toes.

Optimal physical fitness requires both aerobic exercise and muscle-strengthening exercises (preferably done at a separate time). This combination results in better all-around fitness, with greater muscle strength and flexibility, than either type of exercise performed exclusively. In 1990 the American College of Sports Medicine revised its statement on exercise, which serves as a guide for healthy adults attempting to reach and maintain a higher level of fitness. The guidelines recommend continuous strenuous aerobic activity that lasts for twenty to sixty minutes, performed three to five days per week. The amount of time you spend exercising depends on the activity's intensity: the harder you work, the less time you have to put in. Activities with low to moderate intensity, like riding a stationary bicycle, are recommended for those just starting an exercise program. When exercising, be sure to allow five to ten minutes for warmup and cool-down periods, including stretching exercises to prevent injury as well as to maximize your flexibility. Flexibility has been increasingly recognized by experts as helpful in preventing injury. To achieve your potential, try setting goals when you work out, pushing yourself toward, but not all the way to, your limits of endurance. A number of experts now suggest that optimal cardiovascular fitness requires at least three workouts a week in which you burn up 300+ calories a session, or four workouts if you use only 200 calories each time. For women on restricted-calorie weight-loss diets, this level of weekly exercise is a minimum if weight loss is to occur.

Your goal for physical fitness should be personal and should relate to your own needs (see

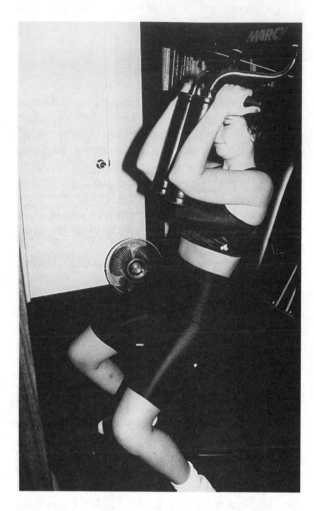

Table 88). People may exercise for relaxation, to increase their muscular flexibility or strength, to improve their heart-lung functioning (see Aerobic Exercise below), to increase motor skills, to alter their body shape (lose inches), or for weight control or weight loss (see Table 90). People may do the same exercises for different reasons, as in adult ballet classes, where the goal may be to strengthen certain muscles, improve flexibility, or develop specific motor skills.

When you decide to begin a program of exercise, you should:

1. Be certain that your exercise plan will not aggravate any chronic physical condition you may have, such as arthritis. Check with your doctor first.
2. Pick an exercise that uses skills different from those you may use at work.
3. Consider choosing an activity you already enjoy or would like to try.

4. Begin exercising gradually and work up slowly to your desired level of fitness.
5. Use equipment that is the right size or weight for your level of skills and physical size.
6. Begin each exercise time with a gradual warm-up period that includes flexibility exercises (i.e., stretching) (at least five minutes) and end your exercise with a cool-down period (also 5 minutes), gradually bringing your body back to rest.
7. Be certain to get enough daily rest.
8. Use common sense in your exercise program. Pay attention to your own body's signals when they tell you to slow down.
9. Never exercise after a heavy meal or after drinking alcohol. If you feel sick or dizzy, stop immediately.
10. Plan an exercise program that includes resistance training (strength training) as well as aerobic activity (endurance training).

After and during exercise, prevent dehydration by drinking water, orange juice, or perhaps one of the commercially available liquids, like Gatorade, which replace salt and other minerals lost in sweat.

If you live in a warm climate and you exercise outdoors, to avoid the possibility of heatstroke, exercise in the early morning or late evening when it is cooler. When the humidity is high (over 80%), exercise cautiously or not at all, as moisture in the air tends to slow sweat evaporation and puts an extra strain on the heart.

If you live in a cold climate and you exercise outdoors in the winter, take sensible safeguards: Cool down very gradually after you have worked up a sweat. Protect yourself against frostbite. If the air is very cold, you may want to put a loose-knit scarf over your mouth to help warm up the air you are breathing in. Or you may try to arrange to use a local school gym during off hours—say, in the early morning or evening hours.

Recently, there has been more interest among women in their percentage of fat in body weight. Prepuberty, normally active boys and girls average 15% of body fat. After puberty, girls climb up to 22% and boys decrease to 10%, assuming equal activity. Female hormones tend to increase these normal fat deposits. The percentage of body fat can be measured most accurately by immersion in a water tank. Women who have

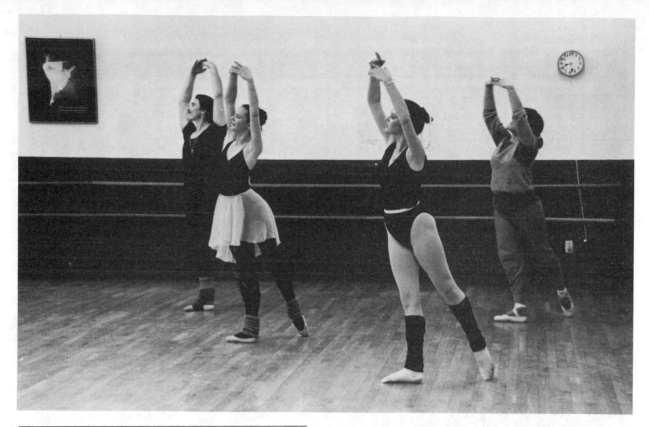

Table 88   GOALS OF EXERCISING

Goal of Exercise	Exercise Program
improved motor skill	an exercise related to desired skill, e.g., backboard practice for tennis, pitching for softball, etc.
increased muscular strength	softball, weight lifting, tennis, karate, Royal Canadian Air Force Exercise Plan
increased muscular flexibility (range of motion in a joint)	stretching movements, such as those done in ballet, gymnastics, yoga, sailing, tennis
increased endurance	any aerobic exercise program, i.e., jogging, cycling, walking briskly, certain kinds of dancing, swimming, skiing
changed shape (lose inches)	gymnastics, modern dance, specific exercise program
weight control or weight loss	any exercise if done in combination with a reduction in calories (weight-loss diet) to lose weight
increased relaxation	isometric exercises, yoga, deep breathing, walking, bicycling, running, horseback riding; any exercise that can be done comfortably without great mental concern about a specific skill

between 18 and 25% body fat appear to be the healthiest, both emotionally and physically. Olympic women gymnasts (who are mostly teenagers) average 14% body fat. Despite claims to the contrary, there is no easy way to "spot reduce" or lose fat selectively from a particular part of the body. In women, fat is added to the thighs and hips first and then to the arms and upper body. Loss of fat occurs in the reverse fashion, from the upper body first and then from the lower body. Exercises for specific parts of the body are excellent for firming and shaping the underlying muscles, and hence, shaping your body—leading to the *appearance* of lost fat—but systemic, whole-body exercise, such as aerobic exercise, is necessary to remove fat. A good resource for learning more about the subject of body fat is *The Fit or Fat Woman* by Covert Bailey.

Older women need exercise for the same reason that younger women do—to maintain aerobic capacity, muscle flexibility, and strength, and to maintain optimum body-fat levels. Exercise also helps to reverse the loss of bone minerals that occurs after menopause. It is not yet known how much exercise is needed to maintain bone integrity. Studies in older people show that exercise can slow the deterioration of the brain and sharpen mental functioning.

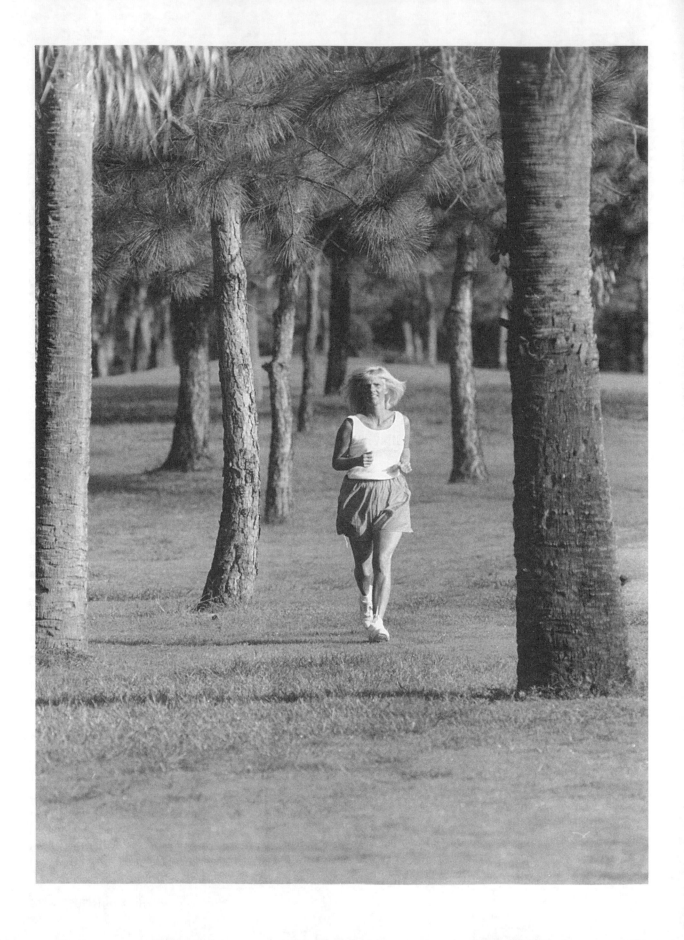

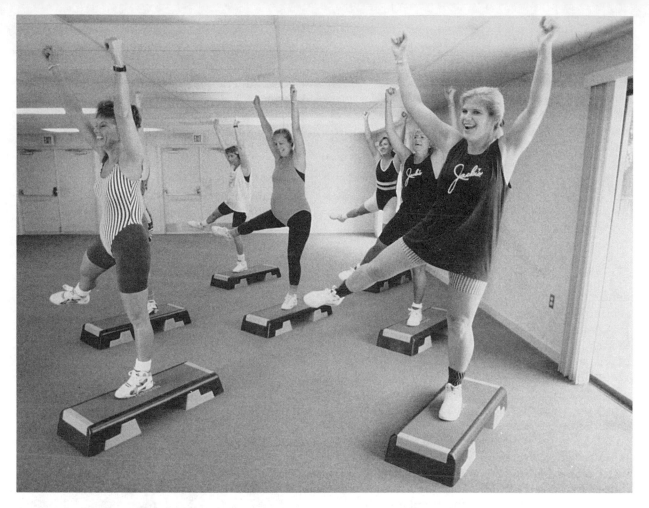

Shortcuts to maintaining a fit body and strong heart just don't exist. "Toning tables" or other table workouts have not been found to increase muscle strength in healthy people, as the tables don't provide the necessary resistance to build muscle capacity. Neither do the electrical muscle stimulators (EMS), which make muscles contract by delivering electrical currents to contact pads on the skin. Especially beware the shortest of shortcuts—pills and injections to help build muscles or run faster. The most frequently used, anabolic steroids, are synthetic versions of the male sex hormone testosterone, which aids in muscle growth. Steroids will work to build muscles but have been linked to medical complications such as heart disease and liver damage.

If you are thinking about acquiring a home gym or fitness center, set practical goals before you purchase expensive equipment, such as an exercise bicycle complete with all the electronic gadgets. The single largest drawback to indoor exercise is boredom; running on a treadmill never could and never will be as interesting as jogging through the woods. As with most exer-

cise routines, sticking to a home exercise program requires some discipline. Be careful to select equipment that fits into your home and budget as well as your exercise needs. Carefully planned, however, a home exercise program may be a practical, efficient use of your time. Paying a personal trainer to supervise your exercise has increased in popularity. There are also personal training software programs available to use at home, as well as many exercise videotapes.

Aerobic Exercise

Aerobic exercise refers to forms of exercise which are designed to strengthen your heart and lungs. Examples of aerobic exercises are walking, swimming, cycling, and running. With proper conditioning, aerobic exercises allow your heart and lungs to utilize oxygen more efficiently; in other words, for a given activity, your heart is able to deliver oxygen through your blood to your body doing less work, as evi-

Table 89   FINDING YOUR TARGET HEART RATE

Age (years)	Target heart rate (beats per minute)
20	120–160
30	114–152
40	108–144
50	102–136
60	96–128

denced by a lowered pulse rate. The concept of aerobic exercise was developed by Dr. Kenneth H. Cooper. A useful book, *The New Aerobics for Women*, by M. Cooper and K. Cooper, fully explains aerobic exercise programs for all age groups of women.

It is important to find your target heart rate when exercising for cardiovascular fitness. You should achieve a sustained heart rate at least equal to your target rate for at least fifteen minutes when exercising. You can check your heart rate by feeling your wrist just below the thumb to get your pulse. Count for 10 seconds and multiply by 6 to find the number of beats per minute. See Table 89 to determine your target heart rate. It is calculated at about 60% to 90% of your maximum heart rate (the fastest your heart can beat). Your maximum heart rate is usually about 220 beats per minute minus your age. Exercising between 60% and 90% of your maximum heart rate is best for cardiovascular conditioning. Remember to always precede exercise with a gentle warm-up that utilizes full range of motion.

Women and Sports

Active participation by increasing numbers of women in many types of athletic competition is a relatively recent trend. Women have been encouraged to enter sporting activities by Title IX of the Federal Educational Assistance Act of 1972, which legalized equal federal financial support for school programming of male and female sports. Sports opportunities for girls and women of all ages are blossoming, which should enable a young girl to develop the kind of preconditioning necessary for participation in skilled athletics as an adult.

One area of special concern to women athletes is the effect of exercise on the menstrual cycle. It is now known that some women, especially professional athletes, develop menstrual irregularities or stop menstruating for several months or more after engaging in a program of strenuous exercise. This is most common in long-distance runners. The reason for this is not clear and does not affect all women. Possibly the stress involved—both physical and emotional—leads to hormone changes that disrupt normal menstrual cycles. When the woman stops or decreases the amount of exercise, her periods usually return to normal.

Sports are not only fun to take part in, they

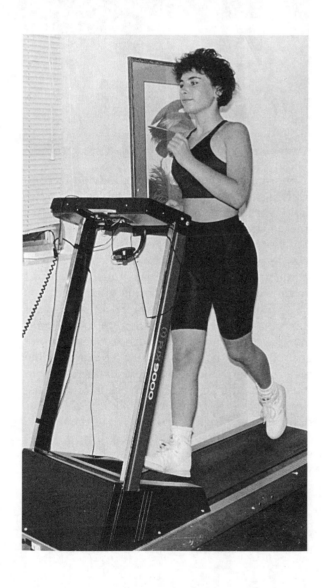

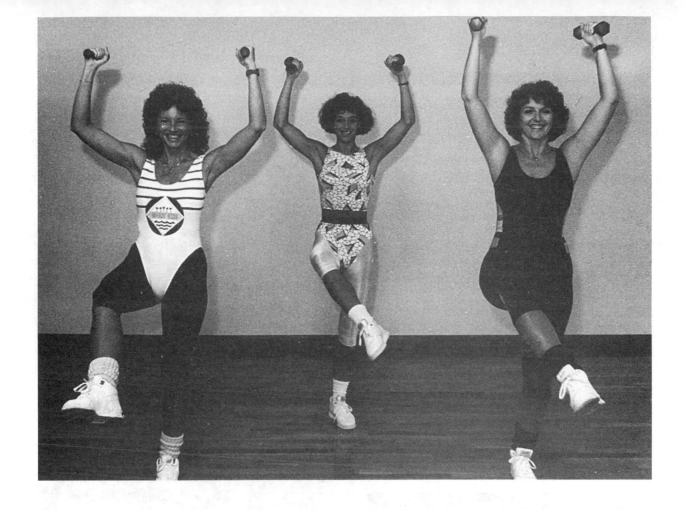

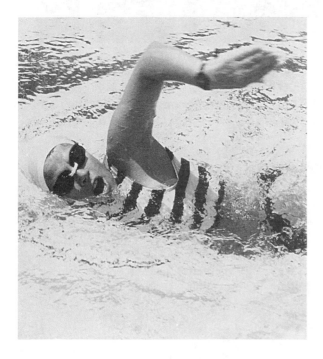

can also be an excellent part of a weight-control or weight-loss program. Table 90 will give you an idea of the number of calories you use up when you participate in certain sports activities.

Exercise and Certain Medical Problems

Exercise, in general, does much to improve your whole body functioning and, in particular, depending on the kind of exercise you do, improves your heart and lung functioning (that is, the oxygen and blood supply to all your tissues), increases your muscle tone and muscle strength, increases bone density, and decreases your body-fat deposits. Because of these and other benefits, exercise can have a direct beneficial effect on many specific conditions and symptoms, among them the following: urinary stress incontinence, diabetes, insomnia, anxiety, nervousness, mild depression, some lung conditions, and some heart and blood vessel problems. If you have any of these problems, be sure to check

Table 90 CALORIE EXPENDITURE FOR SOME COMMON SPORTS ACTIVITIES

Activity	Estimated No. of Calories Used Up per Hour*
Bicycling (5.5 mph)	190–265
Bowling	225–335
Golf (foursome)	240–350
Gymnastics	200–270
Racquetball	620–850
Roller-skating	275–350
Running	400–550
Skiing	460–558
Swimming	400–550
Tennis	330–440
Walking or hiking	230–335

* Range is based on body weight of 110 lbs. to 150 lbs. The exact amount of calories you burn up per hour depends on how much you weigh (the more you weigh, the more calories you burn up per hour of exercise) and on how hard you work at your exercise. Going up a hill when you are bicycling, walking, running, or carrying a back-pack when you are hiking, will increase caloric expenditure.

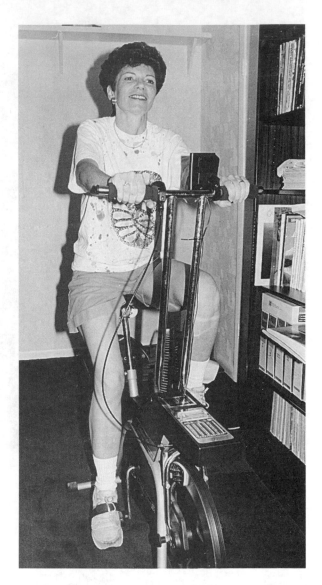

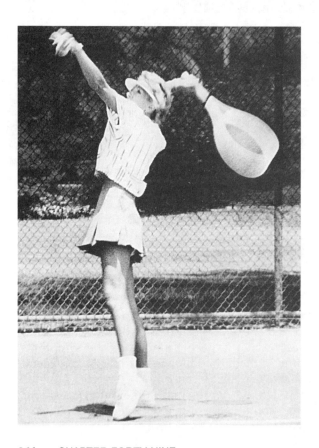

first with your physician as to the appropriate beneficial exercises for you before you begin a vigorous exercise program. Exercise is also important in pregnancy (see Chapter 16).

Resources

American Alliance for Health, Physical Education, Recreation and Dance
1900 Association Drive
Reston, Virginia 22091

Community recreation centers
Senior citizen centers

References for Section Ten

Chapter 47—Staying Healthy

American College of Obstetricians and Gynecologists *Technical Bulletin* 180. Smoking and reproductive health, May 1993.

American College of Obstetricians and Gynecologists *Technical Bulletin* 160. Immunization during pregnancy, Oct 1991.

American College of Obstetricians and Gynecologists, Committee on obstetrics: maternal and fetal medicine, *Committee Opinion* 112. Vitamin A supplementation during pregnancy, Aug 1992.

American College of Obstetricians and Gynecologists, Committee on obstetrics: maternal and fetal medicine, *Committee Opinion* 120. Folic acid for the prevention of recurrent neural tube defects, Mar 1993.

American College of Obstetricians and Gynecologists, Committee on gynecological practice, *Committee Opinion* 128. Routine cancer screening, Oct 1993.

The fifth report of the Joint National Committee on detection, evaluation, and treatment of high blood pressure. *Archives of Internal Medicine* 153:154–183, Jan 25, 1993.

National Cholesterol Education Program. *Second Report of the Expert Panel on Detection, Evaluation, and Treatment of High Blood Cholesterol in Adults*, 1993.

American Cancer Society, *Facts on Lung Cancer*, 1990.

American Cancer Society, *Quit Smoking, The Lives you Save . . . Could be Theirs*. 1987.

Bishop, G. *Health Psychology, Integrating Mind and Body*. Allyn and Bacon, 1994.

Yoder, L. The association between healthcare behavior and attitudes. *Health Values* 9(4):24–29, July/Aug 1985.

Report of the Health Service Task Force on Women's Health Issues. *Public Health Reports* 100(1):75–105, Jan/Feb 1985.

LaRossa, J. Women and coronary heart disease—facts and considerations for intervention. *Women's Wellness* 2(4):Apr 1988.

American Cancer Society, The Health Professional and Cancer Prevention and Detection—1988.

Hogue, C. You can help your OB patients stop smoking. *Contemporary OB/GYN* 130–143, Aug 1987.

Makuc, D. National trends in the use of preventive health care by women. *American Journal of Public Health* 79(1):21–26, Jan 1989.

Smoking and health: a 25 year perspective (editorial). *American Journal of Public Health* 79(2):141–143, Feb 1989.

Fluoridation, then and now (editorial). *American Journal of Public Health* 79(5):561–562, May 1989.

Byrd, J. Passive smoking: a review of medical and legal issues. *American Journal of Public Health* 79(2): 209–213, Feb 1989.

Rosenberg, L. The risk of myocardial infarction in women who smoke. *Journal of the American Medical Association* 253:2965–2969, 1985.

Baird, D. Cigarette smoking associated with delayed conception. *Journal of the American Medical Association* 253:2979–2983, 1985.

Gritz, E. Cigarette smoking: the need for action by health professionals. *CA—A Cancer Journal for Clinicians* 38(4):194–212, July/Aug 1988.

Chez, R. Battered pregnant women. *Genesis* 11 (1): 15–16, Jan/Feb 1989.

Chapter 48—Nutrition

March of Dimes Birth Defects Foundation and International Food Information Council Foundation. *Healthy eating during pregnancy*, Jan 1994.

Galante, V. Nutrition and psychological health. *The Health Psychologist* 16(3):4–8, Winter 1994.

National Institutes of Health. NIH Consensus Statement, *Optimal calcium intake*, 12(4): June 1994.

Bardes, C. Good reasons for checking cholesterol values. *Contemporary OB/GYN* 35–45: June 1994.

U.S. Department of Health and Human Services. *The Surgeon General's Report on Nutrition and Health*. New York: Warner Books, Inc. 1989.

Lecos, C. Planning a diet for a healthy heart. *FDA Consumer*, Mar 1987.

Barber, H. Elevated cholesterol: what the OB/GYN should know. *The Female Patient* 14: 11–12, Aug 1989.

Miller, V. Hypercholesterolemia in women: what are the special considerations? *The Female Patient* 13: 22–32, Apr 1988.

Filstead, W. High-risk situations for engaging in substance abuse, and binge-eating behaviors. *Journal of Studies on Alcohol*, 49(2):136–141, 1988.

Gotto, A. Cholesterol: new approaches to screening and management. *Contemporary OB/GYN* 32(1):56–70, July 1988.

Good fish . . . bad fish, fish oil: fad or find? *Nutrition Action Health Letter* Mar 1989.

Focus on nutrition. *Women's Wellness* 2(1):Jan 1988.

Brody, J. *Good Food Book*. New York: Bantam, 1987.

Chapter 49—Physical Fitness

American College of Obstetricians and Gynecologists *Technical Bulletin* 173. Women and exercise, Oct 1992.

Driscoll, C. Women in sports: guidelines for patient fitness. *The Female Patient* 13:41–51, June 1988.

Bailey, C. & L. Bishop. *The Fit or Fat Woman*. Boston: Houghton Mifflin, 1989.

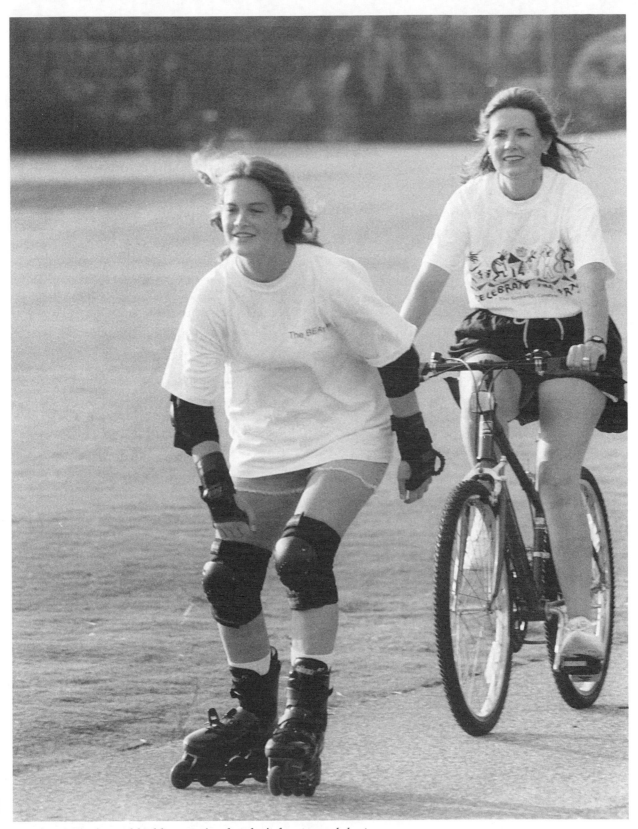

Exercise can be fun and health-promoting, but don't forget your helmet.

WHAT YOUR SYMPTOMS MEAN

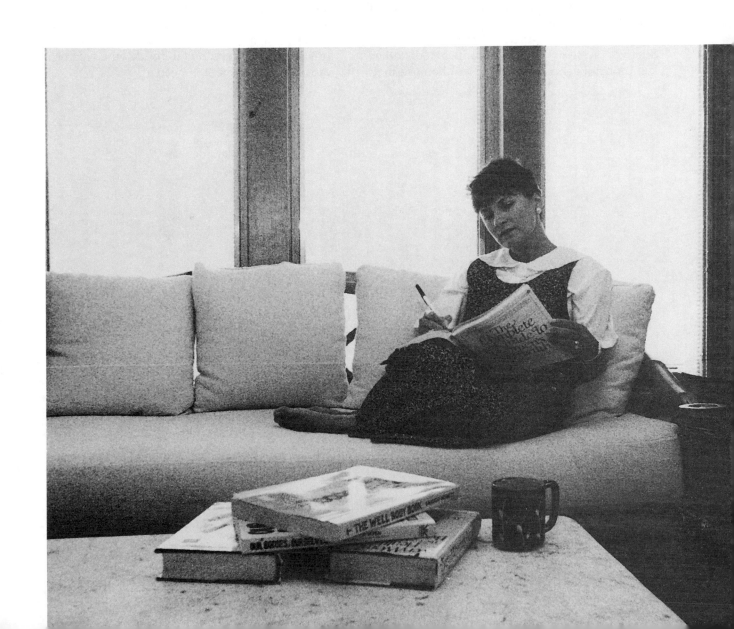

How to Use This Section

This section is about common symptoms—what they mean, what medical care can do, and what you can do to help yourself. Whether you see a general practitioner, a nurse practitioner, a family doctor, an internist, or a gynecologist, there are about one hundred symptoms or areas of concern that women commonly give as the reasons for visiting their clinicians. These problems are listed alphabetically below, along with a reference to the appropriate chapter or chapters in this section where each problem is discussed. Some symptoms, such as irregular menstrual periods and vaginal discharge, are directly related to conditions affecting the female reproductive system. We have included other symptoms (backaches, joint pains) because they bring about high disability in women. Certain chapters in this section deal with conditions (hypertension, migraine headaches) affecting women more frequently than men.

Each chapter begins with basic information about a particular symptom and what the symptom can mean, as well as how pregnancy may be involved. Under the heading *What Medical Care Can Do*, the usual methods of diagnosis and treatment are explained. Finally, under *What You Can Do (Self Care)*, we suggest ways you can handle the problem yourself and suggest when you should seek medical care. Flow charts are provided in each chapter with references to appropriate chapters to help you decide when medical care or self-treatment is needed.

Health Concerns

CHAPTER 50

Acne

Acne, the most common skin problem in women, is a disorder of the hair follicle and oil (sebaceous) glands. It first occurs during puberty and affects about 75% of adolescent women. Certain hereditary predispositions to acne account for the persistence of this condition over many years in some women. Normally secretions from skin glands travel up the hair follicle to the surface. In acne, the hair follicle is blocked, resulting in a build-up of oil and bacteria which ultimately ruptures into the skin. Secondary infections from the skin bacteria then occur, causing pimples and other skin changes characteristic of acne. Pimples and blackheads are the most common finding in acne and may cause cosmetic problems when scarring occurs.

Acne is predominantly a response of the skin gland to androgens, weak male hormones produced in small amounts by the ovaries and adrenal glands in women. During puberty, there is a temporary hormone imbalance favoring a slight increase in the ratio of androgens to estrogens. Psychological factors may also affect the course of acne. In times of stress, our bodies release additional androgens. Among the factors that do not contribute to acne are failure to wash properly, sexual activity, and diets high in sweets.

Acne may be affected by different factors during the woman's life cycle. Some women characteristically have an increase in acne the week prior to menses. Some women who do not ovulate regularly and have irregular, infrequent periods have a disproportionate amount of acne as a result of the increased androgen production in their ovaries. Estrogens, such as found in birth control pills, sometimes alleviate acne by diminishing skin sensitivity to androgens. Withdrawal of birth control pills (oral contraceptives), known popularly as the pill, may produce a worsening of acne in some women. In some women, acne persists past puberty into the twenties, thirties, or even later. Adult acne may be associated with other skin problems like tiny broken blood vessels (telangectasia) or inflamed eyelids (blepharitis).

Frequently in some women the skin improves during pregnancy as a result of the effects of high levels of estrogen. In other women, however, acne becomes worse in pregnancy for reasons not understood.

What Medical Care Can Do

In the nonpregnant woman, topicals such as retinoic acid and benzoyl peroxide, and the oral tetracycline antibiotics are the most effective prescription medicines used to treat moderately severe acne. The use of topical Retin-A (tretinoin) is well established in the treatment of acne; its recent and well-publicized use to improve aging skin and reduce wrinkles is still under study. The drug, which comes as a cream, gel, or liquid, produces rapid cell turnover in the skin glands and should be used sparingly to determine the extent to which skin drying and peeling will occur. Retin-A, a potent derivative of vitamin A, may cause side effects of vitamin overdose, including cracked lips, dry skin, and headache. When taking this drug, minimize exposure to sunlight (your skin will be more susceptible to sunburn) and avoid the use of medicated or abrasive soaps, as well as the use of cosmetics and skin cleansers that have a strong drying effect. Birth defects have not been reported with Retin-A cream. However, you should not use Retin-A during pregnancy or while trying to conceive. Birth defects have been reported with use of chemically similar drugs, like Accutane. Topical preparations containing benzoyl peroxide (Desquam, Persa Gel, etc.) are peeling agents like Retin-A but also have antibiotic activity. Other topicals include antibiotics such as erythromycin and clindamycin. Overexposure to sun, wind, and cold should be avoided when you use these preparations because your skin is more sensitive.

When used to treat acne, tetracycline (or the related drug, doxycycline) is taken for several weeks. As improvement occurs, tetracycline is reduced to a daily dose and ultimately the drug is usually discontinued after several months. In general, long-term antibiotic therapy is best avoided for three reasons: tetracyclines may ultimately lead to the development of antibiotic-resistant bacteria, cause vaginal yeast infections, or reduce pill effectiveness in women on birth control pills. When tetracycline therapy is unsuccessful, topical antibiotics may be tried, but their use remains controversial.

Accutane (isotretinoin), a drug sometimes prescribed for severe cystic acne, can cause severe birth defects in pregnancy. Accutane, which has been prescribed mostly by dermatologists for an estimated 30,000 American women, is being closely monitored by the Food and Drug Administration. An FDA investigator estimated recently that several hundred infants have been born with Accutane-related birth defects. These may include ear deformities, cleft palate, heart defects, and various other abnormalities. Birth defects occur in up to 25% of babies exposed to this drug in utero. Accutane is probably best avoided unless you are not sexually active or are using a highly effective method of birth control such as the pill. If you do take Accutane, you must have a pregnancy test performed prior to starting the drug. Small amounts of Accutane remain in the body for more than two years after treatment, indicating that the risk of birth defects may extend for a prolonged period of time after stopping the drug. Accutane is a potent drug with numerous potential side effects, including decreased night vision, diarrhea, vomiting, conjunctivitis, joint pains, and headaches.

For the woman who uses oral contraceptives as a birth control method or for some other medical reason, the pill may also be used for the treatment of acne. Because of the risks involved, however, the pill should not be used exclusively for the purpose of treating acne. An individual's skin response to taking birth control pills is highly variable and improvement may take as long as six months. There is no way to predict how a woman who has had severe acne as an adolescent will react to pregnancy or to taking the pill. Acne scars may be treated surgically using procedures such as dermabrasion, chemical peeling, or simple scar excision or grafting.

What You Can Do (Self Care)

Exposure to sunlight in small doses is sometimes helpful. Avoid oils, greasy cleansing creams, and other cosmetics. If you use makeup, be certain to wash your hands before applying it. Keep your makeup stored in the refrigerator to limit bacterial growth. Discard old makeup and buy new makeup frequently; unused portions of eye makeup should be discarded after three to four months' use. Don't use anyone else's makeup, only your own. Use an ordinary mild soap, such as Ivory, to keep your skin clean. Neutrogena acne soap may be helpful in preventing secondary bacterial infections. Nonprescription products containing low-dose benzoyl peroxide include Pan Oxyl, Persa Gel, Oxy10, and many others. X-ray treatments for acne are dangerous because they may lead to cancer. Remember that any chronic condition including anemia and poor nutrition may make acne worse. Eat plenty of fresh fruits and vegetables. Avoid a high-fat diet and such foods as chocolate and peanuts. To prevent disfigurement in severe cases, see a dermatologist promptly.

ACNE

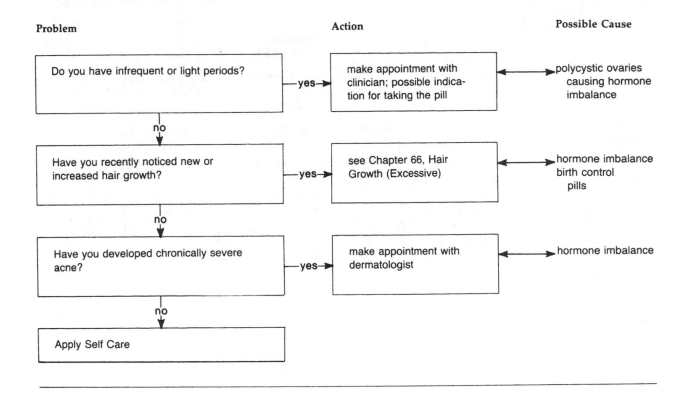

Problem	Action	Possible Cause

Do you have infrequent or light periods? — **yes→** — make appointment with clinician; possible indication for taking the pill ← polycystic ovaries causing hormone imbalance

no ↓

Have you recently noticed new or increased hair growth? — **yes→** — see Chapter 66, Hair Growth (Excessive) ← hormone imbalance birth control pills

no ↓

Have you developed chronically severe acne? — **yes→** — make appointment with dermatologist ← hormone imbalance

no ↓

Apply Self Care

CHAPTER 51

Backache

As many as 25% of women having a routine checkup by their gynecologist complain of backache. Low backache is the most common form of back pain in women; it has numerous causes, most of which are not serious. Some women experience back discomfort every month during menses. This pain is not usually a sign of disease since the uterus normally "refers" pain, or sends pain signals, to the back just as a toothache pain may be referred to the jaw. A popular misconception is that women with a "tilted" uterus are backache prone; pain occurs in this case only if the uterus is held back in this position as a result of disease such as endometriosis. Endometriosis produces severe low abdominal or back pain usually a day or two before as well as during menses. Certain conditions—uterine tumors such as fibroids, ovarian cysts, and pelvic infections of the tube or cervix—may cause low back discomfort at any time during the menstrual cycle. Table 91 tells you what symptoms are also present along with backache with certain conditions. Cancer of the pelvic organs almost never presents itself as backache alone. The backache of kidney infections is felt in the upper back toward the right or left side rather than in the low back and is usually associated with painful or bloody urination.

The terms *back strain* or *lumbosacral strain* usually refer to muscle spasm associated with trauma to the spinal column from your lifting objects that are too heavy or from a sudden spine-twisting turn. Even a bad mattress or poor posture can cause muscle spasms. Whatever the cause, the result is low back pain that is disabling. A much more serious problem that may result from straining your spine is a so-called slipped disc. In this painful condition, adjacent bones in the spine collapse upon each other as a result of rupture of the disc between them. This condition often irritates the spinal nerves, sending shooting pains down the backs of your legs.

Table 91   SYMPTOMS FOUND IN CERTAIN CONDITIONS THAT CAUSE BACKACHE

Condition Causing Backache	Associated Symptom(s)
Tube infection	Low abdominal pain, vaginal discharge, sometimes fever
Ovarian cyst	Low abdominal pain on one side
Endometriosis	Low abdominal pain occurring during and just before period
Cervical infection (cervicitis)	Chronic vaginal discharge
Uterine fibroid	Heavy or irregular menstrual bleeding
Kidney infection	Fever, painful urination, bloody urine

Older women are especially prone to two diseases of the spine: arthritis and osteoporosis. Osteoporosis affects about 30% of women over sixty years of age and is three to five times more common among women than men. This disease is characterized by gradual loss of bone from the spinal column, particularly after menopause, resulting in pain, a loss of height, and susceptibility to fractures. The condition of lower levels of estrogen following menopause has been suggested as a cause of osteoporosis (see Chapter 27). Arthritis of the spine is usually associated with chronic pain or stiffness in other joints, as well as in the spine.

Whatever the cause of backache, the role of stress must be evaluated. Most women have some minor back discomfort at one time or another for which no specific cause is found except tension. People under chronic stress tend to hold their muscles in an increased state of contraction, thereby contributing to back discomfort.

Most pregnant women suffer from at least minor degrees of back discomfort. This discomfort occurs predominantly in the second half of pregnancy as the enlarging uterus places more strain on the back muscles. Occasionally a shooting pain down the back of one or both legs may occur from pressure of the uterus on the pelvic nerves.

What Medical Care Can Do

The physical examination will emphasize your posture, weight, and evaluation of any areas of tenderness along the spine. The lower limbs are usually checked for abnormal reflexes, weakness, or loss of sensation. You will be asked to lie down while the examiner lifts first one leg and then the other. If this maneuver elicits back pain, the problem may be a back strain or disc injury. The latter is usually managed by a bone specialist or an orthopedic surgeon. If pelvic pain accompanies back pain, you may need a referral to a gynecologist.

If back pain persists for several weeks or a slipped disc is suspected, special diagnostic tests are usually done. A traditional test for back pain used to be the myelogram, a somewhat painful X-ray procedure in which dye is injected into the spine. Today, less invasive tests, such as the CAT scan and even newer magnetic resonance imaging, or MRI (see glossary for these), are often performed instead. The MRI gives a detailed picture of the spinal column without the use of spinal injections or X-rays.

Most back problems do not require surgery. Medical treatment for a slipped disc may require some bed rest with or without prescription pain pills or muscle relaxants. Current research is very supportive of strengthening exercises to assist in early return to functional tasks. Local injections with anesthetics sometimes provide immediate pain relief. A specific exercise program for your type of back pain may be obtained by referral to a physical therapist. Other modalities of therapy have had uncertain results. Spinal manipulation, a procedure often done by doctors of osteopathy and chiropractors, may bring temporary relief but is no more effective than conservative measures, such as rest and muscle-strengthening exercises. Regular spinal manipulation does not prevent back-injury progression and could delay diagnosis of a more serious problem, such as a spinal tumor. Acupuncture provides short-term pain relief, but pain ultimately comes back in most cases. Biofeedback has had some limited success, particularly in individuals with chronic tension and anxiety. Finally, TENS, which stands for transcutaneous electrical nerve stimulation, is a treatment that can provide temporary relief of chronic back pain by using a weak electrical current that blocks the transmission of pain signals by providing alternative signals.

What You Can Do (Self Care)

There are several self-care tricks that may help you avoid backache in the first place. Many of them relate to good posture and body positioning. Wear supportive shoes when standing or walking for long periods. Avoid high-heeled shoes, especially in pregnancy. Heels force you to increase your anterior pelvic tilt to maintain your balance and put strain on your back. When lifting something, do not bend over at the waist. Instead squat down close to anything you plan to pick up, including your baby, bending your knees and keeping your back straight. Rise slowly from a bent-knees position, using your leg muscles, not your back. When standing for long periods, shift position from one foot to the other. The use of a footstool to keep one leg flexed at all times relieves back strain. Especially in pregnancy, roll to the side when you want to get up, and push yourself up using your arms. Don't do sit-ups unless both knees are bent. When caring for your baby, work at arm level to avoid bending over. For example, use a changing table or sit at your kitchen table. The pregnant woman who is gaining too much weight puts extra strain on her back, too. Control of weight to an optimum level also helps prevent and perhaps relieve back strain.

Proper positioning and sufficient rest are essentials for relief of back strain. The best rest is achieved by lying down, not sitting. If you lie on your back, do so only with a pillow positioned under your knees. If you choose to rest on your stomach, position a flat pillow under your pelvic area. When resting on your side, pull your knees toward your chest as much as feels comfortable. These positions reduce the anterior tilt of your pelvis and result in a flattening of the lumbar curve of your low back and a gentle stretching of the low-back musculature.

Other suggestions to relieve backache include:

1. Rest—slowing down your activity level even to the point of bed rest usually helps to decrease pain in a few days.
2. Exercise—"pelvic rock" and other back exercises may help backache especially

during pregnancy or during menstruation. Exercises to increase strength of abdominals and back extensor muscles are important in the prevention and treatment of lumbosacral strain. Ask your clinician for specific instructions.

3. Heat—moist heat through baths, showers, or hot packs relieves muscle spasm more effectively than dry heat, such as that provided by commercial heating pads.

4. Analgesics—over-the-counter drugs to relieve pain usually contain acetaminophen (Tylenol, Panadol, etc.) or aspirin. Both drugs have approximately equal ability to relieve pain. What determines the brand name product's potency depends mainly on the *dosage* of the ingredient or ingredients. Aspirin, which has been associated with fetal bleeding and birth defects, should be avoided in pregnancy. Also, aspirin's notorious potential to cause internal bleeding and ulcers (when taken chronically) make it a poor choice in a woman with stomach problems such as chronic indigestion. However, aspirin may be preferred over acetaminophen-containing drugs when backache is caused by arthritis because of aspirin's anti-inflammatory properties. A third type of analgesic, ibuprofen, has anti-inflammatory effects like aspirin and also has been found to be useful in relieving menstrual cramps and related backache. This drug, marketed under trade names like Advil and Nuprin, was the first new nonprescription pain killer to be approved in twenty years by the FDA. Chronic use may be associated with stomach problems similar to those with aspirin as well as rare instances of kidney damage in people with high blood pressure, heart disease, and pre-existing kidney problems. Like aspirin, ibuprofen should be avoided in pregnancy.

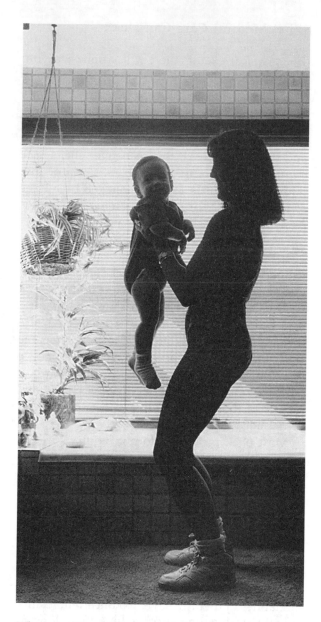

When you lift, protect your back by using your arm muscles, bending your knees, and keeping your back straight.

BACKACHE

Problem	Action	Possible Cause
Does this pain occur only during or just before menses?	—yes→ **see Chapter 79,** Menstrual Periods— Painful	endometriosis

no ↓

Do you have chronic pelvic pain?	—yes→ **see Chapter 83, Pelvic** Pain	uterine fibroid ovarian cyst tube infection

no ↓

Is backache associated with painful or bloody urination?	—yes→ **see Chapter 86, Urinary** Problems—Painful or Bloody Urination	urinary tract infection kidney stone

no ↓

Is backache associated with bleeding in pregnancy?	—yes→ **see Chapters 54 and 55,** on bleeding in pregnancy	threatened miscarriage "bloody show"— early labor placenta previa

no ↓

Is backache associated with painful joints?	—yes→ **see Chapter 73, Joint** Pains	arthritis of the spine

no ↓

Has backache developed gradually in association with or following menopause?	—yes→ **see Chapter 70, Hot** Flashes	osteoporosis

no ↓

Is backache associated with loss of leg sensation, leg weakness, or pain radiating down the backs of your legs?	—yes→ call or make appointment with orthopedic surgeon	slipped disc back strain

no ↓

Is backache getting worse despite pain pills?	—yes→ make appointment with clinician	back strain

no ↓

Apply Self Care

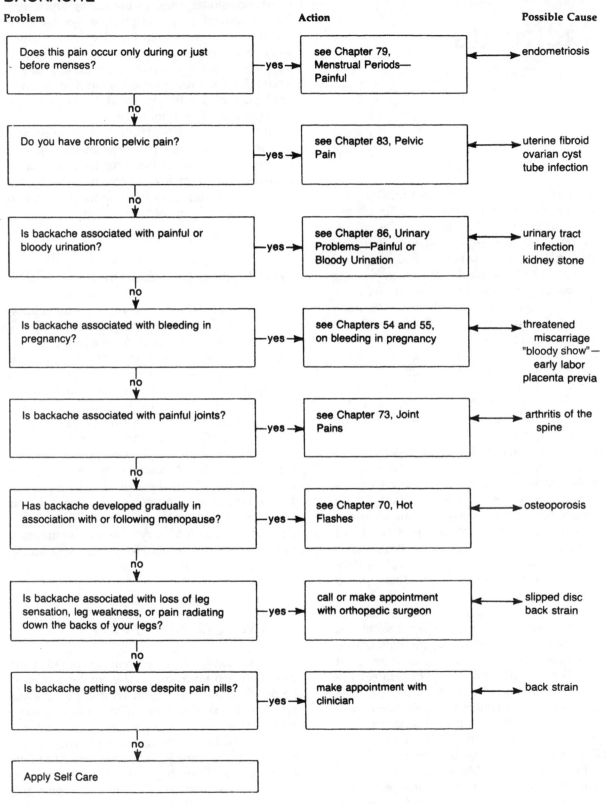

CHAPTER 52

Blackouts

The most common cause of blackouts is fainting, or *syncope*, the medical name for a temporary drop in pulse rate and blood pressure accompanied by a brief loss of consciousness. Pain, low blood sugar, sudden psychological stress, or fright can cause these blackouts. Accompanying symptoms may include blurred vision, sweating, nausea, and, when severe anxiety is present, numbness of mouth and hands from overbreathing (hyperventilation). Aggravating factors in fainting include prolonged sitting or standing, excessive coughing or straining, and collars or neck scarves that are too snug. You can faint during any procedure which stretches the cervix, such as insertion of an IUD, especially if you have never been pregnant.

The second major cause of blackouts in women is rapid blood loss from either external vaginal or rectal bleeding or internal abdominal bleeding as in the case of a ruptured cyst or tubal pregnancy. In women with peptic ulcer disease, tarry (black with the consistency of tar) stools may be the only sign of bleeding within the intestine. Internal bleeding is especially dangerous because it is less likely to be recognized early.

Other causes of blackouts, particularly in women over the age of forty, are heart problems, brain circulatory disorders, and, rarely, seizures. Heart disease is often accompanied by chest pain or shortness of breath. High blood pressure associated with small strokes may produce symptoms such as inability to move the arms or legs, loss of sensation, blurred vision, or difficulty with speech in addition to blackouts. These small strokes are usually temporary. Seizures are differentiated from blackouts by the rhythmic shaking movement that seizures often produce and by the accompanying loss of bowel or bladder control that frequently occurs.

An occasional cause of blackouts which may be overlooked is prescription drugs, such as those used to treat high blood pressure. These drugs may cause a person to faint when the person gets up suddenly from a reclining position. Tranquilizers, antidepressants, barbiturates, and antihistamines may also lead to blackouts if taken in excessive amounts.

In early pregnancy, fainting is common and frequently associated with low blood sugar or vomiting. Fainting in late pregnancy is due to changes in the circulation brought about by the weight of the uterus pressing on the major blood vessels to and from the heart.

What Medical Care Can Do

Your clinician will do a complete examination including taking your blood pressure and pulse rate, which usually varies from 60 to 100 beats per minute. Neurological examination is done if symptoms resemble a stroke or if you have a history of seizures; a referral to a neurologist may be made. In a woman with a suspected heart ailment, referral to a cardiologist may be made. An EKG (cardiogram) is ordered if the heartbeat is irregular or if chest pain is the presenting symptom. Medication to regulate heart rate or to control blood pressure may be needed. In addition to a complete examination, a blood count is done to rule out internal bleeding or chronic anemia. A history of stomach pain may require checking the stool for microscopic bleeding due to an ulcer.

What You Can Do (Self Care)

If you feel faint, lie down or sit down with your head between your knees. Use smelling salts or spirits of ammonia. If you faint easily, always rise from the reclining or sitting position slowly; and avoid sudden turning of your head or wearing tightfitting clothing around your neck, which may increase your susceptibility to fainting episodes. If you hyperventilate, breathe into a paper bag so that you rebreathe your own car-

BLACKOUTS

Problem	Action	Possible Cause

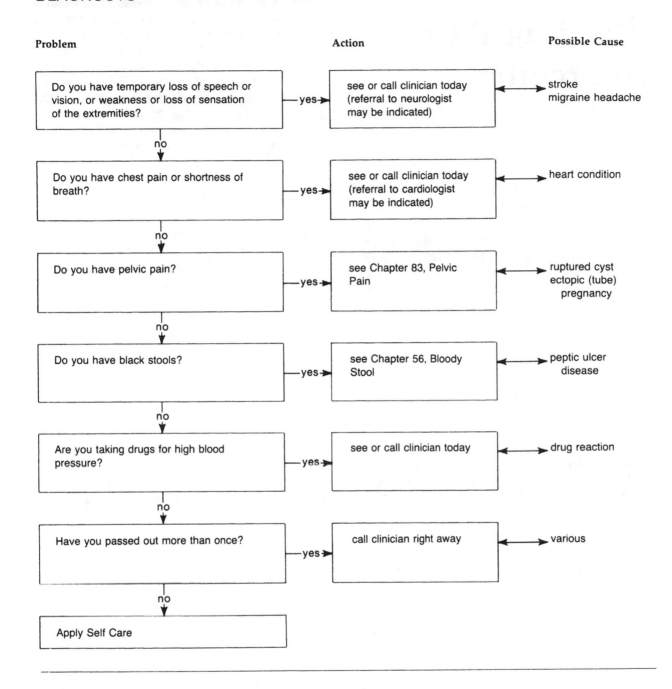

Problem	Action	Possible Cause
Do you have temporary loss of speech or vision, or weakness or loss of sensation of the extremities?	—yes→ see or call clinician today (referral to neurologist may be indicated)	stroke / migraine headache
↓ no		
Do you have chest pain or shortness of breath?	—yes→ see or call clinician today (referral to cardiologist may be indicated)	heart condition
↓ no		
Do you have pelvic pain?	—yes→ see Chapter 83, Pelvic Pain	ruptured cyst / ectopic (tube) pregnancy
↓ no		
Do you have black stools?	—yes→ see Chapter 56, Bloody Stool	peptic ulcer disease
↓ no		
Are you taking drugs for high blood pressure?	—yes→ see or call clinician today	drug reaction
↓ no		
Have you passed out more than once?	—yes→ call clinician right away	various
↓ no		
Apply Self Care		

bon dioxide and thereby prevent fainting. Take any medicines for blood pressure, heart problems, seizure disorders, or diabetes as directed, and avoid overuse of drugs that make you drowsy.

In pregnancy, fainting spells may be reduced by avoiding prolonged sitting and by getting up slowly after lying down. Eat frequent, small meals rather than three large meals a day to prevent rapid changes in blood sugar.

CHAPTER 53

Bleeding After Intercourse

The most frequent cause of bleeding after intercourse is inflammation of the cervix, or *cervicitis*. This condition is usually a chronic one related to glandular changes in the cervix during pregnancy. Acute cervicitis is associated with symptoms of infection such as an irritating vaginal discharge. Bleeding is expected, and is normal, following initial intercourse because of stretching and small tears made in the hymen. Occasionally menses begins at the time of intercourse, so the appearance of blood is really coincidental. Tumors of the cervix, including polyps and cancer, are uncommon causes of spotting or bleeding after intercourse.

During pregnancy, bleeding after intercourse may occur as a result of the increased number of blood vessels and glands covering the cervix. This so-called pregnancy cervicitis is also accompanied by an expected increase in vaginal discharge. Sometimes it is impossible to differentiate between the bleeding caused by cervicitis and the bleeding caused by another disorder or by pregnancy. When bleeding persists, intercourse may need to be temporarily discontinued. Sexual activity does not cause miscarriage. However, in late pregnancy, bleeding due to intercourse may occur if the placenta lies directly over the cervix, a condition known as *placenta previa* (see Chapter 55). This condition necessitates abstinence through the remainder of the pregnancy. Bleeding after intercourse which occurs in the second half of pregnancy should be evaluated promptly by a physician.

What Medical Care Can Do

A pelvic examination and Pap smear are done to diagnose the cause of bleeding. Usually cervicitis is found and a vaginal cream or suppository is prescribed. Cervical growths such as polyps are biopsied. Sometimes no cause for the bleeding can be determined. Persistent bleeding after intercourse may require further follow-up, often including cervical or endometrial biopsies (see Chapters 37 and 40).

What You Can Do (Self Care)

A douche containing povidone iodine (see Chapter 87) may be used nightly for one week. This treatment will often clear up mild cervicitis. It is best to avoid intercourse during this time.

BLEEDING AFTER INTERCOURSE

Problem		Action	Possible Cause
Are you pregnant?	yes →	see Chapters 54 and 55, on bleeding in pregnancy	pregnancy effect cervix infection
no ↓			
Has it been more than a year since your last Pap smear?	yes →	make appointment with clinician	cervix infection or polyp cancer of cervix
no ↓			
Is the bleeding associated with a vaginal discharge?	yes →	see Chapter 87, Vaginal Discharge or Irritation	cervix infection or polyp
no ↓			
Has this happened several times?	yes →	make appointment with clinician	cervix infection or polyp
no ↓			
Apply Self Care			

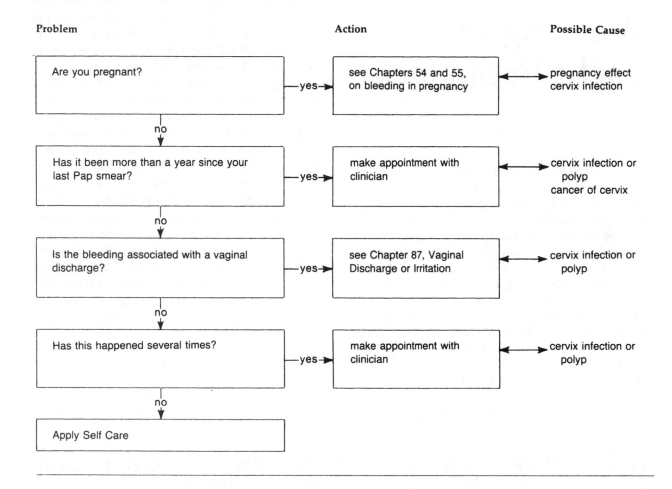

CHAPTER 54

Bleeding in Early Pregnancy

It is possible to mistake what is really bleeding in early pregnancy for your regular menstrual period, especially if the pregnancy is unexpected or unaccompanied by the characteristic symptoms of breast tenderness and morning sickness. So it's smart to consider the possibility of pregnancy whenever your period is unusual for you: very heavy, very light, or delayed. Sometimes what is interpreted as a light period may actually represent implantation bleeding. This bleeding may occur when the fertilized egg implants in the uterus about one week after conception, causing a little spotting for one or two days; implantation bleeding usually poses no threat to the pregnancy.

The three basic causes of bleeding in early pregnancy are: miscarriage (see also Chapter 20); pregnancy occurring outside the uterus, usually in the tube (ectopic pregnancy); and inflammation of the cervix (cervicitis). Cervicitis occurs to some degree in all pregnant women. As a result of the normal increase in mucus secretion, bacteria can flourish and produce a heavy discharge, sometimes accompanied by scant bleeding, particularly following intercourse. Cervicitis may occur at any time during pregnancy and is not dangerous to you or your pregnancy. Miscarriages and ectopic pregnancies account for the majority of moderate to severe bleeding episodes, and over 90% of these disorders occur within the first three months of pregnancy. After this time, you are unlikely to have either of these pregnancy complications.

Miscarriage occurs in 10% to 15% of all pregnancies. This is nature's way of handling things when there is a basic abnormality of the sperm or the egg. Usually a single miscarriage does not hurt your chances for a healthy baby the next time.

Basically there are two types of miscarriage. The first and more usual type, *spontaneous abortion*, causes bleeding and cramping. Severe cramping is caused by strong uterine contractions which dilate the cervix and expel the fetus.

Table 92 FINDINGS ASSOCIATED WITH CONDITIONS CAUSING BLEEDING IN EARLY PREGNANCY (FIRST THREE MONTHS)

Condition	Medical Name	Typical Symptoms	Size of Uterus	Condition of Cervix
Threatening to miscarry	Threatened abortion	bleeding; mild cramping	enlarged	closed
Miscarriage (usual type)	Incomplete or spontaneous abortion	bleeding, often heavy; moderate to severe cramping; tissue may be passed	enlarged	open
Internal miscarriage (uncommon type)	Missed abortion	no bleeding or scant bleeding	normal size or enlarged less than expected	closed
Infection of cervix (mouth of uterus)	Cervicitis	vaginal discharge; bleeding after intercourse	enlarged	closed, discharge present
Pregnancy in tube	Ectopic pregnancy	bleeding, rarely heavy; moderate to severe pain, often on one side; fainting	enlarged minimally, if at all	closed
Hormone imbalance (not pregnant)	Dysfunctional bleeding	bleeding, variable	normal size	closed

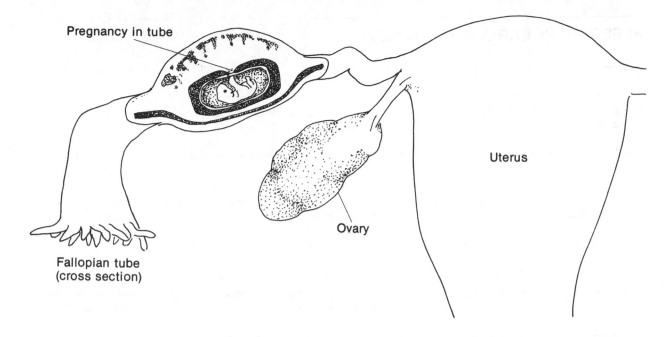

Pregnancy in tube

Uterus

Ovary

Fallopian tube
(cross section)

Figure 51 *An ectopic pregnancy is one that occurs outside the uterine cavity, usually in the Fallopian tube.*

Many women have what is called a *threatened miscarriage*; that is, they have some bleeding with little or no cramping. Bleeding is often in the form of light spotting which may go on for several days before it becomes known whether a miscarriage is going to occur or not.

The second and less common form of miscarriage is the *missed abortion*, in which the fetus, for reasons not well understood, fails to grow and develop normally. Consequently the uterus does not enlarge from one month to the next. The woman has little or no outward signs of problems, such as cramping or bleeding. In fact, her missed abortion may go undetected for several weeks unless pelvic exams are done in early pregnancy to confirm normal uterine growth. After the fourth month of pregnancy (16 weeks from the last menstrual period), failure to "show" or absence of fetal heart tones arouses suspicion of a missed abortion. The condition of missed abortion usually requires a D & C (see Chapter 42) to prevent infection and other complications.

Spotting may also indicate an ectopic pregnancy—that is, a pregnancy that occurs outside the uterus and one in which the fetus cannot survive. Ectopic pregnancy now complicates one pregnancy in fifty and represents the single leading cause of maternal mortality in the United States. In the past twenty years, the number of

diagnosed ectopics has quadrupled, partly due to the continuing epidemic of tube-damaging, sexually transmitted infections and also because of better diagnostic methods. Ectopic pregnancies are most commonly located in one of the Fallopian tubes and cause progressive pelvic pain and internal bleeding (see Figure 51). Tubal pregnancies leak most of the blood out the end of the tube into the abdomen; but some of the blood can trickle down into the uterus, accounting for the spotting characteristic of this condition. The apparent blood loss is deceiving since most of the bleeding occurs inside the body. Fainting commonly occurs. Pelvic inflammatory disease and IUDs are often associated with ectopic pregnancies.

Table 92 presents some of the findings associated with conditions causing bleeding in early pregnancy.

What Medical Care Can Do

The clinician approaches bleeding in early pregnancy by trying to answer three questions: 1) Is the woman in fact pregnant? 2) Is the pregnancy in the uterus? and 3) Is the woman miscarrying? He or she finds the answers through a combination of the pelvic exam, pregnancy testing, and sometimes a pelvic sonogram (see glossary).

BLEEDING IN EARLY PREGNANCY

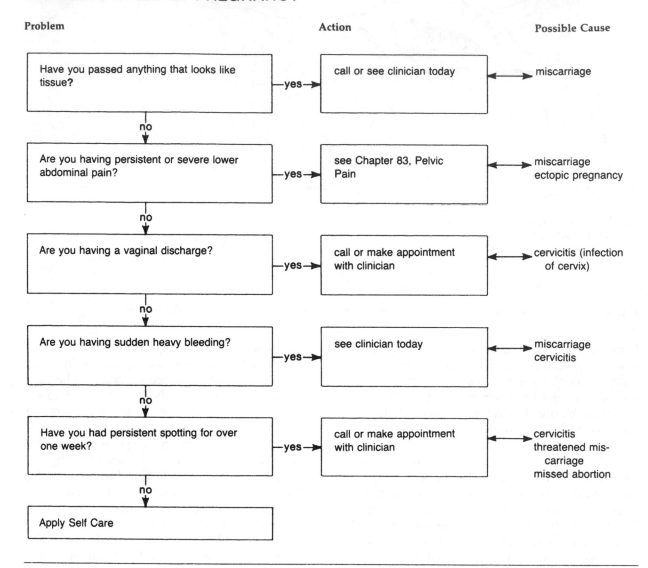

Problem | Action | Possible Cause

Have you passed anything that looks like tissue? —yes→ call or see clinician today ←→ miscarriage

↓ no

Are you having persistent or severe lower abdominal pain? —yes→ see Chapter 83, Pelvic Pain ←→ miscarriage / ectopic pregnancy

↓ no

Are you having a vaginal discharge? —yes→ call or make appointment with clinician ←→ cervicitis (infection of cervix)

↓ no

Are you having sudden heavy bleeding? —yes→ see clinician today ←→ miscarriage / cervicitis

↓ no

Have you had persistent spotting for over one week? —yes→ call or make appointment with clinician ←→ cervicitis / threatened miscarriage / missed abortion

↓ no

Apply Self Care

The speculum exam may simply reveal a yellow discharge around the cervix, the hallmark of cervicitis or cervical inflammation (see Chapter 87). The clinician makes the diagnosis of miscarriage if tissue from the fetus or the placenta is seen coming through the dilated cervix. Usually, bleeding continues after a miscarriage, indicating that some tissue is still inside the uterus and will need to be removed by means of a D & C. In the absence of passage of tissue and severe abdominal pain, bleeding through an undilated cervix usually means you are "threatening" to miscarry. The bimanual examination is done next; and, assuming the uterus is still enlarged, no specific therapy is indicated for threatened miscarriage. Although bed rest is often prescribed and hormone pills and shots were widely used in the past, these measures do not alter the natural course of events if you are going to miscarry.

If the bimanual examination shows that the uterus is becoming smaller rather than growing since the last examination, the doctor may tentatively diagnose a missed abortion in a woman who has had prolonged spotting without the symptoms of a regular miscarriage. The diagnosis may be confirmed by pelvic sonogram before a D & C is done.

If the pregnant woman is spot bleeding and experiences severe pain, especially during the bimanual exam, then the physician will suspect ectopic pregnancy. In the presence of a rapid pulse, low blood pressure, and a low blood count, he or she will perform immediate exploratory surgery, as these are signs of internal bleeding from a "ruptured" ectopic pregnancy—i.e., one that has grown through the wall of the tube, causing it to burst. Today, however, most ectopics are diagnosed before rupture occurs. Distinguishing among ectopic pregnancy, miscarriage, and normal pregnancy complicated by spotting can be difficult, since all three situations initially may be associated with little or no discomfort. Making the right diagnosis is often helped by two types of tests: blood pregnancy tests and pelvic sonograms (also known as *ultrasound*; see glossary).

The pregnancy tests that physicians rely upon in these situations are blood tests that detect HCG (human chorionic gonadotropin), the hormone produced by the placenta in early pregnancy. The initial blood test is reported as either "positive" or "negative" and is sensitive enough to detect pregnancy as early as six days after you conceive. If the blood test is positive and ectopic pregnancy or miscarriage is suspected, the physician then orders a *quantitative* HCG, a blood test to measure the actual amount of hormone present in international units (IUs). By repeating the quantitative HCG in, say, forty-eight hours, the physician can determine if the hormone level is increasing, as it should in a normal pregnancy or dropping (or showing an abnormally small rise), as seen with miscarriage and most ectopic pregnancies.

A sonogram is most useful if it can confirm that the pregnancy is located within the uterus. This is possible as early as three weeks after conception, when a ring-shaped gestational sac can be visualized inside the uterus. The presence of a sac (or of a visible heartbeat, which can be detected two to three weeks later) within the uterus excludes the possibility of an ectopic pregnancy, but is not predictive of whether or not miscarriage will subsequently occur. Such a determination can usually be made using successive quantitative HCG tests.

While seeing the hallmark gestational "ring" within the uterus helps in diagnosing the cause of bleeding, the absence of a ring does not. All three conditions—miscarriage, ectopic pregnancy, and an early normal pregnancy in which the sac has not yet formed—can show up that

way. With such "inconclusive" sonograms, the physician again turns to quantitative pregnancy tests to help distinguish among these situations. A single test may be all that is needed if the hormone level is high (over 2500 IU), which, in the absence of seeing a sac with the more sensitive vaginal probe technique, usually signifies an ectopic pregnancy. A suspected ectopic pregnancy is confirmed by laparoscopy, a short procedure to visualize the internal organs (see Chapter 13). An abnormal rise or drop in hormone level, as measured when the test is repeated in forty-eight hours, indicates either miscarriage or ectopic pregnancy. In this circumstance, a D & C is performed first; if fetal tissue is not found within the uterus, laparoscopy is done. Usually, an ectopic pregnancy can be removed by laparoscopy. If not, the physician makes a regular abdominal incision to do the surgery. In many cases, the involved tube can be preserved. Recently, an anticancer drug called methotrexate has been used to medically treat ectopic pregnancy without the need for surgery. This new alternative treatment has been gaining acceptance and may soon become one of the preferred methods of therapy for this pregnancy disorder.

Pregnancy testing using urine tests may sometimes confuse the evaluation of bleeding in early pregnancy. False-negative tests may result when testing is done very early in pregnancy or if the urine sample is a very dilute one. Urine tests are particularly unreliable as regards ectopic pregnancies, which may test positive only 50% of the time. Again, more sensitive blood tests can accurately establish whether a woman is or recently has been pregnant, and in ectopic pregnancies, these tests will nearly always show some pregnancy hormone present and test positive.

Table 93 shows the steps a doctor goes through to determine and treat the causes of bleeding in early pregnancy.

What You Can Do (Self Care)

If you are planning to become pregnant, keep a calendar record of your periods to help establish when you became pregnant. This information may help your clinician determine normal or abnormal uterine growth. If you develop severe pain, notify your physician. While many women

Table 93   HOW A DOCTOR EVALUATES BLEEDING IN EARLY PREGNANCY

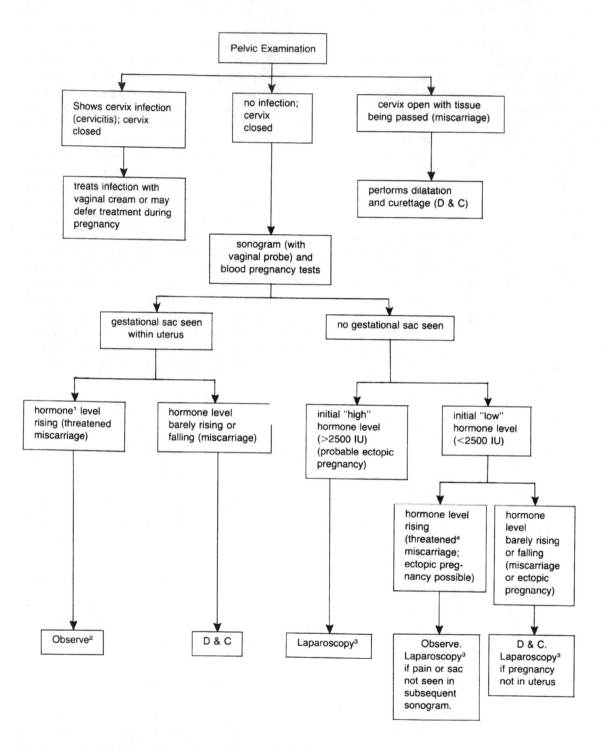

[1] Hormone level means HCG (pregnancy hormone), measured in international units (IU).

[2] Many pregnancies proceed normally. Cause may be cervicitis.

[3] Usually the ectopic pregnancy can be removed by laparoscopy. Otherwise, surgery using a regular abdominal incision is performed.

[4] In very early pregnancy, the gestational sac is not detectable on the sonogram.

have some form of low abdominal cramping in early pregnancy, this condition is rarely severe. You should also report to your health care provider any spotting or passing of tissue. Save any tissue that is passed for microscopic analysis later. Do not feel that activity, sexual or otherwise, contributes to bleeding; it doesn't. Most women who have bleeding in early pregnancy do not miscarry, and those who are going to miscarry will do so regardless of activity.

The limits of tests and the unpredictability of pregnancy outcome when bleeding accompanies early pregnancy makes this symptom a most stressful one. If the outcome is unfavorable, the stress is compounded by the need for surgery. An added frustration is that, presently, treatment is unavailable to stop the ectopic or miscarriage process. For some couples, the grieving process following such pregnancy loss may be particularly profound or prolonged, and counseling may be helpful.

CHAPTER 55

Bleeding in Late Pregnancy

Any bleeding in the second half of pregnancy is potentially serious and may pose a threat to you or your baby. Heavy vaginal bleeding occurs in fewer than 1% of all pregnancies and usually involves a problem with the afterbirth, or *placenta*. A specific cause is not found in more than 50% of bleeding instances. Inflammation of the cervix (cervicitis) is often considered a contributing factor. The passage of a blood-tinged mucus plug, sometimes called a "bloody show," occurs toward the end of the ninth month of pregnancy, is perfectly normal, and often heralds the onset of labor within twenty-four hours.

Of the two problems that often cause bleeding in late pregnancy, the more common and usually less serious is *placenta previa*. Placenta previa means that the placenta is located in front of the cervix instead of in its normal position in the upper uterus. Typically the bleeding occurs on and off for several weeks, starting with minimal amounts but becoming heavier during successive episodes. The bleeding is usually painless. Sometimes the placenta is not directly in front of the cervix (placenta previa) but lies just above it (low-lying placenta). Low-lying placenta is far more common but less likely to cause bleeding than placenta previa. Placenta previa is more likely to happen in women who become pregnant after the age of thirty, who are pregnant with twins, or who have had a previous cesarean birth.

Separation of the placenta from the uterus before labor begins is known as *abruptio placenta*. This condition occurs more often in women over thirty, especially where there is a history of high blood pressure. If the placenta detaches from the uterus, sudden bleeding may occur, accompanied by moderate to severe abdominal pain which feels like a strong, continuous contraction. With further separation, bleeding may be very heavy, and prompt delivery will be required since the fetal oxygen supply becomes threatened. Of all the conditions causing bleeding in late pregnancy, abruptio placenta is the most serious and may require blood transfusions to prevent shock.

What Medical Care Can Do

Immediate treatment of severe bleeding in late pregnancy depends on the overall condition of mother and fetus. Blood transfusions are given when excessive bleeding is indicated by a low blood count, rapid pulse, and dropping blood pressure. When blood loss causes shock, an emergency cesarean section will be done. However, in the great majority of instances, bleeding is not a medical emergency.

The best way to find the cause of bleeding is by means of a sonogram (see glossary). By the use of sound waves, the placenta can be accurately located within the uterus. If the placenta is found to lie over the mouth of the uterus, the diagnosis of placenta previa can be confirmed.

Since both placenta previa and abruptio placenta are likely to occur before the ninth month, the greatest hazard to the fetus is premature birth. Premature infants are likely to have many respiratory problems which may require days or weeks in the newborn intensive care unit. With placenta previa, it is possible to postpone delivery if bleeding does not persist. You may be discharged from the hospital or observed for bleeding in the hospital until approximately the 37th week of pregnancy. At that time, an amniocentesis (see Chapter 20) is performed to determine whether the fetal lungs will tolerate life outside the uterus. The doctor will postpone delivery until that time unless bleeding becomes heavy. A cesarean section is usually done since the fetus cannot be delivered in the normal manner when the placenta blocks the opening of the birth canal. In many instances of low-lying placenta, however, labor proceeds with little or no bleeding; and with the aid of a fetal monitor, vaginal delivery can be allowed.

With abruptio placenta, delivery cannot wait; fetal risks of delayed delivery outweigh the risks of prematurity. Bleeding is unlikely to stop by itself. Delivery is induced by rupturing the membranes and giving a drug (oxytocin) to stimulate contractions. Electronic monitoring is

BLEEDING IN LATE PREGNANCY

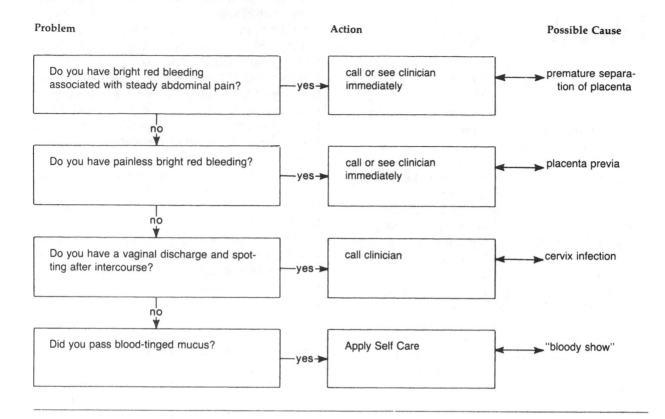

Problem	Action	Possible Cause

Do you have bright red bleeding associated with steady abdominal pain? —yes→ call or see clinician immediately ←→ premature separation of placenta

no ↓

Do you have painless bright red bleeding? —yes→ call or see clinician immediately ←→ placenta previa

no ↓

Do you have a vaginal discharge and spotting after intercourse? —yes→ call clinician ←→ cervix infection

no ↓

Did you pass blood-tinged mucus? —yes→ Apply Self Care ←→ "bloody show"

used to detect abnormalities in the fetal heart rate, and a cesarean section can be done if any problems occur.

What You Can Do (Self Care)

Bleeding in late pregnancy requires medical attention. In most instances, after a preliminary sonogram, you will be advised to rest in bed and to avoid intercourse, the use of tampons, and douching. Ask your doctor exactly what he or she thinks is going on and what the sonogram shows. If placenta previa or a low-lying placenta is excluded as the cause of bleeding, there isn't any proven benefit to your lying in bed or otherwise reducing normal activity. If you have been given certain instructions during an office visit and the bleeding has not recurred, ask the physician on your follow-up visit if the same restrictions will apply. If bleeding, especially without pain, recurs from time to time, ask about having a sonogram to localize the placenta if this has not been done before. If you have heavy bleeding, meet your doctor at the hospital rather than at the office. Usually spotting near your due date is from bloody show, sometimes brought about by a pelvic examination. However, if continuous abdominal pain occurs or if the baby's activity is markedly diminished, see your doctor at once.

CHAPTER 56

Bloody Stool

The alarming experience of seeing blood in the stool occurs at some time or another to nearly all women. Usually the cause is hemorrhoids or an irritation around the anal opening known as a fissure. In these disorders, which are often due to constipation, a few drops of blood may be mixed with the stool or noticed on the toilet paper. Blood in the stool accompanies any cause of chronic diarrhea as a result of the irritation of the intestinal lining (see Chapter 63).

When a large amount of rectal bleeding occurs, more serious disorders of the digestive tract are suspected. Peptic ulcer disease involves either the stomach or small intestine and may be associated with excessive use of aspirin, ibuprofen, coffee, or alcohol, all of which may contribute to heartburn and indigestion. These substances may also contribute to inflammation of the stomach (gastritis), which causes symptoms similar to peptic ulcer. When peptic ulcers or gastritis cause bleeding, the stools may be black or tarry (like tar) in appearance and consistency. Severe bleeding leads to extreme thirst, fainting, weakness, vomiting blood, and ultimately shock. Chronic peptic ulcer disease may cause only the slightest amount of bleeding; it may go unnoticed until a routine blood count shows you are anemic. Intestinal polyps, which may be hereditary, can cause bright red, painless bleeding and are usually benign. Because cancer of the colon and rectum is the second most frequent cancer in women, you should be aware that rectal bleeding is one of its symptoms. Fortunately, cancer is the least likely among the common causes of bloody stool mentioned here. Colon cancer occurs predominantly after the age of fifty and is usually associated with a persistent change in bowel habits, such as constipation or diarrhea.

What Medical Care Can Do

The evaluation of rectal bleeding depends on your overall condition. Heavy, bright red intestinal bleeding from an ulcer, for instance, is a medical emergency requiring blood transfusion and, sometimes, exploratory surgery. In the absence of acute bleeding, a very low blood count may be reason enough for hospitalization. Usually the basic X-rays—upper GI (gastrointestinal) series, lower GI series (i.e., barium enema), and sigmoidoscopy (see glossary for these tests)—can be done on an outpatient basis. Colonoscopy (see glossary), a somewhat newer procedure, enables the physician to examine the entire colon and biopsy abnormal areas. Some physicians recommend this procedure over the barium enema in patients over forty who have bloody stool or other symptoms of bowel disease. Advocates of colonoscopy believe it allows detection of colon cancer at an earlier, more curable, stage. Physicians favoring barium enema as the best diagnostic test point out that this X-ray visualizes the entire colon 95% of the time (compared to 75% for colonoscopy), is less costly, and has a lower risk of complications like perforation of the colon. If you have persistent rectal bleeding, you may want to consult an internist specializing in digestive diseases (gastroen-

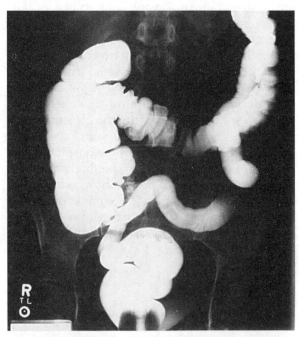

An X-ray of the colon (obtained by barium enema) is used to evaluate various bowel symptoms such as blood in the stool.

BLOODY STOOL

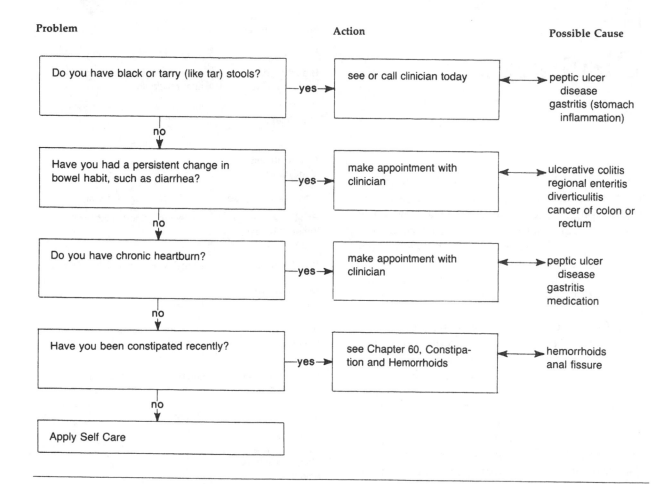

Problem	Action	Possible Cause
Do you have black or tarry (like tar) stools?	—yes→ see or call clinician today	peptic ulcer disease / gastritis (stomach inflammation)
no ↓		
Have you had a persistent change in bowel habit, such as diarrhea?	—yes→ make appointment with clinician	ulcerative colitis / regional enteritis / diverticulitis / cancer of colon or rectum
no ↓		
Do you have chronic heartburn?	—yes→ make appointment with clinician	peptic ulcer disease / gastritis / medication
no ↓		
Have you been constipated recently?	—yes→ see Chapter 60, Constipation and Hemorrhoids	hemorrhoids / anal fissure
no ↓		
Apply Self Care		

terologist) or a surgeon specializing in colon diseases (proctologist).

What You Can Do (Self Care)

If you have hemorrhoids, you can treat occasional episodes of rectal bleeding at home (see Chapter 60). But you should see your doctor for repeated bouts of such bleeding. Use a mirror if there is any doubt as to whether the bleeding is from the rectum or the vagina. Remember that if you take iron, the color of the stool may be black, similar to the tarry stool seen with bleeding ulcers. Stopping the iron should be associated with return to the normal stool appearance within two to three days. Some physicians recommend that women over the age of forty have a stool specimen tested for microscopic bleeding as part of their routine annual examination.

CHAPTER 57

Breast Discharge

A breast discharge may be noticed at many different times in a woman's life from adolescence to menopause (see Table 94). A clear or milky discharge from both breasts is known as *galactorrhea* and is associated with the brain's production of a hormone called prolactin. Galactorrhea is normal during pregnancy, in breast-feeding women, and in adolescents at puberty. Breast discharge may persist up to two years following pregnancy. The symptoms may also be provoked by manual stimulation during sexual activity. A variety of medications may produce galactorrhea, including antihypertensives, antidepressants, and tranquilizers. In addition, either taking or stopping birth control pills can bring on galactorrhea in some women. Chest wall disease such as shingles or chest surgery such as breast biopsy may also cause breast discharge. In women with galactorrhea, gynecologists are very concerned about the possibility of pituitary tumors, an uncommon but serious cause of breast discharge. Such tumors are usually associated with infrequent or absent menstrual periods and sometimes headaches or blurred vision.

In contrast to galactorrhea, conditions originating within the breast itself usually cause breast discharge from only one breast. The discharge may be bloody, green, brown, or yellow. Uncommonly, fibrocystic disease (see Chapter 34) may cause breast discharge. Breast tumors known as papillomas may occasionally produce a bloody discharge. Although a bloody discharge may be associated with cancer, a nonbloody discharge almost never is. Sometimes when it appears that a discharge is occurring from only one breast, manipulation of the opposite breast reveals that the discharge is actually coming from both breasts.

Table 94   POSSIBLE CAUSES OF BREAST DISCHARGE

Normal Causes	Comment
Pregnancy	usually in late pregnancy
Breast-feeding	may persist for up to two years after childbirth
Breast manipulation	may be associated with sexual stimulation

Localized Causes Due to Breast Conditions	Comment
Fibrocystic disease	usually clear or yellow discharge
Papilloma (benign tumor in breast duct)	sometimes bloody discharge
Breast cancer	almost always bloody discharge

Nonlocalized Causes	Comment
Pituitary (brain) tumors	uncommon; associated with lack of or infrequent periods; sometimes headaches
Chest wall surgery such as mastectomy on opposite side	sometimes any form of surgery can cause breast discharge as a result of hormonal changes associated with stress
Chest wall injury such as burns or disease such as shingles	
Birth control pills	also associated with going off the pill
Tranquilizers (such as Thorazine)	
Blood pressure pills (such as Aldomet or Reserpine)	
Antidepressants	
Hypothyroidism (low thyroid)	associated with fatigue, dry skin, cold intolerance, weight gain

What Medical Care Can Do

Tell your physician about any accompanying symptoms you have such as headaches or

Table 95   TESTS TO DIAGNOSE ABNORMAL BREAST DISCHARGE

Test	When Indicated	Purpose of Test
1. Sudan stain (microscopic smear of discharge for fat content)	Often useful except when discharge is bloody	To determine if discharge is milk (galactorrhea) or due to local breast disease (such as pus, cyst fluid)
2. Prolactin (blood test to measure a hormone produced in pituitary gland of the brain)	All cases of milky discharge (galactorrhea)	Screening test for pituitary tumor
3. Thyroid blood tests	Symptoms of low thyroid (weight gain, fatigue, dry skin, cold intolerance); most cases of milky discharge	Detect low thyroid condition
4. Skull X-rays	Headaches or blurred vision *or* lack of or infrequent periods or abnormal prolactin test (elevated level)	Detect pituitary tumor
5. Mammogram (breast X-ray)	Breast lump felt *or* fibrocystic disease *or* discharge from only one breast	Detect breast abnormalities, including cancer
6. Cytology (microscopic smear of discharge to detect cellular abnormalities)	Same as test 5	Same as test 5

blurred vision. You should also tell him or her about any medication you are taking and whether or not you have a history of cystic breast disease. The doctor will test the breast secretion to determine if it contains milk or another, nonmilky substance such as pus from an infection or fluid from a cyst.

During your physical, the doctor will examine your eyes to check for increased intracranial pressure, which, if present, would implicate the rare pituitary tumor. Also, the thyroid is examined because certain thyroid conditions associated with diminished production of thyroid hormone may be associated with galactorrhea.

All women with abnormal galactorrhea should have a prolactin level taken, that is, a blood test of a hormone produced by the pituitary in the brain. If this test shows an increased level of prolactin, an X-ray of the skull is done to look for a pituitary tumor. Keep in mind that there are many harmless conditions that can also cause elevated prolactin levels. However, most women with a breast discharge have a normal prolactin level. When galactorrhea persists, prolactin levels are usually repeated in six months to a year.

If you have a discharge from only one breast, your doctor may recommend that you have a mammogram (see Chapter 34) to check for a cyst or tumor. Cytology, or cellular evaluation, of the breast discharge may be done, especially if the discharge is bloody. Table 95 describes the tests your doctor might use to diagnose abnormal breast discharge, when the tests are indicated, and the purpose of each.

A drug is now available for treatment of breast discharge associated with irregular or absent periods. The drug, Parlodel (bromocriptine), is indicated only after skull X-rays and possibly a CAT scan (see glossary) and other appropriate steps are taken to evaluate the pituitary gland for a tumor. Parlodel has been very successful in establishing regular periods and in stopping breast discharge.

What You Can Do (Self Care)

Breast self-examination is essential and is unlikely to stimulate galactorrhea. Call your doctor if you have any type of breast discharge, especially if it is bloody or associated with cracking, scaling, or irritation around the nipples. Remember that most causes of breast discharge are benign, and even stress itself can be a factor accounting for this symptom.

During pregnancy, the presence of breast milk is no cause for alarm. Some women have very little; others have moderate amounts in the early portion of their pregnancy. Wash away any dried milk with soapy, warm water so your nipples will not become itchy, irritated, or sore.

Table 96 will answer some questions you may have about breast discharge.

Table 96   QUESTIONS COMMONLY ASKED ABOUT BREAST DISCHARGE

Question	Yes	No	Comment
Is a green or yellow breast discharge a sign of infection?		X	These discharges usually accompany benign fibrocystic disease and represent blood pigments.
Is milk secretion from both breasts in a nonpregnant, non-breast-feeding woman a sign of breast disease?		X	Such secretions are due to hormonal changes from a variety of causes.
Can manual stimulation cause breast discharge?	X		Especially during pregnancy and breast-feeding.
Is a bloody nipple discharge usually cancer?		X	The commonest cause is a benign tumor of the breast ducts called a papilloma.
Are tranquilizers a cause of breast discharge?	X		Especially the phenothiazine types, such as Thorazine.

CHAPTER 58

Breast Lump

Breast lumps are among the most common complaints of women who visit gynecologists. Breast lumps may be associated with pain or breast discharge. Localized breast changes such as swelling, redness, skin dimpling, or recent nipple inversion (the nipple turns "inside out") should be investigated promptly by your doctor.

Three conditions must be distinguished in women with breast lumps: fibrocystic disease, fibroadenoma, and breast cancer (see Breast Diseases, Chapter 34). Women with fibrocystic disease may feel many tiny cysts when they examine their breasts, and a consistency of lumpiness or doughiness may be felt (see also Chapter 59). Fibroadenomas are solitary, firm, mobile, benign tumors commonly found in young women in their twenties. Breast cancer often presents itself as a hard, painless lump in one breast. Although breast cancer is rare under the age of thirty and very uncommon before age forty, the disease must be at least considered in any woman with a persistent breast lump. Risk factors include a family history of breast cancer in a close relative such as your sister or mother, first pregnancy after the age of thirty, and menopause after the age of fifty.

What Medical Care Can Do

Breast lumps can be evaluated initially by inserting a small needle, under local anesthesia, into the cavity of the mass and then withdrawing any fluid present into a syringe. This process of fluid removal is called *aspiration*. If the fluid obtained is clear and the lump disappears following aspiration of the fluid, no further treatment is needed except for routine examinations

Table 97   HOW A DOCTOR EVALUATES A LUMP IN THE BREAST

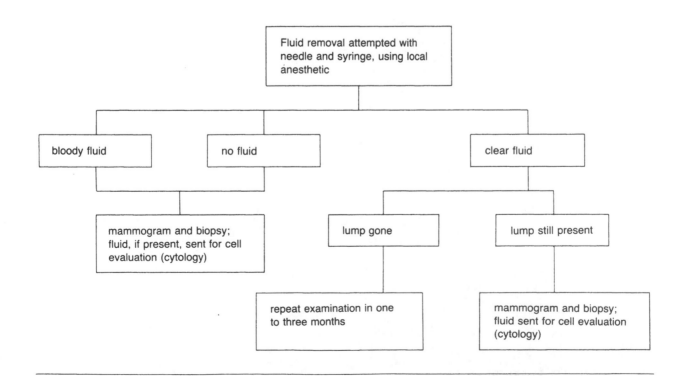

every six months. Such masses are usually due to fibrocystic disease. If the fluid is bloody or the mass is still present after the procedure, mammography (see Chapter 34) and biopsy are indicated. A frequent cause of bloody fluid in a breast lump is a benign tumor called a *papilloma*. But since a breast cancer could also be the cause, the fluid is sent to the lab for cytology (examination of the cell characteristics). Women who have recurrences of cysts previously drained by aspiration will usually need a biopsy to rule out the presence of cancer. Fortunately most biopsies are benign. The biopsies are usually done by general surgeons as opposed to gynecologists and may be done on an outpatient basis. This way, if the biopsy shows a malignancy, there is time to make a decision as to the type of further surgery or treatment indicated.

Table 97 summarizes how a doctor evaluates a lump in the breast.

What You Can Do (Self Care)

The hallmark of prevention of breast disease is the monthly breast self-examination (see Chapter 3), which is best done just after menses or, if you are past menopause, at a regular time every month. If you discover a lump in your breast, call your clinician. You should report any lump, regardless of how indefinite it may seem. If you are over forty, in addition to your self-exam, you should have your clinician examine your breasts approximately every twelve months and have periodic mammograms. (See Table 3, in Chapter 4, and Table 60, in Chapter 34.)

CHAPTER 59

Breast Tenderness

In nonpregnant women, cyclic breast tenderness before a period is common. At least 30% of women between the ages of thirty-five and fifty have tenderness associated with cystic breast changes sometimes known as *fibrocystic disease* (see Chapter 34). Fibrocystic disease means that there are multiple tiny cysts in one or both breasts. This condition, which may produce breast discharge, seems to be hormone dependent and tends to subside as menopause approaches. The vast majority of women with fibrocystic breast disease are not at increased risk for breast cancer (see Chapter 34).

Injury to the breast, which can go unnoticed, also causes breast tenderness and bruising. Black-and-blue areas subside in about two weeks. The presence of a tender lump may arouse fear of cancer. However, breast cancer rarely causes pain unless it is far advanced. Estrogens also cause breast tenderness in some women on birth control pills as well as in women taking Premarin or other estrogens. In general, the pill is associated with less breast pain and fewer breast cysts, which often accompany fibrocystic disease.

Breast tenderness is most commonly associated with pregnancy and breast-feeding. During pregnancy, the breast may feel heavy or may tingle and may be especially tender during examination. Breast infections are most frequent during the postpartum period during breast-feeding, when bacteria from the skin may be introduced into the breasts. Early symptoms of a breast infection are tenderness, redness, and fever.

What Medical Care Can Do

Nonpregnant women with cyclic breast tenderness may be treated with diuretics, although response to this treatment varies. The use of birth control pills may be considered unless there is a history of a breast biopsy showing *atypical cells* or *atypical hyperplasia*. Progestrone pills such as Provera may be tried for breast tenderness and are occasionally effective. Progesterone has not been associated with blood clots. Danazol, another hormonal drug (see Chapter 36), shows promise in alleviating breast tenderness and has been approved by the FDA for this purpose.

Following delivery, the presence of redness around the breast accompanied by fever in breast-feeding women indicates infection. Antibiotics such as penicillin are usually prescribed.

What You Can Do (Self Care)

In nonpregnant women, mild cyclic breast tenderness does not require treatment. A low-salt diet may decrease engorgement of the breasts during the premenstrual period of your cycle. A supportive bra is advisable if you are prone to breast soreness, especially during physical activity such as jogging.

Several reports indicate that fibrocystic breast disease may improve with the reduction or elimination of caffeine and caffeinelike foods from the diet. These studies have shown that women who eliminated caffeine-containing substances, like chocolate, tea, coffee, and cola, from their diet experienced a marked decrease in breast cysts and tenderness. In other research, vitamin E, when taken for two months, has been reported to decrease symptoms of fibrocystic breast disease. Although further research is needed to confirm its effectiveness, taking vitamin E, 400 to 600 units daily, may help reduce your symptoms.

During pregnancy and lactation, the best way to prevent sore breasts is by the use of a supportive bra worn twenty-four hours a day if necessary. During pregnancy, after washing your breasts with soap and water, briskly dry the nipples with a stiff terry cloth towel to help "toughen" the nipples for lactation. If you decide to breast-feed, limit the time spent nursing to no more than ten to fifteen minutes on each breast. If necessary, use breast shields to protect your nipples from cracks, which can lead to breast infections. If breast infection does occur, hot compresses may reduce your symptoms; however, antibiotic treatment is generally necessary if fever occurs. Breast engorgement can be treated with ice packs and a supportive bra.

CHAPTER 60

Constipation and Hemorrhoids

Constipation, a symptom reported twice as often by women as by men, exists when bowel evacuation is delayed several days or when the stool is unusually dry and hard or difficult to pass. The frequency of bowel movements varies greatly among healthy women; it is not necessary to have a bowel movement every day. The chief causes of constipation are improper diet, lack of exercise, certain drugs, excessive use of laxatives, and failure to establish a habit of regular defecation. Specific medical causes of constipation include certain digestive disorders such as irritable bowel syndrome and, less frequently, cancer of the colon, which is usually associated with a marked unexplained change in bowel habits. Low thyroid, or hypothyroidism, may cause constipation; but other symptoms such as fatigue, weight gain, or dry skin are also usually present. During pregnancy, hormone changes produce a relaxation of intestinal muscles, making constipation a frequent problem. Taking iron pills also contributes to constipation in pregnancy as does the pressure from an enlarging uterus.

Hemorrhoids may be a consequence of or

Table 98   DRUGS THAT MAY CAUSE CONSTIPATION

Antacids

Iron preparations

Narcotics (includes any drug containing codeine)

Antihistamines

Water pills (diuretics)

Antidiarrhea drugs

---

contributor to constipation. Hemorrhoids, or piles, are varicose veins located at the anal opening (external hemorrhoids) or just within the anus (internal hemorrhoids). You can't see internal hemorrhoids. Both types may be brought on or aggravated by straining because of constipation. Failure to respond to the urge to defecate because of hemorrhoid pain may lead to further constipation and development of a vicious circle. Common symptoms of external hemorrhoids may include a soft tissue protrusion from the anus with or without itching, pain, or bleeding. Internal hemorrhoids show up as rectal bleeding, often without other symptoms. Hemorrhoids are common during pregnancy, which may help to explain the greater frequency of this condition among women as compared to men.

What Medical Care Can Do

An otherwise healthy woman can take care of common constipation at home. But if you are troubled with diarrhea, pelvic pain, or bloody stool (see these symptom chapters), you might need to consult your clinician. If conservative treatment of hemorrhoids (see below under What You Can Do) is unsatisfactory, there are a number of office procedures which may be tried. These include injecting chemicals into internal hemorrhoids and "freezing" the external hemorrhoids using cryosurgery (see glossary). These procedures may not cure the problem; hemorrhoids can recur. When a blood clot (thrombosis) forms in an external hemorrhoid, the hemorrhoid takes on a bluish appearance and becomes swollen and exquisitely tender. The pain is immediately relieved by surgical removal of the clot under local anesthesia. For severe cases or recurrences, complete external and internal hemorrhoidectomy (removal of hemorrhoids) by a general surgeon is indicated and curative. Sigmoidoscopy and a barium enema (see glossary) are done if the only symptom is rectal bleeding.

What You Can Do (Self Care)

You can take an occasional mild laxative, such as milk of magnesia or Metamucil, for simple constipation. Avoid chronic use of any laxative.

In general these guidelines are the safest approach to treating constipation:

1. Establish a pattern of regular evacuation by responding to the urge to defecate. Even in the absence of this urge, set aside a regular time after a meal for a bowel movement.
2. Drink six to eight glasses of fluid a day.
3. Increase the roughage (fiber) in your diet by eating plenty of fresh fruits, salads, and raw vegetables. Bran, another good source of roughage, can be sprinkled in fruit juice, mixed with another cereal, or eaten as a snack, such as granola bars. Prunes, dates, figs, raisins, and whole wheat bread also add roughage to your diet. These high-fiber foods stimulate muscle activity in the lower bowel and rectum in contrast to dairy products, which may be constipating.
4. Get some exercise each day.
5. Avoid or minimize the use of drugs that may cause constipation (see Table 98).
6. Following childbirth or pelvic surgery when elimination may be painful, the use of a stool softener helps and it is not habit-forming. This will help you maintain regular bowel habits and prevent constipation.

Most of the time you can treat hemorrhoids yourself. Take a warm bath to relieve local pain. Take mineral oil or stool softeners temporarily to facilitate elimination, but avoid harsh laxatives such as castor oil. Over-the-counter ointments and suppositories such as Anusol provide relief of local symptoms. Suppositories may be preferable since external hemorrhoids may be repositioned when the suppository is inserted. Ointments containing anesthetics may cause localized allergic reactions and are best avoided. For a severe bout with hemorrhoids, try Anusol-HC. The HC stands for hydrocortisone, a potent anti-inflammatory ingredient now available over-the-counter in low-dose form. For a stronger version, ask your physician to prescribe Proctofoam HC, Anusol HC cream 2.5%, or Anusol HC 25 mg suppositories. The HC-containing drugs have not been established as safe to use in pregnancy, however.

Table 99 lists common nonprescription laxatives that are presently considered safe to use during pregnancy. Table 100 lists the ones to avoid during pregnancy.

Table 99 NONPRESCRIPTION LAXATIVES PRESENTLY CONSIDERED SAFE TO USE DURING PREGNANCY

Brand Name	Type
Colace	Stool softener
Dialose	Stool softener
Doxinate	Stool softener
Dulcolax	Mild stimulant
Kasof	Stool softener
Metamucil	Bulk laxative (mild)
Milk of magnesia (various brands)	Mild but rapid-acting (2–3 hrs) stimulant
Senokot	Mild and slow-acting (8–10 hrs) stimulant
Senokot S	Mild stimulant plus stool softener
Surfak	Stool softener

Table 100 NONPRESCRIPTION LAXATIVES TO AVOID DURING PREGNANCY

Name	Comment
Castor oil	Strong stimulant, may start uterine contractions
Ex-Lax	Strong stimulant
Haley's M-O	Inhibits vitamin absorption since it contains mineral oil
Mineral oil	Inhibits vitamin absorption
Pericolace	Strong stimulant
Purge	Contains castor oil

CONSTIPATION

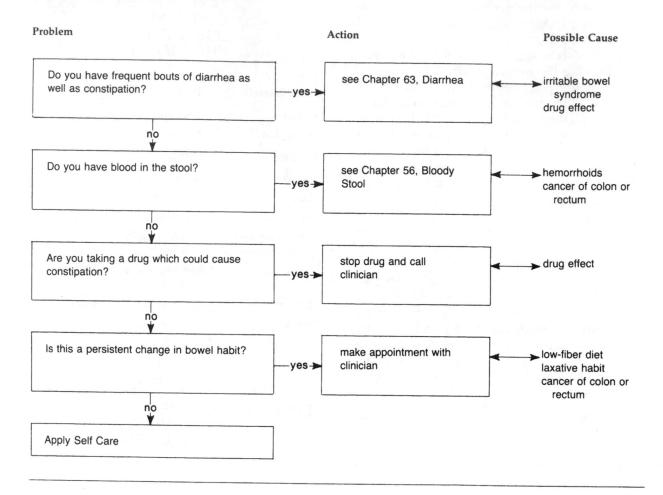

Problem	Action	Possible Cause
Do you have frequent bouts of diarrhea as well as constipation?	see Chapter 63, Diarrhea	irritable bowel syndrome drug effect
Do you have blood in the stool?	see Chapter 56, Bloody Stool	hemorrhoids cancer of colon or rectum
Are you taking a drug which could cause constipation?	stop drug and call clinician	drug effect
Is this a persistent change in bowel habit?	make appointment with clinician	low-fiber diet laxative habit cancer of colon or rectum
Apply Self Care		

CHAPTER 61

Cough

A major factor contributing to this symptom is the increased incidence of women who smoke. Approximately one in three women of reproductive age now smokes cigarettes. Since 1964, when the Surgeon General issued the first report on smoking and health, study after study has identified cigarette smoking as a major cause of serious respiratory disease, including bronchitis, emphysema, and lung cancer. Lung cancer rates among women increased more than sixfold between 1950 and 1990. Cancer of the lung has now overtaken breast cancer as the leading cause of cancer deaths in women.

In his 1989 report, "Reducing the Health Consequences of Smoking: 25 Years of Progress," former Surgeon General C. Everett Koop singled out women, noting that women smokers face a "catastrophic epidemic" of lung cancer in the years ahead. This report and subsequent ones have found that women are quitting smoking slower than men: in 1965, 50% of men smoked, and since then 20% have quit. Among women, 33% smoked in 1965, but only 5% have since stopped. Tobacco use is closely associated with level of education and income, with economically disadvantaged and less educated women much more likely to begin or continue smoking. Despite the vast amount of information about smoking risks, cigarette use in the 1990s continues to be relatively widespread among young women, especially teenagers. Teens often start smoking as early as age thirteen. They also tend to follow their mother's smoking behavior and may disregard their father's if he is a non-smoker.

Cough is the most common symptom of respiratory disease. Coughing is a reflex by which the body tries to get rid of an irritating substance somewhere along the respiratory tract in the throat, breathing tubes (bronchi), or lungs. Cough may be unproductive (that is, nothing is coughed up) as in the dry cough of influenza or may be productive of sputum as in asthma, bronchitis, or pneumonia. Colds and flu, the most common causes of coughing, are discussed in Chapter 65.

More serious respiratory conditions associated with a cough, such as pneumonia, occur when environmental factors decrease natural resistance of the body to infection. Such factors may include viral respiratory tract infections, poor nutrition, chronic alcohol or drug use, chronic fatigue, and cigarette smoking. In addition, industrial exposure to hazardous chemicals such as asbestos may contribute to chronic lung disease.

Cough may be a prominent symptom in bronchitis, pneumonia, emphysema, or lung cancer, all of which may bear a direct relationship to cigarette smoking. Pneumonia, or infection of the lungs, is an acute debilitating illness associated with sudden onset of fever, chills, and yellow sputum production, sometimes accompanied by chest or shoulder pain which increases while the patient takes a breath. Bronchitis is invariably associated with a productive morning cough. Chronic bronchitis associated with cigarette smoking ultimately leads to emphysema, the most common form of chronic lung disease in women. Unlike bronchitis, emphysema involves actual destruction of lung tissue and may be accompanied by progressive shortness of breath. Along with cough, common symptoms of lung cancer are weight loss, bloody sputum, and chest pain. Historically this disease has been more common in men, but women smokers are catching up. In fact, according to government estimates, women smokers will outnumber men who smoke by sometime in the 1990s.

Occasionally cough may be due to conditions unrelated to the respiratory tract. In older women with heart disease, an enlarged heart may cause cough and shortness of breath at night or during exertion. In women taking hormones, including the pill, cough accompanied by bloody sputum, chest pain, and fever may be a sign of blood clots in the lung (pulmonary embolus). Associated findings may include calf pain in instances where a blood clot has traveled to the lungs from an inflamed vein in the leg.

Women who chronically cough may ultimately develop urinary stress incontinence, a condition in which the bladder muscles become weakened as a result of the continuous strain

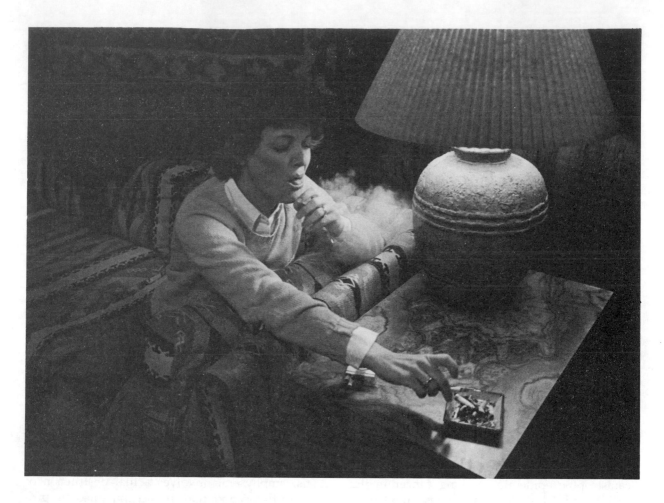

of coughing and allow urine leakage. In addition, coughing tends to place a strain on the ligaments that support the uterus and may contribute to a "dropped," or prolapsed, uterus.

Various reasons are given for the increase in smoking among women. Changing life styles and pressures of work and home which were formerly linked to the male domain have been suggested as contributing factors. So have the cigarette companies, which continue to direct much of their brassy and "newly liberated" pitches directly at women. Women's magazines got a bonanza shortly after cigarette commercials were banned from television. Shortly after the ban, cigarette ads quadrupled in *Cosmopolitan*, *Ladies' Home Journal*, and *Woman's Day* compared to an identical period in the previous year.

During pregnancy, smoking is hazardous to the fetus for several reasons (see also Chapter 31). Many studies have indicated that smoking is associated, for reasons not competely understood, with lower birth weight babies as well as increased number of miscarriages, stillborns, and malformations of the newborn. Among conditions not related to smoking which cause cough, most do not become worse during pregnancy or have harmful effects on the fetus. Asthma, for instance, improves or remains unchanged in most women. Most colds and other respiratory infections are well tolerated in pregnancy by both mother and fetus.

What Medical Care Can Do

The physician initially will check your temperature and examine your throat, heart, and lungs. A chest X-ray and sputum tests may be obtained to diagnose infections such as pneumonia. Where tumor is suspected, the sputum is sent also for cytology, or cellular evaluation. Treatment of pneumonia will usually include penicillin antibiotics. During pregnancy, most medications used for treating pneumonia and asthma are not contraindicated with the excep-

COUGH

Problem	Action	Possible Cause

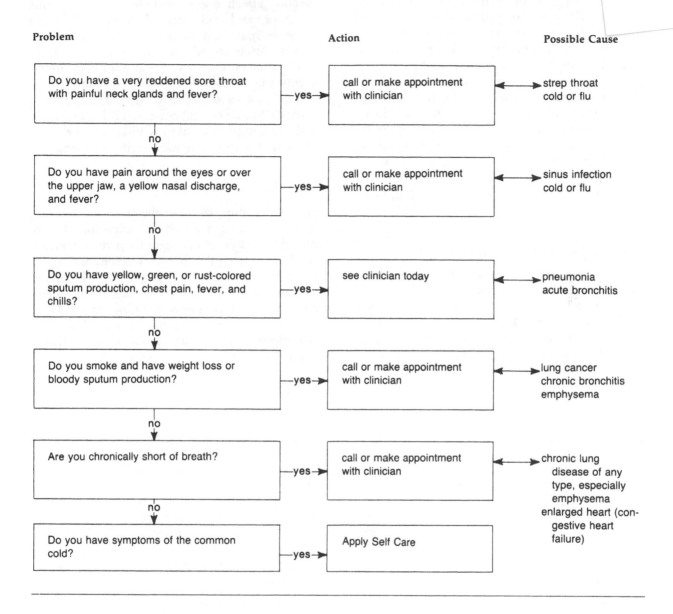

Problem	Action	Possible Cause
Do you have a very reddened sore throat with painful neck glands and fever?	—yes→ call or make appointment with clinician	strep throat / cold or flu
↓ no		
Do you have pain around the eyes or over the upper jaw, a yellow nasal discharge, and fever?	—yes→ call or make appointment with clinician	sinus infection / cold or flu
↓ no		
Do you have yellow, green, or rust-colored sputum production, chest pain, fever, and chills?	—yes→ see clinician today	pneumonia / acute bronchitis
↓ no		
Do you smoke and have weight loss or bloody sputum production?	—yes→ call or make appointment with clinician	lung cancer / chronic bronchitis / emphysema
↓ no		
Are you chronically short of breath?	—yes→ call or make appointment with clinician	chronic lung disease of any type, especially emphysema / enlarged heart (congestive heart failure)
↓ no		
Do you have symptoms of the common cold?	—yes→ Apply Self Care	

tion of potassium iodide, which may produce fetal goiter.

What You Can Do (Self Care)

All infections of the respiratory tract benefit from bed rest, an increase in fluids (especially hot tea or another hot drink) to loosen secretions, and steam inhalation by means of a vaporizer. Avoid cigarettes. When antibiotics are prescribed, take the full amount for the total number of days prescribed. If you have a tendency to chronic infections, bronchitis, or pneumonia, get early medical treatment when respiratory tract infections such as colds develop. When symptoms such as bloody sputum, chest pain, or shortness of breath occur, see your doctor. (See Chapter 65.)

Many programs have been developed to help people stop smoking. If you want to quit, contact your local branch of the American Lung Association, American Cancer Society, or American Heart Association.

You may also want to discuss the use of Nicorette gum with your doctor. This "gum" is held in the mouth and is not really supposed to be chewed. Nicorette provides a slow-release form of nicotine and has been shown to be effective as a temporary aid to the cigarette smoker attempting to give up her habit. Another product consists of a transdermal (skin patch) system (Habitrol, Nicoderm, Nictrol, Prostep) that slowly releases nicotine into the bloodstream. The patches, which are worn daily for several weeks, help reduce the physical craving for nicotine. These products should be used under a doctor's care and may be contraindicated with certain medical conditions including heart disease.

Over-the-counter cough suppressants

Among the many ingredients in over-the-counter cough suppressants, the FDA has found very few to be both safe and effective. They include dextromethorphan (found in Vicks Formula 44, Robitussin, and many other drugstore products) and codeine. Depending upon state law, codeine may be purchased in small doses without a prescription. Other ingredients of uncertain effectiveness include ethylmorphine, camphor, and cod liver oil. Medicated cough lozenges may contain various "medical" ingredients. Antibacterial ingredients contain doses too low to be effective. Local anesthetic ingredients may mask serious disease; hard candy can be just as effective to soothe an irritated throat. Chronic cough, cough with high fever or rash, or cough associated with asthma or bronchitis will normally require medical treatment.

Over-the-counter cough expectorants

Another group of over-the-counter products used in treating a cough, the expectorants, are intended to thin out phlegm to increase sputum production from the lungs. Two common ingredients used are glycerol guaiacolate (guaifenesin) and terpin hydrate. Although neither drug has proven effectiveness according to the FDA, they are included as ingredients in dozens of prescriptions as well as over-the-counter cough and cold remedies.

CHAPTER 62

Depression

Depression, in one form or another, knows no age group. It is today the most common mental difficulty of both children and adults. Men and women both suffer depression, but women are more likely to seek relief from it.

Many studies show that depressed people feel worse and are more limited in their daily activities than those with chronic medical conditions like diabetes and arthritis. Women are at higher risk for depression and the symptom becomes more common with aging. Depression is often

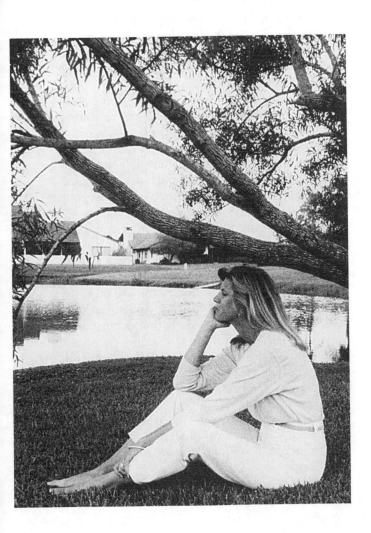

related to a personality style characterized by pessimistic thinking that focuses too much on hopeless feelings instead of the development of an action plan. The high prevalence of sexual and physical abuse also contributes to depression in women as do economic factors, such as poverty. Depression may also accompany times of stress or change in a woman's life, including postpartum, following surgery (especially hysterectomy), or during menopause.

Specific health-related events in a woman's life, such as childbirth, a miscarriage, or a hysterectomy, may also trigger depression. Eighty-five percent of women become depressed, to some degree, at some time during the course of a normal pregnancy, and most experience the so-called postpartum blues.

Depression, along with the feelings and thoughts associated with it, ranges from the individual who occasionally feels blue to the individual who is so immobilized that the only alternatives he or she sees are either staying in bed or taking his or her life. In practice, people who experience depression usually fall into one large grouping we will call *mildly depressed* or another large grouping we will call *severely depressed*.

Mild depression among women is often experienced as a sad, blue, low-down feeling. A depressed woman may lose interest in almost everything, and nothing gives her joy. Some women can't sleep and others can only sleep. She has little energy and a lot of fatigue. There may be present an inability to concentrate, a poor self-image with low self-worth, and a hugely pessimistic attitude. The depressed woman sometimes experiences teary eyes, and occasionally she cries. Some mildly depressed women have thoughts of suicide and occasionally they attempt suicide.

Severe depression has the same symptoms as mild depression only more so. One of the most outstanding symptoms of severe depression is negativism, accompanied sometimes by irrational thinking. The person's appetite may be poor and there may be significant weight loss. The woman will complain of feeling hopeless and worthless. Some women may suffer memory loss. Suicidal thoughts and occasional gestures of suicide are usually present. Explosive anger that borders on rage is often reported. Sometimes the individual's moods will shift from anger to pessimism to a brooding, silent, dark sadness. The individual's moods may swing sometimes rapidly and sometimes slowly from agitated, anxious elation to the darkest depths of depression.

Elavil and Tofranil were two of the first antidepressants developed and two of the most prescribed antidepressants today. In recent years many new similar drugs have come on the market. These include Sinequan, Asendin, Ludiomil, Pamelor, Vivactyl, and certain combination drugs such as Triavil. Most of these antidepressants share similar side effects, including drowsiness, blurred vision, and dryness of the mouth. Less frequent reactions to these drugs include dizziness, heart palpitations, and fainting. In the 1990s the medical treatment of depression was profoundly changed by the development of a new class of drugs called selective serotonin reuptake inhibitors (SSRIs). These include Prozac, Zoloft, and Paxil. SSRIs may have fewer side effects than traditional antidepressants and have proven highly effective.

If an antidepressant or a tranquilizer has been prescribed for you, you should discuss the drug thoroughly with the physician who prescribed it, in order to learn about the medication. Alcohol in most cases must be avoided, and in some cases certain common foods must not be eaten. Antidepressants may interact with one another, with some tranquilizers, with other drugs, and sometimes with certain foods. They may also adversely affect a wide variety of existing medical conditions from thyroid problems to heart disease. Following prolonged use of an antidepressant or a tranquilizer, abrupt stopping of these drugs is to be avoided, because withdrawal symptoms (such as abdominal cramps, vomiting, and insomnia) may result.

Depression can accompany an illness, such as rheumatoid arthritis or hypoglycemia. If you become depressed after starting to take a new drug, be certain to inform your doctor.

The probabilities are that if you have taken the time to read this chapter, you are either not depressed or only mildly depressed. But you may know someone close to you who is severely depressed. If so, she (or he) may need your help; she may not be able to help herself. Although depressed people need a great deal of social support, their extremely negative attitude often causes them to drive away the very people they need—their families and their friends.

The mental health professional never takes the suicidal threats of a severely depressed person lightly; neither should anyone else.

What Medical Care Can Do

The single most important function the physician can perform is to distinguish between mild and severe depression. If the depression is mild, your physician may recommend an antidepressant or may refer you for counseling. If the depression is severe, your physician may refer you to a specialist. The specialist may treat you with medication, counseling, and in some cases hospital treatment.

What You Can Do (Self Care)

1. Research has shown that one of the best treatments for depression is exercise. Try brisk walking, jogging, or swimming, and for detailed information on exercise see Chapter 49.
2. Keep up your daily routine: don't stop. Many people report feeling better during the times they work hardest.
3. If possible, join a women's counseling group. In many cities there is a women's center which has support or counseling groups for women who have undergone mastectomies, are going through a divorce, or are experiencing other traumatic events.
4. Talk to friends and relatives who will give you support. Remember that all people have limits in their ability to help others; a person may want to help you but is only able to go so far—you can and must help yourself.
5. Follow the directions and recommendations of your physician. Take the prescribed medication according to how it is prescribed.
6. If you have premenstrual syndrome, reduce your salt, caffeine, and sugar intake. Vitamin B_6 (50 to 100 mg per day) may help.
7. You can ask for help from any of the fol-

DEPRESSION

Problem		Action		Possible Cause

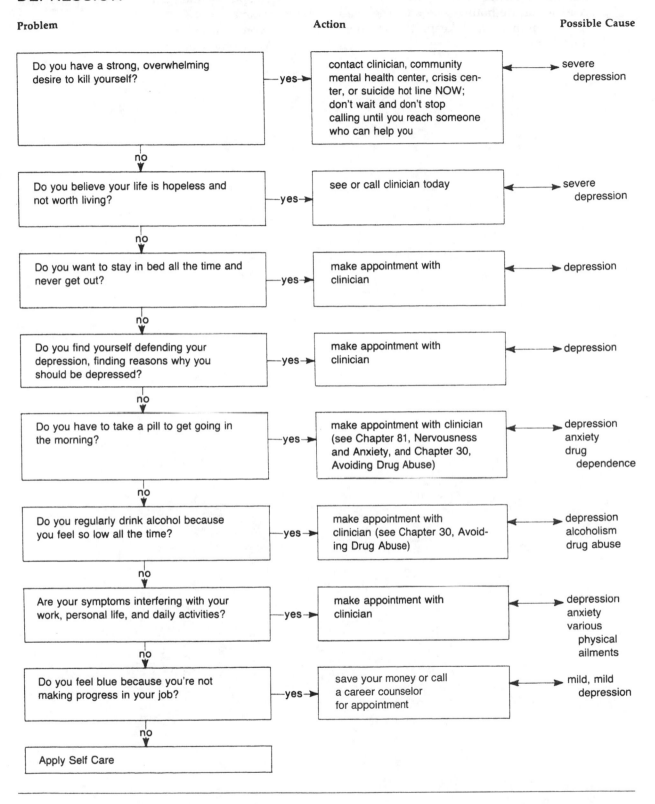

Problem — **Action** — **Possible Cause**

Do you have a strong, overwhelming desire to kill yourself?
—yes→ contact clinician, community mental health center, crisis center, or suicide hot line NOW; don't wait and don't stop calling until you reach someone who can help you ← severe depression

no ↓

Do you believe your life is hopeless and not worth living?
—yes→ see or call clinician today ← severe depression

no ↓

Do you want to stay in bed all the time and never get out?
—yes→ make appointment with clinician ← depression

no ↓

Do you find yourself defending your depression, finding reasons why you should be depressed?
—yes→ make appointment with clinician ← depression

no ↓

Do you have to take a pill to get going in the morning?
—yes→ make appointment with clinician (see Chapter 81, Nervousness and Anxiety, and Chapter 30, Avoiding Drug Abuse) ← depression anxiety drug dependence

no ↓

Do you regularly drink alcohol because you feel so low all the time?
—yes→ make appointment with clinician (see Chapter 30, Avoiding Drug Abuse) ← depression alcoholism drug abuse

no ↓

Are your symptoms interfering with your work, personal life, and daily activities?
—yes→ make appointment with clinician ← depression anxiety various physical ailments

no ↓

Do you feel blue because you're not making progress in your job?
—yes→ save your money or call a career counselor for appointment ← mild, mild depression

no ↓

Apply Self Care

lowing, as appropriate:

Community mental health center.

Crisis or suicide hotline—look up the telephone number and keep it near your telephone.

Mental health association.

Hospital—emergency room; psychiatric unit.

Women's center.

Your physician.

CHAPTER 63

Diarrhea

Acute diarrhea, which lasts only a few days, is often due to simple intestinal infections or to drug side effects. The most common intestinal infection, gastroenteritis or stomach flu, typically begins with fever, vomiting, and stomach pains that may mimic appendicitis. In adults, intestinal infection is usually caused by a *virus*. However, if you have stomach flu following close contact with small children, the source may be *bacterial* gastroenteritis since this form is more prevalent in youngsters.

The most common prescription drugs causing diarrhea—antibiotics—include tetracycline, ampicillin, and cleocin, which are widely prescribed for female pelvic infections. Diarrhea accompanied by fever and abdominal cramping may develop during or several weeks following antibiotic treatment. Over-the-counter drugs which may produce diarrhea include iron, antacids (containing magnesium), and laxatives.

"Traveler's diarrhea" may occur when you are traveling from one country to another, especially when the change involves marked differences in climate, social conditions, or sanitation. This common ailment is usually due to alterations of intestinal bacteria but in some instances results from either bacterial or parasitic infection. Diarrhea from food poisoning, especially common among travelers, occurs from six to forty-eight hours after you have eaten contaminated food or liquid and is often accompanied by vomiting but usually not fever.

Chronic diarrhea, especially when associated with weight loss and weakness, may indicate a serious underlying disease. A "change in bowel habit" is one of cancer's seven warning signs and may indicate colon cancer, the second most frequent malignancy in women after breast cancer. However, 99% of the time changes in bowel habits are due to benign causes, such as inflammatory diseases and what is called *irritable bowel syndrome*.

The principal inflammatory diseases causing chronic diarrhea are *diverticulitis, ulcerative colitis,* and *regional enteritis* (Crohn's disease). Symptoms of diverticulitis vary markedly from occasional mild diarrhea to acute episodes of severe diarrhea, which causes sharp pain in the left lower abdomen.

Ulcerative colitis, which involves the large intestine (colon), and regional enteritis, which involves the small intestine, afflict women more frequently than men. No one knows what causes these diseases, but physicians suspect that chronic stress triggers recurrences of the diseases. Both conditions may be associated with periods of bloody diarrhea, abdominal cramping, fever, and weight loss. Unpredictable periods of lessening and worsening of symptoms occur as well as long periods of freedom from symptoms. These conditions usually begin during the reproductive years but do not adversely affect menses or fertility. However, the effect of childbearing on these diseases may be serious if the disease becomes active or first develops at this time. The long-term effect of pregnancy may be to increase the severity of these two inflammatory conditions. Pregnancy should not be attempted during a flare-up of these conditions. However, unless symptoms are severe, these diseases do not require abortion or sterilization for medical reasons.

There are many names for irritable bowel syndrome, including *functional diarrhea, spastic colon,* and *nervous diarrhea.* Sometimes a set of symptoms for which no physical cause can be demonstrated by lab tests, X-rays, or surgery are lumped under one heading. This is the case with irritable bowel syndrome, which probably represents several separate disorders manifested differently in different women. Some individuals have recurrent bouts of watery diarrhea associated with anxiety or stressful situations and little, if any, abdominal pain. Other women have alternating episodes of diarrhea and constipation along with lower abdominal cramping. In pregnancy, the symptoms of irritable bowel syndrome often subside as a result of an increased tendency toward constipation.

What Medical Care Can Do

The doctor will prescribe antidiarrhea drugs for acute diarrhea unaccompanied by abdominal

DIARRHEA

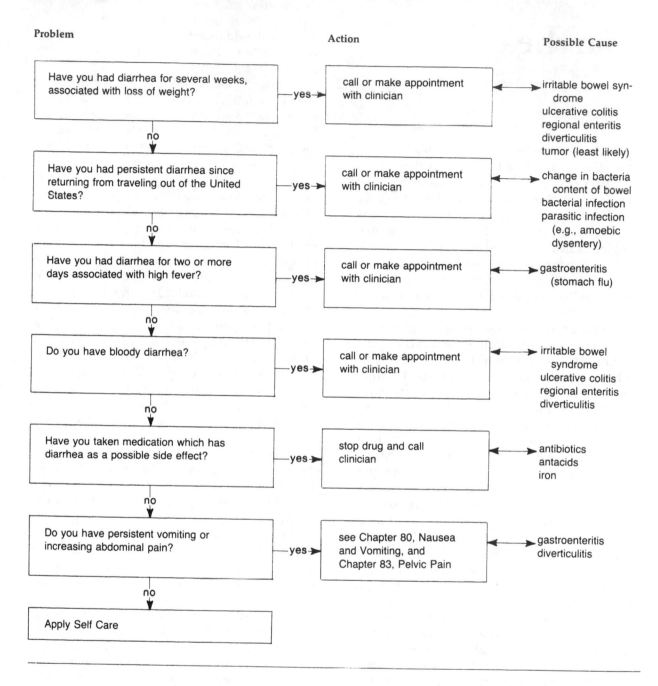

Problem	Action	Possible Cause
Have you had diarrhea for several weeks, associated with loss of weight?	—yes→ call or make appointment with clinician	irritable bowel syndrome / ulcerative colitis / regional enteritis / diverticulitis / tumor (least likely)
↓ no		
Have you had persistent diarrhea since returning from traveling out of the United States?	—yes→ call or make appointment with clinician	change in bacteria content of bowel / bacterial infection / parasitic infection (e.g., amoebic dysentery)
↓ no		
Have you had diarrhea for two or more days associated with high fever?	—yes→ call or make appointment with clinician	gastroenteritis (stomach flu)
↓ no		
Do you have bloody diarrhea?	—yes→ call or make appointment with clinician	irritable bowel syndrome / ulcerative colitis / regional enteritis / diverticulitis
↓ no		
Have you taken medication which has diarrhea as a possible side effect?	—yes→ stop drug and call clinician	antibiotics / antacids / iron
↓ no		
Do you have persistent vomiting or increasing abdominal pain?	—yes→ see Chapter 80, Nausea and Vomiting, and Chapter 83, Pelvic Pain	gastroenteritis / diverticulitis
↓ no		
Apply Self Care		

pain. Hospitalization is not necessary unless you have excessive fluid loss that requires immediate intravenous fluid and mineral replacement. A stool specimen is examined for parasitic or bacterial infection if you recently traveled outside the United States or if you were recently exposed to a child with diarrhea. Bacterial infec-

tions respond well to prescribed antibiotics; viral infections do not.

When diarrhea is chronic, the clinician searches for the underlying cause. He or she can often diagnose cancer of the colon and the inflammatory conditions by an upper GI series and barium enema (see glossary), perhaps with the aid of sigmoidoscopy or colonoscopy (see glossary). If these tests leave some doubt as to the diagnosis, further tests or surgery may be necessary. The physician treats flare-ups of ulcerative colitis and regional enteritis with powerful antiinflammatory drugs called corticosteroids, whose use in pregnancy is felt to be justified. Also, sulfa drugs (sulfasalazine) and a promising new drug, mesalamine (Rowasa—also known as 5-ASA), are used to control these two diseases. Rowasa is presently available only as an enema but should be approved in all forms soon. Occasional complications of these inflammatory conditions, such as intestinal blockage and abscess formation, may require surgery.

Treatment of irritable bowel syndrome is also nonspecific although doctors often prescribe tranquilizers, sedatives, and antispasmodic drugs. Most studies suggest these drugs are minimally effective. It is best to avoid antidiarrhea or antispasmodic drugs during pregnancy since this condition poses no threat to mother or fetus. Therapy with a high-bulk diet and Metamucil is safe and effective for the pregnant woman.

What You Can Do (Self Care)

You can treat most forms of acute diarrhea yourself. Restrict solid foods during the first twenty-four hours, but drink plenty of fluids such as broth and carbonated drinks (such as ginger ale). Eliminate dairy products, especially whole milk and cream. Gatorade, a commercial preparation available in supermarkets, is a good source of mineral and fluid replacement, especially if vomiting occurs.

As diarrhea subsides, you can add small, bland meals while avoiding raw vegetables and fruits, fried foods, sweets, spices, coffee, and al-

coholic beverages. Do not force yourself to eat if you have severe abdominal pain or vomiting.

Women with chronic diarrhea usually require vitamins, extra rest, and some change in the diet. The diet for women with irritable bowel syndrome should be free of milk, milk products, and raw fruits and vegetables. In addition, she may alleviate symptoms by increasing dietary bulk either naturally through the use of bran or other high-fiber foods or by supplementing the diet with Metamucil.

Most of the time an over-the-counter drug is safer, milder, and less expensive than a prescription drug for treatment of diarrhea. For example, Kaopectate is one of the safest drugs for diarrhea because the drug itself is not absorbed.

When traveling outside the United States, take Pepto-Bismol with you. Recent studies indicate that this over-the-counter drug effectively prevents and treats traveler's diarrhea. Take four tablespoons four times a day for the first two weeks of travel. If you are going to a country where medical services are limited, ask your physician to prescribe Lomotil, a common antidiarrhea drug. Also remember to drink bottled water, eat cooked foods, and avoid tap water or ice cubes made from tap water.

Resources

Crohn's and Colitis Foundation of America, Inc.
386 Park Avenue South, 17th Floor
New York, New York 10016
(212) 685–3440

Digestive Disease National Coalition
711 Second Street, N.E., Suite 200
Washington, D.C. 20002
(202) 544–7497

CHAPTER 64

Dizziness and Vertigo

Dizziness means lightheadedness or giddiness. Vertigo refers to the sensation of objects spinning around you—that is, an object your eyes are focused on seems to move out of position. Lightheadedness commonly occurs when you suddenly stand up after sitting or lying down. This form of dizziness, known medically as *orthostatic hypotension*, is due to delayed adjustment of the circulatory system to changes in posture. The effect is more pronounced in pregnancy because the growing uterus compresses the blood vessels to and from the heart. Orthostatic hypotension may also occur in women taking blood pressure medication or having anemia.

More serious causes of dizziness in women include bleeding, high blood pressure, and low blood sugar. Chronic blood loss from an ulcer or heavy menstrual periods produces a low blood count, which may be associated with weakness or dizziness. More rapid losses of blood also cause dizziness such as is found with ectopic pregnancy, in which the bleeding occurs internally and is not apparent immediately. Women with high blood pressure may have no symptoms or they may have occasional headaches or dizziness (see Chapter 69, High Blood Pressure). Hypoglycemia, or low blood sugar, may cause dizziness as well as headache, sweating, hunger, shakiness, and fatigue (see Chapter 75, Lethargy).

Vertigo, a more specific and disturbing symptom than dizziness, may be caused by an ear infection or by hardening of the arteries at the base of the brain, the latter usually occurring in elderly women. Other causes of dizziness and vertigo include drugs, particularly sedatives, tranquilizers, antihistamines, aspirin, and "water pills" (diuretics). The exact cause of dizziness is often not found; however, stress and emotional factors, particularly anxiety and depression, frequently play a role. Hyperventilation may occur when anxious individuals breathe rapidly, leading to dizziness and numbness in the hands and lips. Stress-related migraine headaches may also be associated with dizziness.

What Medical Care Can Do

Dizziness is usually diagnosed after a complete examination. A neurological examination is performed if there is evidence of neurological involvement from your history. The doctor will examine your eyes, which can reveal information about hardening of the arteries elsewhere in the body. A pelvic exam is done to check for uterine enlargement due to pregnancy or fibroid tumors which may cause heavy periods and anemia. Pertinent lab tests may include a blood count, examination of the stool for microscopic bleeding, and a pregnancy test. The clinician may refer you to a neurologist, an ear specialist, or an internist if he or she finds gross abnormalities in the examination of the nervous system, ear, or heart, respectively. In most cases the primary care clinician can deal with this symptom after excluding serious underlying disease.

What You Can Do (Self Care)

Drugs having the side effects of dizziness may need to be reduced in dosage or stopped altogether; consult with your doctor. However, if you are taking blood pressure medication, it may need to be increased. After the age of thirty, have your blood pressure checked annually. Get up slowly from the reclining position. In late pregnancy especially, this is best accomplished by turning to the side and slowly pushing yourself up with your arms. Avoid sweets in your diet because sweets may make you susceptible to hypoglycemia. Persistent dizziness associated with vertigo, suspected bleeding, or ear pain should be reported to your physician.

DIZZINESS AND VERTIGO

Problem	Action	Possible Cause

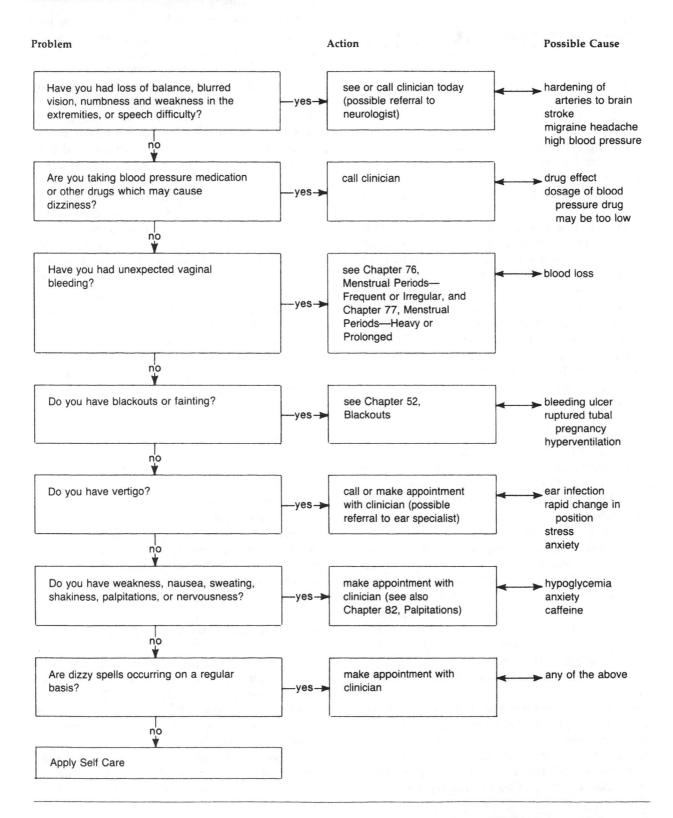

Problem — **Action** — **Possible Cause**

Have you had loss of balance, blurred vision, numbness and weakness in the extremities, or speech difficulty?
→ yes → see or call clinician today (possible referral to neurologist) ← hardening of arteries to brain / stroke / migraine headache / high blood pressure

no ↓

Are you taking blood pressure medication or other drugs which may cause dizziness?
→ yes → call clinician ← drug effect / dosage of blood pressure drug may be too low

no ↓

Have you had unexpected vaginal bleeding?
→ yes → see Chapter 76, Menstrual Periods—Frequent or Irregular, and Chapter 77, Menstrual Periods—Heavy or Prolonged ← blood loss

no ↓

Do you have blackouts or fainting?
→ yes → see Chapter 52, Blackouts ← bleeding ulcer / ruptured tubal pregnancy / hyperventilation

no ↓

Do you have vertigo?
→ yes → call or make appointment with clinician (possible referral to ear specialist) ← ear infection / rapid change in position / stress / anxiety

no ↓

Do you have weakness, nausea, sweating, shakiness, palpitations, or nervousness?
→ yes → make appointment with clinician (see also Chapter 82, Palpitations) ← hypoglycemia / anxiety / caffeine

no ↓

Are dizzy spells occurring on a regular basis?
→ yes → make appointment with clinician ← any of the above

no ↓

Apply Self Care

CHAPTER 65

Fever and Chills

Fever accompanies many illnesses, most of which are benign. Fever generally indicates infection somewhere in the body. Your temperature normally fluctuates on any given day up to as high as 100 degrees. The main significance of fever is not how high it is but what is causing it. This can usually be determined by the accompanying symptoms. Fever accompanied by chills usually means that an infection has spread to the bloodstream.

Common causes of fever which usually get better on their own are shown in Table 101. These include colds and stomach flu. You are probably all too familiar with the cold symptoms: headache, runny nose, sore throat, cough, hoarseness, and muscle aches. A low-grade fever is sometimes present. Influenza, or the flu, often occurs in epidemics and may be a more sudden and serious illness than the cold, producing extreme fatigue. The stomach flu (gastroenteritis) characteristically causes nausea, vomiting, or diarrhea in addition to the other symptoms.

Colds and stomach flu are caused by viruses and therefore do not respond to antibiotics. Although these ailments themselves are not serious, several of their complications are serious; and this is where medical treatment and sometimes antibiotics can help. The common complications of colds and flu in adult women are listed in Table 102. In addition to colds and flu, mononucleosis is a viral condition causing fever, sore throat, tender neck glands, and chronic fatigue. The condition is diagnosed by a blood test and generally runs an uncomplicated course.

Table 103 describes the more serious infections that require a visit to your clinician. These illnesses may become life-threatening if untreated. One of the most common infections in women is pyelonephritis, or kidney infection (see Chapters 85 and 86 on urinary problems).

Another serious cause of fever in women is pelvic inflammatory disease (see Chapter 24, Sexually Transmitted Diseases).

During pregnancy, a high fever may be hazardous to the fetus by causing premature labor. Pregnancy does not significantly increase the susceptibility to illness. However, colds and flu, when complicated by bacterial pneumonia, may be particularly severe in pregnancy. Urinary tract infections are more frequent in pregnancy. However, pelvic inflammatory disease is less common during pregnancy because of the increased amount of cervical mucus, which acts as a barrier to bacteria. Despite the prevalence of varicose veins during pregnancy, the actual incidence of thrombophlebitis is not much different from that in nonpregnant women.

Among fever-causing conditions that are due to pregnancy itself, the most common is premature rupture of the membranes (see Chapter 20). The amniotic sac or fetal membranes may rupture prematurely, usually in the last third of pregnancy. Infection known as *amnionitis* may then occur, is associated with fever, a bad-smelling discharge, and abdominal pain and is potentially very dangerous to the fetus. Except when the pregnancy is less than 34 weeks or so, labor is induced to prevent amnionitis. Childbirth fever sometimes occurs on the third or fourth postpartum day and is usually due to infection of the lining of the uterus (endometritis). This condition happens more commonly when delivery does not occur within twenty-four hours after rupture of the membranes. The symptoms are very similar to amnionitis. Other causes of fever following childbirth are urinary tract infections, breast engorgement or infection, and, much less commonly, thrombophlebitis.

What Medical Care Can Do

The symptoms and physical findings due to febrile conditions (that is, conditions in which fever is present) are numerous. Where the apparent cause seems to be an infection localized, for example, to the urinary tract or uterus, antibiotics are usually started immediately after appropriate cultures are obtained. Uncomplicated cases of colds and flu do not require antibiotics unless strep throat is confirmed by

Table 101 COMMON CAUSES OF FEVER

Cause	Possible Symptoms	Contact clinician if you have:
flu (influenza)	nausea, vomiting, diarrhea, muscle aches, headaches	vomiting of blood or severe abdominal pain lasting more than six hours
cold or upper respiratory infection	sore throat, runny nose, headache, cough	chest pain, shortness of breath, coughing up blood, or stiff neck
mono (mononucleosis)	sore throat and swollen neck glands, slight fever, chronic fatigue	yellow pigmentation of skin or eyes (jaundice) or any cold associated with fatigue that persists

Table 102 COMPLICATIONS OF THE COMMON COLD AND FLU

Complication	Diagnostic Test	Symptoms
pneumonia or bronchitis	chest X-ray	cough productive of green or yellow sputum fever and chills trouble breathing or you are wheezing chest pain especially when breathing
sinus infection	sinus X-ray	nasal discharge which is green or yellow sinus pain, especially around the eyes and over the upper jaw
strep throat	throat culture	very red throat often covered with a yellow or white drainage over tonsils tender neck glands

throat culture or there is a history of chronic lung disease. Antibiotics may also be necessary for certain conditions that can start out as a cold, such as sinus infections, bronchitis, and otitis media. Antibiotics such as amoxicillin, erythromycin, and sulfa drugs are considered first-line agents for treating these types of infections and are the least costly.

When the cause of fever is unclear, screening tests may include a complete blood count (CBC), urinalysis, and chest X-ray. The CBC includes a white blood cell count which measures infection in the body. If you have severe abdominal pain or dehydration along with fever, you may be hospitalized. Occasionally surgery is indicated as in the case of pelvic abscess or appendicitis. Thrombophlebitis also requires hospitalization for initial medical treatment.

What You Can Do (Self Care)

In cases of fever due to colds and stomach flu, symptomatic treatment of such complaints as headache, diarrhea, or nausea is all that is indicated since the condition goes away by itself. (See individual chapters for these symptoms). Getting plenty of rest will assist your body's natural defense mechanisms. Tylenol, or aspirin if you are not pregnant, may be used to lower fever, although temperatures between 100 and 101 degrees are not at all serious in otherwise healthy, nonpregnant individuals. Tepid baths may also bring down a fever without the use of drugs. Avoid smoking if the problem is in the respiratory tract. Gargling with warm salt water is soothing to the throat and often helps decrease throat swelling. You need to replace the fluid lost through sweating when you have a fever. Try drinking a glass of tea, fruit juice, or other beverage at least every two hours. The increased water absorbed will also help to thin out and wash away mucous secretions. Cold steam through the use of a vaporizer is also effective for liquefying secretions and relieving cough. Good nutrition is as important as adequate hydration, because your need for calories increases from a fever, but eat and drink what you feel

Table 103   CAUSES OF FEVER REQUIRING MEDICAL TREATMENT

Cause	Typical Symptoms	How Diagnosed	Comment
pelvic infection (involving tube or ovary)	moderate to severe low abdominal pain persisting for several hours to days; vomiting may occur; vaginal discharge may be present	examination of abdomen and pelvis	diagnosis always presumptive; may be confirmed by laparoscopy or exploratory surgery
kidney infection	burning with urination; backache felt on one or both sides just above the waist; bloody or frequent urination may occur	urinalysis; urine culture	bladder infections cause the same symptoms without fever or backache
appendicitis	moderate to severe low abdominal pain persisting several hours and becoming worse on right side; vomiting usually occurs	examination of abdomen and pelvis	abscess of ovary or tube may cause same symptoms
pneumonia	cough with yellow or green sputum production; chest pain while taking a breath may occur; shortness of breath may occur	examination of the chest; chest X-ray confirms	in women over forty who smoke, these symptoms may be caused by lung cancer
meningitis	headache with stiff neck	spinal tap	relatively rare; flu may mimic these symptoms
thrombo-phlebitis	leg pain; swelling or redness particularly in area of the calf	examination of the lower extremities	associated with prolonged bed rest, use of birth control pills, recent surgery, or childbirth
connective tissue disease (such as lupus erythematosus)	joint pain; rash; chest pains	blood tests	although uncommon, may affect young women; multiple symptoms

like. Don't force yourself to eat when you're nauseated. Resist the temptation to have antibiotics prescribed for the common cold or for influenza unless complications occur.

Common ingredients in many drugstore cold and flu remedies include pain relievers, expectorants (to help bring up secretions), and cough suppressants. Two other ingredients, antihistamines (see glossary) and decongestants (see glossary), are often included in cold remedies to reduce mucous secretions. Decongestants are far more effective in relieving symptoms of nasal and sinus congestion compared to antihistamines. In addition, antihistamines may cause unwanted drowsiness. Ingredients in some common over-the-counter drugs for treating cold and flu symptoms are listed in Table 104. Remember that these drugs treat symptoms but do not cure infection itself.

During pregnancy, avoid all drugs unless they are absolutely necessary (see Chapter 31, Drugs and the Pregnant Woman). Even cold remedies should be used cautiously (if at all) in pregnancy and only after consultation with your doctor. Drugs are necessary if you have a culture that indicates strep throat, a chest X-ray indicating pneumonia, or a sinus X-ray showing sinus infection.

Table 104 COMMON NONPRESCRIPTION COLD AND ALLERGY DRUGS*—WHAT THEY CONTAIN

Brand Name	Antihistamine	Decongestant	Pain Reliever	Expectorant	Cough Suppressant	Alcohol (at least 3% by Volume)
Allerest Headache-Strength Tablets	X	X	X			
Cheracol Plus	X	X			X	X
Chlor-Trimeton	X					
Chlor-Trimeton Decongestant Tablets	X	X				
Comtrex Multi-Symptom Cold Reliever	X	X	X		X	X
Contact Severe Cold and Flu Formula Caplets	X	X	X		X	
Coricidin	X		X			
Coricidin "D" Decongestant Tablets	X	X	X			
Dimetapp Extentabs	X	X				
Drixoral Cold and Flu	X	X	X			
Novahistine Elixir	X	X				X
Robitussin				X		
Robitussin-CF		X		X	X	
Robitussin-DM				X	X	
Robitussin-PE		X		X		
Robitussin Maximum Strength Cough Suppressant					X	
Triaminic Cold Tablets	X	X				
Triaminic Expectorant		X		X		
Triaminic-DM Syrup		X			X	
Triaminicol Multi-Symptom Relief	X	X			X	

* Not containing codeine or other narcotics.

CHAPTER 66

Hair Growth (Excessive)

Excessive hair growth, called *hirsutism*, is a relatively common complaint among women partly because of our cultural stigma against the presence of hair on certain parts of the body. The quantity and distribution of hair depends on genetic, racial, and hormonal factors. Some families have an inherited tendency to more pronounced hair growth due to increased androgen. Androgen is the primary male sex hormone that is normally present in women in small quantities. Slight increases in androgen account for most cases of hirsutism in women. Often such an increase is a physiologic process during puberty or pregnancy when increased hair growth is temporary.

Another cause of hair growth in women of reproductive age is hormone imbalance. This condition results from subtle changes in levels of various female hormones made in the ovaries and in special centers within the brain (pituitary and hypothalmus). Hormone imbalance may be triggered by various things, including stress, or may be due to a biochemical abnormality within the ovary causing cysts to form (polycystic ovary syndrome—see Chapter 78). Hormone imbalance is sometimes associated with irregular or absent periods, acne, obesity, and infertility. Some or all of these factors may be present, but in any case, dark, coarse hair may appear on the face, abdomen, or chest.

During menopause, the drop in estrogen combined with a rise in androgen can account for slightly increased hair growth. Drugs containing estrogen as well as an androgen (testosterone), sometimes prescribed around the time of menopause, may also increase hair growth.

Rarely, an ovarian or adrenal tumor may account for excessive hair growth, sometimes associated with other symptoms, such as hoarseness or clitoral enlargement.

What Medical Care Can Do

Since most causes of increased hair growth are due to inherited or physiologic processes, treatment is usually not indicated. Blood tests may be obtained to rule out the possibility of an ovarian or adrenal tumor. The physician may order birth control pills for treatment of hormonal imbalance when hair growth is extreme, especially if associated with acne. Some birth control pills work because the estrogen in them balances the androgen present. Keep in mind that removing the cause of hirsutism may not lead to loss of unwanted hair.

What You Can Do (Self Care)

Remember that hair growth patterns are inherited characteristics and that changing hair growth patterns normally accompany puberty, pregnancy, and menopause. Since these changes are mild and often temporary, the best treatment may be no treatment at all. Some women, however, try using bleaching solutions to lighten the hair color; this procedure is fine as long as the solution does not irritate your skin. Depilatory creams, such as Neet, and wax treatments may help temporarily but they may also cause skin irritations. Electrolysis by a certified technician is costly and may require several treatments to finally be effective. If you are taking any hormones, ask your doctor if this could be contributing to excessive hair growth.

HAIR GROWTH

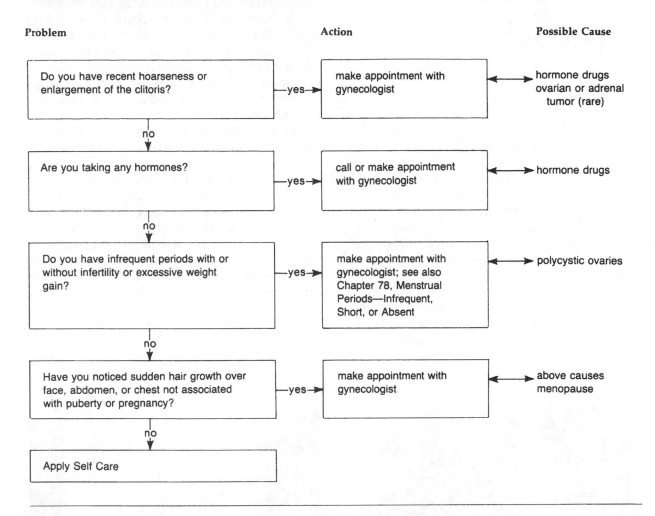

Problem	Action	Possible Cause
Do you have recent hoarseness or enlargement of the clitoris?	—yes→ make appointment with gynecologist	← hormone drugs ovarian or adrenal tumor (rare)
no ↓		
Are you taking any hormones?	—yes→ call or make appointment with gynecologist	← hormone drugs
no ↓		
Do you have infrequent periods with or without infertility or excessive weight gain?	—yes→ make appointment with gynecologist; see also Chapter 78, Menstrual Periods—Infrequent, Short, or Absent	← polycystic ovaries
no ↓		
Have you noticed sudden hair growth over face, abdomen, or chest not associated with puberty or pregnancy?	—yes→ make appointment with gynecologist	← above causes menopause
no ↓		
Apply Self Care		

CHAPTER 67

Headache

Women seek care for headaches four times as often as men do. Headaches may have various causes, such as hunger, sinus infections, sexual activity, head injury, or "TMD" syndrome (see Chapter 73). Infrequently, headache may be due to "organic" causes—i.e., a physical problem inside the head such as a tumor, blood clot (stroke), or ruptured blood vessel (aneurysm). But most often, headache is due to stress, fatigue, or emotional distress. The chronically suppressed desire to express anger is probably the most common psychological reason for headache. When the resulting tension and anger become self-directed, depression is produced and sometimes goes unrecognized as part of the headache's symptoms. According to the National Headache Foundation, 45 million Americans have chronic and recurrent headaches, accounting for 50 million office visits annually at a cost of 400 million dollars spent on over-the-counter pain pills. Fortunately, 85% of chronic headache sufferers can be helped significantly by drugs, biofeedback, and relaxation techniques.

Psychological stress can trigger both *tension headaches* and *migraine headaches*, the two basic types. *Tension headaches* are due to a tightening or contraction of the facial or neck muscles. Typical symptoms include a continuous ache or pressure that feels like a band around the head. The neck muscles may be tender, or pain may radiate to the neck or back. These headaches usually last for several hours and sometimes recur chronically. Tension headaches may be triggered by poor posture, eyestrain, or dental problems.

In *migraine headaches*, throbbing pain often starts on one side of the head and then spreads throughout the face and head. Some migraines

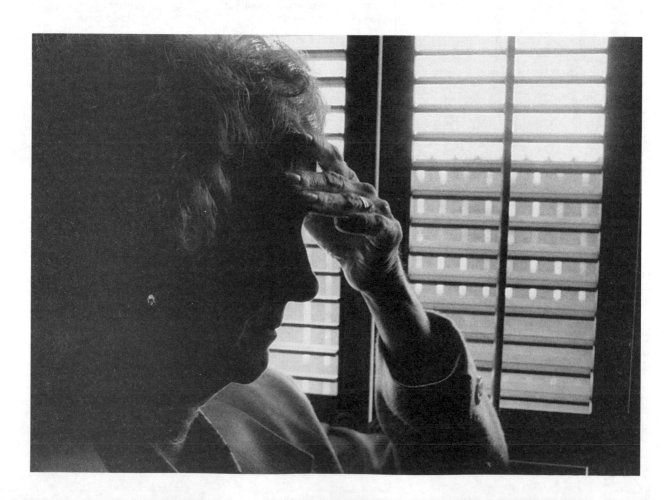

are severe and may last for several days, accompanied by nausea, vomiting, diarrhea, or nasal stuffiness. Migraines affect some women only once a year or less often and other women twice daily. The average frequency is two or three times each month. Migraine headaches, which may be inherited, affect nearly 30% of all women at some time. Among factors that trigger migraines are changing hormone levels. During, before, and after a period, migraines may occur with increased frequency. Women on birth control pills may experience an increase in the severity of preexisting migraine headaches. Use of birth control pills is not advisable if you suffer from frequent migraines.

Cluster headaches, which some experts consider a variant of migraine, cause intense pain on one side of the head, sometimes associated with tearing or a runny nose. Cluster headaches affect men more often than women, cause intense pain for a few minutes up to an hour or two, and occur several times a day for weeks at a time. Then the headaches stop, only to return months or years later.

Certain foods may trigger migraine headaches: alcoholic beverages such as wine; aged cheeses; chocolate; citrus fruits; excessive caffeine; nitrate-containing foods such as cold cuts and hot dogs; and food with monosodium glutamate (MSG), which is often used in Chinese foods. In some women, not eating for several hours may set off a migraine as may any change in the pattern of sleep.

Some people experience warning symptoms just prior to a migraine attack. These symptoms frequently occur the same way each time. Such warning symptoms include some or all of the following: irritability, blurred vision, seeing multicolored or bright lights, or more alarming neurological symptoms such as temporary weakness or speech difficulty.

During pregnancy, particularly in the second half, migraine headaches are less common. Headaches experienced in the latter part of pregnancy may be associated with elevated blood pressure and other symptoms of toxemia (see Chapter 20), such as rapid weight gain and fluid retention.

During menopause, migraine headaches often disappear; however, because of irregular hormone levels during menopause, they may occur for the first time. In such cases, migraines usually subside completely in one to two years.

Women near the menopause on continu[ous] doses of estrogen frequently experienc[e] [in]crease in migraine frequency.

Table 105 shows you the extent to w[hich] [sev]eral factors are involved in tension he[adache] and in migraine headaches.

What Medical Care Can Do

During the history-taking part of your visit, the clinician may ask questions concerning your family, job, and personal relationships since emotional factors play such an important role in headaches. A thorough head and neck and possibly neurological examination will be performed. X-rays of the skull, sinuses, and neck may be indicated. Occasionally an electroencephalogram (see glossary) is obtained. In general, more complex and costly procedures such as CAT and MRI scans (see glossary) are reserved for atypical and very severe headaches.

Medical therapy for both tension and migraine headaches includes analgesics, antidepressants, tranquilizers, and antimigraine drugs. Over-the-counter analgesics contain aspirin, acetaminophen (Tylenol, Panadol, etc.), ibuprofen (Advil, Motrin IB, Nuprin, etc.), or naproxen (Aleve). Prescription pain pills for headache often contain multiple ingredients, including a narcotic such as codeine or a narcoticlike ingredient like proproxyphene (Darvon, Wygesic, etc.). Antidepressants and tranquilizers are discussed in Chapters 62 and 81, respectively.

If your headache is of the migraine type, a specific antimigraine drug such as Cafergot, Ergostat, Midrin, or Sansert may be helpful. Two newer prescription drugs that have shown promise in the treatment of migraine include Stadol NS and Imitrex. Stadol NS is a nasal spray analgesic that may provide pain relief similar to injectable narcotics. Imitrex, available orally or as a self-administered subcutaneous injection, acts by constricting large intracranial blood vessels and usually provides significant relief within one to two hours of a migraine attack. Imitrex should be used cautiously and under close medical supervision as occasional serious side effects have been reported, especially in patients who have heart disease or high blood pressure.

HEADACHE

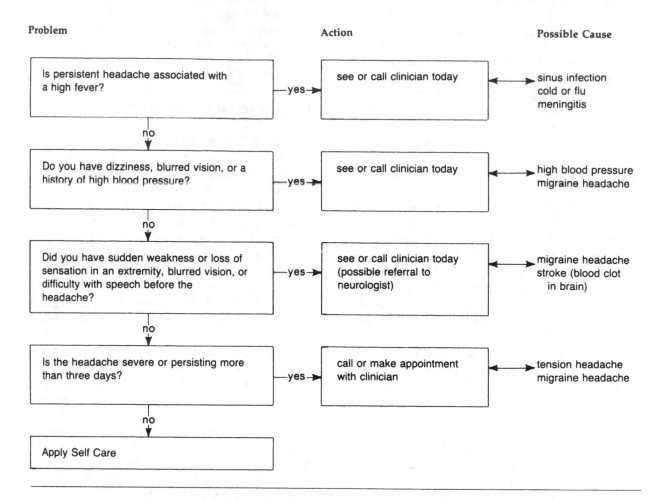

Problem | Action | Possible Cause

Is persistent headache associated with a high fever? — yes → see or call clinician today ← sinus infection / cold or flu / meningitis

no ↓

Do you have dizziness, blurred vision, or a history of high blood pressure? — yes → see or call clinician today ← high blood pressure / migraine headache

no ↓

Did you have sudden weakness or loss of sensation in an extremity, blurred vision, or difficulty with speech before the headache? — yes → see or call clinician today (possible referral to neurologist) ← migraine headache / stroke (blood clot in brain)

no ↓

Is the headache severe or persisting more than three days? — yes → call or make appointment with clinician ← tension headache / migraine headache

no ↓

Apply Self Care

In treating chronic, daily headache (as well as preventing migraine), beta-blockers and antidepressants have been among the most effective drugs. Typical beta-blockers—drugs mainly used to treat high blood pressure and abnormal heart rhythms—include Lopressor and Inderal. Some of the more successful antidepressants in the treatment of chronic headache include Adapin, Elavil, Endep, Prozac, and Sinequan.

A common ingredient in several prescription drugs used to treat tension headache is the barbiturate butalbital. Butalbital is usually combined with one or more over-the-counter ingredients, such as acetaminophen (Axocet), aspirin and caffeine (Fiorinal), or acetaminophen and caffeine (Fioricet). It should be remembered that the butalbital ingredient in these medications may cause drowsiness and can be habit-forming.

What You Can Do (Self Care)

Since emotional factors seem to be associated in most cases of tension and migraine headaches, you can do a lot by just evaluating the stress in your life. Talk about these stresses with your family and close friends. Identify problems and try to take some action. Be sure you are eating enough and as often as needed. Are you working longer hours than your health will allow? Are you setting up unrealistic expectations of yourself? Relaxation exercises, transcendental meditation, and brief counseling have been effective in treating migraines. Biofeedback and acupuncture have also been effective in the short run, but the long-term results are uncertain. Avoid the chronic use of tranquilizers and narcotics. See Chapter 51 for information about over-the-counter analgesics.

Table 105 COMPARISON OF TENSION AND MIGRAINE HEADACHES

Factor	In Tension Headache	In Migraine Headache
pain	continuous bandlike ache or pressure around head	throbbing pain, often limited to one side of the head
duration	lasts a few hours	may last many hours to a few days
accompanying symptoms	none	blurred vision, nausea, diarrhea
occurrence during sleep	rare	sometimes interrupts sleep
caused by psychological stress	often	often
caused by dietary factors	no	sometimes
caused by eyestrain	yes	no
associated with premenstrual tension	occasionally	sometimes
may be inherited	no	yes

For immediate relief, a hot bath may be surprisingly effective. Avoid chronic use of over-the-counter analgesics because these may cause a rebound headache when they are discontinued.

To help prevent migraines, avoid the foods which seem to trigger the attack. If you find that MSG affects you badly and you like eating in Chinese restaurants, don't despair. You can ask that the MSG be withheld from the food you order.

CHAPTER 68

Heartburn and Gas

Psychological stress plays an important role in causing heartburn and gas. Everyone swallows air to some degree when they eat. But anxiety can lead to excessive air swallowing while eating, thus causing belching and burping. Intestinal gas also comes from normal digestion of food, and the amount of intestinal gas varies from individual to individual and with different foods. In addition, spicy foods, excessive alcohol, and certain drugs such as aspirin or antiarthritics are well-known causes of heartburn. Nonsteroidal anti-inflammatory drugs (NSAIDs) require FDA labeling warning about the possible risk of stomach ulceration resulting from chronic use of them. NSAIDs are widely used in the treatment of arthritis and in controlling menstrual pain. What you may not know is that chronic dietary indiscretion (that is, continually eating foods that affect you badly, overeating, drinking alcohol to excess, taking too much aspirin, etc.) can eventually cause stomach inflammation called *gastritis*.

Two of the most common medical conditions associated with heartburn are peptic ulcer disease (erosion of the stomach or duodenal lining) and gallbladder problems. Caused by excessive stomach acids, peptic ulcer disease is commonly associated with a recurrent burning pain felt in the upper middle abdomen under the breastbone; this burning sensation is often relieved by food, milk, or antacids. When a bleeding ulcer develops, the first symptom may be black tarry stools. Gallbladder disease, which is more common among women than men, particularly affects individuals who are over the age of forty and who have a fair complexion. Women who take birth control pills also have a slightly greater frequency of gallbladder disease. The gallbladder is located in the upper abdomen on the right side just beneath the rib cage. When the gallbladder is inflamed, cramping pain in this location, belching, and burping may occur, particularly after fatty or fried foods are eaten. If stones plug the gallbladder ducts, jaundice (see glossary) may develop and is sometimes associated with fever and severe pain. Heartburn affects 60% of pregnant women and usually starts about midway through pregnancy. This heartburn occurs primarily because the growing uterus impinges on the stomach. The increased frequency of gallstones in the pregnant woman is related to her changing hormones. Peptic ulcer disease, however, is rare in pregnancy because acid secretion in the stomach is actually decreased.

What Medical Care Can Do

The clinician will examine your abdomen and evaluate the pattern of your discomfort as well as your dietary habits. When severe or chronic abdominal pain occurs, an upper GI series (see glossary) or stomach X-ray may be obtained, as well as a gallbladder X-ray. These X-rays are contraindicated in pregnancy except in unusual circumstances. A sonogram (see glossary) of the upper abdomen is also helpful in evaluating the gall bladder and pancreas, and avoids the use of X-rays. Stool may be tested for microscopic bleeding.

Treatment of acute conditions, like gallstones, may require surgery, but most digestive disorders can be managed with medication. Peptic ulcer disease is commonly treated with antacids or with newer antiulcer agents like Carafate and Prilosec. Other newer prescription drugs known as H_2-receptor antagonists, such as Pepcid, Tagamet, and Zantac, also have proved useful in treating peptic ulcers. Some lower-dose H_2 antagonists, including Tagamet HB and Pepcid AC, are now available over-the-counter. Modern therapy for peptic ulcer disease often involves using various antibiotics to eradicate the microbe *H. pylori*.

What You Can Do (Self Care)

To prevent heartburn, eliminate or reduce the intake or use of stomach irritants, such as coffee, cigarettes, aspirin, and alcohol. You may also want to try eliminating spicy foods for a while.

Antacids, as well as over-the-counter Tagamet HB or Pepcid AC, may be used successfully to relieve heartburn. Antacids containing simethicone or products containing simethicone alone, such as Mylicon, may be used specifically for gas. This symptom can also be controlled by eating slowly and by avoiding gas-producing foods, like beans, cabbage, cucumbers, and any other foods you find cause gas for you. It is important to look for causes of chronic stress in your life which so often precede the development of an ulcer in the form of recurrent heartburn.

During pregnancy, decrease the size and increase the frequency of meals; and eat a relatively bland diet. Antacids may be used in general with the exception of sodium bicarbonate. If indigestion persists at night, you may sleep with your head propped on pillows or elevate the head of the bed. Avoid drugs, such as tranquilizers, particularly during the first third of pregnancy (see Chapter 31).

HEARTBURN AND GAS

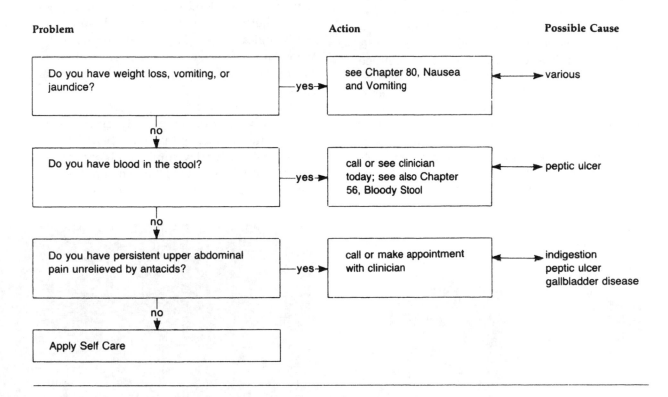

Problem	Action	Possible Cause
Do you have weight loss, vomiting, or jaundice? —yes→	see Chapter 80, Nausea and Vomiting	various
no ↓		
Do you have blood in the stool? —yes→	call or see clinician today; see also Chapter 56, Bloody Stool	peptic ulcer
no ↓		
Do you have persistent upper abdominal pain unrelieved by antacids? —yes→	call or make appointment with clinician	indigestion peptic ulcer gallbladder disease
no ↓		
Apply Self Care		

CHAPTER 69

High Blood Pressure

High blood pressure, called *hypertension*, is being diagnosed in women between the ages of twenty-five and fifty-five with increasing frequency. Hypertension affects 60 million Americans, who spend about $2.5 billion a year on its management. The condition is often identified earlier in women than in men, possibly because women are more likely to have regular checkups, including close blood-pressure monitoring during pregnancies. Hypertension is sometimes called "the silent killer" because it has potentially lethal complications, although most people with high blood pressure feel no ill effects in the early stages. Hypertension that remains uncon-

trolled, however, may lead to severe headaches, blurred vision, damaged blood vessels, and other conditions.

In 85% of women with high blood pressure, no underlying cause for the high blood pressure is found. This situation is known as *essential hypertension*, a disease associated with hardening and narrowing of the walls of the blood vessels, a process that occurs with age. In the other 15% of women with high blood pressure, causes such as kidney disease or the use of certain drugs (e.g., diet pills) account for the high blood pressure. Factors associated with an increased risk of high blood pressure include obesity, a family history of high blood pressure, cigarette smoking, diabetes, elevated blood cholesterol, and psychological stress. High blood pressure is a major cause of stroke, heart disease, and kidney failure, especially when these risk factors are present.

During pregnancy, blood pressure is normally unchanged or temporarily decreased because of the hormones that relax blood vessels. Hypertension may develop by itself or represent continuation of previous high blood pressure. High blood pressure in pregnancy is rarely se-

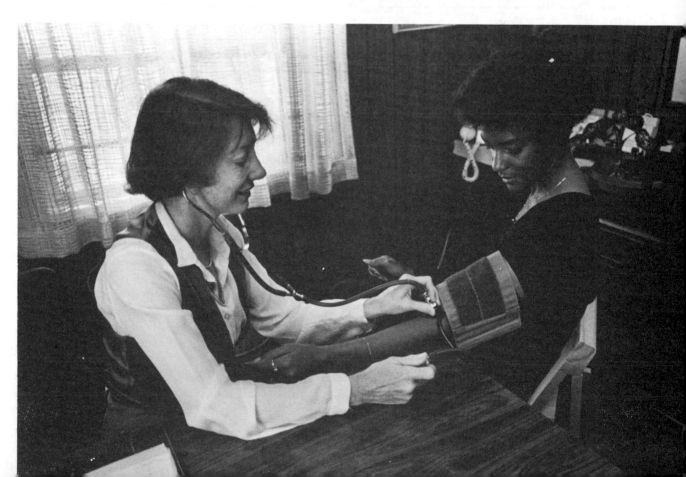

vere enough to warrant abortion. However, sterilization may be medically indicated when blood pressure elevation is especially high or when complications involving the heart or kidneys occur.

What Medical Care Can Do

The clinician will check your blood pressure several times, first in one arm and then in the other, while you are lying down and again while you are sitting. Since blood pressure varies with activity, emotions, and posture, it is important to evaluate blood pressure after you have been sitting or resting quietly for at least five minutes. Several elevated blood pressures are required to confirm a diagnosis of high blood pressure. In general, physicians consider a blood pressure of 120/80 or less normal; 140/90 causes suspicion of hypertension. And elevation to 160/95 or more, even intermittently in the office, almost certainly indicates the presence of at least mild hypertension.

During the physical exam, the clinician examines your eyes to look for blood vessel changes that occur with high blood pressure and evaluates your heart, lungs, and pulse. He may obtain an electrocardiogram (EKG) (see glossary), a chest X-ray, blood tests, and a urinalysis. These tests are often completely normal unless complications of high blood pressure have begun to occur.

Once the physician diagnoses hypertension, standard drugs such as diuretics (water pills) or beta-blockers (e.g., Inderal or Lopressor) may be prescribed. Other therapeutic measures include stopping smoking and increasing exercise. Diuretics lower blood pressure by causing the kidneys to produce more urine, which leads to lower blood volume and a reduced blood pressure. Beta-blockers, which act in part by decreasing cardiac output ("heart work"), are the other first-line drugs. However, beta-blockers should be avoided in women with a history of asthma, heart failure, or diabetes. When first-choice agents are ineffective or contraindicated, other, newer types of medication may be tried to control blood pressure. These include four new drug groups: calcium channel blockers (e.g., Calan), angiotensin-converting enzyme (ACE) inhibitors (e.g., Capoten, Monopril, Prinivil, Vasotec), alpha-blockers (e.g., Minipress, Hytrin),

and alpha/beta-blockers (e.g., Normodyne). Some of these newer, potent drugs are used to treat cardiac conditions, from abnormal heart rhythms to coronary artery disease, and may have potent side effects such as fatigue, depression, and even decreased libido. You may want to discuss these and other newer drugs with your internist if you have high blood pressure. Drug therapy controls but usually does not cure high blood pressure unless a correctable underlying cause is found. In pregnancy, the initial treatment of hypertension consists of bed rest and may necessitate early delivery by induction of labor if high blood pressure becomes severe (see Chapters 20 and 21).

What You Can Do (Self Care)

Nearly half of the people who have high blood pressure don't know they have it, so you should have your blood pressure checked at least once a year after the age of thirty. Reduce as many risk factors as possible. Don't smoke and do keep your weight under control. Certainly, exercise has many benefits, including weight control, but if you are over thirty-five years old, it is advisable to have an exercise stress test before starting on a serious exercise program (see Chapter 49). If you have a family history of high blood pressure, ask your doctor to order cholesterol and triglyceride blood tests to see if dietary changes are needed to reduce the amount of these substances in your body. Be sure to get early treatment of urinary tract infections since kidney damage is associated with the development of subsequent hypertension. If you drink, do so in moderation and avoid consuming more than one ounce of alcohol per day. Women with mildly elevated blood pressure who cut down or stop drinking even this much may lower their blood pressure to the normal range.

It is especially important for women with known hypertension to maintain optimum weight and to reduce salt intake (see Chapter 48). Avoid extra salt in cooking or at the table, or use a salt substitute. Also avoid salty foods, including hard cheeses and lunch meats as well as other processed foods. Read food and over-the-counter drug labels for sodium (salt) content. Discontinue taking birth control pills if high blood pressure develops. Take your blood pres-

HIGH BLOOD PRESSURE

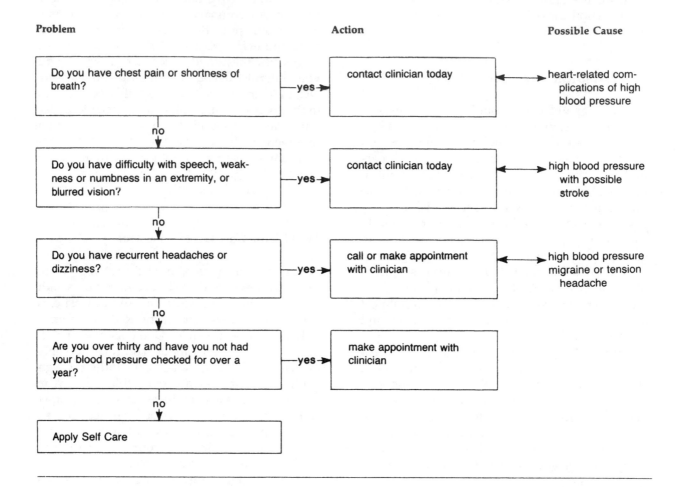

Problem	Action	Possible Cause
Do you have chest pain or shortness of breath?	→yes→ contact clinician today	←← heart-related complications of high blood pressure
↓no		
Do you have difficulty with speech, weakness or numbness in an extremity, or blurred vision?	→yes→ contact clinician today	←← high blood pressure with possible stroke
↓no		
Do you have recurrent headaches or dizziness?	→yes→ call or make appointment with clinician	←← high blood pressure migraine or tension headache
↓no		
Are you over thirty and have you not had your blood pressure checked for over a year?	→yes→ make appointment with clinician	
↓no		
Apply Self Care		

sure medication exactly as prescribed; elevation of blood pressure is likely to recur if you stop your medication. Remember that most diuretics when taken chronically cause potassium salts to be lost in the urine. You can prevent symptoms of potassium depletion (weakness, muscle cramps) by eating high-potassium foods such as bananas, oranges, or cranberry juice or by taking oral potassium supplements prescribed by your doctor.

Lifetime drug therapy is necessary for most individuals with hypertension. The best way to prevent hypertension complications (such as heart disease) in the long run is to adopt a life style that minimizes as many risk factors as pos-

sible, especially in the areas of smoking, obesity, diet, and chronic stress (see Chapter 47). Consider purchasing a blood pressure cuff and learning from your doctor or a nurse how you or a family member can check your blood pressure at home.

For more information about high blood pressure (as well as obesity, high cholesterol, and heart disease), write to the National Institutes of Health at:

National Heart, Lung, and Blood Institute
Information Center
P.O. Box 30105
Bethesda, Maryland 20824-0105

CHAPTER 70

Hot Flashes

A *hot flash* is a reflex circulatory change caused by hormone fluctuations, especially dropping estrogen levels. Blood vessels close to the skin dilate, giving off sensations of warmth and flushing. Most women experience the sudden flush or feeling of warmth over the chest, neck, and face to some degree just prior to and during menopause. The intensity and frequency of hot flashes vary widely, and they often occur at night along with marked perspiration. These episodes, although annoying, are not the least bit harmful. Hot flashes also may accompany surgical removal of the ovaries unless you receive estrogen replacement after the operation (see Chapter 27).

While many people associate hot flashes with menopause, this symptom may have various other causes and may be experienced by men as well as women. In susceptible individuals, hot flashes (the feeling of intense heat) and flushing (the appearance of red splotches, usually in the upper half of the body) may be due to alcohol, physical stimulants, certain tumors, and various chemicals and drugs. The alcohol-induced flush is apparently more common among certain ethnic groups, especially Orientals. Physical stimulation such as drinking a hot liquid or taking a steam bath may produce a flush, which is really no more than an exaggerated physiological response as skin blood vessels dilate in an attempt to lose heat. Some tumors, such as carcinoid tumors, which are usually found somewhere in the digestive tract, may occasionally cause hot flashes in association with diarrhea, palpitations, and other symptoms. And some drugs, such as nicotinic acid, the active ingredient in some cholesterol-lowering drugs, may produce flushing as a side effect. Flushing is also a potential side effect of prostaglandin drugs, which are used to induce abortion and to "ripen" the cervix prior to inducing labor. Other hot flash-producing drugs often prescribed for women include calcitonin-containing products such as Calcimar, which is used to treat osteoporosis; Lupron, a new drug used in the treatment of both endometriosis and fibroids (see Chapter 35); Flagyl, a drug used to treat various vaginal infections; and narcotics such as Demerol and morphine, used to control pain relief after surgery or childbirth.

HOT FLASHES

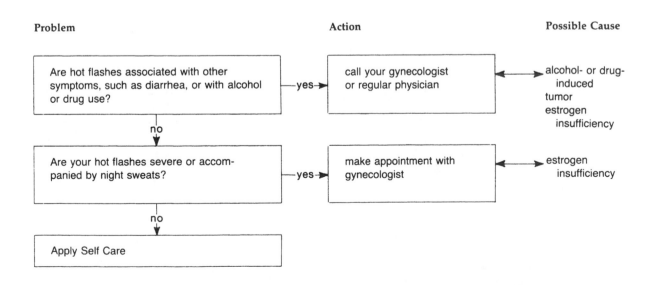

Problem	Action	Possible Cause
Are hot flashes associated with other symptoms, such as diarrhea, or with alcohol or drug use? —yes→	call your gynecologist or regular physician	← alcohol- or drug-induced tumor estrogen insufficiency
no ↓		
Are your hot flashes severe or accompanied by night sweats? —yes→	make appointment with gynecologist	← estrogen insufficiency
no ↓		
Apply Self Care		

What Medical Care Can Do

The physician may be able to diagnose estrogen insufficiency associated with menopause from the pelvic examination if the vagina shows characteristic thinning and paleness. The most reliable blood tests to diagnose the problem are the levels of certain brain hormones—FSH and LH (see glossary). These brain hormones reach a high level in the blood as menopause approaches (see Chapter 26).

The use of estrogen in treating symptoms of menopause is discussed in Chapter 27. The use of tranquilizers to treat hot flashes alone is not recommended. Another drug that may help relieve hot flashes is the anti-hypertensive drug clonidine. Bellergal-S has also been used to relieve hot flashes, but the drug includes a potentially addictive tranquilizer (phenobarbital) and is contraindicated if you have glaucoma, high blood pressure, or coronary artery (heart) disease. All of these drugs have potential side effects, and none works quite as well as estrogen.

What You Can Do (Self Care)

For ease and comfort, wear loose and layered clothing so you can take off outer layers during a hot flash. Some women find it helps to drink a glass of ice water immediately after a hot flash.

It helps to realize that menopausal symptoms do not represent anything wrong and that these temporary symptoms just mark one of the many natural changes which occur in the lifetime of all women. If you are taking hormone replacement, tell your clinician about the occurrence of any side effects of these pills, such as abnormal bleeding.

CHAPTER 71

Insomnia

Occasional insomnia should not worry you because it happens to everyone from time to time. Chronic sleeplessness, however, is a distressing problem that often increases with age and is experienced as trouble falling asleep or staying asleep. Contributing factors include situations of emotional stress at home or at work, medical problems causing pain or other discomfort, or hormonal factors causing night sweats in menopausal women. Insomnia is often linked to common symptoms of depression such as daytime napping, inability to concentrate, loss of appetite, and loss of sexual desire. Some women by necessity or choice arrange their lives so that every minute of every hour is filled with mental and physical activity. The result of this outpouring of energy during the day may be difficulty in sleeping at night.

What Medical Care Can Do

Physicians often prescribe drugs for sleep disorders. These typically may include barbiturates (like Seconal and Nembutal), tranquilizers (like Valium and Librium), and sleeping pills such as Dalmane. Unfortunately any of these drugs may lose their effectiveness with prolonged use, are potentially addicting, and may cause withdrawal symptoms if discontinued abruptly. Such drugs should be avoided in the first trimester of pregnancy and used thereafter only after discussion with your doctor. One of the safest sleeping pills to use in pregnancy is the antihistamine Benadryl, a less potent but more extensively studied drug than many other drugs currently used for this purpose. When depression causes insomnia, the doctor may prescribe antidepressant medication, preferably in combination with some form of counseling to help identify your underlying emotional conflicts. Like tranquilizers, antidepressant medication improves your symptoms only as long as you take the drug.

What You Can Do (Self Care)

Women vary in the amount of sleep needed, which may be more or less than eight hours a night. Some women are "day people" and prefer to go to bed early and rise early. Other women are "night people" who feel better if they sleep during the day and stay awake at night. The important thing is not when or how long, but how well you sleep. Here are some suggestions:

1. Avoid stimulants such as coffee, tea, cola, and amphetamine-type drugs two or three hours (or even longer) before going to bed. Also avoid large meals at this time since the digestive process can interfere with sleep. Some people find that a glass of warm milk is an effective sleep tonic. A hot bath each night before you go to bed may also help you relax.
2. Try to develop regular sleeping habits. Sleep at the same time and the same place every night in a comfortable bed. Plan to get to sleep within a half hour after lying down. Use your bedroom for sleeping and not for working activities.
3. Establish a quiet activity, such as reading, prior to going to bed. Avoid big decisions or family worries at this time. As you go to sleep, develop a habit of thinking of pleasurable plans or events which bring you happiness.
4. Avoid daytime napping.
5. Avoid chronic use of tranquilizers or alcohol to help with insomnia for the reasons mentioned above.
6. Plan for regular, daily exercise (see Chapter 49).

For more information on insomnia and sleep disorders, write to the National Institutes of Health at:

National Heart, Lung, and Blood Institute
Information Center
P.O. Box 30105
Bethesda, Mayland 20824-0105

INSOMNIA

Problem		Action		Possible Cause

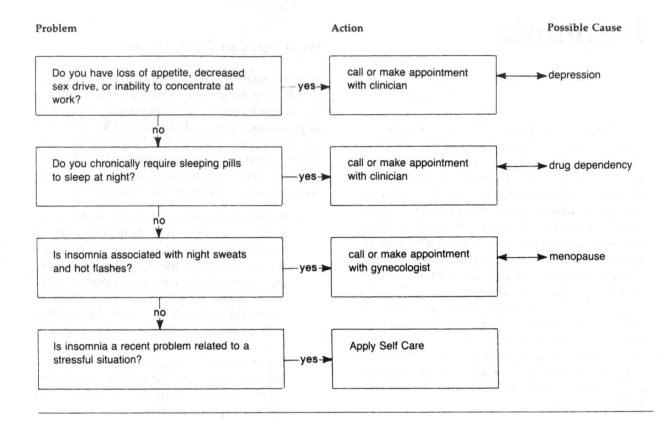

Problem | Action | Possible Cause

Do you have loss of appetite, decreased sex drive, or inability to concentrate at work? —yes→ call or make appointment with clinician ←→ depression

↓ no

Do you chronically require sleeping pills to sleep at night? —yes→ call or make appointment with clinician ←→ drug dependency

↓ no

Is insomnia associated with night sweats and hot flashes? —yes→ call or make appointment with gynecologist ←→ menopause

↓ no

Is insomnia a recent problem related to a stressful situation? —yes→ Apply Self Care

CHAPTER 72

Itching, Rash, and Skin Pigmentation

Common Causes of Itching

One of the most common causes of itching is dry skin. As we grow older, our skin thins and decreases its capacity to retain moisture, causing dry skin. At other times itching may be localized, as in the case of rectal hemorrhoids. Emotional factors also play an important role in itching and, in some instances, may be the only identifiable cause. Other common causes of itching in women fall into three categories: allergy-related conditions, conditions causing vaginal itching, and drug reactions.

Allergy-related conditions

Allergy in the form of itching or rash is one way the body reacts to a foreign substance or an irritant. Hives and contact dermatitis are common skin conditions which may be allergic reactions. Women who acquire contact dermatitis or hives usually have a history of other allergic conditions such as asthma or hay fever.

Hives appear as pink, itchy skin swellings which represent a generalized reaction of the skin to a local irritant such as an insect bite, or to an ingested substance such as strawberries or a drug. Occasionally hives are induced by emotional tension or excitement.

Contact dermatitis is a common type of eczema or skin inflammation causing itching, burning, or stinging from contact with chemicals or other irritants such as poison oak. Skin blisters develop first; then they ooze and ultimately crust and flake in this process. There is always a potential for infection whenever the skin is broken. Your skin may be sensitive to any number of ordinary substances: soaps, detergents, metal, jewelry, creams, and so on. The affected area gives a clue to the cause of contact dermatitis. For instance, a scalp rash may be caused by a hair dye; a rash at the base of one finger could indicate sensitivity to the metal in a ring.

Conditions causing vaginal itching

This itching can be one of the most agonizing symptoms affecting women. The most common cause is a vaginal infection, especially yeast (see Chapter 87). Itching without discharge may represent an allergic reaction to a new soap, vaginal contraceptive foam, or a prescribed vaginal cream or suppository.

Infectious causes of itching without vaginal discharge include lice and scabies. These infestations are characterized by severe itching, often at night, of the pubic area. Although they are not life-threatening, lice and scabies are highly communicable and very much a nuisance. Both conditions are usually acquired through close personal contact though not necessarily through intercourse.

Pubic and scalp lice live on hair and skin; body lice are found in clothing. Lice infection is probably the only disease that is readily acquired from sitting on a contaminated toilet seat. The usual way of getting pubic lice, however, is through close physical contact, especially during intercourse.

Scabies produces itching in warm, moist areas of the body, particularly around the external genitalia. The organism, *Sarcoptes scabiei*, is about the size of a pinhead and burrows in the skin, making little tunnels that look like pencil dots.

In older women, a disorder called vulvar dystrophy is a major cause of intense itching of the external genitalia. Dystrophy causes thinning and shrinkage of the vulva, resulting in painful intercourse. A combination of infections and allergic factors, along with decreasing levels of estrogen, contribute to this condition.

Occasionally chronic vaginal itching may be the first symptom of cancer of the vulva. This disease should be suspected in a woman over the age of fifty when prolonged use of vaginal creams is unsuccessful in relieving her symptoms.

Table 106 summarizes the causes and method of diagnosis of vaginal itching.

Table 106 VAGINAL ITCHING—CAUSES AND DIAGNOSES

Cause of Vaginal Itching	How Diagnosed
Vaginal infection (usually yeast)	microscopic examination of secretions
Skin disease (e.g., psoriasis)	characteristic skin changes not restricted to vulva
Diabetes	glucose tolerance test
Dystrophy of vulva	biopsy of suspected area of vulva
Infestation (scabies, lice)	finding an organism
Allergic reaction	history of use of vaginal hygiene or contraceptive product, new soap, or condom
Psychological stress	emotional factors predominate; other causes ruled out
Cancer of the vulva	biopsy of vulva
Vaginal warts	characteristic appearance (see Chapter 24)

Drug reactions

Itching and rash are the most common forms of drug reaction. Almost any drug may produce nearly any type of rash. The rash may occur suddenly after the drug is taken and involve the entire body. Or the onset may be gradual with the rash beginning on, say, the abdomen. With repeated exposure to a drug, the chance of an allergic reaction is more likely. Sun exposure will increase the chance of a reaction to some drugs, such as diuretics (water pills), barbiturates, mood elevators, tetracycline, and sulfa. The tendency to develop a drug rash following sun exposure is known as photosensitivity.

Birth control pills may occasionally cause a rash, but the principal skin effect is increased pigmentation, that is, darkening of the skin, particularly over the face. This occurs in up to 30% of women on birth control pills. Pigmentation may persist even if the birth control pills are discontinued.

In pregnancy, itching is the most common complaint related to the skin. Itching, sometimes accompanied by a fine, red rash over the abdomen, is more common in the second half of pregnancy. The itching goes away after delivery but may come back with subsequent pregnancies or after birth control pills are started. These symptoms are probably due to increased levels of estrogen.

The most common skin change in pregnancy is an increase in pigmentation which occurs over the face (known as chloasma), nipples, and lower abdomen (*linea nigra*). Chloasma, or increased facial pigmentation similar to that produced by the pill, is known as the *mask of pregnancy* and affects over 50% of pregnant women, particularly brunettes. This type of pigmentation usually fades after pregnancy. Other common skin changes occurring in pregnancy include the formation of stretch marks, or striae, increased size and pigmentation of moles, and increased sweating. About 10% of women develop reddish skin spots on the face, neck, and upper chest. These spots are dilated blood vessels which may have a spidery appearance. Most of these skin spots also disappear after delivery.

What Medical Care Can Do

The clinician will ask you about previous allergy to food or drugs, recent contacts with new chemicals or cosmetics, and a history of skin disease. The diagnosis is usually made from the characteristics and location of the skin lesion. Treatment is often nonspecific, involving antihistamines or sedatives to alleviate itching and antibiotics to prevent secondary bacterial infections. Steroids are reserved for severe cases of hives and contact dermatitis to decrease inflammation. Treatment of vulvar dystrophy, diagnosed by biopsy, includes hormone creams.

What You Can Do (Self Care)

In general, it's essential to follow carefully any medical regimen the physician prescribes for you. If you are treating yourself, start with small amounts of a cream or salve to be sure you are not allergic to it. Stop any drug that seems to produce a local irritation or an allergic response. Don't take a drug which previously caused a rash because subsequent reactions may be more serious. Taking over-the-counter anti-inflammatory cream (hydrocortisone) or antihistamines on a short-term basis may help to control itching.

Some suggestions are given below for specific problems.

Contact dermatitis

Cooling baths to which two tablespoons of baking soda are added may be helpful. Minimize heat and keep the area clean. Avoid scratching irritated skin since bacterial infections can occur. Don't use substances that previously caused skin reactions. Use only hypoallergenic cosmetics or none at all when possible. If you think your detergent may be the cause, wash out your clothes with baking soda, to get rid of the detergent.

Hives

Take cornstarch or oatmeal baths (Aveeno Oatmeal works well and is available over-the-counter with directions), and smooth on calamine lotion after bathing.

Lice and scabies

Be sure all family members and other possible contacts are treated and that all bedding and clothing are laundered or dry-cleaned. Kwell is the drug of choice and a prescription may be called in to your drugstore by a physician. If you use Kwell shampoo, repeat the shampoo in twenty-four hours. If you use Kwell cream or lotion, leave it on for twenty-four hours. Do not use Kwell during pregnancy without physician supervision as it may harm the fetus.

Dry skin

If you have dry skin, never use strong soaps or bubble baths. Small amounts of bath oil, such as Alpha Keri, may be helpful. Excessive bathing should be avoided and may itself cause itching if you have dry skin. Over-the-counter products for dry skin may contain many ingredients, including estrogen, which increases the water-holding capacity of skin. However, the FDA limits the amount of hormone that can be contained in these cosmetics, and they have no effect on the course of dry-skin conditions. Much of the effectiveness of estrogen-containing creams, and any decrease in wrinkles, are due to the cream's base, rather than to the hormone itself.

Pregnancy itching and rash

Oral or topical Benadryl relieves itching; your physician can call your drugstore and order a prescription. Cornstarch baths may also be helpful. A low-fat diet may help by putting less strain on the liver. If yellow pigmentation involving skin or eyes occurs (jaundice), contact your clinician.

Table 107 summarizes the diagnosis and treatment of itching and rash.

ITCHING AND RASH

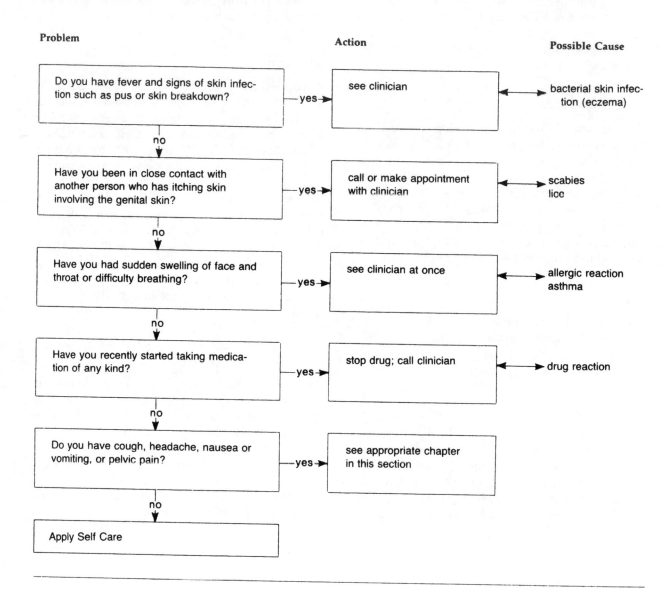

Problem	Action	Possible Cause

Problem

Do you have fever and signs of skin infection such as pus or skin breakdown? — yes → see clinician ← bacterial skin infection (eczema)

no ↓

Have you been in close contact with another person who has itching skin involving the genital skin? — yes → call or make appointment with clinician ← scabies / lice

no ↓

Have you had sudden swelling of face and throat or difficulty breathing? — yes → see clinician at once ← allergic reaction / asthma

no ↓

Have you recently started taking medication of any kind? — yes → stop drug; call clinician ← drug reaction

no ↓

Do you have cough, headache, nausea or vomiting, or pelvic pain? — yes → see appropriate chapter in this section

no ↓

Apply Self Care

Table 107 DIAGNOSIS AND TREATMENT OF ITCHING AND RASH

Condition	Diagnostic Features	Treatment
Contact dermatitis	Recent skin contact with an irritant or allergy-causing substance, e.g., poison oak, detergents, cosmetics	Antihistamines; various topical medications may be prescribed; avoid irritants; cornstarch or baking soda baths
Hives	History of insect bites; drug or food allergies; emotional stress	Antihistamines; cornstarch baths; calamine lotion
Fungus infections (of scalp, hands, feet, body)	Localized chronic scaling and itching patches over part of body involved	Keep skin dry; Tinactin; prescription drugs may be necessary
Drug reaction	Sudden generalized rash following drug use	Antihistamines; avoid drugs
Lice	Intense itching of pubic area	Kwell lotion or cream; wash bedding and clothing
Scabies	Itching, especially at night, often involving genitals; other family members involved	Kwell lotion or cream; wash bedding and clothing
Pregnancy rash	Itching over abdomen with rash	Antihistamines; low-fat diet; cornstarch baths

CHAPTER 73

Joint Pains

Recurrent joint pains in women are usually due to one of the many forms of arthritis which afflict women. Arthritis is an inflammation in the area called the joint, where two bones meet. A capsule containing lubricating fluid encases all the body's joints. Swelling and inflammation within the joint capsule may cause stiffness, rigidity, and pain upon movement. Eventually a scar between the bones may develop, resulting in joint deformity. These processes occur regardless of the cause of the arthritis.

Rheumatoid arthritis, a chronic condition with some family predisposition, afflicts many women and often begins in a woman's reproductive years. The most painful and disabling form of arthritis in women, rheumatoid arthritis typically begins as a chronic nonfebrile (no fever) condition associated with fatigue, loss of appetite, and aching joints. Joint stiffness occurs in the morning but usually subsides during the day. Joints of the hands, feet, and ankles are commonly affected. Occasionally other organs are involved, causing anemia, rash, or diarrhea. This disease is usually progressive but controllable; early treatment may prevent deformities.

Osteoarthritis, a degenerative disease which occurs as a result of aging, is increasingly common after age fifty. The weight-bearing joints, such as the hip and back, are affected as are the joints in the ends of the fingers, which may become enlarged, stiff, and painful. Joint stiffness occurs at the end of the day with osteoarthritis, which is milder than rheumatoid arthritis and does not usually involve other parts of the body.

Infectious arthritis may result from a bacterial infection such as gonorrhea, causing an acute inflammation of one or more joints, sometimes associated with a rash. Joint deformity does not occur.

Systemic lupus erythematosus is the most common of several conditions known collectively as *connective tissue* or *auto-immune disease*. Lupus, as it is sometimes called, affects women almost exclusively, often during the early childbearing years. The cause of lupus, which may affect varied areas of the body such as the skin, blood, and kidneys, is unknown.

Traumatic joint injury due to vigorous exercise or strenuous sports activity may damage the ligaments and tendons. The knees, elbows, and shoulders are most commonly affected. These conditions, as well as muscle strains, must be distinguished from arthritis. Women's joints are more "lax" or looser than men's, which leads to a higher rate of sports injury in women.

Rheumatoid arthritis has no known deleterious effect on pregnancy, fertility, or the fetus. No one knows why rheumatoid arthritis often gets better during pregnancy and then worsens during the postpartum period. Systemic lupus erythematosus has a variable course during pregnancy but becomes worse during the postpartum period in many women. The treatment of lupus requires powerful anti-inflammatory drugs called steroids, which may be necessary during pregnancy to control the disease. Unless severe, lupus is not a medical indication for termination of pregnancy or for sterilization.

One type of joint disorder that particularly affects women is TMD, which stands for *temporomandibular disorders*. (The "TM" joint is located where the mandible or jawbone inserts on each side into the skull.) Symptoms include facial or jaw pain, difficulty opening the mouth or chewing, and various other symptoms, including headaches, dizziness, sinus pain, and ringing in the ears. Contrary to popular belief, a bad bite is an uncommon cause of TMD, which more often results from trauma or nighttime teeth grinding or clenching as a result of emotional stress. Jaw clicks or popping sounds, found in 40% of the population, are not necessarily signs of TMD. Since TMD may affect the teeth, jaw, or facial muscles, a variety of specialists, including dentists, orthodontists, and oral surgeons, may be involved with the diagnosis and treatment of this condition. Only 5% to 10% of the general population have some form of TMD serious enough to warrant treatment. Only 5% to 10% of that group has some persistent pain. The vast majority of TMD problems can be treated conservatively (without surgery).

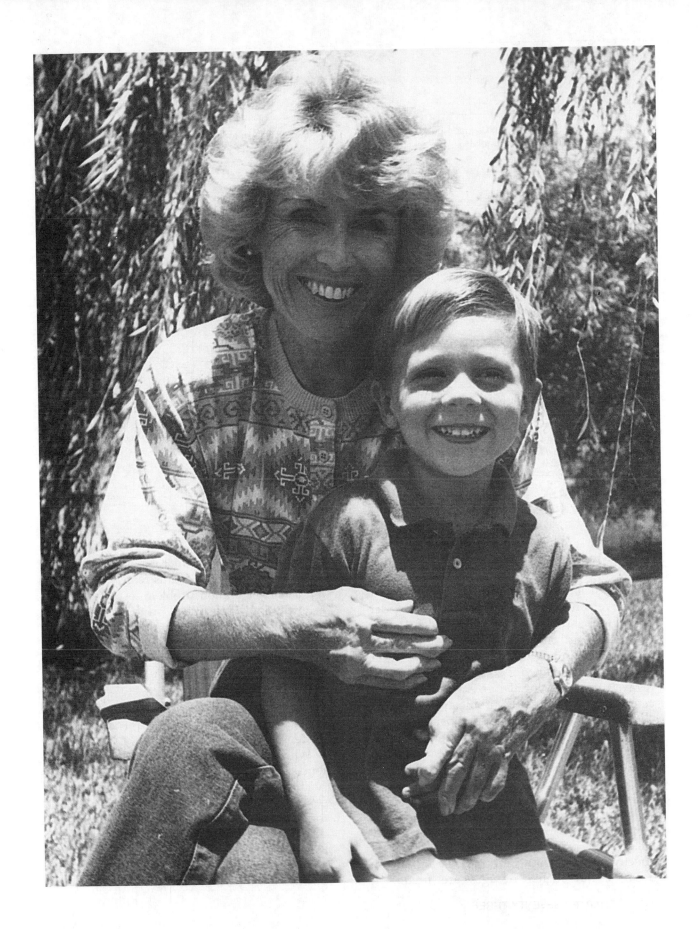

JOINT PAIN

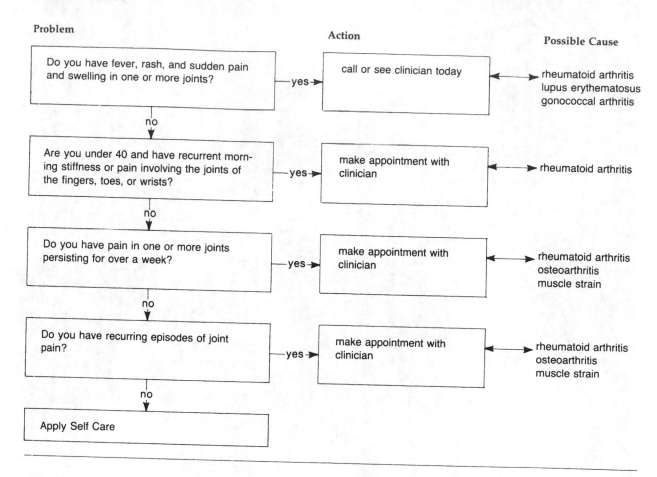

Problem

Do you have fever, rash, and sudden pain and swelling in one or more joints?

—yes→

Action

call or see clinician today

←

Possible Cause

→ rheumatoid arthritis
lupus erythematosus
gonococcal arthritis

no ↓

Are you under 40 and have recurrent morning stiffness or pain involving the joints of the fingers, toes, or wrists?

—yes→

make appointment with clinician

←

→ rheumatoid arthritis

no ↓

Do you have pain in one or more joints persisting for over a week?

—yes→

make appointment with clinician

←

→ rheumatoid arthritis
osteoarthritis
muscle strain

no ↓

Do you have recurring episodes of joint pain?

—yes→

make appointment with clinician

←

→ rheumatoid arthritis
osteoarthritis
muscle strain

no ↓

Apply Self Care

What Medical Care Can Do

The physician will examine the affected joints for movement and localized swelling or tenderness. He or she may order specific lab tests to distinguish arthritis from other disorders or to differentiate among the types of arthritis. A cervix culture is obtained if gonorrhea is suspected. X-rays can determine the extent of disease and can follow the course of chronic arthritis.

Treatment of arthritis varies depending on the cause, and in the case of severe forms a rheumatologist, or specialist in arthritis, may be consulted. The main drugs used to treat arthritis are called nonsteroidal, anti-inflammatory drugs (NSAIDs). The main one, aspirin, is the "gold standard" against which the other, newer drugs are compared for effectiveness and tolerability. All NSAIDs can relieve pain (and are especially effective at controlling menstrual pain) at low dosages, but higher dosages are needed to

achieve the anti-inflammatory effects necessary for treating arthritis. For this reason, side effects are a fairly common problem, especially stomach irritation, which may lead to ulcer formation or intestinal bleeding. For unknown reasons, patients who do not respond to one NSAID may have excellent results with another product. Some NSAIDs that have been available for several years are Clinoril, Motrin, Nalfon, Naprosyn, and Tolectin. More recently approved NSAIDs include Anaprox DS, Ansaid, Cataflam, Feldene, and Orudis.

When NSAIDs do not control arthritis symptoms, the physician turns to other medications such as corticosteroids (commonly referred to simply as *steroids*). These potent anti-inflammatory drugs are used in treating connective-tissue disorders, but because of the many side effects associated with them, they are rarely used over a long period of time to treat arthritis. Like aspirin and other anti-inflammatory drugs, steroids may cause stomach irritation and peptic ulcer. When these drugs are unsuccessful and in severe cases of rheumatoid arthritis, gold injections or penicillamine, a penicillin derivative, may induce remission of the disease. These drugs, too, have potent side effects and variable effectiveness, so they are tried only if other medications fail.

In addition to drug therapy, lightweight removable splints are sometimes used to decrease inflammation and to keep the joints in the normal use position, protecting them against muscle contractions that might lead to deformity. Various physical modalities may be recommended by a physical therapist to assist in reducing pain associated with arthritis. Surgery is a last resort in the treatment of arthritic conditions. Despite exciting developments in orthopedic surgery allowing hip, elbow, shoulder, and knee replacement, no surgeon can guarantee good results every time.

TMD symptoms are often first evaluated by your dentist. He or she may prescribe short-term pain medication or even out your teeth surfaces to help your problem. You may be referred to an orthodontist or other dental specialist or to a maxillofacial surgeon. A removable plastic mouth guard may be prescribed for nighttime teeth clenchers to keep jaw muscles relaxed during sleep. Magnetic resonance imaging offers a relatively new, safe, but expensive technique for seeing bone detail to diagnose structural defects in the TM joint. You may be referred to a specialist for further tests and treatment. If surgery is being considered, arthroscopic surgery is one of the most conservative approaches and allows removal of adhesions in the TM joint through a tiny incision in the jaw.

What You Can Do (Self Care)

Aspirin is the most effective and least costly drug for treatment of arthritis. Inflammation reduction requires larger doses—up to 10 or 15 five-grain tablets per day. Avoid aspirin in pregnancy (see Chapter 31) and in breast-feeding because it increases newborn susceptibility to bleeding. Remember that name brands cost more than generic aspirin. The chance of stomach irritation is reduced by taking aspirin-containing drugs with meals or with a glass of milk. Also worth trying for arthritis self care are the anti-inflammatory drugs containing ibuprofen: Advil, Motrin IB, Nuprin, ketoprofen (Orudis), etc., and naproxen (Aleve). These drugs should not be taken if you are pregnant or nursing a baby, except at the advice of your physician.

Moist heat in the form of hot baths, especially in the morning, is effective as are hot water bottles and heating pads.

A proper balance of rest and exercise is essential. Regular rest is particularly important with rheumatoid arthritis since flare-ups often occur during fatigue. When flare-ups do occur, bed rest is indicated. Exercise can be good or bad depending on the type of arthritis. Since arthritis affects each woman differently, there is no one program suitable for all. The most helpful exercise allows joints to move slowly through their full range of motion with no resistance. Swimming in a heated pool accomplishes this. Isometric exercises for muscles that support or surround the involved joint may be indicated. Avoid exercises or activity which require twisting, bending, jarring, or stooping. Jogging or other strenuous athletics may place strain on the ankle and knee joints. It is important to continue exercises even when pain and stiffness subside. This may prevent an earlier return of symptoms.

No special diet has been shown to relieve arthritic pain in spite of the claims in the numerous books published each year on the subject. It is important to maintain optimum weight (see Chapter 89) so that you avoid excessive stress on weightbearing joints.

Beware of miracle drugs, vitamins, and hormones promising to cure arthritis. These miracle remedies and others, such as copper bracelets, achieve nothing and will only drain you financially. Any "cure" is due to a period of remission which would occur naturally anyway during the course of arthritis. Many times unproven "cures" are promoted as panaceas for all types of arthritis despite the fact that arthritis is caused by many different diseases requiring varying kinds of therapy. Although most of these so-called remedies will not harm you, some are unsafe and may lead you to delay proper treatment until irreversible joint damage has occurred. Despite the benefits and availability of self-care measures, see your doctor promptly when arthritis symptoms develop.

Consider obtaining a second opinion if jaw-repositioning appliances, orthodontics, or surgery are being considered as treatments for TMD. Avoid chewing hard foods as well as chewing gum or ice, or cradling a phone receiver on one shoulder. Consider physical ther- apy, biofeedback, or relaxation therapy to re- duce emotional stress, if present, before turning to more radical and expensive methods to treat TMD.

CHAPTER 74

Leg Aches and Pains

In the nonpregnant woman, leg aches and pains are likely to be related to strenuous exercise, varicose veins, or low back problems. Daily exercise, such as jogging, may lead to aching in both calves as a result of muscle strain. When a person stands for a prolonged period of time, poor circulation in blood vessels returning blood to the heart from the lower extremities (a condition resulting from varicose veins) may cause leg aches or cramps. A tendency toward varicose veins is largely inherited. Varicose veins, which afflict women far more frequently than men, may predispose one to blood clots in the leg (thrombophlebitis) but, unless severe, are not usually considered a contraindication to the use of birth control pills. Low back pain may be associated with pain down the backs of both legs (see Chapter 51). In the postmenopausal woman early signs of diminished circulation to the lower legs may include calf pain brought on by walking and relieved by rest.

During pregnancy, leg cramps may result from varicose veins or from mineral problems—usually a deficiency of calcium or an excess of dietary phosphorus. Since high levels of phosphorus are found in meat, cheese, and milk, increasing the intake of these foods does not prevent and may even worsen this symptom. Leg cramps may occur while the woman is lying down and may awaken her from sleep, particularly after the first three months of pregnancy.

Varicose veins contribute to leg cramps during pregnancy because this growing uterus may affect blood circulation to and from the legs. Varicose veins tend to become worse as pregnancy progresses and may involve the vulva, producing an aching sensation. Severe varicosities afflict fewer than 20% of pregnant women and subside promptly following delivery. With subsequent pregnancies, varicose veins tend to become more severe and produce symptoms earlier.

What Medical Care Can Do

The clinician will examine your legs for signs of inflammation, range of motion, and the presence of varicose veins. X-rays may be necessary to rule out a fracture if trauma has occurred. Often the problem is one of muscle strain, and muscle relaxants or narcotic pain medication may be prescribed. They should be used sparingly and are best avoided completely in pregnancy. Varicose veins may be evaluated by doppler ultrasound, a technique using sound waves to measure blood flow. In nonpregnant women, severe varicose veins may require surgery (often by a procedure called *vein stripping*), while spider veins and smaller varicosities can be treated with superficial laser therapy or with sclerotherapy. With sclerotherapy, the more widely used technique, the physician uses very small needles to inject small veins with a chemical solution. The technique can remove symptoms and improve leg appearance in appropriately selected patients with varicose veins. Compression hose (available over the counter or sometimes prescribed individually) are recommended before and after surgery or sclerotherapy.

What You Can Do (Self Care)

In nonpregnant women, acute muscle pains tend to be temporary, mild, and often related to muscle strain. These conditions are self-curing with time, rest, heat, and drugstore analgesics. Liniments containing methylsalicylate may provide some relief from muscle spasm.

Both pregnant and nonpregnant women with varicosities may benefit from the use of elastic stockings, frequent elevation of the legs, and avoidance of prolonged sitting or standing.

During pregnancy, the application of heat and massage and a diet which moderately restricts high-phosphorus foods may help leg cramps. If leg cramping persists, ask your doctor to prescribe calcium lactate, 600 milligrams, taken three times a day before meals. If necessary, you might ask your physician about the special support devised for pregnant women with severe vulvar varicosities.

LEG ACHES AND PAINS

Problem   Action   Possible Cause

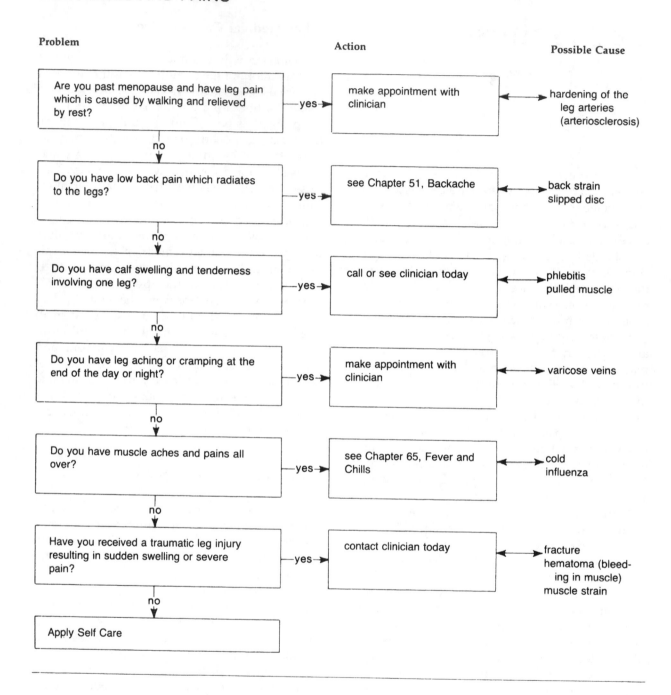

Problem	Action	Possible Cause
Are you past menopause and have leg pain which is caused by walking and relieved by rest? —yes→	make appointment with clinician	← hardening of the leg arteries (arteriosclerosis)
↓ no		
Do you have low back pain which radiates to the legs? —yes→	see Chapter 51, Backache	← back strain slipped disc
↓ no		
Do you have calf swelling and tenderness involving one leg? —yes→	call or see clinician today	← phlebitis pulled muscle
↓ no		
Do you have leg aching or cramping at the end of the day or night? —yes→	make appointment with clinician	← varicose veins
↓ no		
Do you have muscle aches and pains all over? —yes→	see Chapter 65, Fever and Chills	← cold influenza
↓ no		
Have you received a traumatic leg injury resulting in sudden swelling or severe pain? —yes→	contact clinician today	← fracture hematoma (bleeding in muscle) muscle strain
↓ no		
Apply Self Care		

CHAPTER 75

Lethargy

All of us feel lethargic now and then. Most of the time, a little sleep or a little less stress will clear up this fatigue. If it doesn't go away, you may want to consider other causes. Persistent lethargy without apparent symptoms is often due, for example, to depression. Look for these symptoms that suggest depression: decreased ability to concentrate, morning fatigue or headache, loss of appetite, decreased sex drive, and insomnia.

Lethargy may also be a sign of numerous underlying conditions, from the common cold to cancer. Chronic diseases such as arthritis, ulcerative colitis, diabetes, and hypothyroidism (low thyroid) may be associated with lethargy. In a woman of childbearing age, lethargy may be an early symptom of pregnancy. Lethargy associated with fever, sore throat, and tender, swollen lymph nodes may be due to viral infections such as mononucleosis, Epstein-Barr virus (EBV), or infection from the HIV virus that causes AIDS. Blood tests can distinguish among these three conditions. HIV testing should be considered in any woman with risk factors for AIDS (see Chapter 24).

EBV infection has recently been found to be associated with chronic fatigue and lethargy lasting for six months or more and may be associated with swollen lymph glands, muscle weakness, joint pain, and insomnia. For unknown reasons, EBV is twice as common in women as in men. It now appears to be a leading cause of chronic fatigue and debility in some women who were formerly diagnosed as having depression. You should see your doctor if lethargy becomes a chronic symptom, especially if associated with persistent cough, unintended weight loss, persistent pelvic pain, or a change in bowel habits.

In women, two major causes of lethargy are hypoglycemia and anemia. You are probably familiar with hypoglycemia, or low blood sugar, because this condition has been extensively covered in the press in recent years. Hypoglycemia is frequently confused with anxiety or depression since all of these conditions may produce fatigue, headache, mental sluggishness, and an inability to concentrate, as well as palpitations, sweating, hunger, and tremor. Often hypoglycemia afflicts women with premenstrual syndrome (see Chapter 32). In early pregnancy, many women tend to get hypoglycemia as a result of the frequency of nausea and vomiting and because the fetus selectively uses maternal carbohydrates for nutrition and growth at this time.

Anemia resulting from iron deficiency is probably the most frequent medical condition causing fatigue or lethargy in women. This is due usually either to heavy periods or to bleeding somewhere in the digestive tract. In women beyond the menopause, severe iron-deficiency anemia is likely to be due to stomach ulcers or an intestinal tumor.

Iron-deficiency anemia may go unnoticed when it is mild or occurs gradually over several weeks or months. Chronic blood loss results in compensatory adjustments in the body's circulation as well as in increased production of blood cells so that symptoms of lethargy and weakness are minimal. For this reason, your blood count should be checked at least once a year, especially if you are over forty. A hemoglobin of less than 11 grams would be considered moderate anemia.

Iron-deficiency anemia affects well over half of all pregnancies. It is more common in women who have had more than one baby, especially when the pregnancies have been closely spaced. This deficiency happens because the build-up of maternal iron stores following childbirth takes several months. The amount of dietary iron which can be absorbed from the stomach is limited, averaging only about 20% of the ingested amount. During pregnancy, there are increased iron needs. The need for supplemental iron is greatest during the second half of pregnancy and continues through lactation in women who breast-feed.

Sickle-cell anemia (see glossary) tends to become much more severe during pregnancy and predisposes the woman with sickle-cell disease to crisis as well as to increased rates of miscarriage, stillbirth, and premature labor.

LETHARGY

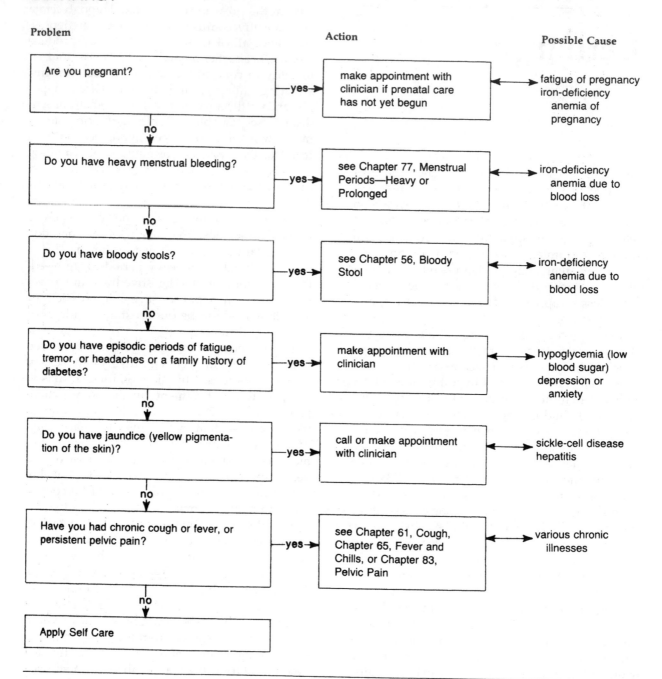

Problem | Action | Possible Cause

Are you pregnant? —yes→ make appointment with clinician if prenatal care has not yet begun ←→ fatigue of pregnancy iron-deficiency anemia of pregnancy

no ↓

Do you have heavy menstrual bleeding? —yes→ see Chapter 77, Menstrual Periods—Heavy or Prolonged ←→ iron-deficiency anemia due to blood loss

no ↓

Do you have bloody stools? —yes→ see Chapter 56, Bloody Stool ←→ iron-deficiency anemia due to blood loss

no ↓

Do you have episodic periods of fatigue, tremor, or headaches or a family history of diabetes? —yes→ make appointment with clinician ←→ hypoglycemia (low blood sugar) depression or anxiety

no ↓

Do you have jaundice (yellow pigmentation of the skin)? —yes→ call or make appointment with clinician ←→ sickle-cell disease hepatitis

no ↓

Have you had chronic cough or fever, or persistent pelvic pain? —yes→ see Chapter 61, Cough, Chapter 65, Fever and Chills, or Chapter 83, Pelvic Pain ←→ various chronic illnesses

no ↓

Apply Self Care

What Medical Care Can Do

Low thyroid conditions, mononucleosis, and other viral conditions are diagnosed by simple blood tests. When you have the symptom of lethargy and no other symptoms, your doctor's evaluation will often concentrate on ruling out hypoglycemia and anemia. With hypoglycemia,

a glucose tolerance test (see glossary) is needed for diagnosis. Anemia is initially evaluated by a complete blood count, including an evaluation of how the blood cells appear under the microscope. With iron-deficiency anemia, the cells are smaller and paler than normal. A blood test for the iron level is the most accurate method of diagnosing this form of anemia. If you have a very low blood count, further tests to evaluate causes of chronic blood loss may require a stool specimen, to test for internal bleeding, and X-rays of the upper and lower intestines (upper GI series and barium enema—see glossary). If the cause of anemia cannot be determined, you may be referred to a hematologist, a specialist in the blood. Usually the cause of anemia is iron deficiency, which is readily treated with iron over several weeks or months (see Chapter 48).

If elective surgery is planned, postpone it until your blood count rises to normal. Transfusions of blood for iron deficiency should not be done to "prepare" you for elective surgery because of the risk of blood transfusions, including hepatitis and transfusion reactions.

What You Can Do (Self Care)

Since working long hours, lack of sleep, or emotional factors play a major part in causing lethargy, look into your own life style to see if you can reduce some of the stress (see Chapter 47).

When possible, minimize the use of sedating drugs, particularly tranquilizers, sleeping pills, and alcohol, all of which are a potential cause of daytime drowsiness. When you have a checkup, make sure you know if your blood count is normal or low. If your hemoglobin (see glossary under complete blood count) is 11 grams or higher, it is most unlikely that your symptoms are due to anemia. If your hemoglobin is below 11 grams, iron-deficiency anemia is probably contributing to your symptoms. This condition can be corrected by simply taking over-the-counter iron preparations such as ferrous sulfate three times a day for three months or more.

Hypoglycemia is sometimes incorrectly diagnosed. If you have a family history of diabetes or if symptoms of hypoglycemia keep recurring, a glucose tolerance test would be advisable. Women with premenstrual syndrome may benefit by avoiding an excess dietary intake of sugar, since sweets may precipitate hypoglycemia, especially during the week before menses.

If you have risk factors for AIDS, consider talking to your doctor about having a blood test for this condition (see Chapter 24).

CHAPTER 76

Memory Loss

Memory is the ability to recall or retain past events. It is critical to the learning of anything new. Memory capacity first interested psychologists in the early 1880s. Currently, there is no one universally accepted model of memory that explains how memory develops, functions, and is altered by the result of trauma, disability, or old age. Our memories can be very general or very detailed. Specific incidences of memory recall include a variety of sensory experiences—touch, smell, sound, a visual picture—as well as the emotional aspects felt while experiencing an event. Obviously, there is a powerful link between emotions and memory. We seem to remember best those events that have an emotional impact on us, like past holidays, unless they are too upsetting, in which case we repress, or subconsciously forget the experience.

Many of the things we do automatically every day, such as driving a car or writing a sentence, involve memory. Memory affects how we perform simple motor activities as well as complicated intellectual tasks. At times we cannot recall how we learned such information, but this knowledge guides our performance in tasks such as taking our daily route to work or cooking a meal without a recipe. Any change in our memory functioning is frightening because we are so dependent on it. Our sense of identity depends on a normal functioning memory. Each of us also has her own unique way of "committing items to memory"—some of us use instant pictures, others use auditory messages, and some use symbols.

Memory ability gradually increases from birth to age thirty, when a gradual decline begins. Most of us will experience a slow loss of memory, with greater recall of past events than current events in old age. In general, it is felt that aging does diminish cognitive functioning and thus memory ability as well. About 5% of older people suffer from severe mental impairment and about 5% from milder impairment. It appears we remember most what we have "practiced most." In other words, automatic habits, such as brushing your teeth, and other daily routines are behaviors that tend to be remembered.

A new entry in the *DSM-IV* (*Diagnostic and Statistical Manual of Mental Disorders*) identifies a decline in cognitive functioning consequent to the aging process that is within normal limits. Individuals with this condition may report problems remembering names or may experience difficulty in solving complex problems.

Anxiety can affect attention, and this commonly influences your memory. When you fear that you can't remember something, you waste time and energy worrying about it instead of concentrating on how to capture the memory. Motivation also influences attention. If you are sincerely interested in remembering something, you are more likely to focus on it and thus retain it.

Depression can affect loss of memory. Depressed adults are often internally focused and do not pay as much attention to outside events; thus, they do not recall them as well. Severe depression can cause memory loss and mental confusion, although memory tends to increase after depression is treated.

The loss of memory and reasoning capacity in adults is called dementia. Common forms include organic brain syndrome, senility, Alzheimer's disease, senile dementia, and presenile dementia. If a psychiatric disorder such as depression or schizophrenia mimics symptoms suggestive of dementia, it is called a pseudo-dementia.

Two major conditions result in mental confusion, memory loss, and intellectual impairment: delirium and dementia. Delirium usually occurs in persons with some underlying medical illness. Common symptoms include drowsiness, confusion, and forgetfulness. Delirium can be caused by illnesses, such as pneumonia, kidney failure, or chronic alcoholism, or by drug reactions. It can be reversed by correcting the underlying medical cause. Dementia occurs in otherwise alert individuals. Its primary characteristics include memory loss and a disturbance in other thinking processes that cause impairment in occupational or social functioning.

Alzheimer's disease (AD) is one of the most frequent causes of irreversible dementia in

MEMORY LOSS

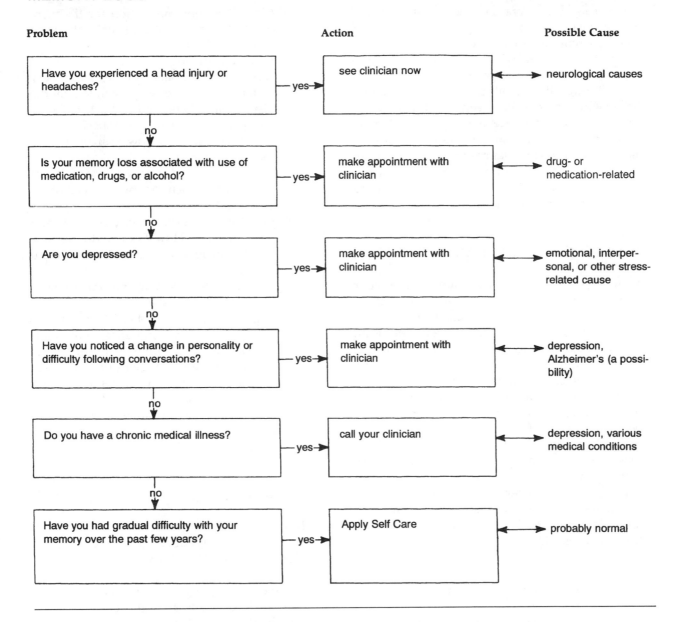

Problem	Action	Possible Cause
Have you experienced a head injury or headaches?	—yes→ see clinician now	← neurological causes
↓ no		
Is your memory loss associated with use of medication, drugs, or alcohol?	—yes→ make appointment with clinician	← drug- or medication-related
↓ no		
Are you depressed?	—yes→ make appointment with clinician	← emotional, interpersonal, or other stress-related cause
↓ no		
Have you noticed a change in personality or difficulty following conversations?	—yes→ make appointment with clinician	← depression, Alzheimer's (a possibility)
↓ no		
Do you have a chronic medical illness?	—yes→ call your clinician	← depression, various medical conditions
↓ no		
Have you had gradual difficulty with your memory over the past few years?	—yes→ Apply Self Care	← probably normal

adults; intellectual impairment progresses gradually from forgetfulness to complete disability. Structural changes are visible in the brain in autopsies of sufferers of Alzheimer's, and it is felt to be an organic process.

Memory impairment has many manifestations during the course of AD. Memory loss becomes pervasive and far more disabling than just misplacing the car keys. Present memory, even information experienced within the last hour, is most affected. This impacts daily cir-

cumstances—bills aren't paid, appointments are missed. As AD progresses, it becomes difficult to remember basic tasks like bringing a shopping list to the grocery store. Eventually the person may develop aphasia (loss of language), apraxia (inability to perform everyday actions), and agnosia (inability to recognize people and objects). Personality characteristics can also be exaggerated; for example, a suspicious person may become paranoid. An estimated 2% to 4% of persons over sixty-five have AD, and the incidence increases with age, affecting about 20% of people over age eighty.

The role of hormones, including estrogen and testosterone, in memory has been the subject of some current research. One recent study indicates that women who had taken estrogen-replacement therapy were less likely to develop AD, although this result is far from fully established. Other studies have suggested that the onset of AD might be delayed or prevented by long-term use of anti-inflammatory drugs such as aspirin, Motrin, Naprosyn, and corticosteroids. There have been no environmental causes reliably linked to AD, although some studies suggest that serious head injury raises the risk.

What Medical Care Can Do

Your physician needs to ascertain whether your loss of memory is due to a medical condition, such as stroke and anemia, and to try to treat the underlying cause. You and your physician may find the cause to be environmental (climatic changes from a move), emotional (depression), or developmental (aging). Often your physician may refer you to a neurologist, psychiatrist, or mental health counselor for further evaluation if he or she cannot find a medical reason. When medical causes are determined, your physician may use appropriate procedures or medications (such as antidepressants). A CAT scan or MRI may be done. In general, the focus of treatment is the specific suspected cause of the memory loss. Research continues to seek an effective treatment for AD.

What You Can Do (Self Care)

1. Set the expectation that you will remember the memory task.

2. Reduce environmental distractions like TV.
3. Maximize your motivation for the memory task. Find a way to make the event meaningful for you.
4. Focus on the event.
5. Examine the demands of the memory task in terms of its sensory channels (audio, visual, kinesthetic or touch). What sense will you use to help remember?
6. Rehearse (practice) how you plan to remember the task.
7. Organize the information into a logical framework (such as by association or grouping).
8. Monitor your performance of the memorized material. How did you do? You can develop insight into your most successful strategies.
9. Frequent use of review and practice helps develop memory skills.
10. Organize yourself to help develop your memory. Use lists and sticky note pads. Set aside a box for immediate tasks (bills) and another for later tasks (letters). Use a bulletin board to leave notes for yourself or others. Reserve a special spot where you always put your purse, keys, or briefcase.

Resources

Alzheimer's Association
919 N. Michigan Avenue, Suite 1000
Chicago, Illinois 60611-1676

The American Health Assistance Foundation
15825 Shady Grove Road, Suite 140
Rockville, Maryland 20850
800-437-2423

CHAPTER 77

Menstrual Periods— Prolonged, Frequent, or Irregular

Normally a woman loses up to four tablespoons of blood during a menstrual period. Sometimes when menstrual flow is a little heavier than usual, the blood will clot. The fact that your blood clots does not necessarily mean that anything is wrong; in fact, it indicates your blood-clotting system is working as it should. Bleeding for more than seven days is considered excessive. Excessive menstrual bleeding is usually produced by conditions that interfere with the uterine mechanism for limiting menstrual blood loss. Benign uterine tumors located within the uterine wall (adenomyosis) or within the uterine cavity (fibroids or polyps) are among the most common causes of heavy periods. These conditions may also cause bleeding between periods. Hormone imbalances, ovary infections, or cancer of the uterus rarely cause heavy periods and are more likely to show up as continuous or irregular on and off spotting. Among nongynecologic causes of heavy periods are hypothyroidism (low thyroid) and abnormalities in blood clotting, such as thrombocytopenia (low platelets). The most common inherited bleeding disorder is called Von Willebrand's disease. This condition, which may cause heavy bleeding at the time of menstruation, as well as bleeding gums or frequent nose bleeds, affects up to 1% of the population.

Regular menstrual cycles depend on a delicate hormonal balance, which may be affected by physical or emotional factors. Most women do not have perfectly regular cycles that are timed like clockwork and always start on the same day of the month. In fact, frequent or irregular menses is the natural state of events at two times during a woman's life—during adolescence and for several years before menopause. During these times, production of the ovarian hormones, estrogen and progesterone, is slightly uneven; estrogen is produced in slightly greater amounts than progesterone. In the adolescent this condition exists because estrogen is the only hormone produced until the ovary matures and secretes progesterone. Menstrual periods may be very irregular and heavy for many months until this normal imbalance corrects itself. In the older woman approaching menopause, the opposite happens. The aging ovary stops producing progesterone first, which results in a relative excess of estrogen that may cause irregular bleeding. Many other temporarily abnormal patterns are associated with stressful events, such as moving to an unfamiliar city, starting a new job, or experiencing serious personal or family problems.

Women taking birth control pills tend to have very regular cycles. Most other women will start their period on a different day of the month each cycle. Some women normally have a period every three weeks; for others, every five weeks is the rule.

Irregular menses may take many forms. Some women experience spotting for several days just before a period. Others notice scant bleeding midway between periods as a result of the normal hormonal changes associated with ovulation. Daily spotting that comes and goes is one of the most common bleeding patterns causing women to consult a gynecologist. Although physical causes such as tumors, infections, and pregnancy must be ruled out, the most common cause of this bleeding pattern is hormone imbalance.

What Medical Care Can Do

In patients with heavy menstrual periods, the clinician may order blood tests to screen for thyroid disease or to check your clotting system. She or he will do a pelvic exam to search for uterine infection, polyps, fibroids, or cancer. If you are premenopausal and your uterus is enlarged, the doctor will order a pregnancy test,

Problem   **Action**   **Possible Cause**

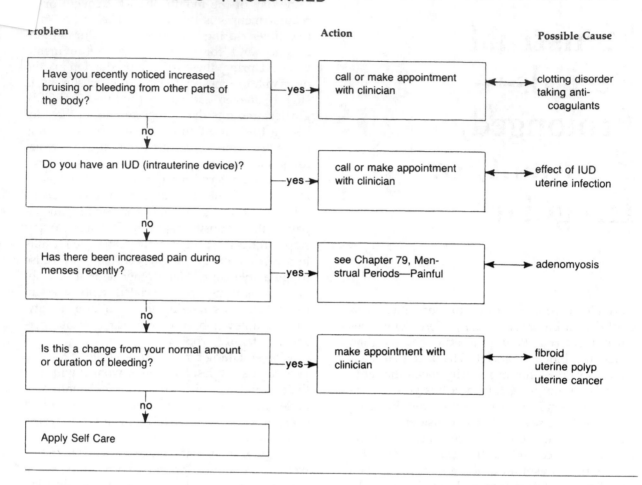

Problem	Action	Possible Cause
Have you recently noticed increased bruising or bleeding from other parts of the body? →yes→	call or make appointment with clinician ←	clotting disorder taking anti-coagulants
↓no		
Do you have an IUD (intrauterine device)? →yes→	call or make appointment with clinician ←	effect of IUD uterine infection
↓no		
Has there been increased pain during menses recently? →yes→	see Chapter 79, Menstrual Periods—Painful ←	adenomyosis
↓no		
Is this a change from your normal amount or duration of bleeding? →yes→	make appointment with clinician ←	fibroid uterine polyp uterine cancer
↓no		
Apply Self Care		

even when your periods are regular. If your blood count indicates anemia and your uterus is enlarged, an endometrial biopsy, a D & C, or a hysteroscopy may be done to establish a definite diagnosis (see Chapter 42). Persistent heavy periods for which no apparent cause is found even after a D & C may cause severe anemia. Often the use of nonsteroidal, anti-inflammatory drugs (see Chapters 79 and 83), such as Anaprox and Ponstel, will cut down on the amount of bleeding as well as reduce menstrual pain. Some women may elect to have a hysterectomy as a definitive treatment for this problem depending upon its severity, their desire for future childbearing, and the degree of debilitation and inconvenience involved.

In patients with irregular menses, a blood pregnancy test may be ordered to diagnose an early pregnancy. A blood count is done to assess the severity of your irregular bleeding. The pelvic examination may reveal the presence of uterine tumors such as polyps or fibroids. In addition to a Pap test, an endometrial biopsy (see Chapter 40) may be performed in any woman over the age of forty with mid-cycle spotting, prolonged periods, or irregular spotting in order to diagnose tumors within the uterus that cannot be felt by examination. Special tests to measure hormone levels are rarely needed unless other problems such as hair growth, excessive weight gain, or breast discharge occur (see Chapters 66, 89, and 57, respectively).

The simplest treatment for irregular periods in a woman who needs contraception is birth control pills. For the woman not needing contraception, a few days of progesterone pills (such as Provera) each month will usually regulate the cycle. Because of rare hazardous fetal effects,

MENSTRUAL PERIODS—FREQUENT OR IRREGULAR

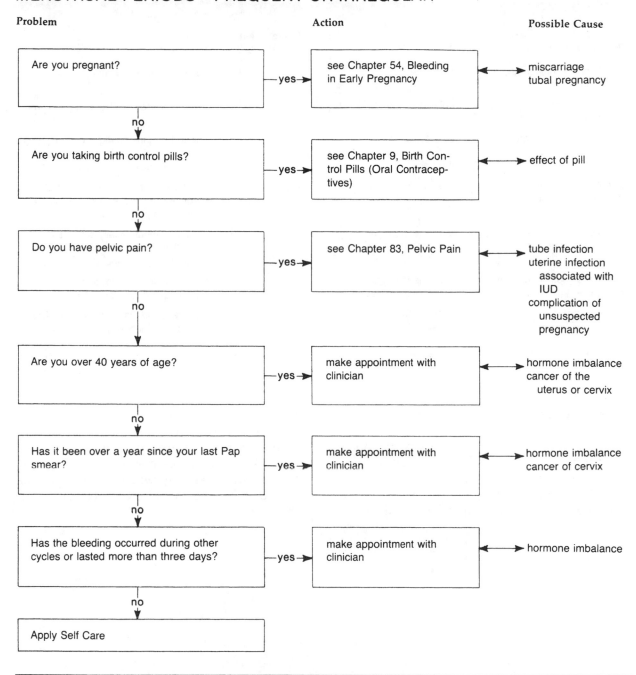

Problem	Action	Possible Cause
Are you pregnant? —yes→	see Chapter 54, Bleeding in Early Pregnancy	miscarriage tubal pregnancy
↓ no		
Are you taking birth control pills? —yes→	see Chapter 9, Birth Control Pills (Oral Contraceptives)	effect of pill
↓ no		
Do you have pelvic pain? —yes→	see Chapter 83, Pelvic Pain	tube infection uterine infection associated with IUD complication of unsuspected pregnancy
↓ no		
Are you over 40 years of age? —yes→	make appointment with clinician	hormone imbalance cancer of the uterus or cervix
↓ no		
Has it been over a year since your last Pap smear? —yes→	make appointment with clinician	hormone imbalance cancer of cervix
↓ no		
Has the bleeding occurred during other cycles or lasted more than three days? —yes→	make appointment with clinician	hormone imbalance
↓ no		
Apply Self Care		

these pills should not be used unless pregnancy has been ruled out. Progesterone therapy, which works best in women with minor degrees of hormone imbalance, is intended to bring on a so-called withdrawal period starting two to seven days after the last progesterone pill, so don't be alarmed by this second period. When uncontrolled by hormone therapy, unscheduled bleeding lasting more than a few days or occurring in two or more cycles requires further investigation, usually an endometrial biopsy or D & C with hysteroscopy (see Chapter 42) to rule out the possibility of uterine cancer.

Table 108   MENSTRUAL CYCLE IRREGULARITIES

Bleeding Pattern	Medical Name	Is Treatment Indicated?	Comment
periods start on different day each month	(normal)	no	some variation is normal
periods occur regularly every three weeks	polymenorrhea	no	unless this pattern is a change for you
spotting midway between periods for one day	ovulatory bleeding ("mittelschmerz" refers to the pain)	no	due to hormone changes during ovulation and sometimes accompanied by a sharp pain
light bleeding for several days before a period	premenstrual spotting	yes	initial treatment usually consists of progesterone (tablets) after ruling out tumors and pregnancy
continuous spotting for over a week (under age forty)	menometrorrhagia or "anovulatory bleeding"	yes	initial treatment usually consists of progesterone (tablets) after ruling out tumors and pregnancy
continuous spotting for over a week (over age forty)	menometrorrhagia or "anovulatory bleeding"	yes	treatment and diagnosis requires endometrial biopsy or D & C
bleeding after the menopause	postmenopausal bleeding	yes	treatment and diagnosis requires D & C or endometrial biopsy

What You Can Do (Self Care)

Lie down or decrease your activity as much as possible. Reduce stress when feasible since this is a major cause of prolonged spotting or irregular bleeding. Take an over-the-counter iron preparation twice daily. A blood count by your physician is the most accurate way to determine your need for iron supplements. If you are taking estrogen, contact your physician. See Chapter 9 on hormonal contraception if you have bleeding while taking the pill. If you have heavy bleeding contact your physician.

CHAPTER 78

Menstrual Periods— Infrequent, Short, or Absent

The interval between menstrual periods normally ranges from 21 to 35 days. Some women normally menstruate no more frequently than every six weeks. As long as your period comes at regular intervals, you need not worry.

Amenorrhea is the term used to describe absent menses and is called *primary amenorrhea* in a woman who has not begun menstruation by age eighteen. Failure to start having periods by age sixteen requires a visit to a gynecologist to make sure there is no abnormality of the reproductive organs. Most women who experience primary amenorrhea are perfectly normal, the problem being just an inherited tendency to begin periods later in life.

The term *secondary amenorrhea* refers to menstrual periods that occur four months or more apart. This condition is much more common than primary amenorrhea. Such delays in menses may occur temporarily because of hormone imbalances related to stressful situations such as emotional problems, crash diets, or marked changes in weight or to the effects of a variety of drugs, including tranquilizers and antidepressants. Women with a condition known as cystic ovaries may have a chronic tendency to have their periods at intervals ranging from every six weeks to every six months. In this form of hormone imbalance, called *polycystic ovary syndrome* (POS), the ovaries cannot regularly secrete the hormones that trigger menstruation. In addition to infrequent periods, POS is associated with in-

fertility (due to irregular ovulation), obesity, and hirsutism (abnormal hair growth).

Women beyond the childbearing years may notice an increased spacing between menstrual periods as a result of declining hormone production. Beginning sometime in the forties, these hormone changes cause shorter, less frequent menstrual periods.

Women who have very little menstrual bleeding are sometimes concerned that they have not had a "good period." In most instances, scant menstrual flow is not abnormal unless it represents an abrupt change from your normal pattern. The amount of bleeding just reflects the thickness of the lining of the uterus that is shed that month. Women with light menses have built up less tissue to shed, so bleeding is less. Short but regular periods do not indicate a health problem or lack of fertility. Women on the pill normally have short periods.

What Medical Care Can Do

In women of childbearing age, the clinician will first rule out pregnancy. Even if there is no evidence of pregnancy during the pelvic examination, he or she will order a pregnancy test for a woman who has not menstruated for many weeks. Blood tests can diagnose pregnancy as early as one week after conception.

The clinician will often order blood tests to measure levels of hormones produced by the pituitary, ovary, and thyroid glands. If this testing shows that hormone imbalance, with or without polycystic ovary syndrome, is the problem, minimum treatment consists of progesterone therapy either by injection or by tablet to bring on a period. The tablet form (synthetic progesterone) should never be taken if you could be pregnant since it may cause birth defects. The pure hormone used in injectable progesterone has not been associated with these defects. In either case, if you are already pregnant, the hormonal medication will not bring on a period.

In most cases of hormone imbalance, progesterone will trigger a period within a week of the last progesterone pill taken. It may be a rather heavy period or just slight spotting, depending on your response. No further treatment is needed except that you should have a period induced at least every four months if you normally have only one or two periods each year. This

MENSTRUAL PERIODS—INFREQUENT, SHORT, OR ABSENT

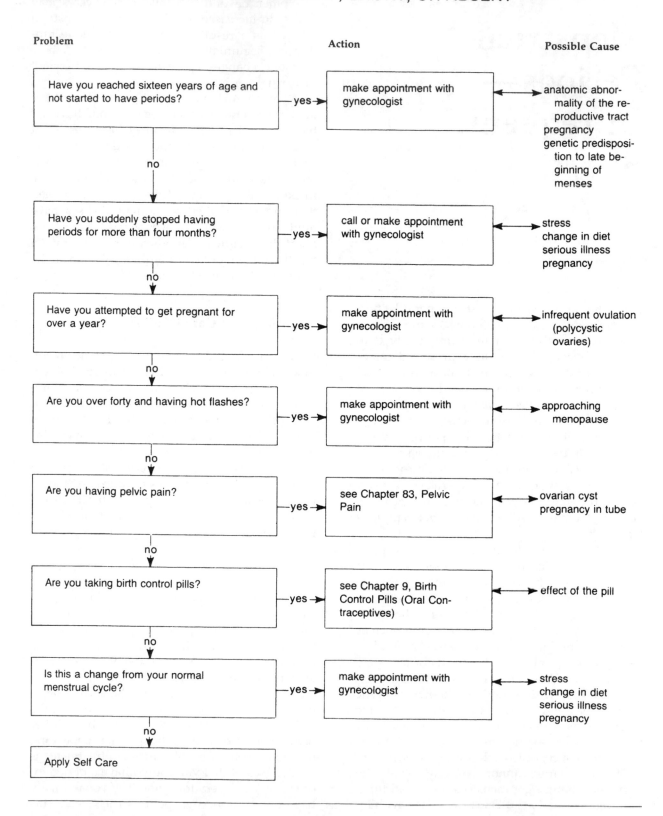

Problem

Have you reached sixteen years of age and not started to have periods?

→ yes → **Action:** make appointment with gynecologist ← **Possible Cause:** anatomic abnormality of the reproductive tract / pregnancy / genetic predisposition to late beginning of menses

↓ no

Have you suddenly stopped having periods for more than four months?

→ yes → call or make appointment with gynecologist ← stress / change in diet / serious illness / pregnancy

↓ no

Have you attempted to get pregnant for over a year?

→ yes → make appointment with gynecologist ← infrequent ovulation (polycystic ovaries)

↓ no

Are you over forty and having hot flashes?

→ yes → make appointment with gynecologist ← approaching menopause

↓ no

Are you having pelvic pain?

→ yes → see Chapter 83, Pelvic Pain ← ovarian cyst / pregnancy in tube

↓ no

Are you taking birth control pills?

→ yes → see Chapter 9, Birth Control Pills (Oral Contraceptives) ← effect of the pill

↓ no

Is this a change from your normal menstrual cycle?

→ yes → make appointment with gynecologist ← stress / change in diet / serious illness / pregnancy

↓ no

Apply Self Care

treatment is recommended because markedly infrequent periods are associated with excessive stimulation of the uterus by estrogen and a slightly greater risk of uterine cancer.

Since failure to ovulate and infertility are sometimes associated with infrequent periods, drugs to stimulate ovulation, such as clomiphene (Clomid), may be given to stimulate ovulation once a period is induced with progesterone. Women with infrequent menses but also desiring contraceptive protection can usually have birth control pills prescribed once a progesterone-induced period begins.

What You Can Do (Self Care)

Infrequent or skipped periods are not uncommon and rarely indicate a serious problem. They may be a warning signal of stress you need to reduce. If you are concerned about possible pregnancy, try free pregnancy screening where available. Urine pregnancy tests, including the drugstore variety, will turn positive starting about fourteen days after conception. If the test is negative, before you take any medications repeat the test in two weeks if there is any possibility of pregnancy.

CHAPTER 79

Menstrual Periods—Painful

Up to 80% of women have some discomfort during their menstrual periods, and painful menstruation (*dysmenorrhea*) is the most common symptom requiring women to take time off from work or school. The discomfort may be experienced as low abdominal cramping or as backache which sometimes radiates to the upper thighs. Menstrual cramps may be accompanied by nausea, vomiting, diarrhea, headache, and irritability. No one knows why pain is particularly severe in some women. Pain thresholds vary from individual to individual and with stressful situations and anxiety.

Although the exact cause of menstrual pain is unknown, hormones called *prostaglandins* probably play an important role. Prostaglandins are found in the menstrual blood and in the uterine wall in increased amounts in women who have painful menses. These hormones cause increased uterine contractions that temporarily cut off the uterine blood supply and produce cramping. Prostaglandins also stimulate the intestines, producing digestive symptoms such as nausea and diarrhea. Another factor contributing to menstrual pain is stretching of the cervix, which occurs when large blood clots are passed.

There are two types of dysmenorrhea, the *primary* form and the *secondary* form. The primary form usually lasts for one or two years and occurs in women who have just begun to menstruate. Hormone imbalance is normal during adolescence, and future fertility is unaffected by this problem. Some spontaneous improvement usually occurs with time, and primary dysmenorrhea subsides almost completely by the late twenties. Childbirth dramatically relieves this form of dysmenorrhea, possibly from stretching of the cervix or from increasing uterine blood supply during pregnancy.

Secondary dysmenorrhea refers to menstrual pain that develops in women who previously had little or no cramping with their periods. This form of dysmenorrhea is much less common than the primary form. It is usually associated with some type of physical abnormality of the reproductive organs, such as benign uterine tumors (polyps, fibroids), pelvic infections, or endometriosis (see Chapter 36). Fibroids or polyps occur inside the uterine cavity and may stimulate forceful uterine contractions in an attempt to expel these tumors during menses. The pain of endometriosis occurs one or two days before the onset of menstrual bleeding. In contrast, pelvic infections often cause pain after menstrual bleeding has begun. Another common cause of painful periods is the intra-uterine device, especially in women who have never been pregnant. Cramps normally diminish a few cycles after IUD insertion, but if menstrual pain persists, removal of the IUD may be necessary.

Although pain anywhere in the body may have a psychological component, physicians have tended to view dysmenorrhea as a psychosomatic illness more often than other painful conditions. But it is now known that painful periods are most often not psychosomatic but are based on physical factors.

What Medical Care Can Do

The treatment of painful menstrual periods depends on the findings during the pelvic exam. If the exam is normal, the woman's pain is usually due to physiological—i.e., normal—dysmenorrhea. In the past, dysmenorrhea was treated with aspirin, or if necessary, with narcotics like codeine. More recently, a group of drugs known medically as nonsteroidal, anti-inflammatory drugs (NSAIDs) have been used increasingly to relieve menstrual pain. Examples of NSAIDs include the prescription drugs Anaprox, Daypro, Motrin, and Naprosyn, as well as a number of similar, less potent, over-the-counter drugs (see below). These drugs all work the same way— they reduce cramps by lowering prostaglandin levels within the uterus. For women desiring contraception, the pill is helpful in relieving menstrual pain while also providing the most effective method of birth control available.

In patients whose pain is unrelieved by medical measures, a procedure called laparoscopy (see glossary) may be performed to check for

MENSTRUAL PERIODS—PAINFUL

Problem	Action	Possible Cause

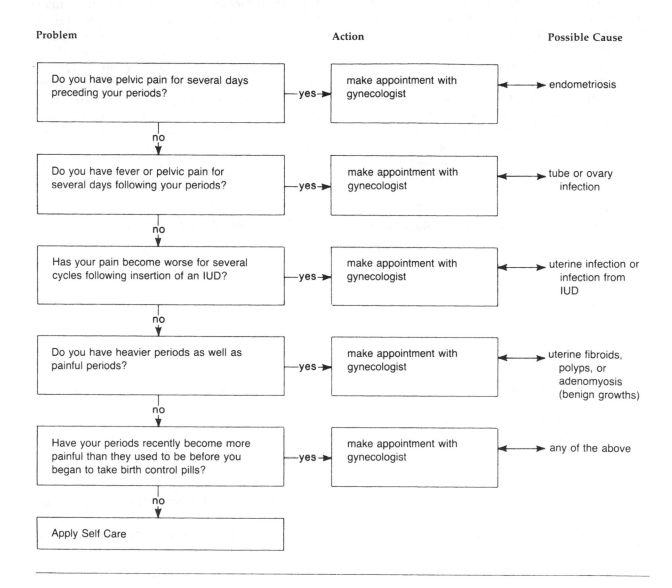

Do you have pelvic pain for several days preceding your periods?
—yes→ make appointment with gynecologist ← → endometriosis

no ↓

Do you have fever or pelvic pain for several days following your periods?
—yes→ make appointment with gynecologist ← → tube or ovary infection

no ↓

Has your pain become worse for several cycles following insertion of an IUD?
—yes→ make appointment with gynecologist ← → uterine infection or infection from IUD

no ↓

Do you have heavier periods as well as painful periods?
—yes→ make appointment with gynecologist ← → uterine fibroids, polyps, or adenomyosis (benign growths)

no ↓

Have your periods recently become more painful than they used to be before you began to take birth control pills?
—yes→ make appointment with gynecologist ← → any of the above

no ↓

Apply Self Care

cysts or endometriosis. Surgery is much more likely to be necessary for the secondary form of dysmenorrhea since it is more commonly associated with physical abnormalities of the reproductive tract.

What You Can Do (Self Care)

The chapter on the female reproductive system (see Chapter 3) will help familiarize you with female anatomy and its functions during the menstrual cycle. Understanding where the pain comes from and how it is produced will help you deal with it. Over-the-counter painkillers include acetaminophen, aspirin, ibuprofen, and naproxen. The latter two are antiprostaglandin drugs (see above) approved for over-the-counter sale by the FDA under various brand names, including Advil, Aleve, Motrin IB, and Nuprin (see also Chapter 51). The antiprostaglandin drugs are indicated for minor aches and pains and especially menstrual cramps since they act in part by reducing uterine contractions. Sexual activity may relieve some of the congestive symptoms that accompany menses. Masters and

Johnson have shown that orgasm, achieved either alone or with a partner, shortly after the onset of menses may reduce pelvic cramping and backache. The use of heat (warm baths, heating pads) and exercise may improve blood flow and decrease pelvic pain. When lying down, keep your legs elevated with a pillow under your knees; or when lying on your side, bring your knees up to your chest. If none of these measures work, request one of the newer anti-inflammatory drugs (see above) from your clinician rather than using narcotics.

In addition to taking physical measures, consider your own feelings toward menstruation. Cultural attitudes convey many negative messages about this natural process. Many women feel uncomfortable, mildly depressed, or unattractive at this time. You can guard against some of the cultural conditioning by simply being aware of it. Do you experience the same feelings with each period? Are there certain triggering factors aside from pain which produce these feelings? Use this opportunity to learn more about your emotional rhythms since this is a time when your level of inner perception and sensitivity is likely to be high.

Table 109 answers some questions you may have about painful periods.

Table 109 QUESTIONS COMMONLY ASKED ABOUT PAINFUL PERIODS

Question	Yes	No	Comment
Does a tilted uterus cause painful menses?		X	A tilted uterus may cause painful menses only if the reason it is tilted is a result of disease, such as endometriosis.
Does hormone imbalance cause painful menses?		X	Painful menses is a sign of fertility and is associated with regular cycles and normal ovulation.
Is alcohol recommended to prevent painful cramps?		X	Alcohol relaxes the uterine muscles only slightly and is of limited benefit.
Is aspirin as good as most other painkillers except narcotics?	X		Because of its prostaglandin-inhibiting properties, aspirin is one of the most effective nonnarcotic analgesics for menstrual cramps.
Are painful periods normal in a woman with normal pelvic findings on examination?	X		Painful periods occur as a result of normal physiologic processes.
Do water pills help?		X	Such pills help primarily with cyclic weight gain and fluid retention.
Do birth control pills usually relieve painful periods?	X		Failure of the pill to relieve painful periods indicates that a physical cause may be present.

CHAPTER 80

Nausea and Vomiting

Although nausea and vomiting may accompany serious disease, these symptoms more often result from minor disorders. Intermittent nausea without vomiting almost never necessitates a visit to your doctor. Persistent vomiting, especially when accompanied by other symptoms such as abdominal pain, does require a physician consultation. Hospitalization may be necessary if vomiting causes excessive fluid loss.

Conditions Causing Nausea and Vomiting

Here is a brief guide to potentially serious conditions that cause nausea and vomiting.

Digestive disorders

Frequently accompanied by abdominal pain, digestive disorders often cause nausea and vomiting. Upper abdominal pain is associated with stomach or intestinal ulcers, gallbladder disorders (cholycystitis), inflammation of the pancreas (pancreatitis), and inflammation of the liver (hepatitis). Lower abdominal pain is associated with appendicitis and intestinal flu (gastroenteritis). Generalized abdominal pain and vomiting may be caused by a ruptured appendix, food poisoning, or blockage of the intestine (bowel obstruction). Among these conditions intestinal flu, a communicable disease spread by a virus, is by far the most frequent and least serious. For more information about digestive causes of nausea and vomiting, refer to Chapter 68, Heartburn and Gas; Chapter 63, Diarrhea; and Chapter 56, Bloody Stool.

Drug reactions

Vomiting is a common side effect of many drugs, particularly the tetracyclines, aspirin, narcotic pain pills, and estrogens, including birth control pills.

Stress

Emotional factors play a role in these symptoms. In some illnesses, such as migraine headaches, it may be difficult to differentiate between physical, psychological, and stress-related factors causing nausea.

Vomiting used to avoid possible weight gain may result in a condition known as *bulimia*, an emotional illness found primarily in teenagers and adult women. In bulimia, periods of binge eating (eating excessive amounts of food at one time) to relieve emotional distress are followed by periods of guilt and remorse about the previous intake of a large amount of food. These feelings are temporarily relieved by self-induced vomiting, excessive exercise, use of laxatives, or a combination of these actions. Treatment involves psychotherapy, control of high-risk situations that stimulate the binge/purge cycle, and acceptance of a realistic weight. Restructuring eating habits and weighing oneself only once a week are stressed. Peer support groups have been found to be very helpful (see Chapter 89).

Pregnancy

Sixty-five percent of pregnant women experience some degree of so-called morning sickness during the first three months of pregnancy. Emotional factors, hormone changes, and a sluggish digestive system may contribute to nausea and vomiting in pregnancy, though the specific cause remains unknown. Although feelings of nausea are most common in the morning, these symptoms may be experienced any time of day. If vomiting is prolonged, dehydration may occur and requires hospitalization.

What Medical Care Can Do

The physician will ask how long you've had nausea and vomiting and how your diet affects the symptoms. Eating fried foods, for example, often brings on a gallbladder attack which gives

NAUSEA AND VOMITING

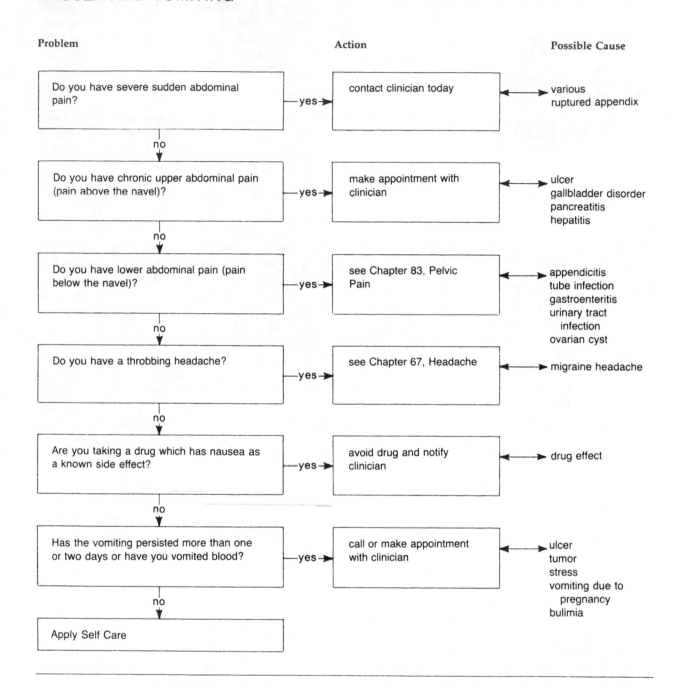

Problem	Action	Possible Cause
Do you have severe sudden abdominal pain? —yes→	contact clinician today	various / ruptured appendix
↓ no		
Do you have chronic upper abdominal pain (pain above the navel)? —yes→	make appointment with clinician	ulcer / gallbladder disorder / pancreatitis / hepatitis
↓ no		
Do you have lower abdominal pain (pain below the navel)? —yes→	see Chapter 83, Pelvic Pain	appendicitis / tube infection / gastroenteritis / urinary tract infection / ovarian cyst
↓ no		
Do you have a throbbing headache? —yes→	see Chapter 67, Headache	migraine headache
↓ no		
Are you taking a drug which has nausea as a known side effect? —yes→	avoid drug and notify clinician	drug effect
↓ no		
Has the vomiting persisted more than one or two days or have you vomited blood? —yes→	call or make appointment with clinician	ulcer / tumor / stress / vomiting due to pregnancy / bulimia
↓ no		
Apply Self Care		

you pain, belching, and nausea. If vomiting is more prominent than abdominal pain, the doctor knows that pregnancy, a drug reaction, food poisoning, or intestinal flu is more likely. Vomiting of blood is an emergency requiring hospitalization and is often due to stomach ulcers (see Chapter 68, Heartburn and Gas).

Your doctor may prescribe antinausea drugs such as Compazine or Phenergan. These drugs come in rectal suppository form, which is preferable if vomiting accompanies nausea. But before taking any medication for morning sickness, especially in the first three months of pregnancy, discuss alternatives (for example, dietary measures) to drug treatment with your doctor.

Bulimia has been variously treated with antidepressant drug therapy, nutritional counseling, stress management, and psychotherapy. Women with this condition usually respond to a lower dose of antidepressant than is used in truly depressed patients.

What You Can Do (Self Care)

During pregnancy, nausea is sometimes relieved by your lying down immediately after meals. Meals should be frequent and small enough to keep your stomach from becoming completely empty or overly stretched out. If morning sickness occurs, try eating plain soda (saltine) crackers or dry toast before you get up. Get up slowly, avoiding sudden movements. Avoid greasy, fried, or spicy foods. Eat whatever appeals to you. It may help to eat only cold foods, or to eat solids and drink liquids an hour apart. Sometimes small amounts of apple juice, grape juice, or noncola carbonated beverages between meals help to lessen nausea. You can take your vitamins and iron after you get through this period of your pregnancy since they may contribute to an upset stomach. Whenever possible, avoid taking drugs, especially in the first three months of pregnancy.

A woman afflicted with or with a tendency toward bulimia may find it helps to keep a diary recording when and what she eats, how often she vomits, and when she uses purgatives or laxatives. This information may help to make her aware that a problem exists or to set targets for gradual reduction in unwanted behavior. Professional counseling is usually recommended.

Nonpregnant women can apply the same dietary recommendations as for pregnant women. In recovering from illness, start nourishment with hot beverages (tea or clear broth) or cold beverages (iced tea, apple juice, cola, or ginger ale). Avoid drugs, such as aspirin, which may cause nausea. If vomiting persists for several days or you vomit blood, call your clinician.

CHAPTER 81

Nervousness and Anxiety

Nervousness is another name for anxiety. Everyone experiences anxiety in one form or another during their daily lives. Chronic anxiety is one of the most common mental health problems in the United States today.

Anxiety is good when it mobilizes the body for action. Controlled anxiety is the force which drives many people to accomplish their life's goals. Anxiety is often the fire behind the drive of creative, successful people. Without that driving force of controlled anxiety, the work of the world would not get done.

Sometimes anxiety may become a problem. When it does, there is usually a remedy readily available to bring it under control. Here are some forms anxiety may take.

Generalized anxiety is often experienced as trembling, jitteriness, or shakiness. Some women report a sensation like feeling their muscles jumping under their skin. Others experience anxiety as a tight band around the head or muscle tension in the limbs. Many people feel knots in their stomachs or backaches. Anxiety may be experienced as a fear or dread, which may be mistaken for depression. The anxious woman cannot relax; she feels tense and has trouble sleeping, eating, indulging in sex, working, and conducting her normal activities. This is mild anxiety.

Some women experience anxiety as a reaction to a drug, such as diet pills (amphetamines) or Reserpine (a drug used to control blood pressure), to caffeine (in coffee, tea, cola, and chocolate), or to an alcoholic drink. Occasionally anxiety signals the onset of a disease, such as hyperthyroidism (overactive thyroid), in which the thyroid gland produces excessive amounts of thyroid hormone. And many women report anxiety as part of premenstrual syndrome (see Chapter 32). Often, when the situation causing the anxiety is corrected or settled, the anxiety will disappear.

When anxiety or panic is felt, regardless of your situation or circumstances, it is called spontaneous anxiety or spontaneous panic depending on the degree of intensity. If anxiety occurs only in specific situations, it is called situational anxiety. Anxiety or panic results from a well-defined perceived threat. A panic attack is an intense state of fear that occurs for no apparent reason. The attack can occur over a period of several minutes or hours and can strike suddenly. Most attacks do not last for more than half an hour. A *panic attack* must include at least four of the following symptoms:

1. Palpitations, pounding heart, or accelerated heart rate.
2. Sweating.
3. Trembling or shaking.
4. Sensations of shortness of breath or smothering.
5. Feeling of choking.
6. Chest pain or discomfort.
7. Nausea or abdominal distress.
8. Feeling dizzy, unsteady, lightheaded, or faint.
9. Derealization (feelings of unreality) or depersonalization (detached from oneself).
10. Fear of losing control or of going crazy.
11. Fear of dying.
12. Paresthesia (numbness or tingling sensations).
13. Chills or hot flashes.

Agoraphobia is anxiety about being in places or situations from which escape might be difficult or embarrassing or in which help may be perceived as unavailable. This anxiety typically leads to an avoidance of situations such as being at a mall, on a bridge, or in an elevator. This anxiety may become so severe that it is difficult to function in one's daily job or routine. Specific phobias result from a persistent fear of specific situations, such as air travel, or of objects, such as dogs or cats.

Obsessive-Compulsive Disorder (OCD) often coexists with depression or with anxiety disorders, including phobias or panic disorders. OCD is characterized by repetitive, persistent thoughts or compulsive ritualistic behaviors, or both. For example, a person with a bacteria phobia might engage in repetitive hand-washing. Obsessions and compulsions may interfere with normal ac-

NERVOUSNESS AND ANXIETY

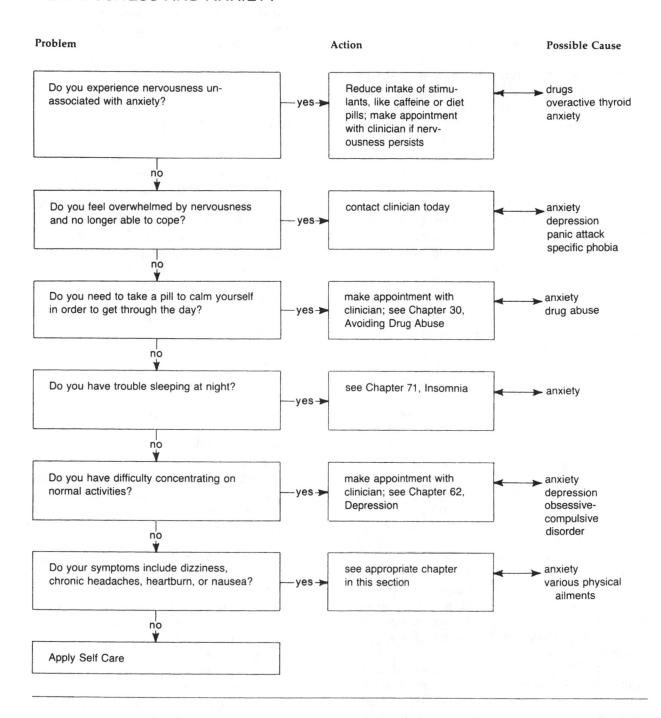

Problem	Action	Possible Cause
Do you experience nervousness unassociated with anxiety? —yes→	Reduce intake of stimulants, like caffeine or diet pills; make appointment with clinician if nervousness persists	drugs overactive thyroid anxiety
↓ no		
Do you feel overwhelmed by nervousness and no longer able to cope? —yes→	contact clinician today	anxiety depression panic attack specific phobia
↓ no		
Do you need to take a pill to calm yourself in order to get through the day? —yes→	make appointment with clinician; see Chapter 30, Avoiding Drug Abuse	anxiety drug abuse
↓ no		
Do you have trouble sleeping at night? —yes→	see Chapter 71, Insomnia	anxiety
↓ no		
Do you have difficulty concentrating on normal activities? —yes→	make appointment with clinician; see Chapter 62, Depression	anxiety depression obsessive-compulsive disorder
↓ no		
Do your symptoms include dizziness, chronic headaches, heartburn, or nausea? —yes→	see appropriate chapter in this section	anxiety various physical ailments
↓ no		
Apply Self Care		

tivities or cause extreme emotional distress or anxiety, especially if the ritualistic thought or behavior cannot be carried out. Adults with this condition usually recognize their obsessions or compulsions as excessive and unreasonable, yet feel compelled to engage in them. Treatment involves counseling, often with behavioral modification and medications. Luvox, a new medication approved in 1995 for treatment of OCD, as well as Prozac and Pamelor have been found to be helpful.

What Medical Care Can Do

If your physician cannot find a medical reason for your anxiety, then it is assumed to be psychological. Your physician and you after discussing your anxiety may discover that it is tied to and caused by a recent situation such as divorce, having to move, or sending a child off to school. Sometimes your physician may prescribe a tranquilizer to be taken over a short period of time and may recommend some short-term counseling. Counseling may involve relaxation techniques such as hypnosis, biofeedback training, meditation; family or group counseling; and, if your physician feels you are physically able, jogging, swimming, or any of the aerobic type exercises (see Chapter 49).

The most commonly prescribed drugs for nervousness and anxiety are tranquilizers belonging to the benzodiazepine group, which include such drugs as Valium, Tranxene, Xanax, Librium, and Ativan. Tranquilizers belonging to this group are considered controlled substances and potentially addictive. For this reason, these drugs should be used only for brief treatment which, preferably, should include some form of counseling. Other anti-anxiety drugs, such as Mellaril and Thorazine, may also be used when anxiety is severe or associated with loss of contact with reality (e.g., hallucinations). One relatively new drug for treating anxiety, Buspar, has the possible advantage of not being a controlled substance with addictive potential.

If you are depressed, standard tranquilizers such as Valium may cause deeper depression. Some people who tend to be chronic worriers or have phobic or obsessive thoughts may be helped by certain antidepressant drugs (see Chapter 62).

Tranquilizers may have pronounced additive effects causing marked sedation when taken at the same time as certain pain pills, alcohol, sleeping pills, or antidepressants. According to a recent study by the Institute of Medicine, some tranquilizers have additional hazards not previously recognized. Because of the long time required for the body's elimination of drugs like tranquilizers, chronic use may cause drug dependency (see Chapter 30). Also, unexpected toxic interactions with alcohol can occur when people take a drug like Valium for sleep and then drink alcoholic beverages the next day without realizing they still have high blood levels of the tranquilizer.

What You Can Do (Self Care)

1. Try to identify the situation which, when you think about it, makes you anxious.
2. Consider actions that would lessen the threat, and try them out (for example, attend childbirth preparation classes to deal with the stress of labor and delivery; eliminate or reduce caffeine intake if nervousness alone is the problem).
3. Avoid potentially dangerous ways of coping with anxiety—smoking, alcohol, drug dependence, overeating, undereating.
4. Express your feelings to someone you trust and can talk with comfortably. This unburdening of feelings often leads to a relief of anxious feelings.
5. Try relaxation techniques or meditation. Both or either often provides relief. Classes in yoga or stress reduction are often available through community programs.
6. If your doctor feels you are physically able to do so, try jogging, swimming, or any of the aerobic type exercises (see Chapter 49).
7. If nervousness regularly precedes menses, try reducing dietary salt to lessen this and other symptoms of premenstrual syndrome.
8. Avoid unnecessary stress—eliminate as many nonessential activities as possible from your daily routine.
9. If your anxiety persists or becomes chronic, seek out a competent mental health professional.
10. You can ask for help from any of the following, as appropriate:
    Community mental health center—most are required to maintain service twenty-four hours a day, seven days a week.

Mental health association—they can refer
   you.
   Health department—they can refer you.

Anxiety Disorders Association of America
6000 Executive Boulevard, Suite 513
Rockville, Maryland 20852

Recovery, Inc.
802 N. Dearborn Street
Chicago, Illinois 60610

CHAPTER 82

Palpitations

Palpitations refer to fluttering sensations in the chest which occur when your heart skips a beat or beats rapidly. Palpitations are usually due to stress, fatigue, emotional factors, or drugs rather than to heart disease. Fear of heart disease may actually cause palpitations to become worse. Although palpitations alone are unlikely to indicate heart disease, you should see your doctor if you experience repeated episodes of palpitations associated with chest pain or shortness of breath. Among the most common causes of palpitations in women are excessive use of alcohol, cigarettes, or caffeine. Diet pills, water pills, decongestants containing ephedrine, and certain antidepressant drugs may cause these symptoms. An overactive thyroid (hyperthyroidism) can also cause palpitations along with weight loss, nervousness, shakiness, and heat intolerance. Palpitations are common in pregnancy and are especially noticeable when you lie down.

A rather common diagnosis today among healthy people in their thirties and forties is *mitral valve prolapse* (MVP). This generally harmless condition, found more frequently in women than in men, may cause palpitations and, occasionally, chest pain, especially during fatigue or stress. MVP is due to a "floppy" heart valve that gives rise to a benign, characteristic heart murmur. Many people with MVP have the murmur but no symptoms. MVP usually does not progress, but antibiotics are recommended as a precaution against heart-valve infection if you have an operation or dental surgery. MVP usually does not require medical treatment, but if palpitations increase in frequency, drugs to regulate heart rhythm, such as Inderal, are prescribed and work well to control symptoms.

What Medical Care Can Do

The clinician will evaluate your pulse for rate and regularity. He or she will examine your thyroid closely and may order thyroid blood tests. If you have chest pain or shortness of breath, the doctor will also obtain an electrocardiogram (EKG) (see glossary) and perhaps a twenty-four-hour Holter monitor, which records the workings of your heart as you participate in your normal daily activities. Or your doctor may choose to evaluate your heart by means of a stress test, which involves recording heart activity with an EKG as you go through increasingly strenuous exercises on a treadmill. The science of stress testing is far from exact, and many stress tests show heartbeat irregularities in perfectly healthy women. Only if palpitations are frequent and associated with symptoms of heart disease will the doctor prescribe drugs to control heart rhythm.

What You Can Do (Self Care)

If you have episodes of rapid heartbeat, try taking your pulse to determine the rate. You can learn to take your own pulse by placing the tips of your fingers across the wrist of the opposite hand on the thumb side to feel for the heartbeat. The normal pulse varies from 60 to 100 beats per minute during rest. If you exercise daily, your normal pulse rate may be less than 60. The two things to note about your pulse are its rate and rhythm. The rate is determined by counting the number of beats during one minute (or you can count for 15 seconds and multiply by four). The rhythm should feel regular. If the rhythm is irregular or if the rate is over 100 after you have rested for five minutes, then you should call your doctor. You should also see your doctor if you take heart pills or are on antiarrhythmic drugs to control heart rate. You can often control uncomplicated palpitations yourself, however, by avoiding stimulants such as caffeine, cigarettes, alcohol, and diet pills. When these episodes occur, sit down or change your activity from something stressful to something you like to do. Get as much sleep as possible, as well as regular exercise. Recurrent episodes warrant a visit to the physician's office if for no other reason than reassurance since most of the time palpitations are not due to heart disease.

PALPITATIONS

Problem	Action	Possible Cause

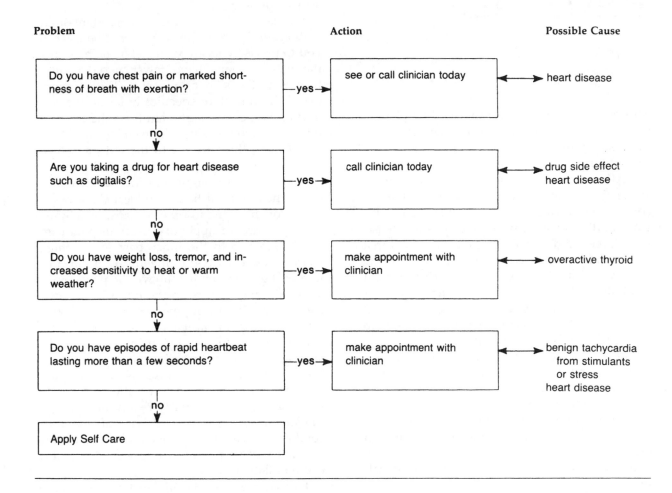

Problem

Do you have chest pain or marked shortness of breath with exertion?

—no→

Are you taking a drug for heart disease such as digitalis?

—no→

Do you have weight loss, tremor, and increased sensitivity to heat or warm weather?

—no→

Do you have episodes of rapid heartbeat lasting more than a few seconds?

—no→

Apply Self Care

Action

—yes→ see or call clinician today

—yes→ call clinician today

—yes→ make appointment with clinician

—yes→ make appointment with clinician

Possible Cause

heart disease

drug side effect
heart disease

overactive thyroid

benign tachycardia
from stimulants
or stress
heart disease

CHAPTER 83

Pelvic Pain

This chapter covers the complicated problem of severe or chronic pelvic pain. The subject is complicated because there are so many abdominal organs that can be the source of this pain. We're not talking about the pain related to your menstrual cycle or to the passing discomfort that accompanies, say, a bout with diarrhea. Rather, we want to discuss some possible causes of intense, unrelieved abdominal discomfort—pain that will definitely require a visit to your physician at some point. Unless you are entering labor, it is unlikely that you will experience severe or chronic pelvic pain. But if you do, it's important that you evaluate your own pain—it may help your physician pinpoint a difficult diagnosis.

Sudden acute pain lasting more than six hours in a previously healthy individual is usually serious. It may require prompt surgical treatment or evaluation by an internist. You may be referred for a consultation with a general surgeon since many causes of low abdominal pain are not due to gynecological disease. Even so, your gynecologist may be the first doctor you see.

When you do see the doctor, he or she will want to know *if the pain started abruptly or gradually* and how it has progressed. Sudden severe pain with little or no vaginal bleeding may accompany a ruptured tubal pregnancy or ovarian cyst. The pain subsides after rupture since the tube or ovary is no longer distended. Most other gynecologic causes of pain start more gradually.

The physician will also ask about *the character of the pain*, since the type of pain gives clues to its cause. Distention (stretching) of organs such as one of the Fallopian tubes (as in a tubal pregnancy) or the uterine cervix (as in a miscarriage) will cause a colicky pain. This kind of pain comes in sharp, intermittent waves during contractions of the muscles of the involved organ. A ruptured ovarian cyst or tubal pregnancy that spills fluid into the pelvic cavity can cause severe, steady pain. Adhesions (see glossary) within or between organs may form after previous abdominal surgery, and they cause a dull ache or pulling pain.

Location of the pain, too, is important information for the clinician. It may not be easy for you to precisely locate your pelvic pain because the pelvic organs have fewer nerve endings than, say, the skin or muscles. The physician may help you more specifically locate the pain during the pelvic exam. Pain from the ovary or tube, for example, is usually well localized to an area two to three inches to the left or right of the midline (an imaginary line extending down from the navel; see Figure 45) and within an inch above the pubic hairline. Pain located above this region often is due to other organs, usually the large intestine or appendix. Ovarian pain commonly radiates to the inner part of the thigh. Uterine pain is located in the lower midline portion of the abdomen just above the pelvic bone. This pain may radiate to the buttocks or lower back, especially during menses. Bladder disease often causes pain similar to uterine pain but is usually accompanied by urinary symptoms, such as a burning sensation when you urinate. Vaginal disease rarely causes abdominal pain. Whether the pain is felt on both sides of the lower abdomen (bilateral) or only on one side (unilateral) is important. Pelvic inflammatory conditions involving the tube and ovary tend to be bilateral. Cysts and tubal pregnancies tend to cause unilateral pain.

Finally, the doctor will need to know *other symptoms that are associated with the pain*. It is helpful to your doctor if you can tell him or her the relationship of your pelvic pain to each of five specific physical events:

1. *Relationship to menses*. If you skipped your last period or you are having unscheduled vaginal bleeding, pregnancy disorders such as miscarriage or ectopic pregnancy (see Chapter 54) are more likely. Pain occurring just before and during menses suggests a common disorder such as endometriosis (see Chapter 36) or adenomyosis (see Chapter 77). Pain beginning a few days after a period starts may be from an inflammatory process since your natural physiologic barrier to infection is temporarily removed at menses.

2. *Relationship to diet and digestion.* The absence of vomiting, diarrhea, or bloody stools tends to exclude the digestive tract as a cause of the pain.
3. *Relationship to bladder function.* The absence of painful urination, bloody urine, and frequent urination tends to exclude disease of the urinary tract and bladder.
4. *Relationship to fever and chills.* The absence of fever and chills rules against the likelihood of serious pelvic inflammatory conditions, such as acute tube infections or ruptured pelvic abscess, as well as other severe, nongynecologic infections.
5. *Relationship to intercourse.* Abdominal pain that increases with intercourse may indicate pelvic inflammatory disease or endometriosis.

Pain during early pregnancy may be associated with any of the causes of pelvic pain previously mentioned. After the first three months of pregnancy, pain is due mostly to pressure produced by the enlarging uterus. Pressure over the pelvic bones causes a variety of pains which may be sharp, dull, or stabbing and may radiate to the legs, hips, or vagina. A particularly common form of pelvic discomfort in late pregnancy is *round ligament pain*, due to stretching of these supporting ligaments found along both sides of the uterus. This type of pain may be more pronounced on one side, sometimes mimicking a kidney stone or appendicitis when severe. However, there are no accompanying symptoms such as fever, vomiting, or bleeding. One of the most serious causes of acute pain in late pregnancy is abruptio placenta (see Chapter 55).

Probably the most common pains in the second half of pregnancy occur as a result of uterine contractions. The differences between real and false labor, both of which may be quite painful, are summarized in Table 111. Knowledge of the signs of labor can be one of the most important aspects of childbirth education, since premature labor and delivery contribute, more than any other factor, to newborn respiratory distress and death during the first month of life. Premature labor (see Chapter 21) usually occurs spontaneously but may also occur following bleeding (abruptio placenta, placenta previa; see Chapter 55) or in association with high blood pressure (toxemia) or premature rupture of the membranes (see Chapter 20).

Acute Lower Abdominal Pain— What Medical Care Can Do

The cause of acute abdominal pain can often be identified from an evaluation of the pain as described above. Diseases of the urinary tract are usually excluded by a urinalysis in the office. The possibility of appendicitis requires hospitalization until the correct diagnosis can be confirmed. A surgical consultation is routine when nongynecologic disease is considered in the diagnosis of acute abdominal pain.

During the physical exam the doctor is concerned with deciding if you need surgery. The abdominal exam is all-important in the diagnosis of appendicitis but gives less information as to the exact source of gynecologic conditions causing pain. The speculum exam is essential in diagnosing miscarriage because tissue is visualized as it is passed through the dilating cervix. The presence of a uterine discharge seen during the speculum exam is consistent with pelvic inflammatory disease but does not prove the diagnosis. When a ruptured ectopic pregnancy is suspected, a culdocentesis (see glossary) is performed to rapidly detect the presence of internal bleeding, a potentially life-threatening situation. In ectopic pregnancy, the bimanual exam may provide little additional information to the gynecologist because severe pain makes relaxation of the abdominal wall impossible.

The common lab tests that evaluate low abdominal pain include: complete blood count (CBC), urinalysis, pregnancy test, cervical culture (transgrow), abdominal and kidney X-rays, and a sonogram.

The treatment of acute pelvic pain will often require surgery unless an infection, such as a tube or an intestinal inflammation, is suspected. In this case, antibiotics are often given while your condition is observed in the hospital.

Among the surgical approaches in treating abdominal pain is dilatation and curettage (D & C) (see Chapter 42), which is the best treatment for a miscarriage. A laparoscopy (see glossary) is done when an ectopic pregnancy or ovarian cyst is suspected. If the diagnosis is mistaken, a laparoscopy may prevent an unnecessary incision and longer surgical recovery time. A laparotomy (see glossary) is usually indicated when the doctor diagnoses internal bleeding, a ruptured pelvic abscess, or some other condition requiring emergency surgery.

Table 110 FINDINGS ASSOCIATED WITH VARIOUS CAUSES OF ACUTE LOWER ABDOMINAL PAIN

Finding	Cause of Acute Lower Abdominal Pain					
	Infection of Tube or Ovary	Miscarriage	Rupture of Tubal Pregnancy or of Ovarian Cyst	Urinary Tract Infection	Appendicitis	Intestinal Inflammation (Colitis, Diverticulitis)
Pain location	Bilateral	Midline	Unilateral	Variable	Variable at first, shifts to lower right side	Variable
Fever	Yes	Sometimes	No	Yes	Yes	Yes
Missed periods	No	Yes	Sometimes	No	No	No
Bleeding	No	Yes	No	No	No	No
Foul vaginal discharge	Yes	No	No	No	No	No
Diarrhea	Sometimes	No	No	No	Sometimes	Yes
Urinary symptoms (burning) and urinalysis shows infection present	No	No	No	Yes	No	No

Table 110 summarizes the findings associated with various causes of acute lower abdominal pain.

Acute Lower Abdominal Pain— What You Can Do (Self Care)

If severe pain persists for several hours, get early medical attention. Do not eat or use an enema as long as the pain is severe. If you are pregnant, learn the signs of labor (see Table 111) and get prompt medical attention if pain is accompanied by bleeding or markedly decreased fetal movement.

Chronic Lower Abdominal Pain— What Medical Care Can Do

Chronic pelvic pain—pain lasting six months or more—may be hard to diagnose and cause a great deal of worry. Usually, the cause isn't anything life-threatening, but it may very well threaten a woman's fertility or take time away from work, and consequently be a source of great frustration. Chronic pain is the major reason cited for one out of every eight hysterectomies performed in the United States today. Women with this symptom tend to be in their thirties or forties and many have seen more than one physician or pain clinic while seeking a correct diagnosis or cure.

The approach to treating chronic pelvic pain begins with a detailed history and careful physical examination that attempts to pinpoint the pain's exact location and determine the cause. If an immediate diagnosis can be made, medical treatment by the gynecologist may include hormones, antibiotics, vaginal creams, and pain medication. The pain may be due to a nongynecological cause requiring referral to a specialist such as a urologist, an internist, or an orthopedic surgeon. Emotional stress and distress are often associated with chronic pelvic pain. Depression, insomnia, and sexual problems (such as loss of desire) all may complicate this symptom, either as a cause or as a result of it. For this reason, some women who have experienced pelvic discomfort for months at a time find it useful to work with a psychologist or other counseling professional. Biofeedback, self-hypnosis, and stress management may also help.

In patients who fail to respond to initial medical therapy, further evaluation may be accomplished by diagnostic laparoscopy, a procedure that allows the doctor to see all the pelvic organs as well as the appendix and upper abdomen (see Chapter 13). Your gynecologist may videotape this procedure and show it to you later. Visualizing the cause of pelvic pain is sometimes helpful, although in 25% of cases, the laparoscopy findings are negative—i.e., everything looks normal. Common gynecological conditions causing chronic pelvic pain include pelvic inflammatory disease, endometriosis and adenomyosis (see Chapters 24, 36, and 77, respectively), as well as pelvic adhesions. Adhesions (see glossary) are an unpredictable cause of pelvic pain as some individuals with adhesions have pain while others, for unknown reasons, do not. Whether caused by tubal infections or prior surgery, adhesions can be removed with a knife, electrocautery, or by using a laser (see Chapter 41). In older women, usually those over sixty, chronic pain may be related to loss of pelvic support and associated with uterine prolapse or the presence of a cystocele (see Chapter 28).

Surgery is only one of the available therapies for chronic pelvic pain. Surgery, including hysterectomy with or without removal of the ovaries, is discussed in Chapter 45. It should be pointed out here, however, that such surgery generally may be avoided (and if performed may be unsuccessful) unless a physical cause for the pain is present. Despite the fact that less radical surgical treatments than hysterectomy are available and can usually be tried first, approximately 100,000 hysterectomies are performed annually in the United States for this symptom. Some of these are unnecessary. Medical alternatives for treating chronic pain that have had some success include acupuncture, TENS (transcutaneous electrical nerve stimulation; see glossary), and trigger-point injections, in which specific areas are injected with a local anesthetic. Chronic narcotic use should be avoided in the treatment of chronic pelvic pain. Instead, your physician may prescribe one of the nonnarcotic painkillers called NSAIDs (nonsteroidal, anti-inflammatory drugs). These drugs are also used to treat arthritis (see Chapter 73) and often help in relieving chronic pain without the risk of being habit-forming. Another alternative consists of a new and unique prescription medication for chronic pelvic pain called Ultram. This recently approved drug has a potency similar to that of some narcotics, but is not a "scheduled" drug. Ultram does not have anti-inflammatory action and tends to avoid the side effects, like intestinal bleeding or ulcer formation, sometimes associated with such drugs.

Table 111 SIGNS OF LABOR

Factor	Real Labor	False Labor
Intensity of discomfort	increases	remains the same
Time between contractions	gradually shortens	remains long
Regularity of contractions	regular	irregular
Location of discomfort	entire uterus and back	lower abdomen and groin
Effect of alcohol or other sedatives	unaffected	often relieved
Cervix opening	cervix dilated	cervix not dilated
Effect of previous childbirth	none	increases likelihood
"Bloody show"	often associated	not associated

CHRONIC PELVIC PAIN

Problem	Action	Possible Cause

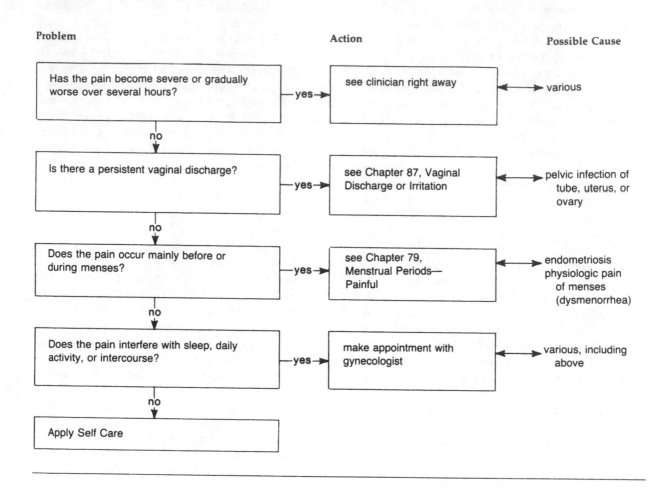

Problem	Action	Possible Cause
Has the pain become severe or gradually worse over several hours? → yes →	see clinician right away	← → various
↓ no		
Is there a persistent vaginal discharge? → yes →	see Chapter 87, Vaginal Discharge or Irritation	← → pelvic infection of tube, uterus, or ovary
↓ no		
Does the pain occur mainly before or during menses? → yes →	see Chapter 79, Menstrual Periods—Painful	← → endometriosis physiologic pain of menses (dysmenorrhea)
↓ no		
Does the pain interfere with sleep, daily activity, or intercourse? → yes →	make appointment with gynecologist	← → various, including above
↓ no		
Apply Self Care		

Chronic Lower Abdominal Pain— What You Can Do (Self Care)

Keep a record of your pain—when it occurs, its location, what makes it better or worse. Bring your record with you to the next office visit. Avoid whatever makes the pain recur. Many pains for which no cause is determined go away on their own. Pelvic inflammation responds to rest and temporary abstinence from sexual intercourse. Bladder infections also improve faster if intercourse is avoided and if you drink fluids during treatment. To help relieve the pain, try a heating pad over the abdomen or back. If an antibiotic or other medication has been prescribed, take the full amount even if symptoms begin to improve before you complete the prescription (see Chapter 29). Take Tylenol, or other analgesics containing acetaminophen, in preference to aspirin-containing drugs; aspirin often causes stomach irritation. See also Chapter 51 for further discussion of over-the-counter analgesics (pain pills). Pain often produces emotional stress, and this stress then makes the pain worse; and a vicious circle is created. Make your health a high priority by allowing extra time for rest periods, including a good night's sleep.

CHAPTER 84

Swelling and Fluid Retention

In women the most common cause of generalized swelling (edema) is premenstrual fluid retention. Women in their thirties and forties are particularly affected. The addition of several pounds of water which occurs gradually during the two- to ten-day length of time before menses may cause a variety of symptoms including swollen legs, breast fullness, pelvic ache, headache, nervousness, irritability, insomnia, and loss of concentration. These symptoms peak in intensity just before menses and cease abruptly after the onset of bleeding. There is wide variation in the symptoms experienced among women. These symptoms comprise part of premenstrual syndrome (PMS).

Both the physical and emotional symptoms of PMS appear to have some biochemical basis related to the high level of hormones in the second half of the menstrual cycle, when the estrogen level is higher. Research indicates that an important factor is the ability of estrogen to partially block salt and water excretion by the kidneys. As a result, the body retains fluid. Increased retention of fluid within the intestines helps to account for the frequency of diarrhea and cramping experienced by some women. Fluid retention involving the pelvic organs may have positive or negative effects. Some women experience congestion of the pelvic veins and feel this congestion as a dull, low abdominal aching pressure. Congestion around the vulva, on the other hand, may stimulate increased clitoral or vaginal awareness associated with greater sexual desire or responsiveness.

Women taking birth control pills (see Chapter 9) sometimes have fewer and milder premenstrual symptoms compared to women using other contraceptive methods or none at all. This difference is due, perhaps, to the fact that the fixed ingredients of the pill prevent the slightest hormonal imbalance from occurring and because most birth control pills in current use contain relatively low dosages of estrogen. Premenstrual fluid retention and weight gain often subside after two or three months of birth control pill use.

Abdominal swelling unaccompanied by fluid retention elsewhere in the body is often due to a digestive problem. Gas, indigestion, and air swallowing cause temporary bloating and are likely to occur at times of psychological stress. A serious digestive disorder causing abdominal swelling is usually associated with abdominal pain, jaundice, vomiting, or bloody stool. In the gynecologic area pregnancy and ovarian tumors are the principal causes of abdominal swelling.

Pregnancy is associated with fluid retention of much greater magnitude than that of premenstrual swelling, although the symptoms produced in each case may be strikingly similar. Characteristically, swelling, or *edema*, is worse at the end of the pregnancy when the total amount of excess water retained may amount to 6½ quarts or more. About half of the water content is found in the fetus, bag of waters, and placenta. The rest is distributed to the mother's tissues, especially to the blood, breasts, and uterus. The mother's feet and legs usually swell the most because the growing uterus compresses the large veins that return blood from the lower extremities to the heart. When you lie down on your side, the uterus no longer blocks these vessels and swelling tends to go down. This is why at night more frequent urination occurs as fluid from the legs is available for excretion by the kidneys.

In pregnancy generalized edema involving the hands and face, as well as the legs, may be an abnormal finding signifying hypertension or high blood pressure, especially when the edema is accompanied by headaches, blurred vision, or dizziness. Rapid accumulation of water of more than five pounds in any given week may be the first sign of hypertension even before generalized swelling occurs.

What Medical Care Can Do

The treatment of premenstrual tension depends on the severity and type of symptoms experienced. The physician's medical management for premenstrual fluid retention consists primarily of water pills (diuretics). With many of these drugs, when taken chronically, potassium salts are lost in the urine and must be replaced with foods rich in potassium, such as bananas, oranges, or cranberry juice, or by potassium supplementation in the form of pills. Depletion of potassium may cause weakness and muscle cramps. Water pills are also used to control blood pressure. Because of the possibility of side effects, water pills should be used sparingly when taken for relief of fluid retention or premenstrual syndrome. For more information on PMS see Chapter 32.

If you are pregnant, you should avoid drug therapy if possible. The use of water pills for treating uncomplicated leg swelling in pregnancy is not effective and is potentially hazardous to your unborn. The occasional use of certain diuretics for the pregnant woman with high blood pressure may be necessary.

What You Can Do (Self Care)

Your body retains water to dilute dietary salt, so restriction of salt is one of the most important steps in reducing fluid retention (see Chapter 48). The week before your period, avoid adding salt in cooking and don't eat salty foods, such as processed lunch meats, or highly seasoned foods. Drinking large amounts of water "to flush the kidneys and rid salt" from your body sounds like a good idea but has limited practical benefit in reducing symptoms of fluid retention. If you are on the pill, consider a change to a lower estrogen dose pill or to a mini-pill (see Chapter 9). In addition to rest and a nutritious diet (see Chapter 48), recreation and activity, especially sexual activity, relieve vascular congestion as well as emotional tension in many women.

During pregnancy, bed rest is the most effective way to reduce water retention. Elevate your legs whenever possible during the day. Fitted support hose may help. The restricted use of salt to control edema in pregnancy is controversial. Fluid retention and weekly weight gain are the result of many complex hormonal factors involving more than how much salt a woman takes in her diet. Although some women are particularly sensitive and respond to high salt intake with swelling, most do not and will not find symptomatic relief by restricting salt. Attempts to completely eliminate salt from your diet may, in fact, be hazardous to the fetus and are not recommended in pregnancy.

SWELLING AND FLUID RETENTION

Problem	Action	Possible Cause

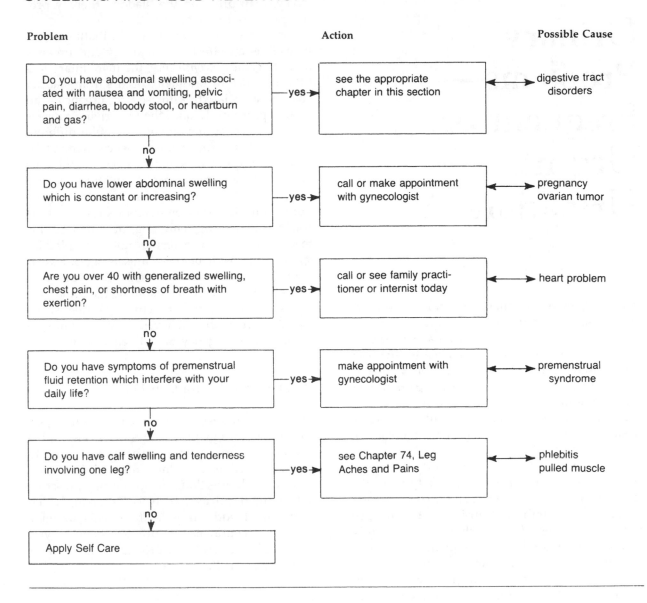

Problem: Do you have abdominal swelling associated with nausea and vomiting, pelvic pain, diarrhea, bloody stool, or heartburn and gas? — yes → Action: see the appropriate chapter in this section ← Possible Cause: digestive tract disorders

no ↓

Problem: Do you have lower abdominal swelling which is constant or increasing? — yes → Action: call or make appointment with gynecologist ← Possible Cause: pregnancy ovarian tumor

no ↓

Problem: Are you over 40 with generalized swelling, chest pain, or shortness of breath with exertion? — yes → Action: call or see family practitioner or internist today ← Possible Cause: heart problem

no ↓

Problem: Do you have symptoms of premenstrual fluid retention which interfere with your daily life? — yes → Action: make appointment with gynecologist ← Possible Cause: premenstrual syndrome

no ↓

Problem: Do you have calf swelling and tenderness involving one leg? — yes → Action: see Chapter 74, Leg Aches and Pains ← Possible Cause: phlebitis pulled muscle

no ↓

Apply Self Care

CHAPTER 85

Urinary Problems— Frequent or Urgent Urination

If you experience frequent urination, called *urinary frequency*, or the sudden urge to urinate, called *urinary urgency*, you may have a urinary tract infection. Such infection usually involves some discomfort as well—either a burning sensation during urination or a dull pain in the lower abdomen toward the end of urination. A bladder infection (cystitis) may cause a constant desire to void (urinate) even when the bladder is nearly empty.

In the absence of painful or bloody urination, frequent or urgent urination is likely to result from other conditions, especially *urethral stenosis* and *cystocele*. Urethral stenosis, or stricture, refers to narrowing of the urethra. In women this condition occurs relatively frequently and from various causes. Urethral stenosis may be present from birth and first show up in adolescence or even earlier. At other times, this problem results from previous infection (such as gonorrhea—see Chapter 24), or it first develops after menopause from estrogen-deficiency related changes in the urethra (see Chapter 26). A cystocele (see Chapter 28) refers to a vaginal hernia or bulge that develops from a weakening of the vaginal muscles, especially in postmenopausal women. Cystoceles cause symptoms of urinary frequency and urgency because complete emptying of the bladder is prevented.

Frequent urination without urgency may be due to excessive fluid intake, anxiety, alcohol, beverages containing caffeine, or diuretics (water pills), all of which increase urine formation. In addition, any pelvic mass, including a pregnancy, may press on the bladder, thereby producing more frequent urination.

Emotional stress can be a contributing cause, as well as an effect, of frequency and urgency and of *urgency incontinence*, the involuntary loss of urine. Such incontinence occurs from bladder spasms associated with severe urgency and clears up promptly once the underlying cause is treated. Urgency incontinence is quite different from another form of incontinence called *stress incontinence*, which is not associated with urinary frequency or urgency. With stress incontinence, the involuntary loss of urine occurs during physical (not emotional) stress, such as coughing, sneezing, laughing, or running. This form of incontinence results not from bladder spasms but from bladder muscle weakness or damage (for example, from childbirth) that prevents the bladder from containing the urine during strenuous physical activity. While stress incontinence is often relieved by surgery or special exercises, urgency incontinence is not.

What Medical Care Can Do

The physician does a pelvic exam to exclude pelvic tumors, pregnancy, or cystocele. He or she will also obtain a urinalysis or urine culture to check for bladder or kidney infection. In the absence of such infection, the doctor may prescribe antispasmodic drugs, such as Ditropan, which relaxes the bladder muscle. If you have urgency or stress incontinence or urethral stenosis, you may need a referral to a urologist (bladder and kidney specialist).

What You Can Do (Self Care)

Urinary frequency and urinary urgency are usually temporary symptoms or are related to dietary or emotional factors which you may be able to minimize. Bladder reconditioning—i.e., voiding by the clock at increasingly longer intervals—is very helpful for some individuals. Symptoms of stress incontinence may be reduced by a special exercise (called Kegel's exercise). (See Chapter 28, under Urinary Stress Incontinence, for instructions on how to do this exercise.) If incontinence becomes worse or per-

URINARY PROBLEMS—FREQUENT OR URGENT URINATION

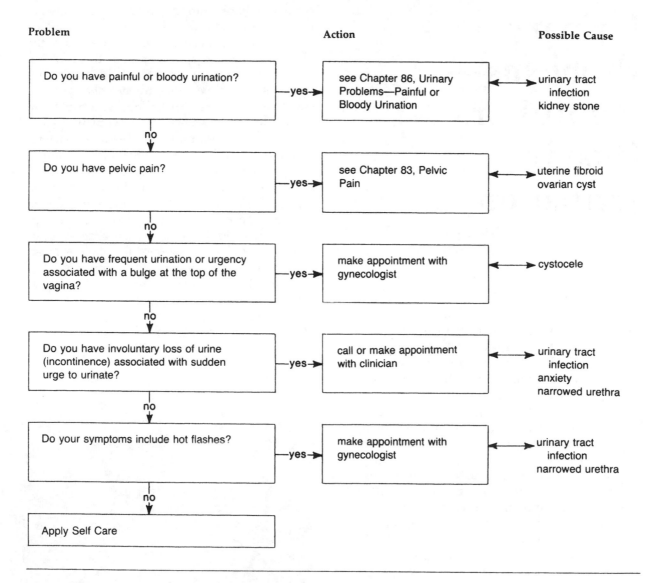

Problem

Do you have painful or bloody urination?

    no

Do you have pelvic pain?

    no

Do you have frequent urination or urgency associated with a bulge at the top of the vagina?

    no

Do you have involuntary loss of urine (incontinence) associated with sudden urge to urinate?

    no

Do your symptoms include hot flashes?

    no

Apply Self Care

Action

— yes → see Chapter 86, Urinary Problems—Painful or Bloody Urination

— yes → see Chapter 83, Pelvic Pain

— yes → make appointment with gynecologist

— yes → call or make appointment with clinician

— yes → make appointment with gynecologist

Possible Cause

urinary tract infection
kidney stone

uterine fibroid
ovarian cyst

cystocele

urinary tract infection
anxiety
narrowed urethra

urinary tract infection
narrowed urethra

sists or if you have bloody or painful urination, see your physician. Special pads for urinary incontinence are now available at drug-stores. They can be used when incontinence would be an embarrassment, such as during exercise.

CHAPTER 86

Urinary Problems— Painful or Bloody Urination

Painful or bloody urination is usually due to a urinary tract infection. Such infections affect women far more frequently than men because the urethra, which connects the bladder to the outside of the body, is located very close to the vagina and anus, both of which are sources of bacteria. Because of poor hygiene or during intercourse, childbirth, or gynecologic surgery, bacteria may enter the urethra and eventually cause infection of the lower or upper urinary tract (see Figure 52).

Lower urinary tract infections may involve the urethra (*urethritis*) or bladder (*cystitis*). Women with symptoms of these infections account for 1% of all physician office visits in the United States—more than 5 million trips to the doctor, at a cost of nearly $1 billion annually. But the impact of these infections is even greater. Left undiagnosed or improperly treated, they can become a significant cause of chronic kidney damage years later.

Cystitis will cause painful and sometimes bloody, frequent, or urgent urination. When the only symptom is a burning sensation on urination, urethritis is more likely to be the cause. No one knows why some women are more prone to urinary tract infections. Bladder infections often result from sexual activity and are sometimes known as *honeymoon cystitis* since they frequently occur among young women who have just become sexually active. A two- to fourfold increased risk of cystitis has been reported in some diaphragm users. Presumably this occurs due to the diaphragm's compression of the urethra. By interfering with normal bladder emptying, the diaphragm may predispose women to infection after intercourse, when small numbers of bacteria are normally introduced into the bladder. In some diaphragm users, this problem may be due to inappropriately large diaphragm size. In some women, the presence of a cystocele (see glossary) may make her susceptible to chronic infection because of the woman's inability to completely empty her bladder. Bacteria may grow rapidly in the urine which remains.

When cystitis spreads beyond the bladder, then upper urinary tract or kidney infection (*pyelonephritis*) occurs. Kidney infections, unlike bladder infections, are associated with symptoms such as weakness, nausea, backache, fever, and chills. Kidney infections, like bladder infections, usually respond rapidly to antibiotics. Occasionally kidney infections become chronic and result in kidney damage.

During pregnancy, hormonal changes cause a general relaxation in the muscle tone of the uri-

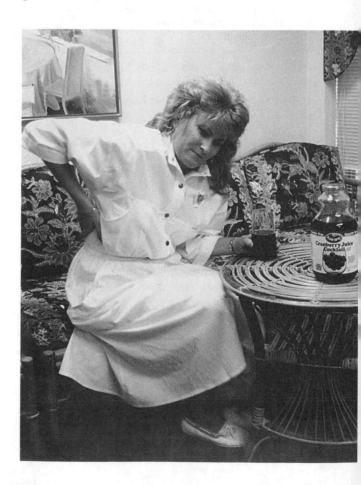

Figure 52
The female urinary system.

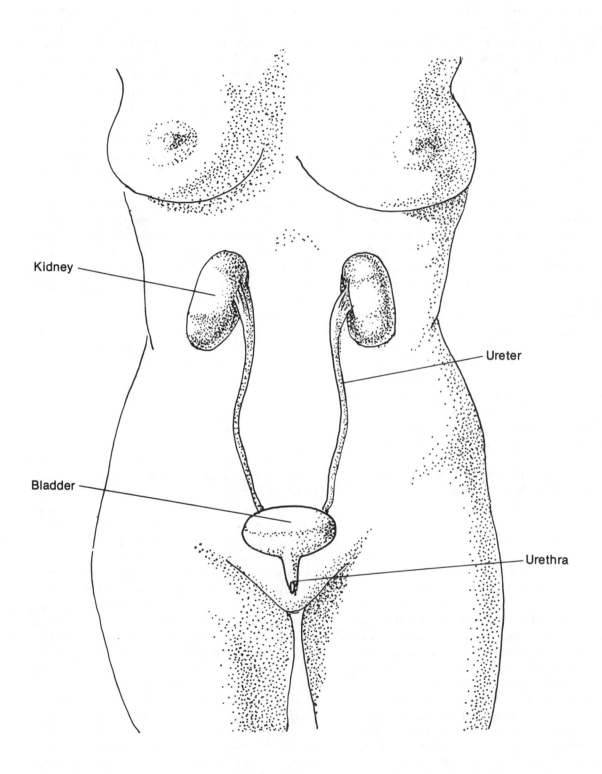

Kidney

Ureter

Bladder

Urethra

nary system, resulting in retention of urine in the two ureters (the *ureter* is the tube carrying urine from each kidney to the bladder) and bladder. This urine retention makes the woman susceptible to symptomless bacterial growth. For this reason, physicians may routinely perform urine cultures during pregnancy, because kidney infections may be associated with premature labor.

Various types of *urethritis* (unassociated with a bladder infection) comprise the other type of lower urinary tract infection. The urethra contains numerous tiny pockets and crevices which make it an easy target for infection. Several small pockets may form one large pouch, called a *diverticulum*, which may collect urinary debris. Swelling and inflammation of this diverticulum may prevent adequate drainage and result in one form of chronic urethritis. Sexually transmitted infections that involve the urethra, including gonorrhea, account for another type of urethritis. A third type of urethritis, known as *urethral syndrome*, is characterized by urethritis-like symptoms, such as painful, frequent urination, with no apparent cause. Various explanations for this difficult-to-diagnose syndrome have included allergy, slight trauma during sex, insufficient estrogen, and chlamydia infection. This form of urethritis differs in one basic way from garden-variety bladder and kidney infections: the urine is "sterile"—i.e., it contains no bacterial growth when tested for infection.

It is now apparent that bladder and kidney infections are sometimes misdiagnosed as urethral syndrome because of the way physicians used to define a "positive" urine culture. Previously, a strict definition was adhered to: a culture was positive if it contained more than 100,000 bacterial colonies. Anything short of this number was considered "negative" and not due to infection. Recent studies, however, indicate that in up to one-third of women with bladder and kidney infections, the urine culture will show a bacterial colony count of less than 100,000. It is important to keep this in mind if you have symptoms of bladder infection (painful, frequent, sometimes bloody urination) and your doctor does *not* want to treat you with antibiotics because of a low culture count. With such symptoms and a urinalysis showing white cells, it may be best to get treated.

Painful urination alone is not always associated with infection of either the urethra or the bladder. Various other conditions, including herpes infections, vaginal infections, intercourse, and chemical irritation from vaginal medication or contraceptive products, may cause discomfort during urination. In these conditions, urinary discomfort is usually felt over the lower vulva as a result of contact with the urine—not as a localized stinging at the bladder opening (urethra), characteristic of urethritis and cystitis. Sometimes, however, the symptom of painful urination is not quite so clear-cut. In menopause, for example, lowered estrogen levels may cause thinning of the urethra and bladder lining and give rise to painful urination that may mimic a bladder infection.

Persistent bloody urine, which may indicate a kidney stone or tumor in the urinary tract, as well as persistent symptoms of painful urination, require evaluation by a urologist. One of the more difficult disorders to diagnose and treat is *interstitial cystitis*, a chronic condition causing pain in the bladder area, the urge to urinate often, and frequent voiding at night. The cause of this noninfectious condition, which causes the bladder to become chronically inflamed, is poorly understood.

What Medical Care Can Do

The doctor will do a pelvic exam and may test for gonorrhea and chlamydia if venereal infection is suspected. He or she will diagnose a urinary tract infection by urinalysis (see glossary) and urine culture. A newer screening method uses a paper strip that changes color in less than a minute when dipped in infected urine. But the most accurate diagnostic technique is the urine culture, which takes twenty-four to seventy-two hours for the results. The culture tells which bacteria are causing the infection, and the doctor will know which antibiotic will destroy the bacteria. To collect a urine sample for a urine culture, here is what you do: first, you separate the lips of the vagina and clean the urinary opening with mild soap and water; next, you urinate a small amount into the toilet bowl; and then you urinate a portion of the urine into the sterile container. This process is known as a *clean-catch midstream* collection; and the specimen is much more reliable than a specimen collected from

URINARY PROBLEMS—PAINFUL OR BLOODY URINATION

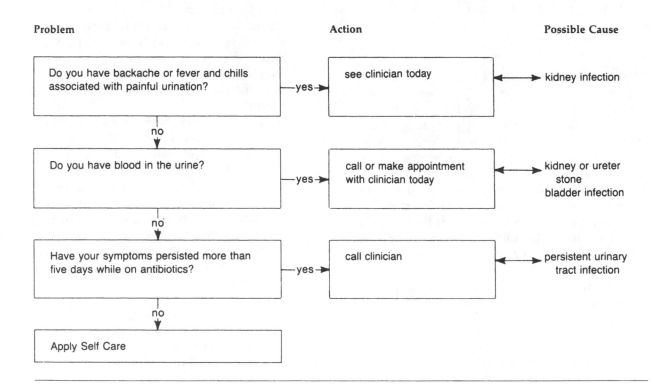

Problem	Action	Possible Cause

Do you have backache or fever and chills associated with painful urination? —yes→ see clinician today ←→ kidney infection

no↓

Do you have blood in the urine? —yes→ call or make appointment with clinician today ←→ kidney or ureter stone / bladder infection

no↓

Have your symptoms persisted more than five days while on antibiotics? —yes→ call clinician ←→ persistent urinary tract infection

no↓

Apply Self Care

simply urinating into a cup, which may cause contamination of the urine specimen. When a urine culture reveals no bacterial growth, the physician must consider other causes of painful urination, including sexually transmitted diseases, vaginitis, and chemical irritants.

The physician may refer you to a urologist if urinary tract infections occur chronically. An IVP (intravenous pyelogram—see glossary) is a kidney X-ray which may be ordered by a physician to check for signs of previous kidney infection, kidney stones, or slight anatomic variations in the urinary tract which sometimes make a person susceptible to infection. *Urethroscopy* and *cystoscopy* are procedures to examine the inside of the urethra and bladder and may help identify and treat certain urethra and bladder problems, including urethral diverticulum, interstitial cystitis, and bladder cancer. This may be done in the doctor's office or as an outpatient surgical procedure.

The treatment of urinary tract infection always involves taking antibiotics, for several days for first-time lower-tract infection, and usually for ten days or more for kidney infections.

Recently, single-dose treatment regimes have been reported as effective. Some of the drugs currently favored for treating uncomplicated bouts of cystitis include trimethoprim (e.g., Proloprim, Trimpex), nitrofurantoin (e.g., Macrobid, Macrodantin), and sulfa (e.g., Azo Gantrisin, Azo Gantanol). These recommendations are based on cure rates, cost, and the relatively few side effects associated with these drugs. Ampicillin is less often prescribed today because of increased bacterial resistance to the drug. Persistent bladder and kidney infections may require a course of antibiotics lasting several months. Newer drugs for treating recurrent or resistant infections include Noroxin and Cinobac, as well as more traditional drugs such as Macrodantin, Bactrim, and Septra. Certain antibiotics may also be prescribed for long periods during pregnancy, when changes in the urinary system make a woman susceptible to the growth of bacteria.

If you have a long history of multiple bladder or kidney infections, your doctor may prescribe antibiotics as a preventative to be taken once before or immediately after intercourse. Hospitalization may be required for treating kidney infections that occur in pregnancy or for recurrent infections among nonpregnant women not responding to oral antibiotics.

What You Can Do (Self Care)

Drink plenty of fluids to help flush out the urinary tract. Drinking cranberry juice acidifies the urine, which helps prevent bacterial growth within the urinary tract. Take antibiotics exactly as prescribed even though your symptoms subside in three or four days. It is a good idea to have a repeat urine culture two weeks after your treatment begins to make sure that the infection is cleared up. A consultation with a urologist is advisable when urinary tract infections persist despite antibiotic therapy.

Here are suggestions that will help you to prevent urinary tract infections:

1. Don't hold your urine for prolonged periods; respond to the urge to urinate.
2. Be sure to wash the external genitalia each time you bathe or shower.

3. Urinate soon after intercourse.
4. After a bowel movement, be sure to wipe from front to back to avoid contamination of the urinary tract.
5. Avoid the use of urethral irritants, such as vaginal perfumes and bubble baths. Continue to use vaginal contraceptive cream or foam (if this is your birth control method) since these products kill bacteria as well as sperm.
6. During pregnancy, have a urine culture ordered if you have a history of urinary tract infections. Many women do not realize that prenatal urine evaluations in the doctor's office, while checking for protein or sugar, may not include a test for infection.
7. If you use a diaphragm and have a history of frequent cystitis, check with your doctor to see if you could be fitted for the next smaller size without loss of contraceptive effectiveness.

Table 112 answers some specific questions about urinary tract infections.

Table 113 summarizes some information about the causes of chronic bladder and urethral infections in women.

Table 112 QUESTIONS COMMONLY ASKED ABOUT URINARY TRACT INFECTIONS

Question	Yes	No	Comment
Are kidney or bladder infections contagious?		X	They are not transmitted by intercourse, unlike venereal infection. However, gonorrhea may produce symptoms like a bladder infection such as burning with urination.
Is a kidney stone the commonest cause of bloody urination after urinary tract infection?	X		The stone may become lodged in the ureter (the tube between the kidney and bladder) and produce severe back or abdominal pain on one side.
Can chronic kidney damage cause high blood pressure?	X		High blood pressure may occur after multiple kidney infections.
Is kidney damage common?		X	Most urinary tract infections are limited to the bladder and urethra.
Should a previously prescribed antibiotic be taken for a urinary tract infection?		X	Although the symptoms may be the same, different infections may be caused by different bacteria and will require different antibiotic treatment.
Does wearing a tampon delay recovery from a urinary tract infection?		X	There is no effect on the course of the infection.
Are periods of increased sexual activity associated with an increased frequency of bladder infections?	X		Bacteria from the vagina may be mechanically introduced into the urethra (the tube through which urine passes from the bladder to the outside of the body).
Are bladder infections more common during and after menopause?	X		Estrogen loss during and after menopause makes the tissues more vulnerable to bacteria.
Is painful and frequent urination always a sign of a bladder or kidney infection?		X	Chemical irritation and vaginal herpes infections also cause these symptoms.

Table 113 CAUSES OF CHRONIC BLADDER AND URETHRAL INFECTIONS IN WOMEN

Cause	Source of Infection	Where Infection Occurs	Treatment
resistant bacteria	insufficient or wrong antibiotic	bladder or urethra	antibiotics for several weeks
cystocele (weakening or hernia of bladder wall)	incomplete bladder-emptying due to cystocele	bladder	surgery (in some cases)
diverticulum (pocket in urethra)	small amounts of bacteria chronically pocketed in diverticulum	bladder or urethra	surgery
venereal infection involving urethra (gonorrhea or chlamydia)	sexual intercourse with infected partner	urethra	antibiotics

CHAPTER 87

Vaginal Discharge or Irritation

Vaginitis is an inflammation of the vagina, often accompanied by pain, itching, discharge, and odor. These symptoms may be most unpleasant. Vaginal discharge is most often due to an infection, while irritation alone is often due to allergic reactions to various substances such as vaginal contraceptions, condoms, and deodorant sprays. Vaginal infections are among the most common reasons for a visit to a gynecologist and now account for more than 5 million clinician visits each year. Various explanations for the frequency of vaginal infections include changing patterns of sexuality and contraceptive practices. Increased use of the pill has brought about a decline in the use of condoms, which protect women from infections carried by male sex partners. Freer sexual practices increase the risk of vaginal infections, especially when a person, male or female, has multiple sexual relationships. Some causes of vaginal discharge may be sexually transmitted diseases such as herpes, chlamydia, and gonorrhea (see Chapter 24). At other times vaginal infection may result from a medical problem such as diabetes.

All vaginal infections are caused by an overgrowth of microscopic organisms which normally inhabit the healthy vagina in small numbers. Conditions that decrease your resistance to infection as well as environmental factors, such as the pill or antibiotics, can interfere with your body's natural hormonal or bacterial balance and allow such infections to occur. Sometimes the infections recur, especially if there is more than one organism involved. These are called *mixed infections*. Chronic vaginitis can cause painful intercourse, either by decreasing lubrication or by irritation of the vulva itself.

When vaginal infections are chronic, there is usually inflammation of the cervix as well, the cervix often being secondarily infected. On the other hand, infection within the cervix, such as gonorrhea or a uterine infection associated with the use of an IUD, may be the primary cause of vaginal discharge.

The most common vaginal infections are discussed below.

Yeast infections, also known as *monilia* or *candidiasis*, are the most common type of vaginal infection. Yeast infections are caused by an overgrowth of a funguslike organism, usually *Candida albicans*. This organism is normally present in small amounts in the vagina as well as in the mouth and digestive tract. Monilia causes a white discharge which looks like cottage cheese. The most common symptom is intense itching of the external genitalia. Symptoms may vary from mild irritation to severe redness and swelling of the vulva. There may also be painful urination or pain during intercourse. Monilia is more common during pregnancy and in women taking hormones, including birth control pills. It is also more frequent when antibiotics are being taken because of the imbalance of normal bacteria that occurs. Chronic monilia may be the first sign of diabetes, and chronic yeast infections that also involve the mouth (oral thrush) may be associated with immunocompromised states including AIDS. Consult your physician about testing for these conditions. Although monilia is the most common cause of vulvar itching, many other causes of itching or rash unassociated with a discharge may be confused with monilia (see Chapter 72).

Vaginal creams or suppositories provide the standard treatment of yeast infections and are effective about 80% to 90% of the time. The most effective drugs include miconazole (Monistat products), clotrimazole (Gyne-Lotrimin and Mycelex-G products), and newer drugs that contain either butoconazole (Femstat), tioconazole (Vagistat), or terconazole (Terazol). Some of these products have recently become available over-the-counter, including Gyne-Lotrimin, Monistat 7, and Mycelex 7. Each of these products is available as a seven-day vaginal cream. Recently, a new prescription oral medication called Diflucan has been approved for the treatment of vaginal yeast infections. Simpler than vaginal creams or inserts, a single Diflucan tablet (150 mg) taken as an oral dose is usually effective. However, side effects may be somewhat more common than with vaginal preparations, and initial studies showed that among Diflucan users 13% experienced headache and 7% nausea. In addition, there have been rare cases of serious hepatic toxicity, mainly in patients with already existing serious medical conditions. Diflucan appears, on balance, to offer an attractive alternative, especially for patients with chronic yeast infections or those who do not respond to the usual first-line vaginal preparations. Chronic or recurring yeast infections should be treated with a second dose or a different drug from this group of vaginal products prior to more potent treatments such as oral ketaconazole (Nizoral), which has been associated with serious liver damage in a few patients. Steps to prevent yeast infections are discussed below.

Trichomonas infection is diagnosed in at least 4 million men and women in the United States each year, making it one of the most frequent of sexually transmitted diseases. Caused by a bacterialike organism called *Trichomonas vaginalis*, "trich," as it is commonly called, produces a yellow-green, bad-smelling discharge associated with itching and burning. Because the organism can survive in the urinary tract, painful urination also may be an occasional symptom. However, Trichomonas infections produce little or no symptoms in nearly 50% of women. Trich is almost always acquired through sexual contact and accounts for 10% to 30% of patient visits to VD clinics throughout the United States. This microbe is found in 30% to 40% of male partners of infected women but in nearly 85% of female partners of infected men. In addition, gonorrhea is twice as likely to be found among women with Trichomonas infections, making a test for gonorrhea advisable. While it is theoretically possible for a Trichomonas infection to be acquired through the use of infected towels, bathing suits, or other moist objects, such transmission, if it occurs at all, is extremely rare. Trichomonas infections may be an occasional cause of preterm labor. However, the drug of choice, metronidazole (Flagyl) is not advised for pregnant women in the first three months due to a small risk of birth defects. Male partners of women with this vaginal infection are often symptom-free carriers of trich and should be treated.

Bacterial vaginitis (bacterial vaginosis) is an extremely common infection among women of reproductive age. It causes a gray, milky, or yellow discharge often associated with an unpleasant odor. This infection has had a number of different names (which seem to change every few years), including *Hemophilus vaginitis, Gardnerella vaginalis*, nonspecific vaginitis, and most recently, bacterial vaginosis. In this type of vaginitis, itching is less prominent and odor may be quite unpleasant, especially after intercourse. This is due to a chemical reaction between the bacteria causing this infection and alkaline secretions in semen, which combine to produce amines, chemical compounds with a characteristic, fishy odor. Like yeast infections, bacterial vaginosis may recur and become chronic and difficult to cure. Traditional treatments, such as ampicillin, tetracycline, and vaginal creams containing sulfa, have been found to be ineffective. Current therapy calls for either an oral antibiotic (Flagyl or Cleocin) or a vaginal antibiotic cream (Cleocin or Metrogel). This form of vaginitis is sometimes sexually transmitted. Male partners are not routinely treated as they are with trichomonas infections, unless the infection does not respond to initial treatment.

Atrophic vaginitis, a condition which is not really an infection but is more an irritation, is a result of the thinning of the vaginal tissue, a thinning that occurs from a decline in the estrogen produced by the ovaries after menopause. The vagina becomes dry and inflamed and sometimes is associated with discharge. As a result of this condition, the vaginal tissues are less able to fend off bacteria. The tissues are also more susceptible to abrasion during intercourse, which, in turn, increases susceptibility to infection. Atrophic vaginitis may occur before menopause in women who have had surgical removal of the ovaries.

Noninfectious causes of vaginal discharge sometimes occur. The adolescent woman will probably experience a profuse watery discharge prior to or following the beginning of menstruation as a result of the hormonal surge that occurs at puberty. During the reproductive years, some vaginal discharge is considered physiologic, a normal consequence of ovulation especially in women who have had one or more pregnancies. Increased glandular secretions from the cervix may also occur normally as a result of taking birth control pills. Unlike vaginitis, physiologic discharges occur without odor and are perfectly harmless.

VAGINAL DISCHARGE OR IRRITATION

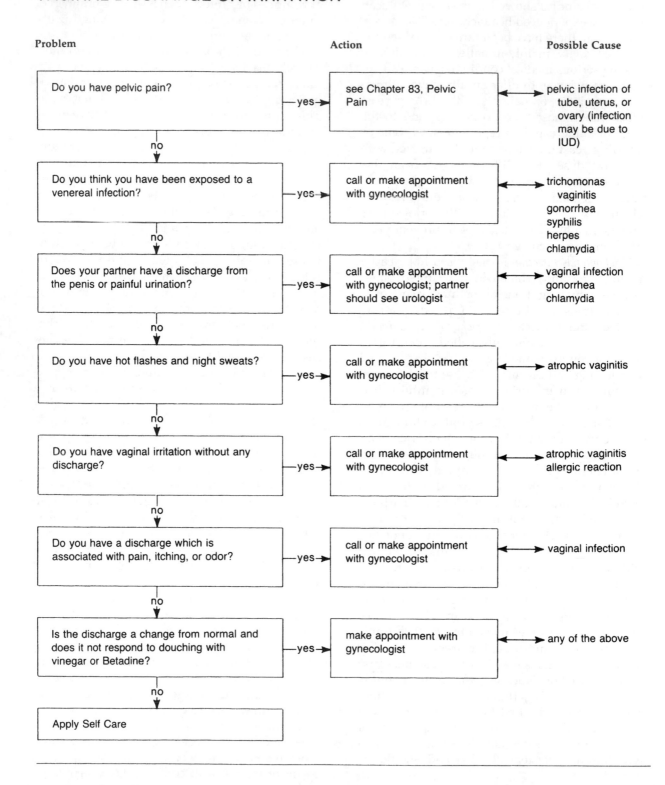

Problem	Action	Possible Cause
Do you have pelvic pain?	—yes→ see Chapter 83, Pelvic Pain	← pelvic infection of tube, uterus, or ovary (infection may be due to IUD)
↓ no		
Do you think you have been exposed to a venereal infection?	—yes→ call or make appointment with gynecologist	← trichomonas vaginitis gonorrhea syphilis herpes chlamydia
↓ no		
Does your partner have a discharge from the penis or painful urination?	—yes→ call or make appointment with gynecologist; partner should see urologist	← vaginal infection gonorrhea chlamydia
↓ no		
Do you have hot flashes and night sweats?	—yes→ call or make appointment with gynecologist	← atrophic vaginitis
↓ no		
Do you have vaginal irritation without any discharge?	—yes→ call or make appointment with gynecologist	← atrophic vaginitis allergic reaction
↓ no		
Do you have a discharge which is associated with pain, itching, or odor?	—yes→ call or make appointment with gynecologist	← vaginal infection
↓ no		
Is the discharge a change from normal and does it not respond to douching with vinegar or Betadine?	—yes→ make appointment with gynecologist	← any of the above
↓ no		
Apply Self Care		

What Medical Care Can Do

Be sure to avoid douching for twenty-four to forty-eight hours prior to the office visit because the diagnosis of vaginal discharge is made on the basis of the pelvic examination and the results from a glass slide of vaginal secretions (*wet smear*). Cultures for gonorrhea and chlamydia and a blood test for syphilis may be obtained if exposure to venereal disease is suspected. Mild physiologic discharge does not need any treatment at all. Excessive discharge without infection is sometimes treated by cautery of the cervix (see glossary), or by using a freeze technique, called cryosurgery (see glossary). If the discharge is due to a uterine or an ovarian infection, the physician will prescribe an appropriate antibiotic.

If a vaginal infection alone is diagnosed, specific antibiotic or local vaginal therapy is prescribed. Treatment of the main types of vaginitis is discussed in Table 114. When the exact cause of a vaginal infection cannot be found, the clinician may then treat for *nonspecific vaginitis*. Treatment in this case is essentially based on a trial-and-error approach, which is less likely to be effective than when a specific cause of vaginitis is diagnosed from the wet smear.

What You Can Do (Self Care)

The sexually active woman should keep in mind that unusual vaginal discharge could represent a veneral disease. If you have any question of exposure to VD or if symptoms persist or recur, see your doctor.

If you have symptoms of a vaginal yeast infection—symptoms that you recognize from having been diagnosed and treated previously by your clinician—you may want to consider using one of the nonprescription products now available for treatment of vaginal yeast infections. However, if symptoms don't improve in two to three days, consult your physician.

A single-ingredient douche occasionally may be used as adjunctive therapy in the treatment of vaginitis. However, douching has few medical advantages in most situations and should be avoided in pregnancy. There are no proven benefits from routine douching, and the technique can aggravate existing infection by forcing bacteria from the vagina into the uterus and fallopian tubes. Multi-ingredient drugstore douches and related "feminine hygiene products" cannot in general be recommended for self-treatment of vaginitis.

When medication has been prescribed, use it as directed; the major cause of recurrence of an infection is failure to take the full course of treatment. If several weeks go by and new symptoms occur, see your doctor for a checkup since you may have a different problem. Do not use a tampon when vaginal cream or suppositories have been prescribed because the tampon may soak up the medication. A sanitary napkin may be worn during treatment and may make you feel more comfortable. A hair blower may help dry irritated areas after you bathe or shower.

If you have been treated for a sexually transmitted disease, be sure your partner(s) is/are treated. Also, it is a good idea to use condoms for at least six months after treatment to lessen the chance of a reinfection.

If you have chronic yeast infections and you are taking birth control pills, try going off the pill. This helps some women but not others. On the other hand, the IUD may be associated with chronic bacterial infections. Sometimes the only way to find out if your IUD is causing vaginitis is to have it removed.

Here are some tips to help prevent vaginitis:

1. Be sure to clean the inside folds of the vulva where bacteria are likely to grow. Keep the vulva as dry as possible since infection thrives on moisture and heat. This means avoiding nylon-crotch pantyhose, panty girdles, tight pants or jeans, and other tightfitting clothing as much as possible. Wear cotton rather than synthetic (nylon, rayon, etc.) underwear, or wear underpants that have at least a cotton crotch.
2. Avoid strong detergent soaps and feminine hygiene deodorants and sprays. Allergic reactions may occur.
3. After a bowel movement, wipe toward the back, away from the vagina, to avoid carrying bacteria or yeast into the vagina.
4. Avoid the unnecessary use of antibiotics, especially for colds. If antibiotics are prescribed and you tend to get yeast infections, ask your doctor to prescribe a vaginal antifungal agent as well.
5. A diet low in carbohydrates and sweets

Table 114 TREATMENT OF VAGINAL INFECTIONS (VAGINITIS)

Type of Infection	Typical Drugs to Treat This Infection	Minimum Treatment Period	Comment
Monilia (yeast)	Femstat (vaginal cream)	3 days	Longer treatment periods than the "minimum" may be necessary when infection is severe or chronic. In some cases, treatment may last two or more weeks.
	Gyne-Lotrimin (vaginal cream or tablets)	7 days	
	Monistat 3 (vaginal tablets)	3 days	
	Monistat 7 (vaginal cream or tablets)	7 days	When vaginal tablets are used, Mycolog cream or one of the vaginal creams listed are sometimes applied to the vulva (outer vagina) as well.
	Mycelex 7 (vaginal cream or tablets)	7 days	
	Mycelex G-500 mg (500 mg vaginal tablet)	1 day	Femstat 3, Gyne-Lotrimin, Monistat 7, and Mycelex 7 are now available over-the-counter. Some of these products come with prefilled, disposable applicators.
	Terazol 3 (vaginal cream or tablets)	3 days	
	Terazol 7 (vaginal cream)	7 days	
	Vagistat (vaginal ointment)	1 day	
	Mycolog (cream or ointment) or Mytrex (cream or ointment)	several days-2 weeks	
Trichomonas ("trich")	Flagyl (pills)* (relief of symptoms sometimes helped by certain vaginal preparations—see Table 115)	1 or 7 days (1 day regime uses higher dosage)	Avoid alcohol—interacts with Flagyl to cause vomiting. Partner should also be treated. Avoid Flagyl in pregnancy.
Bacterial Vaginosis	Cleocin (pills or cream)	7 days	Cleocin may sometimes cause severe diarrhea. Cleocin cream should be available soon.
	Flagyl (pills)*	7 days	Flagyl—see comments above under trichomonas infections.
	Metrogel (gel)	5 days	Partner may need to be treated if infection persists after you have been treated.
Atrophic (estrogen-deficiency related) (For information on oral estrogen therapy for atrophic vaginitis, see Chapter 27.)	Estrace (vaginal cream) Ogen (vaginal cream) Ortho Dienestrol cream Premarin (vaginal cream)	variable (at least 1 week)	All of these drugs contain estrogen and should be avoided if you might be pregnant or if you have had breast cancer. Less estrogen is absorbed with vaginal as opposed to oral products; however, the same precautions apply (see Chapter 27).

* Other equivalent brands include Metryl, Satric, and Protostat.

may help cut down on yeast infections by reducing the amount of yeast in the large intestine. This reservoir of yeast may be a source of reinfection. Avoiding constipation, which also allows intestinal yeast to flourish, is important for women with chronic infections.

6. Avoid using tampons for 12 hours or more as bacterial growth and infection is more likely.

Table 115 COMMON SINGLE-INGREDIENT DOUCHES*

Brand Name	Ingredient	Use
Betadine Disposable Medicated Douche	Povidone-iodine	Disposable units.
Betadine Medicated Douche	Povidone-iodine	Use with douche bag or bulb syringe which you supply.
Massengill	Vinegar	Disposable bottles.
Massengill Medicated	Povidone-iodine	Disposable bottles.
Summer's Eve	Vinegar	Disposable units.

* Available without prescription for relief of minor vaginal irritation or itching or occasionally to supplement primary treatment of vaginitis (due to yeast, bacteria, Trichomonas, or "nonspecific" causes). Avoid douching during pregnancy.

CHAPTER 88

Vaginal Lump

A lump in the vaginal area is a fairly common but upsetting finding, especially when the cause is unknown. Be assured that over 99% of vaginal lumps are benign. Most lumps are painless and are usually discovered inadvertently. Sometimes a woman or her sex partner feels the cervix for the first time and mistakes this part of the anatomy for a tumor.

Small, soft, nontender masses, usually no larger than a grape, are likely to be *retention cysts*. These fluid-filled solitary growths may occur anywhere within the vagina or vulva where glands are found; they are formed when gland ducts opening into the vagina or vulva are blocked. A vaginal cyst may also result from previous episiotomy repair (sewing up of the cut made at childbirth). Retention cysts must be distinguished from hair follicle infections, which are solitary tender areas that often drain intermittently and usually subside in a few days.

A larger type of cyst originating from one of the Bartholin's glands is found at the base of the vagina and typically measures 1 to 2 inches in diameter (see Figure 53). Like retention cysts, Bartholin's cysts are soft and nontender, but they have a much greater tendency to become infected and form an abscess.

Another cause of vaginal lumps is vaginal wall hernias called *cystoceles* and *rectoceles* (see Chapter 28). Cystoceles occur in the front vaginal wall whereas rectoceles are found in the back vaginal wall. These bulges are common in women who have given birth to several large babies; the result of such births is a stretching of the muscles supporting the vagina, bladder, and rectum. Associated symptoms may include vaginal pressure or ache, difficulty emptying the bladder, urinary stress incontinence, difficulty with elimination, or difficulty with penetration during intercourse.

Occasionally venereal warts, called *condylomata* (see Chapter 24), are responsible for the complaint of vaginal lumps. These lumps occur singularly or in groups as wartlike growths rarely larger than the tip of a pencil. Of all the vaginal lumps discussed here, condylomata are the only ones that increase in size and number during pregnancy.

In the postpartum period, the most common cause of vaginal lumps is painful complications of the episiotomy repair, including blood clot formation (hematoma) and infection.

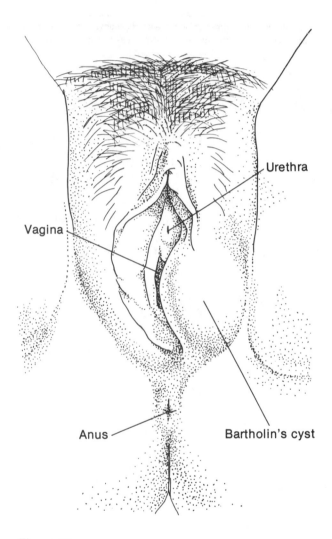

Figure 53
Blockage of the Bartholin's gland on either side of the vulva may result in the formation of a painless cyst. If the cyst becomes infected and forms an abscess, surgery may be required to drain the abscess.

What Medical Care Can Do

The pelvic examination readily distinguishes the causes of the vaginal lumps mentioned. Occasionally a biopsy is done under local anesthesia if a cancerous lump is suspected, but finding a lump that is cancerous is uncommon.

Small cysts rarely require treatment unless they cause pain during intercourse or chronic discomfort. If removal is necessary, it is usually done under local anesthesia in the office. Bartholin's cysts often need to be drained if they become enlarged or infected. Because of the high recurrence rate even after drainage of Bartholin's cysts, a more extensive procedure in the operating room is sometimes necessary.

Condylomata will need to be treated with various chemicals, creams, cautery, or laser surgery (see Chapter 24).

What You Can Do (Self Care)

To begin with, use a mirror to examine yourself. Is the lump tender or leaking pus? Report any change or enlargement of a vaginal growth to your doctor. Painful inflammation of hair follicles, episiotomies, or Bartholin's glands responds to hot tub baths, which reduce pain and swelling. These infections may then drain on their own without need for medical treatment.

A cystocele and a rectocele appear as a swelling of the front and back vaginal wall, respectively, and become visibly enlarged when you strain down. These protrusions require surgery only when symptoms are severe. Cystoceles and rectoceles are less likely to develop or become worse if you maintain optimum weight, avoid strenuous lifting, and prevent chronic cough such as is associated with heavy cigarette smoking.

VAGINAL LUMP

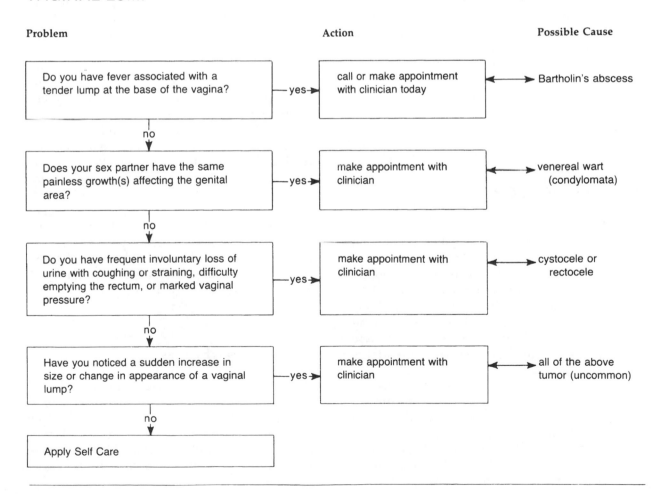

Problem	Action	Possible Cause
Do you have fever associated with a tender lump at the base of the vagina?	—yes→ call or make appointment with clinician today	Bartholin's abscess
↓ no		
Does your sex partner have the same painless growth(s) affecting the genital area?	—yes→ make appointment with clinician	venereal wart (condylomata)
↓ no		
Do you have frequent involuntary loss of urine with coughing or straining, difficulty emptying the rectum, or marked vaginal pressure?	—yes→ make appointment with clinician	cystocele or rectocele
↓ no		
Have you noticed a sudden increase in size or change in appearance of a vaginal lump?	—yes→ make appointment with clinician	all of the above tumor (uncommon)
↓ no		
Apply Self Care		

CHAPTER 89

Weight Gain and Weight Loss

In a society which stigmatizes being overweight, some women take great risks to follow fashion's dictate to look thin by going on crash diets or participating in the latest fad diet. Many of these often unusual dieting techniques may be deceptively effective at first, because they get rid of body water rather than fat stores. The water rapidly reaccumulates, however, once you return to normal eating patterns. *Yo-yo dieting*—the cycle of losing and gaining weight over and over—may be harmful according to recent research. In fact, it is estimated that less than 6% of all weight-reduction techniques are both safe and effective. The reality is: to lose weight, you must eat less or exercise more, or both.

Excessive Weight Gain

Obesity, defined as being 20% over your ideal weight, is the number one nutrition problem in the United States today. Women consistently outnumber men two to one in obesity and exceed men in amount of weight gained. In a 1995 study involving middle-aged women, body weight and mortality from all causes were found to be directly correlated. Even women who were slightly overweight showed increased mortality over lean women.

Weight guidelines for American adults are currently being revised by the U.S. Department of Health and Human Services. The new height and weight table will apply to both men and women, but will no longer consider a weight gain in middle age as "normal." This reflects current research that being overweight adds to your risk of developing heart disease, diabetes, and certain cancers.

Proposed guidelines by the federal government (and currently being used by many medical professionals) will translate recommended weights into a recommended body mass index (BMI) of about 18.9 to 24.9 for men and women of all heights and ages (you calculate the BMI by multiplying weight in pounds by 700 and dividing the result by the square of your height in inches). Current research indicates that weight-related health problems will start to show up when your BMI exceeds 25. Some health professionals define obesity for women as a BMI that exceeds 27.3.

Psychological factors often impede attempts at weight loss. Women who have dieted successfully and then regained the lost weight may experience an intense negative sense of their own worth or may feel hopelessly out of control in managing their weight. On the other hand, women who are depressed or under stress may resort to overindulgence as a means of coping, even though this strategy is self-defeating.

Not everyone slightly overweight needs to go on a diet. Most slightly overweight women (that is, less than 20% over ideal body weight) are not a medical risk as a result of their weight. Chronic or yo-yo dieting is not only unnecessary and frustrating among the slightly overweight, but might ultimately result in a net weight gain. For some women, losing a few additional pounds to reach an ideal weight may be next to impossible. In such women, the cause of overweight is not necessarily overeating in the first place but rather a genetic tendency toward a lower metabolism or increased formation of fatty tissue. Sometimes it is best to accept your weight and concentrate on exercise to "firm up." Not everyone can diet and become extremely thin—your body may just not be built for it.

Excessive Weight Loss

The problem of weight loss is much less common than that of weight gain. Any unplanned weight loss amounting to 10% or more of your usual weight over three to six months could well be due to a medical problem. Although the clinician must rule out the possibility of serious illnesses, such as cancer or diabetes, more often

Table 116 SUGGESTED WEIGHTS FOR HEIGHTS*

Height (without shoes)		Weight (without clothing)					
		Low		Average		High	
Feet & Inches	m**	lb	kg**	lb	kg**	lb	kg**
5'	1.52	100	45	109	50	118	54
5'1"	1.55	104	47	112	51	121	55
5'2"	1.57	107	49	115	52	125	57
5'3"	1.60	110	50	118	54	128	58
5'4"	1.63	113	51	122	55	132	60
5'5"	1.65	116	53	125	57	135	61
5'6"	1.67	120	55	129	59	139	63
5'7"	1.70	123	56	132	60	142	65
5'8"	1.73	126	57	136	62	146	66
5'9"	1.75	130	59	140	64	151	69
5'10"	1.78	133	60	144	65	156	71
5'11"	1.80	137	62	148	67	161	73
6'	1.83	141	64	152	69	166	75

* From *The Healthy Approach to Slimming*, American Medical Association, 1978.
** A meter (m) = 39.37 inches. A kilogram (kg) = 2.2 pounds (lb).

sudden weight loss results from a change in eating habits that, in turn, results from nervousness, anxiety, or depression.

Eating Disorders

Eating disorders—anorexia nervosa, bulimia, chronic overeating—result from maladaptive assumptions concerning food and weight gain. Those with eating disorders do not recognize emotions as valid; such people usually have low self-esteem and distorted perceptions about their weight and body image. Eating disorders usually develop around the age of puberty but may not be recognized until later in adulthood.

In anorexia and bulimia (see Chapter 80), low weight is perceived as crucial for self-esteem. The anorexic controls food intake to the point where weight loss is very great (losing usually at least 20% of original body weight) and menstruation may stop. The anorexic may become so malnourished that she requires hospitalization.

Treatment of both anorexia and bulimia requires medical evaluation of the patient's nutritional status as well as individual counseling. Peer support groups and group psychotherapy are also helpful after initial treatment. Members benefit from role modeling by those who have successfully overcome their eating disorders. Treatment for any eating disorder usually involves a period of several years.

Resource

For an information packet on eating disorders, send a self-addressed, stamped envelope to:

National Eating Disorders Organization (NEDO)
Laureate Hospital
6655 S. Yale Avenue
Tulsa, Oklahoma 74136

Excessive Weight Gain During Pregnancy

A gain of more than 20% over ideal weight for height is excessive. Weight gain should not be equated with good nutrition. Obesity may result from eating calorically rich but nutritionally poor food such as pastries, potato chips, and sweet drinks. On the other hand, excessive weight gain sometimes occurs as a result of physiologic fluid retention in women eating well-balanced diets.

A weight gain of two to five or more pounds in one week is due largely to fluid. It takes an extra thousand calories a day to gain just two pounds a week from food overindulgence alone. Sudden fluid retention of more than five pounds in one week—a common finding in toxemia (high blood pressure during pregnancy)—warrants a call to your physician. Lesser amounts of weight increase are usually due mostly to an increased amount of normal fluid retention. Fluid is eliminated in the first week postpartum when an average weight loss of twenty pounds occurs. The remaining weight loss normally takes approximately three months.

Markedly excessive weight gain (that is, thirty-five to fifty pounds) increases the risk of developing high blood pressure or diabetes during pregnancy. Furthermore, in women who weigh close to two hundred pounds, the risk of the delivery itself, especially by cesarean section, is increased. In addition, postpartum bleeding, anesthesia complications, and vaginal tearing from childbirth are more likely to occur.

Too Little Weight Gain During Pregnancy

Some women delivering healthy babies gain only ten to twelve pounds each pregnancy. However, a gain of less than 15% of ideal weight for height often results from chronic illness, a nutritionally deficient diet, or severe vomiting during early pregnancy, all of which use up protein stores. During the last six months of pregnancy, weight loss or gain of less than two pounds per month puts the fetus at risk for low birth weight. Toxemia is actually more common among women who gain too little weight than for those who gain too much. Subnormal weight gain is associated with closely spaced pregnancies and is more frequent among adolescents for whom prepregnancy nutrition is often inadequate.

What Medical Care Can Do

The treatment of overweight or obesity in the nonpregnant woman is basically up to the woman's own resourcefulness, although her physician should check her blood pressure and check her urine for sugar to screen for diabetes. Many physicians have difficulty dealing with obese patients, partly because nutrition often receives minimal attention in medical training.

Partly because of the demand for weight loss, this area of health care has attracted more than its share of unproven remedies and, at times, outright quackery. The use of hormones such as thyroid in otherwise healthy women and hormone injections containing HCG (human chorionic gonadotropin) has no medical basis in the treatment of weight loss. The consumer should be aware of weight loss clinics that promise quick results and is better advised to stay with established weight control groups, such as Weight Watchers, or to consult a registered dietitian.

The use of diet pills remains controversial, although their use on a limited basis and within a general program of nutritional counseling and exercise has received increasing medical credibility recently. Most of these pills are related to the amphetamines and all are restricted drugs that may be habit-forming. Among those with lesser potential for abuse are diet pills containing phentermine, such as Adipex-P and Fastin. Fenfluramine (Pondimin), a similar drug, differs somewhat from the other prototype diet pills and appears to produce more central nervous system depression than stimulation. The use of diet pills, including their side effects, should be carefully discussed with your physician, but these products may be of some benefit in short-term treatment of obesity.

For some women, a medically supervised, very low calorie (VLC) diet may be considered. Unlike the "liquid protein" diets popular in the 1970s, the VLC diets of the 1990s have two built-in safety features: medical supervision and the use of high-quality protein, which appears to make such diets safer. VLC diets have become quite popular because of their ability to produce rapid weight loss; however, it is not yet clear whether the weight will stay off long-term. Unfortunately, early studies have indicated that about 70% of weight loss on VLC diets is gained back within two years. Still, VLC diets offer women who are substantially overweight (at least 20 to 30% over ideal body weight, usually representing an excess of fifty pounds or more) an opportunity to lose weight rapidly. The better programs also include an educational component and some form of behavioral modification to reinforce good eating and exercise habits. To be successful, a total maintenance program after the weight loss is of critical importance.

VLC diets are marketed under programs such as Health Management Resources, Medibase, Medifast, and Optifast. Typically, these diet programs are divided into three phases, with the first phase consisting of twelve weeks of 800 calories or less per day in the form of a liquid formula taken three to five times a day. Medical screening usually includes an EKG, chest X-ray, and blood tests. Contraindications to VLC diets may include recent heart attack, diabetes, serious liver disease, and pregnancy. Side effects may include fatigue, constipation, dizziness, and hair loss. In the second phase, lasting two weeks to four months, calories are gradually increased through both food and a liquid supplement. The third phase, maintenance, may be optional but is the most important part of the program because it determines whether modified eating habits will be sustained in the future. During the maintenance phase, which should last at least twelve months, periodic behavioral-modification classes begun earlier in the program continue.

VLC programs are expensive: they may easily cost more than $500 per month when all costs are included. Insurance coverage is variable and not likely to pay for the entire program. Yet, for some women who have been unsuccessful with previous diets, such programs may be of such medical benefit as to outweigh the costs involved. Some commercial programs, such as NutraSystems and Jenny Craig, provide packaged meals and individual counseling. Other programs, like Weight Watchers, use a more gradual approach to weight loss along with group support, and avoid prepared food supplements. In either case the greatest challenge arises when you leave the program and are on your own again. It's easy to find yourself resorting to "old eating habits." Remember that successful dieting means a complete change of eating style, which is difficult at best. Be certain to use all the educational and emotional resources available to you.

The clinican's evaluation of weight loss in the nonpregnant woman can involve numerous tests and X-rays unless there are accompanying symptoms which point to a specific cause, such as diabetes. If you have fever, anemia, or loss of appetite unassociated with nervousness or depression, hospitalization is sometimes necessary.

For weight loss that can be classified as anorexic, the woman must first be treated for possible medical problems, and then she may require one of various alternative psychological therapies.

The pregnant woman's weight is carefully monitored. During prenatal visits, the clinician determines fetal growth by measuring the height of the uterus (see Figure 15 in Chapter 16) and by assessing weight gain. Inadequate weight gain may be associated with abnormal fetal growth (see Chapter 16). If you have gained too quickly, the doctor will screen for hypertension by testing your urine for protein and checking your blood pressure. High blood pressure in pregnancy (see Chapter 20) cannot be prevented or treated by restricting calories. Medical therapy consists of bed rest and occasionally drugs to control blood pressure. Again, in the area of weight gain, most of the treatment is up to you.

What You Can Do (Self Care)

If unplanned weight loss is associated with depression or nervousness, refer to Chapters 62 and 81 for suggestions for self care. Otherwise, consultation with your physician is advisable.

Self-treatment of overweight and obesity means recognizing that a tendency to be overweight will require lifetime changes in eating patterns. Your goal should be to establish a healthful eating plan which you can stick to permanently. The best way to lose weight is to establish a life style in which you eat less and exercise more. Completely avoid the use, for the purpose of losing weight, of diet drugs, including amphetamines, thyroid, hormone shots (for example, HCG), and water pills. These drugs are unsafe when used to lose weight, and they interfere with a healthy change of dietary habits. Recently advertised "starch inhibitors" and "fat burners" have not been carefully investigated to prove their effectiveness.

Concerning a weight-loss diet, the amount you eat is sometimes more important than the specific kinds of food you eat. You can get fat

WEIGHT GAIN

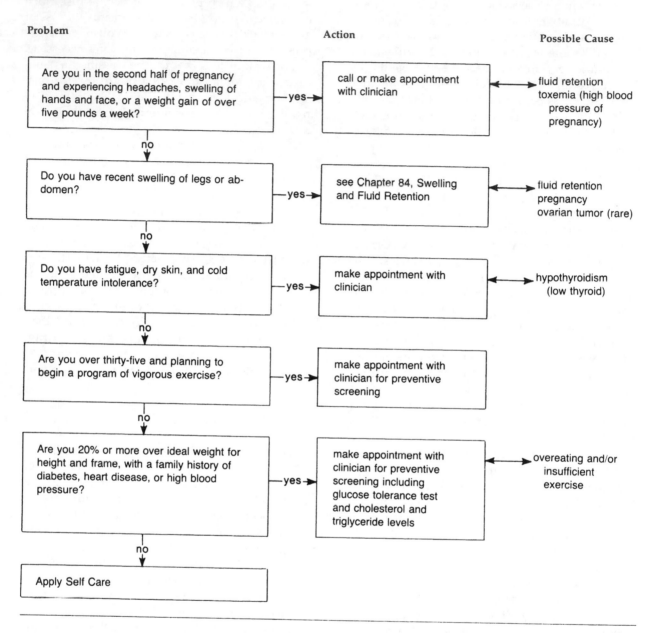

Problem	Action	Possible Cause
Are you in the second half of pregnancy and experiencing headaches, swelling of hands and face, or a weight gain of over five pounds a week?	—yes→ call or make appointment with clinician	← fluid retention toxemia (high blood pressure of pregnancy)
↓ no		
Do you have recent swelling of legs or abdomen?	—yes→ see Chapter 84, Swelling and Fluid Retention	← fluid retention pregnancy ovarian tumor (rare)
↓ no		
Do you have fatigue, dry skin, and cold temperature intolerance?	—yes→ make appointment with clinician	← hypothyroidism (low thyroid)
↓ no		
Are you over thirty-five and planning to begin a program of vigorous exercise?	—yes→ make appointment with clinician for preventive screening	
↓ no		
Are you 20% or more over ideal weight for height and frame, with a family history of diabetes, heart disease, or high blood pressure?	—yes→ make appointment with clinician for preventive screening including glucose tolerance test and cholesterol and triglyceride levels	← overeating and/or insufficient exercise
↓ no		
Apply Self Care		

on a high-protein diet, for instance, if you eat too much, since excess calories can be converted to glucose and stored as fat. Most successful weight-loss diets are designed to have you eat smaller quantities of most of the foods you are presently eating. You need to retrain your appetite to be satisfied with less food in the interest of your future health. If you find yourself feeling starved on a diet, then suddenly binge eating (eating large amounts of food at one time) to relieve your feelings of hunger, then your diet may be too low in calories or carbohydrates. If you frequently feel the need to vomit after binge eating, contact your clinician as frequent vomiting can have harmful physiological effects. (See Chapter 80).

For most women, it is unrealistic to expect a weight loss by dietary measures alone since a major part of overweight and obesity is due to low energy expenditure. Certain activities expend more calories than others. For example, running and swimming burn up about twice as many calories as walking or playing golf (see Table 90 in Chapter 49). Exercise should be regular and vigorous as opposed to occasional and strenuous. Duration of activity is more important than the exertion put into it. In tennis, for example, activity is intermittent, involving only a fraction of the total game-playing time. You will burn fewer calories in this instance as compared to a sport where activity is continuous. Women over thirty-five who are about to start an exercise program should first have a medical examination.

Nutrition research tells us that gradual weight loss is far more likely to be maintained than rapid weight loss. A realistic goal is to lose one or, at the most, two pounds per week. There are 3500 calories in each pound of stored fat; so you need to consume 500 fewer calories each day to lose one pound a week. Once you attain your ideal weight in pounds, multiplying this weight by 15 gives the number of calories you need each day to maintain this weight. The number 15 refers to the number of calories per pound of body weight needed by a woman who leads a moderately active life in order to keep her weight the same; this total will vary somewhat depending on the amount of exercise the woman engages in.

If on your present diet you are maintaining your weight (that is, not gaining or losing) and you want to determine how many calories a weight-loss diet for you should contain, do the following:

1. First estimate the number of calories presently in your diet. To do this, keep a record of everything you eat, including the amounts, over a period of several days or a week and, using a calorie counter, add up the calories. Divide the total by the number of days.
2. Then subtract 500 calories per day. This reduction in calories will allow for a weight loss of about one pound a week if you maintain your same physical activity level.

Your new diet should allow for a variety of foods from the five basic food groups (see Table 87 in Chapter 48). A 1300-calorie diet plan is shown in Table 117. The number of calories shown are average amounts. You can vary the foods and servings as long as you make your choices in the right proportion from each food group and you do not exceed the total number

Table 117 1300-CALORIE DIET PLAN, BASED ON THE BASIC FOOD GROUPS

	Food Group*	Calories**
Breakfast	Fruit	80
	Bread-Cereal	70
	Milk	90
		240
Mid-Morning	Bread-Cereal	70
Lunch	Fruit	40
	Vegetable	50
	Bread-Cereal	70
	Meat	140
		300
Mid-Afternoon	Fruit	40
	Milk	90
		130
Dinner	Vegetable	80
	Bread-Cereal	70
	Meat	210
		360
Evening	Bread-Cereal	70
	Fruit-Vegetable	40
	Milk	90
		200
Total Calories for Day		1300

  * See Table 87 for examples of foods from each group.
 ** Calories from protein: 325 (25%)
    Calories from carbohydrate: 728 (56%)
    Calories from fat: 247 (19%)

of calories. For example: for breakfast you could have, for the "fruit" choice, about 6 oz. of orange juice or a small banana; for dinner, for the "bread-cereal" choice, you could have a slice of bread or a little less than half a cup of cooked spaghetti. In general, a diet of 1200 calories or more does not require vitamin supplementation in healthy women. Diets below 1000 calories per day may leave you tired or vulnerable to illness.

Eat regular meals, eat slowly, scale down portions, and avoid high-calorie snacks. Learn the amount of calories in *everything* you eat. There are many books on the market that give the calorie content of hundreds of basic foods, and some books list the foods by brand name. Don't worry about small differences in calorie values among similar amounts of the same food. Remember, however, that processing often changes the total calorie count for some foods; for example, canned fruits packed in a heavy syrup have more calories than either juice-packed fruits, with no sugar added, or the same fresh fruits. (See Chapter 48 for more information about nutrition.)

Pregnancy is not a time to diet, especially during the last half, which is a critical time for fetal brain development. During this time, inadequate protein or carbohydrate intake may be harmful to the intellectual development of the fetus. Women who are markedly overweight prior to pregnancy, however, may need to limit their weight gain to fifteen to twenty-five pounds (see Chapter 16).

Resources

The following are resources for diet groups; write for information about groups near you, or look in your telephone directory.

Overeaters Anonymous
383 Van Ness Avenue, Suite 1601
Torrance, California 90501

Weight Watchers International
500 N. Broadway
Jericho, New York 11753

References for Section Eleven

American College of Obstetricians and Gynecologists *Technical Bulletin* 100. Urinary incontinence, Jan 1987.

American College of Obstetricians and Gynecologists *Technical Bulletin* 212. Early pregnancy loss, Sep 1995.

American College of Obstetricians and Gynecologists *Technical Bulletin* 150. Ectopic pregnancy, Dec 1990.

American College of Obstetricians and Gynecologists *Technical Bulletin* 135. Vulvovaginitis, Nov 1989.

American College of Obstetricians and Gynecologists *Technical Bulletin* 134. Dysfunctional uterine bleeding, Oct 1989.

American College of Obstetricians and Gynecologists *Technical Bulletin* 68. Dysmenorrhea, Mar 1983.

American College of Obstetricians and Gynecologists *Technical Bulletin* 129. Chronic pelvic pain, June 1989.

Impact of perfectionism and need for approval on the brief treatment of depression: The National Institute of Mental Health treatment of depression collaborative research program revisited. *Journal of Consulting and Clinical Psychology* 63(1):125–132, 1995.

Over-the-counter H_2-receptor antagonists for heartburn. *The Medical Letter on Drugs and Therapeutics* 37(960), Oct 27, 1995.

Skaer, B., Therapeutic use of sumatriptan in the treatment of migraine. *The Female Patient* 20:19–28, Aug 1995.

Valaitis, S. Surgery for genuine stress incontinence *Contemporary OB/GYN* 65–80.

National Women's Health Report. Vaginal yeast infections *Alternative Therapies* 4, May/June 1995.

To douche or not to douche? Many gynecologists do not agree. OB Gyn News, *Gynecology* 6a, May 15, 1995.

Macguire, J. *Your Guide to a Better Memory*. New York: Berkley Books, 1995.

Poon, L., ed. *Clinical Memory Assessment of Older Adults*. American Psychological Association, 1986.

Gruetzner, H. *Alzheimer's*. New York: John Wiley and Sons, Inc., 1992.

Popkess, S. Holistic self-care model for permanent weight control. *Journal of Holistic Nursing* 11(4):41–55. Dec 1993.

St. Jeor, S. The role of weight management in the health of women. *Journal of the American Dietetic Association* 93(9):1007–1012, Sep 1993.

French, S. Consequences of dieting to lose weight: effects on physical and mental health. *Health Psychology* 13(3):195–212, 1994.

Manson J. Body weight and mortality among women. *The New England Journal of Medicine* 333(11):677–685, Sep 14, 1995.

Adler, D. Using drugs appropriately in Crohn's disease. *Drug Therapy* 49–61, Mar 1989.

Mickley, D. Evaluating common eating disorders—10 questions to ask your patient. *The Female Patient* 13: 33–36, Aug 1988.

Julian, T. Chronic pelvic pain, Part I: workup and diagnosis. *The Female Patient* 14(2):28–50, Feb 1989.

Julian, T. Chronic pelvic pain, Part II: treatment strategies. *The Female Patient* 14(3):19–37, Mar 1989.

Sand, P. Cryosurgery versus dilatation and massage for the treatment of recurrent urethral syndrome. *Journal of Reproductive Medicine* 34(8):499–504, Aug 1989.

Fantel, J. Common urologic problems: a management update. *The Female Patient* 14:31–42, Jan 1989.

Soper, D. Cystitis: timesaving protocol for diagnosis and management. *The Female Patient* 14:67–79, Apr 1989.

Fletcher, S. Interstitial cystitis: detection and management. *Medical Aspects of Human Sexuality* 22(11):59–67, Nov 1988.

Bent, A. Urethral syndrome: diagnosis and management. *Medical Aspects of Human Sexuality* 84–86, Mar 1989.

Eschenbach, T. Advances in diagnostic testing for vaginitis and cervicitis. *Journal of Reproductive Medicine* 34(8):555–565, Aug 1989.

Pelosi, M. Vaginitis: update on diagnosis and treatment. *The Female Patient* 14:84–98, May 1989.

Speroff, L. *Clinical Gynecologic Endocrinology and Infertility*, 4th ed. Baltimore: Williams and Wilkins, 1989.

Rakel, R., ed. *Conn's Current Therapy*. Philadelphia: Saunders, 1989.

Tretinoin (retin-A) for aging skin. *The Medical Letter on Drugs and Therapeutics* 30, July 1988.

Goodman, C. Relieving back pain in women. *The Female Patient* 13:17–27, Feb 1988.

Gant, N. Recurrent spontaneous abortion. *Williams Obstetrics*, 17th ed. Supplement 21: Dec/Jan 1989.

Clark, S. Bleeding during early pregnancy. *The Female Patient* 14:71–82, Feb 1989.

Leach, R. Modern management of ectopic pregnancy. *Journal of Reproductive Medicine* 34(5):324–338, May 1989.

Clark, S. Bleeding during late pregnancy. *The Female Patient* 14:89–102, Apr 1989.

Smith, K. Hypertension in women: a management guide for the OB/GYN. *The Female Patient* 14:19–30, July 1989.

Jones, J. The Epstein-Barr "chronic fatigue" syndrome: evaluation guidelines. *The Female Patient* 13:60–67, Sep 1988.

Nashel, D. Standard therapy for rheumatic arthritis. *Drug Therapy* 111–117, June 1989.

Lieberman, M. The role of self-help groups in helping patients and families cope with cancer. *CA-A Cancer Journal for Clinicians* 38(3):162–168, May/Jun 1988.

Adler, T. What you should know about ulcerative colitis. *Drug Therapy* 62–66, Feb 1989.

Mead, P. Vaginitis that fails to respond to treatment. *Contemporary OB/GYN* 73–88, Jan 1989.

Caprini, J. Varicose veins: an approach to treatment decisions. *The Female Patient* 13(10):49–61, Oct 1988.

DeBenedette, V. A brief guide to popular weight loss programs. *Your Patient and Fitness* 3(1):12–15, July/Aug 1989.

APPENDICES

APPENDIX A

Health History Profile

The Health History Profile is explained more fully in Chapter 4. Be certain to mark those items that apply to you and, when you see your clinician, be sure to mention them.

1. **Current Problems**—be sure to mention if you have noticed any of the following recently:

   pelvic pain
   irregular bleeding
   vaginal discharge or itching
   breast pain, lump, or discharge
   hot flashes or night sweats
   loss of urine with coughing or sneezing
   fatigue, weakness, or fainting
   frequent or severe headaches
   chronic cough
   chest pain or palpitations

   shortness of breath
   swelling of hands, feet, or ankles
   frequent, painful, or bloody urination
   painful intercourse
   loss of sexual desire
   inability to reach orgasm or difficulty in reaching orgasm
   indigestion, stomach trouble, or ulcer————s
   nausea, vomiting, or bloating
   diarrhea or constipation
   hemorrhoids, rectal itching or bleeding

2. **Menstrual History**

   Started at age _____ Length of cycle _____ days (from start of one period to start of next period)
   Number of days period usually lasts _____ Date last normal menstrual period started _____
   Flow: light _____ medium _____ heavy _____ excessive _____
   Periods regular? yes _____ no _____
   Have you started menopause? yes _____ no _____
   Pain or cramps? yes _____ no _____ sometimes _____
   Do you ever bleed between periods? yes _____ no _____

3. **Contraceptive History**

   Current method (type and dose of birth control pill, if applicable) _____
   _____
   Previous method(s) _____
   _____

4. **Pregnancy History**—include miscarriages and abortions

Year	Length of pregnancy	Baby's weight at birth	Girl or boy	Hours of labor	Hospital (name & city)	Was anesthesia used?

Mention any of these complications:

1) prenatal hospitalizations such as for toxemia (high blood pressure in pregnancy)
2) special prenatal tests such as oxytocin stress test
3) premature births or stillbirths
4) prolonged labors or cesarean sections
5) newborn complications including congenital abnormalities or need for newborn intensive care
6) postpartum complications requiring antibiotics, blood transfusions, or prolonged hospital stay

5. **Previous Conditions**—mention if you have ever had any of the following:

high blood pressure	anemia	asthma, bronchitis, or pneumonia
heart disease	epilepsy	abnormal Pap smear
stroke	migraine headache	infection of female organ
phlebitis or blood clot	hepatitis	ovarian cyst
diabetes	gallbladder disease	fibroid (uterine tumor)
cancer	breast disease	kidney or bladder infection
thyroid disease	German measles (rubella)	

6. **Previous Hospitalizations**—give a review of your previous serious illnesses

	1	2	3
Type of operation or illness			
Date hospitalized			
Name and location (city) of hospital			
Doctor(s)			

7. **Family History**—it is important to mention any family history of the following:

heart disease	breast or uterine cancer	stroke
high blood pressure	twins	diabetes
bleeding disorder	kidney disease	birth defects, including mental retardation and Down syndrome (formerly called Mongolism)
epilepsy	thyroid problems	

8. **Medication History**

Drug allergies _____

Current medications and dosages _____

_____

APPENDIX B

Glossary

adhesion(s): bands of fibrous tissue that abnormally bind together two body structures. Adhesions within the abdomen may result from previous abdominal surgery or from prior infection, especially involving the pelvic organs.

afterbirth: the placenta and fetal membranes expelled from the uterus after childbirth (see *placenta*).

amniocentesis: a procedure for removing a small amount of amniotic fluid from the uterus during pregnancy. After the skin is numbed with a local anesthetic, a small needle attached to a syringe is inserted into the uterus through the abdomen to obtain the fluid. The fluid may be tested for chromosomal or other genetic abnormalities (usually between sixteen and eighteen weeks) or may be used to assess the fetal condition and gestational age (in late pregnancy). (See Chapters 11 and 20.)

anaphylaxis (or *anaphylactic reaction*): an allergic reaction usually caused by a drug (for example, penicillin), with symptoms ranging from itching and hives to more severe manifestations such as difficult breathing, throat swelling, or loss of consciousness (*anaphylactic shock*). Such reactions characteristically occur within minutes of taking the drug, regardless of dose, and may require immediate medical treatment.

antibody (pl. *antibodies*): a substance formed in the blood in an attempt to counteract or neutralize a foreign body such as a virus. For example, a woman who has had rubella (German measles) develops antibodies which protect her from getting the disease a second time. In other viral infections, such as herpes, antibodies lessen but do not prevent subsequent infections. Rh negative women may develop antibodies after a pregnancy in which the baby is Rh positive. In this case the production of antibodies may be harmful in a subsequent pregnancy (see Chapter 20).

antihistamine(s): a family of drugs found in many prescription and nonprescription cold and hay fever remedies.

atherosclerosis (or *arteriosclerosis*) ("hardening of the arteries"): the aging process within blood vessels, making a person susceptible to heart disease, stroke, and other circulatory disorders.

atypical cells: cells which appear slightly abnormal when studied under a microscope. Such cells may be associated with infection in the cervix (*cervicitis*) or with early precancerous changes in the cervix (*dysplasia*).

barium enema (or *lower GI series*): a procedure for examining the large intestine (colon) by means of X-rays, often obtained to evaluate chronic pelvic pain or bowel problems. An enema and/or laxative is given the night before the X-rays are taken to prepare the colon and make the X-ray picture more distinct. In this procedure the X-ray dye (barium) is introduced by means of a small tube inserted into the rectum. After the procedure, the barium is expelled and usually a laxative is given to help get rid of remaining barium. (See also *GI* and *upper GI series.*)

biopsy: removal of tissue for microscopic diagnosis. Biopsy of the vulva, vagina, cervix, or endometrium can readily be done as an office procedure, usually with minimal discomfort. Breast biopsy, a more extensive procedure than the others mentioned, is usually performed in a hospital, often as an outpatient procedure.

birth canal: the passageway formed during labor by the dilated cervix and the vagina.

Braxton-Hicks contractions: slight uterine cramping or contractions that come and go throughout pregnancy, particularly during the last trimester.

breakthrough bleeding: bleeding, at a time other than a menstrual period, that sometimes results from taking estrogen-containing drugs, including birth control pills.

breast biopsy: see *biopsy.*

carcinoma-in-situ: a cancer which involves only the surface cells and which does not invade the underlying tissue.

catheterization of bladder: placement of a small rubber tube through the urethra and into the bladder to drain urine from the bladder. Catheterization is sometimes necessary during labor or in the first few days after childbirth when bladder emptying may temporarily become difficult. After abdominal or vaginal surgery the catheter, attached to a collection bag, may need to be left in for up to several days (see Chapter 41).

CAT scan (computerized axial tomography): a highly sophisticated, painless procedure that uses a computer to produce two-dimensional X-rays of the body, especially the brain. The test helps to diagnose a variety of conditions, especially tumors.

cauterization: see *cautery of cervix.*

cautery of cervix (cauterization): superficial burning of the lower end of the cervix by means of heat (*electrocautery*) or by freezing (*cryosurgery*). Usually done as treatment for mild to moderate dysplasia or for mild inflammation of the cervix accompanied by vaginal discharge.

CBC: see *complete blood count.*

cervicitis: inflammation or infection of the cervix, sometimes associated with a chronic discharge.

chemotherapy: treatment of cancer or other conditions by the use of special drugs.

chlamydia: a type of bacteria-like microorganism responsible for certain sexually transmitted infections including some cases of nongonococcal urethritis (see Chapter 24).

cholesterol: a fatty substance present in the blood and in certain fatty foods. A high cholesterol level in the blood may make a person susceptible to heart disease. Cholesterol level in the blood may be influenced by heredity and is usually controllable by diet.

chromosomes: structures within cells that contain the genetic material (genes) which determine inherited characteristics (see Chapter 11).

climacteric: the several years preceding menopause when certain physical, emotional, and hormonal changes may occur (see Chapter 26).

colonoscopy: a procedure to examine the entire colon by means of a long, flexible instrument with a built-in lens and light source (colonoscope) that is inserted into the rectum. Colonoscopy may be used instead of an X-ray (barium enema) as an initial test in the evaluation of rectal bleeding, or the procedure may be used in addition to the barium enema when further investigation of a digestive problem or symptom is needed.

colostrum: a thin, white breast discharge that normally precedes the production of breast milk and is secreted from the breast during the last few weeks of pregnancy.

colposcopy: a procedure for looking at and diagnosing abnormalities of the cervix through a special magnifying instrument called a colposcope. In a woman with an abnormal Pap smear this procedure, done in the doctor's office, allows the gynecologist to take a biopsy of the cervix from the most abnormal-appearing area.

complete blood count (CBC): a blood test for evaluation of the blood elements (red blood cells, white blood cells, and platelets). The parts of the CBC known as the *hemoglobin* and *hematocrit* are each a measure of the number of red blood cells. An elevated white blood count is often a sign of infection somewhere in the body, while a low red blood count indicates anemia. A CBC is ordered routinely before major surgery and during most hospital admissions.

condylomata (venereal warts): wartlike growths found on the external genitalia and caused by a sexually transmitted virus (see Chapter 24).

cone biopsy: an operation to remove a cone-shaped segment of tissue from the lower part of the cervix to diagnose the extent of cancerous or precancerous changes (*dysplasia*) (see Chapter 37).

cryosurgery: see *cautery of cervix.*

culdocentesis: a procedure to diagnose the presence of internal bleeding such as from a tubal (ectopic) pregnancy which has ruptured. In this emergency procedure, a needle attached to a syringe is inserted through the upper vagina into the abdominal cavity. The diagnosis is confirmed if blood is withdrawn into the syringe. (See Chapter 54.)

cystitis: bladder infection. Cystitis may cause painful or bloody urination as well as a frequent and urgent need to urinate (see Chapters 85 and 86).

cystocele: a vaginal hernia which causes a bulge in the upper vaginal wall and which becomes more pronounced during any activity involving straining (see Chapters 28 and 85).

cystoscopy: a procedure for looking at the inside of the bladder through a telescopelike instrument called a cystoscope. Cystoscopy is performed by a urologist (doctor specializing in diseases of the urinary system).

D & C (dilatation and curettage): a minor operation involving widening (dilatation) of the cervix opening and curettage (scraping and removing tissue) inside the uterus with a surgical instrument called a curette (see Chapter 42).

decongestants: a family of drugs intended for relief of congestion of the nose, throat, and sinuses due to upper respiratory infections (colds and flu) and certain allergic conditions.

DES (diethylstilbestrol): the term DES refers both to a group of synthetic estrogen-containing drugs and to one of those drugs called diethylstilbestrol (see Chapter 38).

descensus: see *prolapse.*

diabetes: a chronic hormone disorder associated with high blood sugar and sometimes inherited.

dilatation and curettage: see *D & C.*

diuretics: see *water pills.*

diverticulitis: inflammation of the small pockets (diverticula) in the wall of the colon. This condition produces cramping, abdominal pain, and diarrhea (see Chapter 63).

doptone: a device that uses sound waves to allow the clinician to hear the fetal heartbeat. The doptone can reliably pick up the fetal heart sounds by the fifth month of pregnancy and sometimes earlier.

dysplasia: abnormal microscopic appearance of cells obtained by taking a biopsy of the cervix. Although dysplasia may go away by itself in some instances, it can slowly progress over several years, from mild dysplasia to more severe forms of dysplasia or even to cervical cancer if left untreated (see Chapter 37).

ECG: see *electrocardiogram.*

ectopic pregnancy (or *tubal pregnancy*): pregnancy which occurs and develops outside the uterus, usually within one of the Fallopian tubes. Ectopic pregnancies often cause abnormal bleeding or pelvic pain (see Chapters 54 and 83).

edema: fluid retention within tissues, often producing swelling. Sometimes edema is normal as in pregnancy-related leg edema.

EEG: see *electroencephalogram.*

EKG: see *electrocardiogram.*

electrocardiogram (ECG, EKG): a graphic tracing of the electric current associated with contractions of the heart muscle. The ECG is used to diagnose various heart ailments.

electrocautery: see *cautery of cervix.*

electrocoagulation: burning of tissue using an electric current (see *tubal ligation*) (see Chapter 43).

electroencephalogram (EEG): recording of the brain's electrical signals (brain waves). The EEG is used to diagnose various conditions of the nervous system, including brain tumors.

endometrial ablation: a new, still-experimental technique intended as an alternative to hysterectomy as a treatment for persistent menstrual bleeding. The procedure is performed with a hysteroscope, through which is introduced either an electrocautery device or a laser. The hysteroscope is directed into the uterus by way of the vagina, and the uterine lining (endometrium) is cauterized—i.e., burned. This results in scarring, which stops all uterine bleeding either temporarily or permanently.

endometrial aspiration: a procedure for removing cells lining the uterus (see *endometrium*) for diagnostic purposes (see Chapter 40).

endometrial biopsy: a procedure, done in the doctor's office in which tissue lining the uterus (see *endometrium*) is removed for diagnosis (see Chapter 40).

endometrium: the inner lining of the uterus.

episiotomy: the small cut in the perineum which may be made at the time of childbirth to widen the birth canal (see Chapter 19).

estrogen: principal hormone produced by the ovary. Estrogens play an important part in regulating the menstrual cycle and in the growth, development, and maintenance of the entire female reproductive system (see Chapter 3). Synthetic estrogen is used in most birth control pills and in drugs to treat certain symptoms associated with menopause (see Chapter 27).

fetal distress: a sign that the fetal oxygen supply may be less than optimal. Fetal distress in labor indicates the baby could be in danger (although it is often not in danger despite these signs) and may need prompt delivery if the distress is severe (see Chapter 21).

fibroadenoma: a relatively common, painless, benign breast tumor (noncancerous).

fibroids (leiomyomata): muscle tumors of the uterus which are almost always benign (see Chapter 35).

FSH (follicle stimulating hormone): a hormone secreted by the pituitary gland in the brain. By its interactions with hormones made in the ovary, FSH plays an important role in regulating the menstrual cycle (see Chapter 3).

galactorrhea: secretion of milky fluid from the breasts that is unassociated with pregnancy or the postpartum period (see Chapter 57).

gastroenterologist: an internist who subspecializes in diseases of the digestive system.

genes: components of chromosomes containing the genetic material determining inherited characteristics (see Chapter 11).

gestational age: the number of weeks of fetal growth or duration of pregnancy calculated from the last menstrual period. Term pregnancy is approximately 40 weeks. (See Chapter 16.)

GI: gastrointestinal (of the stomach and the intestines). See *barium enema* (lower GI series) and *upper GI series*.

glucose tolerance test (GTT): a series of blood tests obtained over three (or sometimes five) hours to diagnose diabetes or hypoglycemia (low blood sugar) (see Chapter 75).

goiter: a chronic enlargement of the thyroid gland not due to a tumor. Sometimes goiter is associated with excess thyroid hormone production (see *hyperthyroidism*; see Chapters 81 and 82).

HCG (human chorionic gonadotropin): the hormone produced by the placenta in early pregnancy. All pregnancy tests are based upon the detection of this hormone in the urine or blood (see Chapter 16).

hematocrit: see *complete blood count*.

hemoglobin: see *complete blood count*.

high-risk pregnancy: a pregnancy in which one or more conditions exist prior to the pregnancy, or develop during the pregnancy, that place the fetus (and sometimes the mother) at increased risk for complications (see Chapter 20).

hyperthyroidism (overactive thyroid): a condition with various causes in which abnormally high amounts of thyroid hormone are produced. Symptoms include nervousness, loss of weight, palpitations, rapid pulse, trembling, and intolerance to heat. (See Chapters 81 and 82.)

hyperventilation: very rapid or deep breathing which may cause tingling of the face and fingers, dizziness, and fainting.

hypoglycemia: low blood sugar (see Chapter 75). Symptoms include headache, weakness, dizziness, nausea, and nervousness.

hypothyroidism (underactive thyroid): a condition with various causes in which abnormally low amounts of thyroid hormone are produced. Symptoms include dry skin, weight gain, and sluggishness (see Chapter 75).

hysterectomy (total, partial, or radical): surgical removal of the uterus including the cervix. The word *total* before hysterectomy is usually dropped since subtotal hysterectomy, in which the surgeon removes the upper uterus but not the cervix, is rarely performed. When hysterectomy is done without removal of the tubes and ovaries (a separate operation), the procedure is sometimes called *partial hysterectomy*. *Radical hysterectomy* is a more extensive operation performed for cancer of the uterus (endometrium) or cervix in which the upper vagina and nearby pelvic lymph nodes are removed as well as the uterus and cervix.

hysterosalpingogram (HSG): an X-ray of the uterus and tubes showing their inside appearance, including any blockages within these structures (see Chapter 13).

hysteroscopy: a new procedure using a thin, telescopelike instrument similar to the laparoscope for examining the inside of the uterus. Performed in the physician's office or in an outpatient setting, hysteroscopy can be used for evaluation of bleeding problems (sometimes combined with D & C), for infertility evaluation, or for removal of an IUD or of small uterine growths such as polyps and small fibroids.

intravenous pyelogram (IVP): X-rays of the urinary system (kidneys, ureters, and bladder) often obtained to help evaluate pelvic or back pain, bloody urine, chronic kidney infection, or high blood pressure. Shortly before the procedure a dye visible in X-rays is injected into the vein and becomes concentrated in the urinary system minutes later.

jaundice: a yellow coloration of the skin or of the white part of the eyes, usually due to liver damage and the resulting buildup of bile pigments in the blood. Jaundice is usually caused by liver disease but sometimes represents a reaction to drugs.

lactation: the production of breast milk which occurs a few days after childbirth.

laparoscopy: an operation performed through a small incision in the navel. The surgery can be done for diagnosis (for example, to evaluate the cause of pelvic pain) or for tubal sterilization (see Chapter 43).

laparotomy: an operation performed through an incision in the abdomen. The incision is usually four to five inches long except for the mini-laparotomy (see Chapter 43), which involves an incision of less than two inches.

leukorrhea: a white, not necessarily infectious, discharge from the vagina. Some leukorrhea is normally present and usually becomes increased around the time of ovulation.

LH: see *luteinizing hormone.*

linea nigra ("black line"): a line of increased skin pigmentation that develops during pregnancy and extends from the navel to the pubic hairline.

lower GI series: see *barium enema.*

low thyroid: see *hypothyroidism.*

luteinizing hormone (LH): a hormone, produced by the pituitary gland, which helps to regulate the menstrual cycle.

magnetic resonance imaging (MRI—also known as nuclear magnetic resonance): a relatively recent and painless, but expensive, procedure that uses a powerful magnetic field and a computer to create cross-sectional or "slice" pictures of the inside of the body. Unlike the CAT scan, this procedure uses no radiation or contrast dyes and can provide images in any plane or axis. The test is used to diagnose neurological diseases, musculo-skeletal disorders, and especially, in gynecology, to diagnose tumors, infections, and endometriosis.

mammogram: breast X-ray used mainly to help diagnose and screen for breast cancer (see Chapter 34).

mastectomy: one of several types of breast removal operation usually performed for cancer of the breast (see Chapter 34).

meconium: brown coloration of the amniotic fluid (bag of waters) seen during labor and caused by a fetal bowel movement (stool). The presence of meconium in some instances indicates fetal distress (see Chapter 21).

menarche: the first menstrual period of a girl in puberty.

menopause: the time in a woman's life when the ovaries produce decreasing levels of hormones and menstrual periods have ceased for at least one year (see Chapter 26).

mini-laparotomy (or *mini-lap*): a type of sterilization operation performed through a small incision (less than two inches) in the lower abdomen (see Chapter 43).

miscarriage: the expulsion of a fetus from the womb before the fetus is developed enough to survive, usually accompanied by cramping and bleeding (see Chapter 54).

monoclonal antibody: a purified concentration of antibody that reacts with one specific spot or receptor site on a molecule. Such antibodies are used by laboratories to determine the presence and amount of a specific substance, such as human chorionic gonadotropin (HCG), which is measured in pregnancy tests.

myomectomy: an operation on the uterus to remove one or more benign muscle tumors (fibroids) (see Chapter 35).

oophorectomy: an operation to remove one or both ovaries.

osteoporosis: a chronic condition especially common in postmenopausal women in which the calcium in bones gradually becomes depleted and makes the woman susceptible to fractures (see Chapters 27 and 51).

overactive thyroid: see *hyperthyroidism.*

partial hysterectomy: see *hysterectomy.*

perineum: the area between the vulva and rectum (see Chapter 3). An episiotomy (a cut which may be made to widen the birth canal during childbirth) involves a small incision in the perineum (see Chapter 19).

pessary: a device made of rubber or plastic or other synthetic material to lift up and support the uterus. A pessary may be used as an alternative to hysterectomy or other surgery to treat prolapse of the uterus (see Chapter 45).

photon absorptiometry: a test used to screen for osteoporosis by measuring bone density. A light beam is passed through bone (often the radius bone in the forearm) and a detector on the other side measures the beam's intensity as it emerges. A computer converts the photon absorption data and gives bone mineral content in grams per centimeter.

pigmentation: skin coloration. Darkening of the skin (increased pigmentation) in pregnancy often involves the face, nipples, and navel.

placebo: a pill with no active ingredients, given for its suggestive effects. The effects of a placebo, if any, are due to the expectations of the person taking it.

placenta: the organ which supplies oxygen and other nutrients to the fetus. One side of the placenta is attached to the uterus and remains in contact with the mother's circulation while the other side maintains contact with the fetal circulation through the umbilical cord (see *afterbirth*).

postpartum: the six-week time period following childbirth.

procto exam: see *sigmoidoscopy.*

progesterone: a major sex hormone produced by the ovary. This hormone plays an important role in regulating the menstrual cycle and in preparing the uterine lining (endometrium) each month for implantation of a fertilized egg. Progesterone is found in all birth control pills and in some intrauterine devices (IUDs). Progesterone is sometimes given to regulate the menstrual cycle or to treat certain conditions such as endometriosis. In pregnancy, the placenta produces large amounts of progesterone, which plays an important role in maintaining pregnancy.

prognosis: the predicted or expected probable course (outcome) of a disease.

prolapse (of the uterus): a condition in which the uterus has dropped down slightly, compared to its usual position, as a result of weakening of the surrounding muscles. Sometimes as a result of childbirth injuries and especially after menopause, some degree of symptomless uterine prolapse occurs (see Chapter 28).

pyelonephritis: a kidney infection. Unlike a bladder infection (see *cystitis*), kidney infections usually cause fever, chills, and backache (see Chapter 51).

quickening: perception of movement of the fetus beginning around the fifth month of pregnancy.

radical hysterectomy: see *hysterectomy.*

rectocele: a vaginal hernia which causes a bulge in the lower (back) vaginal wall and which becomes more pronounced during any activity involving straining (see Chapter 28).

regional enteritis: a chronic condition in which the small intestine becomes inflamed. This disease is associated with intermittent bouts of diarrhea and abdominal cramping (see Chapter 63).

rooming-in: a hospital procedure allowing for the newborn and mother to share the same room for all or part of the day. This arrangement provides for feeding on demand and gives the mother a chance to care for her baby. Fathers are usually allowed to visit both mother and baby often as well.

salpingectomy: surgical removal of the Fallopian tube. If both tubes are removed, the operation is known as bilateral salpingectomy (unilateral salpingectomy if only one tube is removed).

sedative: a drug that reduces nervousness and anxiety and often produces some drowsiness. Tranquilizers are typical sedatives, but many other types of drugs such as antihistamines found in many cold remedies may have sedative properties (see Chapter 30).

sickle-cell anemia: an inherited type of anemia, mostly affecting black people, in which the blood cells take on a sickle shape and become destroyed more rapidly than normal. Symptoms include episodes of joint and leg pains. A blood test can detect individuals who have or are carriers of this disease.

sigmoidoscopy (or *procto exam, proctological exam*): a procedure for looking at the lining of the lower colon (sigmoid) by means of an instrument with a built-in lens and light source (sigmoidoscope) which is inserted into the rectum.

sonogram: see *sonography.*

sonography (ultrasound): a painless technique using sound waves (as opposed to X-rays) for visualizing internal organs. The resulting picture is called a sonogram. Sonography may be used to diagnose various gynecologic conditions such as ovarian cysts. In the pregnant woman sonography can be very useful in determining gestational age, assessing fetal growth, and diagnosing certain birth defects (see Chapter 16).

spina bifida: a birth defect involving the spinal column, in which part of the spinal cord or the membranes which cover

it may protrude through the spinal column. Spina bifida may be crippling or fatal depending upon the extent and location of the defect in the spinal column. This birth defect may be diagnosed prenatally (see Chapter 11).

stillbirth: the birth of a fetus that is dead prior to delivery, after the twentieth week of pregnancy.

stress test (cardiovascular): a test to assess a person's overall fitness, especially the condition of the heart. The test involves a series of graduated exercises (running in place, etc.) during which the heart's rate and rhythm are measured.

stress test (oxytocin challenge test [OCT]): a test to assess the overall condition of the fetus during pregnancy (see Chapter 20).

Tay-Sachs disease: a hereditary disease, usually fatal in early childhood, found almost exclusively among Jews of central eastern Europe or their descendants. Carriers of this disease, which may cause mental retardation and blindness, may be identified by genetic screening (see Chapter 11).

TENS (transcutaneous electrical nerve stimulation): an electrical device that applies a low-level electrical stimulus to the skin and helps to block painful nerve impulses.

total hysterectomy: see *hysterectomy.*

toxemia: high blood pressure during pregnancy (see Chapter 20).

tubal ligation (or *tubal sterilization*): any operation involving the Fallopian tubes which results in permanent contraception. The tubes may be tied with suture or thread ("ligated"), burned (electrocoagulated), or mechanically blocked with clips or bands (see Chapter 43).

ulcerative colitis: a chronic condition of the large intestine causing symptoms of cramping pain and bouts of bloody diarrhea (see Chapter 63).

underactive thyroid: see *hypothyroidism.*

upper GI series: a procedure for examining the esophagus, stomach, and small intestine by means of a series of X-rays. Flavored barium is drunk just before the X-rays are taken. The barium (an X-ray dye) shows up on the X-ray, outlining the upper digestive tract. This series is often done to evaluate upper abdominal pain or chronic indigestion that may be due to an ulcer.

ureter: one of the two tubes that carry urine from the kidneys to the bladder (see Figure 41).

urethritis: inflammation of the urethra, a condition associated with painful and frequent urination (see Chapters 85 and 86).

urgency incontinence: involuntary loss of urine associated with symptoms of a urinary tract infection, especially the sudden and frequent urge to urinate (see Chapter 28).

urinalysis: analysis of the urine to detect blood, sugar, protein, or other abnormalities. Microscopic examination of the urine to look for white cells (pus) may not be done routinely as part of the urinalysis in routine office checkups unless it is requested.

urinary stress incontinence: involuntary loss of urine when the bladder muscles are stressed as during coughing, sneezing, laughing, running, or other strenuous activity (see Chapter 28).

varicose veins: prominent, sometimes swollen veins usually occurring in the lower extremities. Such veins tend to have weak or improperly functioning valves so that circulation is impaired. Varicose veins may temporarily arise in pregnancy and become worse as a result of pressure from the enlarging uterus against the major veins that return blood from the legs and lower abdomen to the heart (see Chapter 74).

water pills: a class of prescription drugs, known as *diuretics*, which are used to treat high blood pressure, certain heart and kidney ailments, and sometimes simple fluid retention (see Chapter 84).

wet smear (vaginal smear): microscopic evaluation of vaginal secretions. This procedure is usually done to diagnose types of vaginitis (see Chapter 87).

APPENDIX C

Further Reading

General

The New Our Bodies, Ourselves. The Boston Women's Health Book Collective Staff. Peter Smith Publisher, 1996. The first and best-known comprehensive discussion of women's health issues written for the consumer.

The American Medical Association Home Medical Adviser. Random House, 1996. Comprehensive and authoritative general medical reference.

Your Good Health. W. I. Bennett, ed. Harvard University Press, 1989. A guide with good general information, including excellent sections on heart disease, cancer, and aging.

Self Renewal. D. T. Jaffe. Fireside, 1984. Excellent approach to stress management.

Peace, Love, and Healing. B. Siegel. HarperCollins, 1990. Compassionate words from a true healer.

American Cancer Society Cancer Book. A. Holleb, ed. Doubleday, 1992. Another authoritative work.

The New Good Housekeeping Illustrated Guide to Women's Health. K. Cox. Hearst Books, 1995. Good for general health concerns.

The Battered Woman's Survival Guide: Breaking the Cycle. J. Statman and J. Berliner. Taylor Publishing Co., 1995.

The Verbally Abusive Relationship. P. Evens. Bob Adams, Inc., 1992.

Healing and the Mind. B. Moyers. Doubleday, 1993. A thoughtful exploration of the connectedness between mind, emotions, and health.

Total Health for Women. M. Torg and the editors of *Prevention* magazine. Health Books, Rodale Press, Inc., 1995.

The New York Times Guide to Personal Health. J. Brody. Avon Books, 1983.

Anxiety, Phobias and Panics. R. Peurifoy. Warner Books, 1995.

Overcoming Panic Attacks. Whole Person Associates, Pfeifer-Hamilton Publishers, 1990.

Pregnancy

A Child Is Born. L. Nilson. Bantam, 1993. A well-photographed look at fetal development.

Being Born. S. Kitzinger. Putnam, 1992. Another beautifully photographed book about fetal development.

What to Expect When You're Expecting. A. Eisenberg, H. Murkoff, and S. Hathaway. Workman Publishing Co., 1995. An easy-to-read book that discusses pregnancy month by month, in a simple format, from conception through postpartum.

The Pregnant Woman's Comfort Book. J. Louden. HarperCollins, 1995. A warm and readable book that encourages emotional self-care throughout pregnancy and early parenthood.

Mother Massage. E. Stillerman. Dell Trade Paperback, 1992. Specific massage techniques for pregnancy, labor, and postpartum and infant massage are presented.

The Joy of Twins and Other Multiple Births. P. Novotny. Crown Trade Paperbooks, Inc., 1994.

Getting Organized for Your New Baby. M. Bard. Meadowbrook Press, 1995. Helpful discussion and checklists for pregnancy and early child care.

The Baby Book—Everything You Need to Know About Your Baby from Birth to Age Two. W. Sears and M. Sears. Little, Brown and Co., 1994.

Mothering the Mother: How a Doula Can Help You Have a Shorter, Easier and Healthier Birth. M. Klaus. La Leche League, 1992.

The National Directory of Bereavement Support Groups and Services. M. Wong, ed. ADM Publishing, 1996.

Preparation for Birth: The Complete Guide to the Lamaze Method. B. Savage and D. Simkin. Ballantine Books, 1987.

Giving Birth: How It Really Feels. S. Kitzinger. Farrar, Straus and Giroux, 1989. A discussion of the emotional aspects of childbirth focusing on all types of birth, such as cesarean section, vaginal delivery after a C-section, and difficult labors.

The Complete Book of Pregnancy and Childbirth. S. Kitzinger. Alfred A. Knopf, 1989. This comprehensive book covers conception, pregnancy changes, birthing options, pregnancy care providers, relaxation techniques, and hospital procedures.

Natural Childbirth the Bradley Way. S. McCutcheon-Rosegg and P. Rosegg. Plume, 1996.

The Cesarean Birth Experience: A Practical and Comprehensive and Reassuring Guide for Parents and Professionals. B. Donovan. Beacon Press, 1986.

Positive Pregnancy Fitness: A Guide to a More Comfortable Pregnancy and Easier Birth Through Exercise and Relaxation. S. Olkin. Avery Publishing Co. Inc., 1987.

Essential Exercises for the Child-Bearing Year. E. Noble. New Life Images, 1995.

The Birth Partner's Handbook. C. Jones. Meadowbrook Press, 1989. A discussion of how a partner can help deal with childbirth pain, enhance bonding, promote a positive labor and delivery, and maintain a supportive role during and after pregnancy.

Infant Massage: A Handbook for Loving Parents. V. S. McClure. Bantam Books, 1989.

First Feelings: Milestones in the Emotional Development of Your Baby and Child. S. I. Greenspan and N. T. Greenspan. Penguin Books, 1989.

A New Life: Pregnancy, Birth and Your Child's First Year. J. T. Queenan and C. N. Queenan. Little, Brown and Co., 1992.

Infants and Mothers: Differences in Development. T. B. Brazelton. Bantam, Doubleday, Dell Publishing Group, Inc., 1983. From the first week to the twelfth month of life, Dr. Brazelton discusses the average baby, the quiet baby, and the active baby and their behaviors, followed by helpful comments for parents.

The Magic Years. S. Fraiberg. Simon & Schuster, 1996. This descriptive classic discusses a child's emotional and physical development from birth to six years of age; it is fun and insightful to read.

The Womanly Art of Breastfeeding. La Leche League International. Plume Books, 1991. A classic.

Successful Breastfeeding: A Practical Guide for Nursing Mothers. N. Dana and A. Price. Meadowbrook Press, 1985.

Breastfeeding Your Baby. S. Kitzinger. Knopf, 1992.

The Adoption Resource Book. L. Gilman. HarperCollins, 1992.

Beating the Adoption Game. C. D. Martin. Harcourt, Brace and Co., 1988. A wide-ranging discussion of adoption, including agencies, prospective parent résumés, opening birth records, and other practical issues.

When Pregnancy Fails: Families Coping with Miscarriage, Stillbirth and Infant Death. S. Borg and J. Laster. Beacon Press, 1981.

After a Loss in Pregnancy: Help for Families Affected by Miscarriage, Stillbirth, or the Loss of a Newborn. N. Benezin. Simon & Schuster, 1982.

How to Go On Living After the Death of a Baby. L. Peppers and R. Knapp. Peachtree Publishers Ltd., 1985.

Gynecology

Infertility: Your Questions Answered. H. Jacobs. Birch Lane Press, 1995.

Breast Cancer, The Complete Guide. Y. Hirshaut. Bantam Books, 1993. Comprehensive and well written, therapy oriented.

What to Do If You Get Breast Cancer. L. Komarnicky, A. Rosenberg and M. Betancourt. Little, Brown and Co., 1995. Comforting advice for women with breast cancer.

Breast Cancer: What Every Woman Should Know. R. Baron-Faust. Hearst Books, 1995.

No More Hysterectomies. V. Hufnagel and S. Golant. Plume, 1989. A woman physician tells the truth about hysterectomy and the many alternatives to this surgery. Excellent.

Understanding Your Body. F. Stewart, et al. Bantam, 1987. Excellent gynecology reference, especially for clinicians, such as nurse practitioners.

Womancare. J. Patterson and L. Madaras. Avon Books, 1984. A comprehensive gynecological guide by a woman physician.

The Gynecological Sourcebook. M. Rosenthal. Lowell, 1995.

Nutrition

Jane Brody's Good Food Book. J. Brody. Bantam, 1987. Sound nutrition advice from one of the best medical writers in the business.

The Food Pharmacy. J. Carper. Bantam, 1989. Well-researched information on how foods affect your health.

How to Lower Your Cholesterol and Beat the Odds of a Heart Attack. G. C. Griffin. Fisher Books, 1989. Recipes and advice from two experts.

Fat Is a Feminist Issue. J. Orbach. Berkley, 1987. A helpful guide for compulsive overeaters.

Controlling Cholesterol. K. Coopers. Bantam Books, 1989.

Brand Name Fat and Cholesterol Counter. American Heart Association. Times Books, 1994.

The Complete and Up-to-Date Fat Book. K. Bellerson. Avery Pub., 1996.

The Mount Sinai School of Medicine Complete Book of Nutrition. V. Herbert. St. Martin's Press, 1990. A comprehensive guide to all aspects of nutrition.

The New Fit or Fat. C. Bailey. Houghton Mifflin, 1991.

Nutrition for a Healthy Pregnancy. E. Sommer. Henry Holt and Company, 1995.

Fitness

Peak Fitness for Women. Newby-Fraser. Human Kinetics, 1995. A book that encourages all forms of exercise and inspires women to reach for their best fitness level.

The Weight Watchers Complete Exercise Book. J. Roberts. Macmillan, 1995. Includes a personal fitness planner and a well-founded approach to exercise.

The Healthy Heart Walking Book. American Heart Association. Macmillan, 1995. Nutrition and walking are both addressed in this book, which includes a walking diary and goals for walking.

Aerobic Walking, The Weight-Loss Exercise. M. Malkin. John Wiley and Sons, Inc., 1995.

Twenty-Minute Yoga Workouts. American Yoga Association. Ballantine Books, 1995.

Family Fitness Handbook. B. Glover and J. Shepherd. Penguin Books, 1989. A well-rounded discussion of parent and child fitness and fun, including sports programs, fitness as a factor in dealing with stress, and planning for strength and flexibility exercises.

Fitness Walking for Women. A. Kashiwa and J. Rippe. Berkley Publishing Group, 1987.

Sports Illustrated Running for Women. J. Heinonen. Winner's Circle Books, Time, Inc., 1989.

Smart Exercise. C. Bailey. Houghton Mifflin, 1996.

The Complete Sports Medicine Book for Women. Revised for the '90s. M. Shangold. Fireside, 1992. One of the best all-around books of its type.

Teenagers

Reviving Ophelia: Saving the Selves of Adolescent Girls. M. Pipher. Ballantine Books, 1995.

Career Choices: A Guide for Teens and Young Adults. M. Bingham and S. Stryker. Able Pub., 1990.

The What's Happening to My Body? Book for Girls. L. Madaras. Newmarket Press, 1988. This gives easy-to-read, honest, sensitive, and comprehensive information about emotional and physical experiences of puberty.

Choices: A Teen Woman's Journal for Self-Awareness and Planning. M. Bingham, J. Edmondson, and S. Styker. Advocacy Press, 1993. A pleasant and helpful book for young teenage girls in planning career goals, understanding nutritional and other health needs, and organizing their life's priorities.

You and Your Adolescent. L. Steinberg. HarperCollins, 1991.

The Middle Years and After

Estrogen: The Facts Can Change Your Life. L. Nachtigall. HarperCollins, 1991. A well-documented guide to estrogen therapy by a woman physician.

Making the Estrogen Decision. Y. Henkel. Fawcett Book Group, 1993.

Estrogen: Yes or No? M. Notelovitz. St. Martin's Press, 1993.

Is It Hot or Is It Me? G. Sand. HarperCollins, 1993.

Managing Your Menopause. W. Utian and R. Jacobowitz. Simon & Schuster, 1991.

Perimenopause: Preparing for the Change. N. Teaff and K. W. Wiley. Prima Publishing, 1994.

Choice Years. J. Paige and P. Gordon. Fawcett Book Group, 1993.

The Silent Passage. G. Sheehy. Pocket Books, 1993.

What Every Woman Should Know: Staying Healthy After 40. L. Nachtigall and J. R. Heilman. Warner Books, 1995.

Complete Guide to Aging and Health. M. Williams. Harmony Books, 1995.

Alzheimer's: A Caregiver's Guide and Sourcebook. H. Gruetzner. John Wiley and Sons, 1992.

Midlife Health. A. P. Kahn and L. H. Holt. Avon, 1989. Good discussion of women's health problems at midlife.

Sexuality

The Art of Sensual Loving. A. Stanway. Carroll and Graf Publishers, 1989.

Healing the Incest Wound: Adult Survivors in Therapy. C. Courtois. W. Norton & Co., 1996.

Woman's Experience of Sex. S. Kitzinger. Penguin Books, 1985. Deals with a multitude of issues surrounding sex, such as sexual assault, sexual life stages, coping with sexual problems, and children and sex.

Women and Love. S. Hite. St. Martin's Press, 1989. Results of a questionnaire from a woman's point of view on subjects not covered in the original Hite report, such as how women feel about love, relationships, marriage, and monogamy.

The New Gourmet Joy of Sex: A Cordon Bleu Guide to Love Making for the Nineties. A. Comfort. Simon & Schuster, 1993. Enjoyable reading about the variety possible in sexual behavior.

More Joy: A Lovemaking Companion to the Joy of Sex. A. Comfort. Mitchell Beazley Publishers Ltd., 1987.

Men Who Hate Women and the Women Who Love Them. F. Foward and J. Torres. Bantam, 1987. Excellent book for women in relationships with angry, controlling men.

Private Zone. F. Dayee. Warner Books, 1985. Excellent book for parents and children to read together.

Women's Sexual Health. R. Steinberg and L. Robinson. Primus, 1995.

AIDS

The Invisible Epidemic: The Story of Women and AIDS. G. Corea. HarperCollins, 1992.

The Essential HIV Treatment Fact Book. L. Pinsky, P. H. Douglas, and C. Metroka. Pocket Books, 1992.

What Everyone Can Do to Fight AIDS. A Garwood. Jossey-Bass Publishers, 1995.

The HIV Drug Book. B. Kearney. Pocket Books, 1995.

AIDS: The Ultimate Challenge. E. Kubler-Ross. Macmillan, 1993. Questions and case studies of AIDS victims of all ages.

Drugs

Perfect Daughters: Adult Daughters of Alcoholics. R. Ackerman. Health Communications, Inc., 1989.

Drug Comparison Handbook. R. Reilly. Skidmore-Roth Publishing, 1995.

The PDR Family Guide to Women's Health and Prescription Drugs. Medical Economics Co., 1994.

The Complete Drug Reference, 1996. Consumer Reports Books. 1995.

Getting Better: Inside Alcoholics Anonymous. N. Robertson. Fawcett, 1989. A woman journalist recounts her path to recovery.

Physicians' Desk Reference. 50th ed. Medical Economics Co., 1996. Known as the PDR, this bestseller is annually updated to include the latest manufacturers' information about nearly all prescription drugs.

Physicians' Desk Reference for Nonprescription Drugs. 17th ed. Medical Economics Co., 1996. Information about nonprescription drugs, organized like the PDR above.

Codependent No More. M. Beattie. Hazelden Foundation, 1987.

Beyond Codependency and Getting Better All the Time. M. Beattie. Hazelden Foundation, 1989. Both of these books deal with the effects of alcoholism on the family and discuss ways to cope with it as individuals and to break the cycle of dependency between generations.

''It Will Never Happen to Me!'' C. Black. Ballantine Books, 1987. An easy-to-read book about the feelings of growing up in an alcoholic family. This discusses the problems of children of alcoholic parents.

APPENDIX D

Resource Groups

For information about—	Contact—	Chapter
abortion	National Abortion Federation 1436 U Street, N.W., Suite 103 Washington, DC 20009 800-772-9100	44
abortion	Planned Parenthood Federation of America, Inc. 810 Seventh Avenue New York, NY 10019 (212) 541-7800	44
adoption	National Adoption Information Clearinghouse 5640 Nicholson Lane, Suite 300 Rockville, MD 20852 (301) 231-6512	44
AIDS—drug trials	National Institute of Allergy and Infectious Diseases 800-HIV-0440 (9 A.M. to 7 P.M., EST)	24
alcohol abuse	Alcoholics Anonymous Grand Central Station P.O. Box 459 New York, NY 10163	30
alcohol abuse in relative or friend	Al-Anon Family Group Headquarters, Inc. P.O. Box 862 Midtown Station New York, NY 10018-0862	30
alternative birth settings	National Association of Parents and Professionals for Safe Alternatives in Childbirth (NAPSAC) P.O. Box 646 Marble Hill, MO 63764-9725	15
Alzheimer's disease	Alzheimer's Association 919 N. Michigan Avenue, Suite 1000 Chicago, IL 60611-1676 (312) 335-8700 or 800-272-3900 (referral service line)	76
anxiety	Anxiety Disorders Association of America 6000 Executive Boulevard, Suite 513 Rockville, MD 20852 (301) 231-9350	81
arthritis	Arthritis Foundation 1314 Spring Street, N.W. Atlanta, GA 30309 800-283-7800	73
birth centers	National Association of Childbearing Centers 3123 Gottschall Road Perkiomenville, PA 18074	15

For information about—	Contact—	Chapter
birth control	Planned Parenthood Federation of America, Inc. 810 Seventh Avenue New York, NY 10019 (212) 541-7800	10
birth defects; inherited disease	March of Dimes Birth Defects Foundation 1275 Mamaroneck Avenue White Plains, NY 10605 (914) 428-7100	11, 31
breast-feeding	La Leche League International 1400 N. Meacham Road Schaumburg, IL 60173 (708) 519-7730	19
breast-feeding	International Lactation Consultants (ILCA) 200 N. Michigan Avenue Chicago, IL 60101 (312) 541-1710	19
cancer	Cancer Information Service national toll-free telephone number: 800-422-6237	various
cancer	Office of Cancer Communications National Cancer Institute Building 31, Room 10A–16 Bethesda, MD 20892	various
cancer	American Cancer Society, Inc. 1579 Clifton Road, N.E. Atlanta, GA 30329 (404) 320-3333	various
cancer	Cancer Research Foundation 700 Princess Street, Suite 5 Alexandria, VA 22314 800-227-2732	various
child abuse	National Child Abuse Hotline and Referral Service 1-800-422-4453	25
childbirth education	(See Table 26, Childbirth Education Organizations)	14
cholesterol screening	Heart, Lung, and Blood Institute Information Center P.O. Box 30105 Bethesda, MD 20824-0105 (301) 251-1222	48
cosmetic surgery	American Society of Plastic and Reconstructive Surgeons, Inc. 444 East Algonquin Road Arlington Heights, IL 60005 800-635-0635	46
C-section	C/SEC c/o Norma Shulman 22 Forrest Road Framington, MA 01701	21
C-section	International Cesarean Awareness Network (ICAN) 1304 Kingsdale Avenue Redondo Beach, CA 90278 (310) 542-6400; call for local number	21

For information about—	Contact—	Chapter
dental care	American Dental Association Bureau of Health Education and Audiovisual Services 211 East Chicago Avenue Chicago, IL 60611 (312) 440-2500	47
DES	Office of Cancer Communications National Cancer Institute Building 31, Room 10A–16 Bethesda, MD 20892	38
DES	DES Action USA 1615 Broadway Oakland, CA 94612 (510) 465-4011	38
diabetes	American Diabetes Association, Inc. 149 Madison Avenue New York, NY 10016 (212) 725-4925	various
digestive problems	Crohn's and Colitis Foundation of America, Inc. 386 Park Avenue South New York, NY 10016 (212) 685-3440	63
digestive problems	Digestive Disease National Coalition 711 2nd Street, N.E., Suite 200 Washington, DC 20002 (202) 544-7497	63
digestive problems	National Eating Disorders Organization (NEDO) Laureate Hospital 6655 S. Yale Avenue Tulsa, OK 74136	80
domestic violence	National Health Resource Center on Domestic Violence 383 Rhode Island Street, Suite 304 San Francisco, CA 94103 (415) 252-8900	25
drug-abuse prevention	National Clearinghouse for Alcohol and Drug Information P.O. Box 2345 Rockville, MD 20847-2345 (301) 468-2600 or 800-729-6686	30
endometriosis	Endometriosis Association 8585 N. 76th Place Milwaukee, WI 53223 800-992-ENDO	36
exercise	American Alliance for Health, Physical Education, Recreation and Dance 1900 Association Drive Reston, VA 22091 (703) 476-3400	49
exercise	American College of Sports Medicine P.O. Box 1440 Indianapolis, IN 46206	49
general health	American Public Health Association 1015 Fifteenth Street, N.W. Washington, DC 20005 (202) 789-5600	47
headaches	National Headache Foundation 5252 N. Western Avenue Chicago, IL 60625	67

For information about—	Contact—	Chapter
health services; selecting a doctor, etc.	(See Table 1, Resources for Finding Health Care Alternatives)	2
heart problems	American Heart Association 7320 Greenville Avenue Dallas, TX 75231	47
high blood pressure	National Heart, Lung, and Blood Institute Information Center P.O. Box 30105 Bethesda, MD 20824-0105	69
home safety; proper use of prescription and nonprescription drugs	Council on Family Health 225 Park Avenue South, 17th Floor New York, NY 10003 (212) 598-3617	47
hysterectomy	Hysterectomy Educational Resources and Services (HERS) 422 Bryn Mawr Avenue Bala Cynwyd, PA 19004 (610) 667-7757	45
incontinence	National Association for Continence P.O. Box 310 Spartanburg, SC 29305-8310	28
incontinence	Interstitial Cystitis Association 38 Cedar Lane Ossining, NY 10562 (914) 923-1916	86
infertility	RESOLVE, Inc. 1310 Broadway Somerville, MA 02144-1731 (617) 643-2424	13
infertility	The American Fertility Society (American Society for Reproductive Medicine) 1209 Montgomery Highway Birmingham, AL 35216 (205) 978-5000	13
lung conditions and smoking	American Lung Association 1740 Broadway New York, NY 10019 (212) 315-8700	61
lupus	American Lupus Society 3914 Del Amo Boulevard, #922 Torrance, CA 90503	73
lupus	Lupus Foundation of America 4 Research Place, Suite 180 Rockville, MD 20850 800-558-0121	73
menopause	National Institute on Aging Information Center P.O. Box 8057 Gaithersburg, MD 20898	26
menopause	North American Menopause Society University Hospital Cleveland Dept. OB/GYN 2074 Abington Road Cleveland, OH 44106 (216) 844-3334	26

For information about—	Contact—	Chapter
mental health and counseling services	National Mental Health Association 1021 Prince Street Alexandria, VA 22314-2971 (703) 684-7722	47
midwives	American College of Nurse-Midwives 818 Connecticut Avenue, N.W., Suite 900 Washington, DC 20006	15
midwives	Midwives' Alliance of North America (MANA) P.O. Box 175 Newton, KS 67114 (316) 283-4543	15
nutrition	Community Nutrition Institute 910 17th Street, N.W. Suite 413 Washington, DC 20006	48
nutrition	The American Dietetic Association 216 W. Jackson Boulevard Chicago, IL 60606	48
nutrition	Department of Foods and Nutrition American Medical Association 535 N. Dearborn Street Chicago, IL 60610	48
osteoporosis	National Osteoporosis Foundation 1150 17th Street, N.W., Suite 500 Washington, DC 20036	27
panic attacks	Recovery, Inc. 802 N. Dearborn Street Chicago, IL 60610 (312) 337-5661	81
PMS	PMS Access P.O. Box 9326 Madison, WI 53715 800-222-4PMS	32
PMS	Madison Pharmacy Associates Natural Hormone Replacement Therapy P.O. Box 9641 Madison, WI 53715 800-558-7064	32
pregnancy (and other areas of women's health)	American College of Obstetricians and Gynecologists Resource Center 409 12th Street, S.W. Washington, DC 20024-2188 (202) 638-5577	16
pregnancy	National Center for Education in Maternal and Child Health 2000 15th Street, N., Suite 701 Arlington, VA 22201-2617 (703) 524-7802	16
pregnancy loss	The Compassionate Friends, Inc. National Headquarters P.O. Box 3696 Oak Brook, IL 60522 (708) 890-0010	18
pregnancy loss	SHARE—Pregnancy and Infant Loss Support Group Inc. St. Joseph's Health Center 300 1st Capitol Drive St. Charles, MO 63301	18

For information about—	Contact—	Chapter
pregnancy loss	AMEND c/o Maureen Connelly 4324 Berrywick Terrace St. Louis, MO 63128 (314) 487-7582	18
pregnancy loss	Pregnancy and Infant Loss Center 1421 E. Wayzata Boulevard, Suite 40 Wayzata, MN 55391 (612) 473-9372	18
quitting smoking	American Cancer Society, Inc. 1599 Clifton Road, N.E. Atlanta, GA 30329 (404) 320-3333	61
quitting smoking	American Heart Association 7320 Greenville Avenue Dallas, TX 75231 (214) 373-6300	61
sexual assault	National Clearinghouse on Marital and Date Rape (510) 524-1582	25
sexuality and sex counseling	American Association of Sex Educators, Counselors and Therapists 435 N. Michigan Avenue, Suite 1717 Chicago, IL 60611	22
sexuality and sex counseling	Sexuality Information and Education Council of the U.S. 130 W. 42nd Street, Suite 350 New York, NY 10036	22
sexually transmitted diseases (including AIDS)	Centers for Disease Control 1600 Clifton Road, N.E. Atlanta, GA 30333 (404) 639-3534	24
sexually transmitted diseases	STD Hotline 800-227-8922	24
sexually transmitted diseases	American Social Health Association P.O. Box 13827 Research Triangle Park, NC 27709	24
sterilization	Association for Voluntary Sterilization, Inc. 79 Madison Avenue New York, NY 10016 (212) 561-8000	43
sterilization	Planned Parenthood Federation of America, Inc. 810 Seventh Avenue New York, NY 10019 (212) 541-7800	43
stress	The Midwest Center for Stress and Anxiety, Inc. 106 N. Church Street, Suite 200 Oak Harbor, OH 43449	47
twins	Twins Magazine P.O. Box 12045 Overland Park, KS 66282 (913) 722-1090	20
twins	Center for the Study of Multiple Birth 333 East Superior Street Chicago, IL 60611 (312) 266-9093	20

For information about—	Contact—	Chapter
weight loss	Overeaters Anonymous 383 Van Ness Avenue, Suite 1601 Torrance, CA 90501 (310) 618-8835	89
weight loss	Weight Watchers International (516) 939-0400	89
women's health	American College of Obstetricians and Gynecologists Resource Center 409 12th Street, S.W. Washington, DC 20024-2188	various
women's health	National Women's Health Network 514 10th Street, N.W., Suite 400 Washington, DC 20004 (202) 347-1140	various
women's health	National Women's Health Resource Center 2440 M Street, N.W., Suite 325 Washington, DC 20037	various
women's health	Older Women's League (OWL) 666 11th Street, N.W., Suite 700 Washington, DC 20001 (202) 783-6686	various

APPENDIX E

Breast Self-Examination

A woman should perform a breast self-examination regularly as most breast cancers are first detected by the woman herself. The earlier cancer is detected, the better the results of treatment. According to the American Cancer Society, every woman should perform this examination once a month.

The best time to do this examination is about a week after your menstrual period. During this time of your cycle you are less likely to have breast tenderness. Also, the week after menstruation you are less likely to experience cystic breast changes that some women regularly get before a period. After menopause or hysterectomy you should perform the breast self-examination at a convenient time each month. If you do find a breast lump, do contact your doctor so a definite diagnosis can be made. Fortunately the great majority of breast lumps evaluated turn out to be benign.

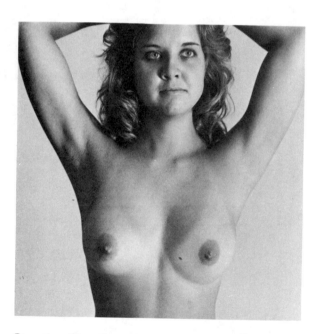

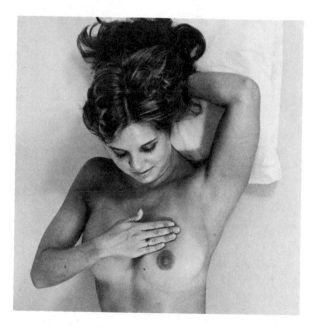

Step 1. Start by standing in front of a mirror and inspect both breasts for anything unusual such as dimpling of the skin or a distinct change in breast size or shape since your last examination. Do this first with your arms at your sides and then with your arms raised above your head.

Step 2. While lying down with your left hand underneath your head, examine your left breast using your right hand. Use the flat of your fingers (not the tips) to feel one area of your breast at a time. Move your fingers back and forth in a circular motion as you examine each area, pressing firmly enough so that the breast tissue moves back and forth under the skin. You will be feeling for a lump or thickening in your breast.

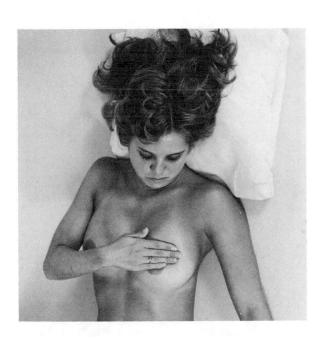

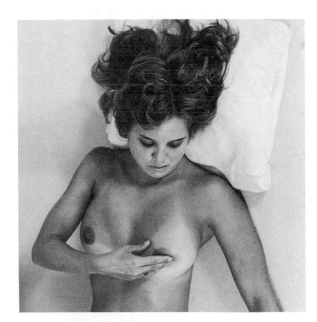

Step 3. Now repeat step 2 but keep your left hand at your side.

Step 4. With your arm still down examine and gently squeeze the nipple and the area around the nipple and note whether there is any discharge. Repeat steps 1–4 as you examine your right breast.

INDEX

Index

hot flashes, 17, 219–220, 221–222, 431–432
    estrogen therapy and, 221–222
    insomnia and, 221
    menstrual cycle irregularities and, 458
human chorionic gonadotropin, 16
human papilloma virus (HPV) infection, 207–209, 271, 274
hymen, 12
hypertension. *See* high blood pressure
hyperventilation, 380, 414. *See also* blackouts
hypoglycemia, 414, 447
    dizziness and, 414
    lethargy and, 447, 448, 449
hypothalamus, 15
hysterectomy, 315–322
    abdominal, 316
    alternatives to, 319–320
    for bleeding problems, 318, 319
    for cancer of cervix, 276, 319
    for cancer of ovary, 283, 319
    for cancer of uterus, 284, 319
    chance of having, 315
    for endometriosis, 268, 318, 319
    for fibroid tumors, 264, 265, 319
    indications for, 316, 318, 319
    long-term effects of, 321–322
    partial, 315–316
    for pelvic inflammatory disease, 205–206, 319
    pelvic pain and, 475
    for prolapse of the uterus, 230, 319
    radical, 316
    recovering from, 321
    removal of ovaries and, 315–316
    risks of, 321
    total, 315, 316
    types of, 315–316
    vaginal, 315, 316
    when to avoid, 319–320
hysterosalpingogram, 78, 79, 264
hysteroscopy, 82, 265, 290, 292, 299, 318, 319, 454

I

incontinence, urinary, 230–231, 480–481
indigestion, 280, 426–427
    pregnancy and, 112
infant massage, 149
inferility, 77–89
    age over thirty and, 77
    artificial insemination and, 80, 83
    birth control pills and, 54
    cervical mucus and, 82
    cryopreservation and, 87

emotional factors in, 77, 83
endometriosis and, 80, 267
estrogen therapy and, 82
fertility drugs and, 81–82
fibroid tumors and, 265
fimbrioplasty and, 80
frequency of, 77
Gamete Intra-Fallopian Transfer (GIFT) procedure and, 85–86, 88
hysterosalpingogram and, 78, 79
hysteroscopy and, 82
Intrauterine insemination (IUI) and, 83
In Vitro Fertilization (IVF) and, 83–84, 85, 88
IUD and, 46
laparoscopy and, 78, 79
laser surgery and, 80
male evaluation and, 82–83
menstrual cycle irregularities and, 81, 457, 458
microsurgery and, 80
ovulation problems and, 81
polycystic ovaries and, 81, 278, 423, 457, 458
sperm banks and, 87
surrogate mothers and, 88–89
temperature chart and, 81
thyroid problems and, 81
treatment of, 77–89
tube infections and, 78–80
venereal disease and, 78
insomnia, 433–434
intercourse. *See* sexual intercourse; sexuality
internist, 2, 3
interstitial cystitis, 484
intrauterine devices (IUDs), 12, 45–47, 58–59, 319, 380, 460, 461, 490, 491
intrauterine insemination. *See* infertility
iron, 343–345, 349, 351
    deficiency anemia, 344–345, 447, 448
    preparations, 349–350
    supplements in pregnancy, 349
irritable bowel syndrome. *See* spastic colon
itching. *See* skin problems; vaginal discharge and infection
IUDs. *See* intrauterine devices

J

joint pains, 440–444

K

Kegel's exercise, 230, 480
kidney disease
    high blood pressure and, 380, 428, 429

nonspecific urethritis. *See* nongonococcal urethritis

non-stress test (NST), 164–165

Norplant, 56–57

nurse-midwife, 3

nurse practitioner, 3

nutrition, 341–356. *See also* diet
   anti-cancer foods, 354–355
   body metabolism and, 350–351
   breast-feeding and, 116–118
   calcium in the diet, 222–223, 350
   carbohydrates, 342
   cholesterol, 342–343, 346, 347, 348
   fats, 342, 343, 346, 347, 348
   fiber, 343, 402
   food additives, 352–354
   food groups, 350
   food labeling, 352
   iron, 343, 344–345, 349–350, 351
   megavitamins, 345–349, 350
   menopause and, 356
   minerals, 343, 345, 346–349, 355, 356
   obesity and, 350–351
   optimal weight and, 350–351
   osteoporosis and, 223
   pregnancy and, 107, 116–118
   proteins, 341
   salt, 352–354, 478
   snacks, 353–354
   vitamins, 343–349
   weight gain and, 350–351

O

obesity. *See* weight gain (excessive)

Obsessive-Compulsive Disorder (OCD), 466–468

obstetrician-gynecologist, 2, 3

office visit, 20–28

oral contraceptives. *See* birth control pills

oral hygiene, 339

osteoporosis
   backache and, 222, 376, 379
   dietary calcium and, 350, 355–356
   estrogen therapy and, 222–223
   exercise for, 224
   new drugs for, 223–224

ovary
   anatomy of, 13
   cancer of, 279–280
   cysts and tumors of, 81, 279–281, 376, 379, 420, 474
   examination of, 26

   surgical removal of, 206–207, 267, 316

overdue pregnancy, 163–164, 168, 173
   induction of labor and, 173–174

ovulation, 15, 17
   painful, 17
   test kits, 81, 108
   vaginal discharge and, 489

oxytocin, 173–174

oxytocin challenge test. *See* contraction stress test

P

painful menstruation. *See* menstrual periods—painful

pain in abdomen, 280. *See also* diarrhea, nausea, heartburn, and pelvic pain

pain pills, over-the-counter, 378, 461

palpitations, 466, 470–471

pancreatitis, 463, 464

panic attack, 466

Pap smear, 22, 23, 270–274, 276
   abnormalities of, 270–272
   age to start having, 24
   cancer of uterus and, 270
   classification of, 271–272
   false positives and negatives, 273
   frequency of having, 22
   human papilloma virus and, 272, 274
   technique of performing, 22–24

pelvic examination, 22–27
   recommended frequency of, 23
   self-examination, 11–13, 22

pelvic inflammatory disease, 205–206
   backache and, 376
   ectopic pregnancy and, 207
   pelvic pain and, 206, 474
   pregnancy and, 205–207
   vaginal discharge and, 206

pelvic pain, 472–476. *See also* menstrual periods—painful
   adhesions and, 472
   appendicitis and, 473, 474
   endometriosis and, 266–267
   fibroid tumors and, 264, 265
   intestinal problems and, 462, 472–473, 474
   kidney infection and, 482–487
   miscarriage and, 384–389, 473, 474
   ovarian cysts and, 278–280
   pelvic inflammatory disease and, 205–207, 474
   tubal pregnancy and, 384–389, 474
   urinary tract infection and, 474, 482–487

nausea and vomiting during, 109, 463
nutrition and, 107–108, 116–118
overdue, 163–164, 168, 173
palpitations during, 470
pelvic pain during, 472, 473, 474
physical changes during, 111–116
postmaturity and, 163–164
preconceptional counseling, 107–108
pregnancy-induced hypertension. *See* high
    blood pressure
premature rupture of membranes during,
    161, 173, 416
preterm labor, 170–172, 390
Rh disease and, 157–158, 168
rubella and, 66, 158
sex and, 121, 193
sexually transmitted diseases and, 194–209
smoking and, 107, 156, 404
sonogram, use during, 69–70, 109–110. *See
    also* sonography
stretch marks and, 113
swelling and fluid retention during, 157, 477
syphilis and, 202
teenagers and, 120
toxemia and, 157
toxoplasmosis and, 160
travel and, 121
tubal. *See* ectopic pregnancy
twins and, 16, 81, 162
urinary tract infections and, 482–486
urination, frequency during, 112
vaginal birth after cesarean (VBAC), 176–177
vaginal discharge during, 488
varicose veins and, 113, 445, 446
venereal warts and, 208–209
video display terminals and, 121
vitamins and, 345, 349
warning signs of, 111
weight gain (excessive) during, 498–499
weight gain (insufficient) during, 498–499
work and, 121–122
pregnancy hormone. *See* human chorionic
    gonadotropin
pregnancy tests, 108–109
premature labor. *See* preterm labor
premature rupture of membranes, 161
premenstrual syndrome, 254–256, 449, 477
prepaid health care groups. *See* health mainte-
    nance organizations
prepared childbirth. *See* childbirth education
preterm labor, 170–172, 276, 391
preventive health. *See* health maintenance

progesterone, 15, 16, 50, 266
    to bring on menstrual period, 457
    treatment of irregular menstrual periods and,
        454–456
prolapse of uterus, 26, 229–230
prostaglandins, 460
puberty. *See also* adolescence
    hair growth and, 420

Q
quickening. *See* fetus

R
rape. *See* sexual assault
rash. *See* skin problems
rectal bleeding. *See* bleeding (rectal)
rectal exam, 26
rectocele, 24, 229, 494
regional enteritis, 411, 412, 413
Retin-A, 373
Reviving Ophelia (Pipher), 19
Rh antibodies. *See* Rh disease
Rh disease, 157–158, 168
    induction of labor, 174
rheumatoid arthritis, 440, 442
Rh negative blood. *See* Rh disease
RhoGAM. *See* Rh disease
rhythm method of birth control. *See* natural
    family planning
ritodrine, 171
rooming-in, 154
RU-486, 314
rubella. *See* German measles
ruptured membranes, 124, 161
    induction of labor and, 174

S
salpingitis. *See* pelvic inflammatory disease
salt (dietary), 352–354, 399, 429
scabies, 435, 437, 438, 439
self-examination, 11–15, 22
    breast, 13–15, 22
    pelvic, 11–13, 22
semen analysis, 82–83
sex hormones
    estrogen, 15, 16, 17, 50
    progesterone, 15, 16, 50
sex selection, 72
sex therapy, 191–192

bladder surgery, 229, 231
cone biopsy, 272–273
cosmetic surgery, 323–329
dilatation and curettage (D & C), 299–300
hysterectomy, 315–322
hysteroscopy, 82, 265, 290, 292, 299
informed consent, 292–293
laparoscopy, 78–80, 266–267, 279, 290–292, 301–303, 388
laser surgery, 80, 290–291
outpatient surgery, 297–298
plastic surgery, for blocked tubes, 80. *See also* cosmetic surgery
procedures before, 293–294
recovering in the hospital, 294–296
recovery room, 294
second opinion programs, 292
sterilization operations, 301–308
termination of pregnancy, 310–314
tubal ligation, 301–308
vaginal repair, 229
vasectomy, 301
surgical incision
horizontal (bikini), 316
vertical, 317
swelling and fluid retention, 477–479
menstrual cycle and, 477
syphilis, 201–203
pregnancy and, 202

T

tampons
toxic shock syndrome and, 257
use after urinary tract infection, 487
Tay-Sachs disease, 66, 68–69, 70, 71, 73
teenage pregnancy, 119–120
temperature chart, infertility and, 81
temporomandibular disorders (TMD), 422, 440, 443, 444
termination of pregnancy, 310–314
termography, 260
"test tube" baby, 83–84
threatened abortion. *See* miscarriage
thrombophlebitis, 416, 417, 418, 445
thyroid problems
breast discharge and, 396
constipation and, 400
lethargy and, 448
menstrual problems and, 453, 457
nervousness and, 466
TMJ. *See* temporomandibular disorders (TMD)

toxemia of pregnancy. *See* high blood pressure
toxic shock syndrome, 257
toxoplasmosis, 160
tranquilizers, 408, 467–468. *See also* drug abuse
trichomonas vaginal infection, 201, 489, 490, 492, 493. *See also* vaginal discharge or infection
tubal ligation, 301–309. *See also* sterilization operations
surgery to reverse, 80
tubal pregnancy. *See* ectopic pregnancy
tube infection. *See* pelvic inflammatory disease
"tummy tuck," 327
twins, 16, 81, 162
fertility drugs and, 81
premature labor and, 170
"tying" tubes. *See* tubal ligation

U

ulcer, of stomach, 426, 463, 464
ulcerative colitis, 393, 411, 412, 413
ultrasound. *See* sonography
umbilical cord sampling, 72
urethra, 12, 23
infection and, 484, 487
stricture of, 480
urethritis, 204–205
urinary problems. *See* bladder and kidney problems
urination—frequent or urgent, 480–481
urination—painful or bloody, 482–487
urinary stress incontinence, 230–231
cough and, 230, 403
urinary tract infection, 474, 480, 487. *See also* bladder infection; kidney infection
pelvic pain and, 377
uterus, 12
anatomy of, 12–13
cancer of, 282–284
enlargement of, 25
examination of, 25–26
fibroid tumor of, 264–265
infection of, 46
prolapse of, 26, 229–230
"tilted", 25–26, 376

V

vaccinations, 340
vagina, 12, 22–26. *See also* vaginal discharge or infection; vaginal lump
anatomy of, 12–13